Blueprints
Q&As for Step 2

Blueprints
Q&As for Step 2

Series Editor:

Michael S. Clement, MD, FAAP
Mountain Park Health Center
Clinical Lecturer in Family and Community Medicine
University of Arizona College of Medicine
Consultant, Arizona Department of Health Services
Phoenix, Arizona

Aaron B. Caughey, MD, MPP, MPH
Assistant Professor, Division of Maternal-Fetal Medicine
Department of Obstetrics & Gynecology
University of California, San Francisco
Division of Health Services and Policy Analysis
University of California, Berkeley
Berkeley & San Francisco, California
Obstetrics & Gynecology

Jeffrey L. Foti, MD, FAAP
Attending Pediatrician, Bill Holt Pediatric
  Infectious Disease Clinic
Phoenix Children's Hospital
Phoenix, Arizona
Clinical Assistant Professor, University of Arizona
  School of Medicine
Tucson, Arizona
Pediatrics

Deirdre J. Lyell, MD
Assistant Professor, Obstetrics & Gynecology
Stanford University School of Medicine
Attending Physician
Stanford University Medical Center
Stanford, California
Obstetrics & Gynecology

James Brian McLoone, MD, DFAPA
Chairman, Department of Psychiatry and
Director, Psychiatry Residency Training Program
  and Medical Student Clerkship

Banner Good Samaritan Medical Center
Clinical Professor of Psychiatry
University of Arizona College of Medicine—Phoenix
  Campus
Phoenix, Arizona
Psychiatry

Edward W. Nelson, MD
Professor of Surgery
University of Utah School of Medicine
Attending Surgeon
University of Utah Medical Center
Salt Lake City, Utah
Surgery

Janice P. Piatt, MD
Medical Director, Bill Holt Pediatric Infectious
  Disease Clinic
Associate Director, Pediatric Clinic
Phoenix Children's Hospital
Phoenix, Arizona
Pediatrics

Brenda L. Shinar, MD
Assistant Program Director
Department of Internal Medicine
Banner Good Samaritan Medical Center
Phoenix, Arizona
Clinical Professor of Internal Medicine
University of Arizona College of Medicine
Tucson, Arizona
Medicine

Susan H. Tran, MD
Resident Physician, Obstetrics
  & Gynecology
Kaiser San Francisco Hospital
San Francisco, California
Obstetrics & Gynecology

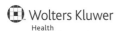 Wolters Kluwer | Lippincott Williams & Wilkins
Health
Philadelphia · Baltimore · New York · London
Buenos Aires · Hong Kong · Sydney · Tokyo

Acquisitions Editor: Nancy Anastasi Duffy
Managing Editor: Cheryl W. Stringfellow
Marketing Manager: Jennifer Kuklinski
Production Editor: Kevin Johnson
Compositor: International Typesetting and Composition
Printer: Data Reproductions Corp

Library of Congress Cataloging-in-Publication Data

Blueprints Q&As for step 2 / editor, Michael S. Clement.
    p. ; cm.
  Includes index.
  ISBN-13: 978-0-7817-7820-6
  ISBN-10: 0-7817-7820-4
  1. Medicine—Examinations, questions, etc.   2. Physicians—Licenses—United States—Examinations—Study guides.   I. Clement, Michael S.   II. Title: Blueprints Q & As for step 2.
III. Title: Blueprints Q and As for step 2.
  [DNLM: 1. Clinical Medicine—Examination Questions.   2. Case Reports—Examination Questions.   WB 18.2 B6578 2008]
  R834.5.B582 2008
  610.76—dc22

                                                                                                2007013858

DISCLAIMER

Care has been taken to confirm the accuracy of the information present and to describe generally accepted practices. However, the authors, editors, and publisher are not responsible for errors or omissions or for any consequences from application of the information in this book and make no warranty, expressed or implied, with respect to the currency, completeness, or accuracy of the contents of the publication. Application of this information in a particular situation remains the professional responsibility of the practitioner; the clinical treatments described and recommended may not be considered absolute and universal recommendations.

The authors, editors, and publisher have exerted every effort to ensure that drug selection and dosage set forth in this text are in accordance with the current recommendations and practice at the time of publication. However, in view of ongoing research, changes in government regulations, and the constant flow of information relating to drug therapy and drug reactions, the reader is urged to check the package insert for each drug for any change in indications and dosage and for added warnings and precautions. This is particularly important when the recommended agent is a new or infrequently employed drug.

Some drugs and medical devices presented in this publication have Food and Drug Administration (FDA) clearance for limited use in restricted research settings. It is the responsibility of the health care provider to ascertain the FDA status of each drug or device planned for use in their clinical practice.

To purchase additional copies of this book, call our customer service department at **(800) 638-3030** or fax orders to **(301) 223-2320**. International customers should call **(301) 223-2300**.

Visit Lippincott Williams & Wilkins on the Internet: http://www.lww.com. Lippincott Williams & Wilkins customer service representatives are available from 8:30 am to 6:00 pm, EST.

Contributors

Sarah Beaumont, MD
Chief Resident, Internal Medicine/Pediatrics
Banner Good Samaritan Medical Center
Phoenix Children's Hospital
Phoenix, Arizona
Medicine

Ryan Bradley
Class of 2004
University of California, San Francisco
San Francisco, California
Obstetrics & Gynecology

Brendan Cassidy, MD
Pediatric Ophthalmologist
Phoenix Children's Hospital
Phoenix, Arizona
Pediatrics

Randal Christensen, MD, MPH
Clinical Assistant Professor
University of Arizona
Tucson, Arizona
Faculty Physician
Phoenix Children's Hospital
Phoenix, Arizona
Pediatrics

Melvin L. Cohen, MD
Director of Medical Education
Phoenix Children's Hospital
Phoenix, Arizona
Clinical Professor, Pediatrics
University of Arizona School of Medicine

Tucson, Arizona
Pediatrics

Rafe C. Connors, MD
Resident, Department of General Surgery
University of Utah School
 of Medicine
Salt Lake City, Utah
Surgery

Tracy L. Crews, MD
Chief Resident, Psychiatry
Banner Good Samaritan Medical Center
Phoenix, Arizona
Psychiatry

Tala Dajani, MD
Fellow, Pediatric Endocrinology
Phoenix Children's Hospital
Phoenix, Arizona
Pediatrics

Darren G. Deering, DO
Chief Resident, Department
 of Internal Medicine
Banner Good Samaritan Medical Center
Phoenix, Arizona
Medicine

Derek Deibler, MD
PGY-3 Psychiatry Resident
Banner Good Samaritan Medical Center
Phoenix, Arizona
Psychiatry

Stephen J. Fenton, MD
Resident, Department of General Surgery
University of Utah School of Medicine
Salt Lake City, Utah
Surgery

Kimberly A. Gibson, MD, MPH
Resident, Department of Obstetrics
 & Gynecology
Kaiser Permanente, San Francisco
San Francisco, California
Obstetrics & Gynecology

M. Rosanna Gray-Swain, MD
Resident, Department of Obstetrics
 & Gynecology
Washington University
St. Louis, Missouri
Obstetrics & Gynecology

Joel A. Hahnke, MD
Pediatric Chief Resident
Phoenix Children's Hospital
Phoenix, Arizona
Pediatrics

Ronald C. Hansen, MD
Chief, Pediatric Dermatology
Phoenix Children's Hospital
Phoenix, Arizona
Pediatrics

John R. Hartley, DO, FAAP
Attending Physician, General Pediatrics
Phoenix Children's Hospital
Phoenix, Arizona
Pediatrics

Amy E. Helmer, BA
Class of 2004
University of California, San Francisco
San Francisco, California
Obstetrics & Gynecology

Michelle Huddleston, MD
Clinical Assistant Professor, Pediatrics
 and Internal Medicine
University of Arizona School of Medicine

Tucson, Arizona
Attending Pediatrician and
Clinical Director of Adolescent Clinic
Phoenix Children's Hospital
Phoenix, Arizona
Pediatrics

John Kashani, DO
Office of Medical Toxicology
Banner Good Samaritan Medical Center
Phoenix, Arizona
Pediatrics

Adam R Koelsch, MD
Chief Resident, Department of Psychiatry
Banner Good Samaritan Medical Center
Phoenix, Arizona
Psychiatry

Frank LoVecchio, DO, MPH
Medical Director
Banner Good Samaritan Poison
 Control Center
Maricopa Medical Center, Department
 of Emergency Medicine
Phoenix, Arizona
Pediatrics

Margaret R. Moon, MD, MPH
Director, General Pediatrics Outpatient Clinic
Phoenix Children's Hospital
Phoenix, Arizona
Pediatrics

J. Robb Muhm, Jr., MD, MBA
Clinical Assistant Professor
University of Arizona School of Medicine
Tucson, Arizona
General Pediatrician
Phoenix Children's Hospital
Phoenix, Arizona
Pediatrics

Elizabeth Baytion Munshi, MD
PGY-3 Psychiatry Resident
Banner Good Samaritan Medical Center
Phoenix, Arizona
Psychiatry

Kay C. Pinckard-Hansen, MD, FAAP
Faculty, General Pediatrics Department;
Teaching Attending Physician; and
Pediatric Consultant, Rehabilitation Program
Phoenix Children's Hospital
Phoenix, Arizona
Pediatrics

Michael Recht, MD, PhD
Director of Hematology
Director, The Hemophilia Center
Division of Hematology/Oncology
Phoenix Children's Hospital
Phoenix, Arizona
Pediatrics

Mukesh Sahu
Class of 2004
University of California, San Francisco
San Francisco, California
Obstetrics & Gynecology

Adam Schwarz, MD
Clinical Associate Professor of Pediatrics
University of Arizona School of Medicine
Director, Education Program
Division of Pediatric Critical Care
Phoenix Children's Hospital
Phoenix, Arizona
Pediatrics

Brian L. Shaffer, MD
Resident, Department of Obstetrics & Gynecology
University of California, San Francisco
San Francisco, California
Obstetrics & Gynecology

Tressia Shaw, MD
Chief Resident, Internal Medicine/
  Pediatrics
Banner Good Samaritan Medical Center
Phoenix Children's Hospital
Phoenix, Arizona
Medicine

Lishiana Solano-Shaffer, MD
Resident, Department of Obstetrics
  & Gynecology
Kaiser Permanente, Oakland
Oakland, California
Obstetrics & Gynecology

Paul C. Stillwell, MD
Director, Pediatric Pulmonology
Physician in Chief
Phoenix Children's Hospital
Phoenix, Arizona
Pediatrics

Jeffrey Weiss, MD
Chief, Section of General Pediatrics
Phoenix Children's Hospital
Phoenix, Arizona
Professor, Clinical Pediatrics
University of Arizona School
  of Medicine
Pediatrics

Mark Yarema, MD, FRCPC
Fellow, Department of Medical Toxicology
Banner Good Samaritan Medical Center
Phoenix, Arizona
Pediatrics

Acknowledgments

MEDICINE

There are many people who helped to make this project a reality. Thank you to my contributors, Darren Deering, Sarah Beaumont, and Tressia Shaw. Thank you to my mentors and colleagues at "Good Sam," Dr. Alan Leibowitz, Dr. Bob Raschke, Dr. Michelle Park, and Dr. Grant Hertel. Thanks to Kate Heinle at Blackwell Publishing for her advice, and to Frank Wallace for his computer genius. Most of all, thanks to my wonderful family for their love, encouragement, and support of my endeavors, and to my husband, Ron, who completes me.

Brenda L. Shinar

There are several people I would like to thank: first of all, my family, whose love and unwavering support have made me the person I am today; my friends, who put up with me during this project; Sarah and Tressia for being there when the going gets tough; Donna, for having the first faith in me as a physician and as a friend; Barb and Kristin— for *everything* you have done for me through the years; and to "J. Crew" for all the happiness you have brought into my life. This project is dedicated to my parents—words can never repay the gifts that you have given me.

Darren G. Deering

First, I would like to thank Brenda Shinar for her guidance in this project. Without the help of my "sisters" Tressia and Doreen, this task would have been impossible. A special thanks goes to Donna for her support, guidance, and friendship. Last but not least, I thank my parents, Matthew, Jackson, and my husband, Doug.

Sarah Beaumont

There are many people who have been great influences in my life. I would especially like to thank my wonderful colleagues and friends Sarah, Darren, Donna, and Jodi. Thanks to Brenda Shinar for including me in this project. But most of all, I would like to acknowledge my family—thanks Mom, Dad, and Amy for always believing in me and supporting my endeavors.

Tressia Shaw

OBSTETRICS & GYNECOLOGY

We would all like to thank the staff at Blackwell Publishing, particularly Kate Heinle and Nancy Duffy for involving us in this project. I would also like to thank my friends and family for their support and encouragement. In particular, Mom and Dad, Mommaroonie and Pops, Mike & Viv, the girls, Rob & Rosaline, Kim & Mike, Nancy, Ethan, Samara, Soyoung & Cameron, Donna & Doug, Linda, Tina, Patricia, the Bhirridge, the Kaiser SF residents and staff, and of course, my guys, Pi and The Bun, who make the journey meaningful.

Susan H. Tran

This project is dedicated to the medical students, residents, faculty and staff at Stanford Medical Center and the Brigham and Women's Hospital, and most of all to Jacob, Isabel, and Max.

Deirdre J. Lyell

I would like to acknowledge my colleagues, including the residents and faculty in the Departments of Obstetrics and Gynecology at UCSF and the Brigham and Women's Hospital, Peter Callen, Mary Norton, and Gene Washington, whose support makes my work possible. I also thank my mother, father, Ethan, Samara, Big & Mugsy, my new family—Ngan, Lieu, Mike, Vivian, Rob, Kim & Nancy, and Mamy, whose unflagging support during all of my projects keeps me on task and productive. This book is dedicated to The Bun and his college education.

Aaron B. Caughey

PEDIATRICS

Phoenix Children's Hospital, Pediatric Radiology Archives, for supplying a majority of the radiological images used in this book. David Carpientieri, M.D., Pathologist, Phoenix Children's Hospital, for assistance in obtaining and supplying images used in this book. This book is dedicated to Louis and Maria, for your continued love and support.

Jeffrey L. Foti

PSYCHIATRY

A heartfelt thanks to Melissa Hardy for her patience, perseverance, and humor assisting with the preparation of the text and to our Psychiatry residents and medical students at Good Samaritan for their inquisitiveness and fresh thinking.

James B. McLoone

SURGERY

The goal of this review was to provide the appropriate scope and quality of information to adequately prepare students for the surgical portions of the USMLE Step 2 exam. The extent to which that goal has been accomplished is entirely attributable to the efforts of my resident authors, Rafe and Steve, and our faculty reviewers, Michelle and Courtney. Most important, we are all indebted to Mary Mone, our collaborator, counsel, and conscience throughout.

Edward W. Nelson

Contents

Abbreviations

μU	micro international unit
5-FU	5-fluorouracil
5-HIAA	5-hydroxyindoleacetic acid
17-OH	17 hydroxy
AAA	abdominal aortic aneurysm
ABC	airway, breathing, circulation
ABG	arterial blood gas
ABI	ankle brachial index
AC	abdominal circumference
ACAS	Asymptomatic Carotid Atherosclerosis Study
ACE	angiotensin-converting enzyme
ACOSOG	American College of Surgeons Oncology Group
ACS	abdominal compartment syndrome
ACTH	adrenocorticotropic hormone
AD	Alzheimer's disease
ADD	attention deficit disorder
ADH	antidiuretic hormone
ADHD	attention deficit hyperactivity disorder
AED	automatic external defibrillator
AF/AV	anteflexed, anteverted
AFB	acid-fast bacillus
AFI	amniotic fluid index
AFP	alpha-fetoprotein
AGA	appropriate for gestational age infant
AHA	autoimmune hemolytic anemia
AI	aortic insufficiency
AIDS	acquired immunodeficiency syndrome
AIHA	autoimmune hemolytic anemia
All	allergies
ALL	acute lymphocytic leukemia
ALS	amyotrophic lateral sclerosis
ALT	alanine aminotransferase
AMA	advanced maternal age
AML	acute myelogenous leukemia
AN	acanthosis nigricans

ANA	antinuclear antibody
Anti-HBC	antibody to hepatitis B core
AOM	acute otitis media
AP	anteroposterior
APC	adenomatous polyposis coli
APOE	apolipoprotein E
APTT	activated partial thromboplastin time
APUD	amine precursor uptake and decarboxylation
ARDS	adult/acute respiratory distress syndrome
AROM	artificial rupture of membranes
AS	aortic stenosis or ankylosing spondylitis
ASAP	as soon as possible
ASCUS	atypical squamous cells of undetermined significance
ASD	atrial septal defect
ASO	anti-streptolysin O
AST	aspartate aminotransferase
ATN	acute tubular necrosis
AV	arteriovenous, atrioventricular
AVM	arteriovenous malformation
AV	node atrioventricular node
AZT	zidovudine
b-hCG	beta human chorionic gonadotropin
BAL	bronchoalveolar lavage
BAL	dimercaprol
BE	base excess
BID	twice a day
BMI	body mass index
BMP	basic metabolic panel
BP	blood pressure
BPD	biparietal diameter, bronchopulmonary dysplasia
BPH	benign prostatic hypertrophy
BPM	beats per minute
BPP	biophysical profile
BRAT	banana, rice, applesauce, toast

BRBPR	bright red blood per rectum	D&C	dilation and curettage
BRCA-1 and 2	breast cancer gene mutations 1 and 2	D&E	dilation and evacuation
BTL	bilateral tubal ligation	d	day
BUN	blood urea nitrogen	DA	dopamine; duodenal atresia
BW	body weight	DCIS	ductal carcinoma in situ
C	Celsius; centigrade	DDAVP	vasopressin
Ca	calcium	DDH	developmental dysplasia of the hip
CA	coronary artery	DEA	Drug Enforcement Agency
CABG	coronary artery bypass graft	DES	diethylstilbestrol
c-Abl	nonreceptor tyrosine kinase protein	DEXA	dual-energy X-ray absorptiometry
CAD	coronary artery disease	DHEA	dehydroepiandrosterone
CAH	congenital adrenal hyperplasia	DHEAS	dehydroepiandrosterone sulfate
cAMP	cyclic adenosine monophosphate	DI	diabetes insipidus
CAP	community-acquired pneumonia	DIC	disseminated intravascular coagulation
CBC	complete blood count	DID	dissociative identity disorder
CBT	cognitive behavioral therapy	DIP	distal interphalangeal (joint)
cc	cubic centimeter	DKA	diabetic ketoacidosis
CCU	coronary care unit	dL	deciliter
CDC	Center for Disease Control	DLB	dementia with Lewy bodies
CEA	carcinoembryonic antigen	DM	diabetes mellitus
CF	cystic fibrosis	DMSA	2,3 dimercaptosuccinic acid
CHF	congestive heart failure	DNA	deoxyribonucleic acid
CI	cardiac index	DSM	diagnostic and Statistical Manual
CIN II	cervical intraepithelial neoplasia grade 2	DTaP	diphtheria, tetanus, acellular pertussis
Cl	chloride	DTR	deep tendon reflex
CLL	chronic lymphocytic leukemia	DUB	dysfunctional uterine bleeding
cm	centimeter	DVT	deep venous thrombosis
CML	chronic myelogenous leukemia	EBV	Epstein-Barr virus
CMP	complete metabolic panel	ECF	extracellular fluid
CMV	cytomegalovirus	ECG	electrocardiogram
c-myc	protooncogene	ECHO	echocardiogram
CNS	central nervous system	ECMO	extracorporeal membrane oxygenation
CO	cardiac output	ECT	electroconvulsive therapy
CO_2	carbon dioxide/bicarbonate	ED	emergency department
COPD	chronic obstructive pulmonary disease	EDC	estimated date of confinement
CPAP	continuous positive airway pressure	EGD	esophagogastroduodenoscopy
CPK	creatine phosphokinase	ECG	electrocardiogram
CPK-MB	creatine phosphokinase MB isoenzyme, creatinine phosphokinase-myocardial	ELISA	enzyme-linked immunosorbent assay
		EMBx	endometrial biopsy
CPM	central pontine myelinolysis	EMG	electromyogram
CPPD	calcium pyrophosphate dihydrate	EMS	emergency medical service
CPR	cardiopulmonary resuscitation	ENT	ears, nose, and throat
Cr	creatinine	EPS	extrapyramidal symptoms
CRF	corticotropin-releasing factor	ER	emergency room
CRP	C-reactive protein	ERCP	endoscopic retrograde cholangiopancreatography
CSF	cerebrospinal fluid		
CST	contraction stress test	ERU	endorectal ultrasound
CT	computed tomography (cat scan)	ESR	erythrocyte sedimentation rate
CTA	computed tomography angiography	EtOH	ethanol, alcohol
CVA	cerebral vascular accident	ETT	endotracheal tube
CVP	central venous pressure	F	Fahrenheit
CXR	chest X-ray	FEV_1	forced expiratory volume in 1 second

FFP	fresh frozen plasma
FHR	fetal heart rate
FIGO	International Federation of Gynecology and Obstetrics
FiO_2	fraction of inspired oxygen
FL	femur length
FLM	fetal lung maturity
FNA	fine-needle biopsy
FOBT	fecal occult blood testing
FSGN	focal segmental glomerulonephritis
FSH	follicle-stimulating hormone
FTA-ABS	fluorescent treponemal antibody absorption
FTT	failure to thrive
g	gram
G	gravida
G6PD	glucose 6-phosphate dehydrogenase
GA	gestational age
GABA	gamma-aminobutyric acid
GAD	generalized anxiety disorder
GAS	group A streptococcus
GBS	group B streptococcus
GCS	Glasgow Coma Score
GDM	gestational diabetes mellitus
GE	gastroesophageal
GER	gastroesophageal reflux
GERD	gastroesophageal reflux disease
GHB	gamma hydroxybutyrate
GI	gastrointestinal
GIFT	gamete intra-fallopian tube transfer
GnRH	gonadotropin-releasing hormone
GTD	gestational trophoblastic disease
GU	genitourinary
H_2	histamine 2 receptor
HA	headache
HAART	highly active anti-retroviral therapy
HAV	hepatitis A virus
HBSAb	hepatitis B surface antibody
HBSAg	hepatitis B surface antigen
HC	head circumference
HCC	hepatocellular carcinoma
hCG	human chorionic gonadotropin
HCM	hypertrophic cardiomyopathy (also called HOCM)
HCO_3	bicarbonate
Hct	hematocrit
HCV	hepatitis C virus
HDL	high-density lipoprotein
HEENT	head, eyes, ears, nose, throat
HELLP	hemolysis, elevated liver enzymes, low platelets
her-2 neu	human epidermal growth factor receptor-2
HgbA1C	hemoglobin A1C
HHV-8	human herpes virus-8
HIDA scan	hydroxy iminodiacetic acid scan
HIPAA	Health Insurance Portability and Accountability Act
HIV	human immunodeficiency virus
HMG-CoA	hydroxy-methylglutaryl-coenzyme A
HNPCC	hereditary nonpolyposis colon cancer
HOCM	hypertrophic obstructive cardiomyopathy
HPF	high power field
HPI	history of present illness
HPP	history of present pregnancy
HPV	human papillomavirus
HR	heart rate
HRT	hormone replacement therapy
HSG	hysterosalpingography
HSV	herpes simplex virus
HT	serotonin
HTLV-1	human T-cell lymphotropic virus-1
HUS	hemolytic uremic syndrome
HVA	homovanillic acid
I^{131}	iodine 131
IAP	intraabdominal pressure
IBD	inflammatory bowel disease
ICP	intracranial pressure
ICSI	intracytoplasmic sperm injection
ICU	intensive care unit
Ig	immunoglobulin
IGF	insulin growth factor
IL	interleukin
IM	intramuscular
INH	isoniazid
INR	international normalized ratio
IPTH	intact parathyroid hormone
IPV	inactivated polio
IQ	intelligence quotient
ITP	immune thrombocytopenic purpura
IUD	intrauterine device
IUFD	intrauterine fetal demise
IUGR	intrauterine growth restriction
IUI	intrauterine insemination
IUP	intrauterine pregnancy
IV	intravenous
IVC	inferior vena cava
IVDA	intravenous drug abuse
IVF	in vitro fertilization
IVH	intraventricular hemorrhage
IVIG	intravenous immune globulin
IVP	intravenous pyelography

J	Joules	mIU	milli-International Unit
JNC-VII	joint national commission VII	mm	millimeter
JRA	juvenile rheumatoid arthritis	mmHg	millimeters of mercury
K	potassium	mmol	millimole
Kcal	kilocalorie	MMR	measles, mumps, rubella
KCL	potassium chloride	MMSE	mini-mental state examination
KG	kilogram	MR(I)	magnetic resonance (imaging)
KOH	potassium hydroxide	MRA	magnetic resonance angiography
k-ras	protooncogene	MS	multiple sclerosis
KUB	kidneys, ureters, bladder (a plain abdominal X-ray)	MTC	medullary thyroid cancer
		MTP	metatarsophalangeal (joint)
L	lumbar	NA	sodium
L	liter	NaHCO$_3$	sodium bicarbonate
LAD	left anterior descending	NASCET	North American Symptomatic Carotid Endarterectomy Trial
Lb	pound		
LCIS	lobular cancer in situ	NBT	nitroblue tetrazolium test
LDH	lactate dehydrogenase	NE	norepinephrine
LDL	low density lipoprotein	NEC	necrotizing enterocolitis
LES	lower esophageal sphincter	ng	nanogram
LFTs	liver function tests	NG	nasogastric
LGA	large for gestational age infant	NGT	nasogastric tube
LH	luteinizing hormone	NJ	nasojejunal
Li	lithium	NKDA	no known drug allergies
LMP	last menstrual period	NLD	necrobiosis lipoidica diabeticorum
LP	lumbar puncture	NMS	neuroleptic malignant syndrome
LSD	D-lysergic acid	n-myc	protooncogene
LSO	left salpingo-oophorectomy	NPO	nil per os (nothing by mouth)
LUQ	left upper quadrant	NPV	negative predictive value
LV	left ventricle	NS	normal saline
LVAD	left ventricular assist device	NSABP	National Surgical Adjuvant Bowel and Breast Project
LVH	left ventricular hypertrophy		
m	meter	NSAID	nonsteroidal anti-inflammatory drug
MAC	membrane attack complex	NST	nonstress test
MALT	mucosa-associated lymphoid tissue	NT	nontender
MAOI	monoamine oxidase inhibitor	O$_2$	oxygen
MCH	mean corpuscular hemoglobin	OA	osteoarthritis
MCHC	mean corpuscular hemoglobin concentration	OCD	obsessive-compulsive disorder
		OCP	oral contraceptive pill
MCP	metacarpophalangeal (joint)	OCT	oxytocin challenge test
MCV	mean corpuscular volume	1,25 OH$_2$D$_3$	1,25-dihydroxyvitamin D
MDMA	ecstasy	OME	otitis media with effusion
MEN	multiple endocrine neoplasia	OPSI	overwhelming
mEq	milliequivalent	OR	operating room
mg	milligram	OSA	obstructive sleep apnea
Mg	magnesium	OTC	over the counter
mg/dL	milligram per deciliter	p	para; parity
MGUS	monoclonal gammapathy of undetermined significance	P	pulse
		PA	posterior-anterior
MHC	major histocompatibility complex	PA	pulmonary artery
MI	myocardial infarction	paO$_2$	partial pressure of O$_2$ in arterial blood
MIBG	metaiodobenzylguanidine	Pap	papanicolaou (smear)
min	minute	PCo$_2$	arterial carbon dioxide pressure

PCOD	polycystic ovarian disease	PTL	preterm labor
PCOS	polycystic ovarian syndrome	PTSD	posttraumatic stress disorder
PCP	phencyclidine; Pneumocystis carinii pneumonia; primary care physician	PTT	partial thromboplastin time (same as aPTT)
PCR	polymerase chain reaction	PTU	propylthiouracil
PCWP	pulmonary capillary wedge pressure	PVC	polyvinyl chloride
PD	parkinson's disease	PVD	peripheral vascular disease
PDA	patent ductus arteriosus	QD	once per day
PE	physical exam/pulmonary embolus	QID	four times per day
PEEP	positive end expiratory pressure	R	respirations
PET	positron emission tomography	RA	rheumatoid arthritis; room air
PFT	pulmonary function tests	Rb	retinoblastoma
PGE1M	prostaglandin E1M – Cytotec/ misoprostol	RBC	red blood cells
		RCC	renal cell carcinoma
PGE2	prostaglandin E2	RDW	red cell distribution width
PGF2a	prostaglandin F2-alpha	REE	resting energy expenditure
PGynHx	past gynecologic history	REM	rapid eye movement
pH	hydrogen ion concentration	RET	rearranged during transfection oncogene
PICU	pediatric intensive care unit	RF	rheumatoid factor
PID	pelvic inflammatory disease	RL	ringer's lactate
PIP	peak inspiratory pressure; proximal interphalangeal (joint)	RNA	ribonucleic acid
		ROM	rupture of membranes
PLTS	platelets	RPR	rapid plasma reagin
PMDD	premenstrual dysphoric disorder	RR	respiratory rate
PMHx	past medical history	RSO	right salpingo-oophorectomy
PMN	polymorphonuclear (white blood cell)	RSV	respiratory syncytial virus
PNS	parasympathetic nervous system	RUQ	right upper quadrant
PO	per os (by mouth)	RV	right ventricle
PO_2	arterial oxygen pressure	RVAD	right ventricular assist device
pO_2	oxygen partial pressure	S	sacrum
PO_4	phosphate	s	seconds
POBHx	past obstetric history	SAB	spontaneous abortion
POC	products of conception	SAD	seasonal affective disorder or social anxiety disorder
POMC	pro-opiate melanocorticotropin		
PPD	purified protein derivative	SaO_2	arterial oxygen saturation
PPROM	preterm premature rupture of membranes	SBE	subacute bacterial endocarditis
		SBO	small bowel obstruction
PPV	positive predictive value	SCC	squamous cell carcinoma
PROM	premature rupture of membranes	SCD	sequential compression device
PR	per rectum	SCFE	slipped capital femoral epiphysis
PRN	as necessary	SG	Swan Ganz
PSA	prostate-specific antigen	SGA	small for gestational age infant
PSC	primary sclerosing cholangitis	SIADH	syndrome of inappropriate antidiuretic hormone
PSGN	Poststreptococcal glomerulonephritis		
PSHx	past surgical history	SICU	surgical intensive care unit
PT	prothrombin time	SIDS	sudden infant death syndrome
PTC	percutaneous transhepatic cholangiography	SLE	systemic lupus erythematosus
		SMI	seriously mentally ill
PTH	parathyroid hormone	SMR	sexual maturity rating
PTHC	percutaneous transhepatic cholangiography	SNS	sympathetic nervous system
		SPEP	serum protein electrophoresis
PTH-rp	parathyroid hormone-related peptide	SROM	spontaneous rupture of membranes

SRU	solitary rectal ulcer	TPN	total parenteral nutrition
SSE	sterile speculum exam	TRH	thyroid-releasing hormone; thyrotropin-releasing hormone
SSI	superficial skin infection		
SSRI	selective serotonin reuptake inhibitors	TSH	thyroid-stimulating hormone
STD	sexually transmitted disease	TSS	toxic shock syndrome
SVE	sterile vaginal exam	TSST	toxic shock syndrome toxin
SVR	systemic vascular resistance	TTE	trans-thoracic echocardiogram
SVT	supraventricular tachycardia	TTN	transient tachypnea of the newborn
T	temperature; thoracic	TTP	thrombotic thrombocytopenic purpura
T_3	triiodothyronine	TURBT	transurethral resection bladder tumor
T_4	thyroxine	TURP	transurethral resection of the prostate
TAB	therapeutic abortion	UA	urinalysis
TAH-BSO	total abdominal hysterectomy and bilateral salpingo-oophorectomy	UC	ulcerative colitis
		UGI	upper gastrointestinal tract
TB	tuberculosis	U/L	International Units per liter
TBSA	total body surface area	UPEP	urine protein electrophoresis
TBW	total body water	URI	upper respiratory infection
TCA	tricyclic antidepressant	US	ultrasound
TD	tardive dyskinesia	UTI	urinary tract infection
TEE	trans-esophageal echocardiogram	VDRL	Venereal Disease Research Laboratory
TEF	tracheoesophageal fistula	V_E	minute ventilation
TFT	thyroid function test	VLDL	very low density lipoprotein
TIBC	total iron-binding capacity	VMA	vanillylmandelic acid
TIA	transischemic attack	V/Q	ventilation/perfusion
TID	three times per day	VS	vital signs
TIPSS	Transjugular Intrahepatic Porto-Systemic Shunt	VSD	ventricular septal defect
		V_T	tidal volume
TM	tympanic membrane	VTE	venous thromboembolism
TNF	tumor necrosis factor	VZIG	varicella-zoster immunoglobulin
TNM	tumor/node/metastasis	VZV	varicella zoster virus
TOA	tubo-ovarian abscess	WBC	white blood cells
Tob	tobacco	WPW	Wolff-Parkinson-White syndrome
TP	total protein	XR	X-ray

Normal Ranges of Laboratory Values

U.S. traditional units are followed in parentheses by equivalent values expressed in SI units.

Blood, Plasma, and Serum Chemistries

Acetoacetate, plasma—<1 mg/dL (0.1 mmol/L)	
Alanine aminotransferase (ALT) (Pediatrics)	2–40 IU/L
Alanine aminotransferase (ALT, GPT at 30 C) (Ob/Gyn)	8–20 U/L
Albumin	3.8–5.4 g/dL
Alkaline phosphatase	42–362 IU/L
Alpha-fetoprotein, serum—0–20 ng/mL (0-20 µg/L)	
Aminotransferase, alanine (ALT, SGPT)—0–35 U/L	
Aminotransferase, aspartate (AST, SGOT)—0–35 U/L	
Ammonia, plasma—40–90 µg/dL (23–47 µmol/L)	
Amylase (Pediatrics)	21–86 IU/L
Amylase, serum (Ob/Gyn)	25–125 U/L
Amylase, serum (Medicine)	0–130 U/L
Anti-nuclear antibody	<1:40
Antistreptolysin O titer (school-aged child)	170–330 Todd units
Antistreptolysin O titer—<150 units	
Arterial blood gas, child	
pH	7.35–7.45
pCO_2	35–40 mm Hg
pO_2	90–95 mm Hg
HCO_3	22–26 mEq/L
Ascorbic acid (vitamin C), blood—0.4–1.5 mg/dL (23–86 µmol/L); leukocyte—<20 mg/dL (<3.5 µmol/L)	
Asparatate aminotransferase (AST, GOT at 30 C)	8–20 U/L
Aspartate aminotransferase (AST)	10–41 IU/L
Bicarbonate	22–28 mEq/L
Bicarbonate, serum—23–28 mEq/L (23–28 mmol/L)	
Bilirubin, serum (Medicine, Surgery)	
Total—0.3–1.2 mg/dL (5.1–20.5 µmol/L)	
Direct—0–0.3 mg/dL (0–5.1 µmol/L)	
Bilirubin, serum (adult) Total/Direct (Ob/Gyn)	0.1–1.0 mg/dL//0.0–0.3 mg/dL
Bilirubin, total (Pediatrics)	0.2–1.1 mg/dL
Blood gases, arterial (room air)	
Po_2—80–100 mm Hg	

P_{CO_2}—35–45 mm Hg
  pH—7.38–7.44
C-reactive protein (CRP)   <0.3 mg/dL
Calcium (Surgery, Pediatrics)   8.8–10.8 mg/dL
Calcium, serum (Ca^{2+}) (Ob/Gyn)   8.4–10.2 mg/dL
Calcium, serum (Medicine)   9–10.5 ng/dL (2.2–2.6 mmol/L)
Carbon dioxide content, serum—23–28 mEq/L
  (23–28 mmol/L)
Carcinoembryonic antigen—<2 ng/mL (2 µg/L)
Carotene, serum—75–300 µg/dL (1.4–5.6 µmol/L)
CD4 absolute count/% (12 months–6 years)
  No suppression   >1000/µL/>25%
  Moderate suppression   500–999/µL/15%–24%
  Severe suppression   <500/µL/<15%
Cerebrospinal fluid, child (CSF)
  WBC   0–7 WBCs/µL
  RBC   0 RBCs/µL
  Glucose   40–80 mg/dL
  Protein   5–40 mg/dL
Ceruloplasmin, serum—25–43 mg/dL (250–430 mg/L)
Chloride   95–105 mEq/L
Chloride, serum—98–106 mEq/L (98–106 mmol/L)
Cholesterol   <170 mg/dL
Cholesterol, serum   Rec: <200 mg/dL
Cholesterol, total, plasma—150–199 mg/dL (3.88–5.15 mmol/L),
  desirable
Cholesterol, low-density lipoprotein (LDL), plasma—≤130 mg/dL
  (3.36 mmol/L) desirable
Cholesterol, high-density lipoprotein (HDL), plasma—≥40 mg/dL
  (1.04 mmol/L), desirable
Complement, serum
  C3—55–120 mg/dL (550–1200 mg/L)
  Total—36–55 U/mL (37–55 kU/L)
Copper, serum—70–155 µg/dL (11.0–24.3 µmol/L)
Creatine kinase (CPK) (Pediatrics)   10–70 U/L
Creatine kinase, serum (Medicine)   30–170 U/L
Creatine kinase, serum (Ob/Gyn)   Female: 10–70 U/L
Creatinine, serum (Pediatrics)   0.6–1.2 mg/dL
Creatinine, serum (Medicine)   0.7–1.3 mg/dL (61.9–115.0 µmol/L)

Delta-aminolevulinic acid, serum—15–23 µg/dL
  (1.14–1.75 µmol/L)
Electrolytes, serum
  Sodium (Na^+)   136–145 mEq/L
  Chloride (Cl^-)   95–105 mEq/L
  Potassium (K^+)   3.5–5.0 mEq/L
  Bicarbonate (HCO_3^-)   22–28 mEq/L
  Magnesium (Mg^{2+})   1.5–2.0 mEq/L
Ethanol, blood—<50 mg/dL (11 nmol/L)
Fibrinogen, plasma—150–350 mg/dL (1.5–3.5 g/L)
Folate, red cell—160–855 ng/mL (362–1937 nmol/L)
Folate, serum—2.5–20.0 ng/mL (5.7–45.3 nmol/L)

Follicle-stimulating hormone, serum/plasma

Female: premenopause 4–30
  mIU/mL
    midcycle peak 10–90 mIU/mL
    postmenopause 40–250
    mIU/mL

Glucose, plasma—fasting, 70–105 mg/dL (3.9–5.8 mmol/L;
  2 hours postprandial <140 mg/dL (7.8 mmol/L)

Glucose, serum

Fasting: 70–110 mg/dL
2-h postprandial: <120 mg/dL

HIV viral load

<50 copies/mL

Homocysteine, plasma—male: 4–16 μmol/L; female: 3–14 μmol/L

Immunoglobulins
   IgG—640–1430 mg/dL (6.4–14.3 g/L)
      IgG_1—280–1020 mg/dL (2.8–10.2 g/L)
      IgG_2—60–790 ng/dL (0.6–7.9 g/L)
      IgG_3—14–240 mg/dL (0.14–2.40 g/L)
      IgG_4—11–330 ng/dL (0.11–3.30 g/L)
   IgA—70–300 mg/dL (0.7–3.0 g/L)
   IgM—20–140 mg/dL (0.2–1.4 g/L)
   IgD—<8 mg/dL (0.1–0.4 mg/L)
   IgE—0.01–0.04 mg/dL (0.1–0.4 mg/L)
Iron, serum—60–160 μg/dL (11–29 μmol/L)
Iron binding capacity, serum—250–460 μg/dL (45–82 μmol/L)

Lactate dehydrogenase, serum (Ob/Gyn)

45–90 U/L

Lactate dehydrogenase, serum (Medicine)

60–100 U/L

Lactic acid, venous blood—6–16 mg/dL (0.67–1.80 mmol/L)

Lead, blood (Pediatrics)

<5 μg/dL

Lead, blood (Medicine)

<40 μg/dL (1.9 μmol/L)

Lipase

16–63 IU/L

Lipase, serum—<95 U/L

Luteinizing hormone, serum/plasma

Female: follicular phase 5–30
  mIU/mL
midcycle 75–150 mIU/mL
postmenopause 30–200 mIU/mL

Magnesium

1.5–2.0 mEq/L

Magnesium, serum—1.5–2.4 mg/dL (0.62–0.99 mmol/L)
Manganese, serum—0.3–0.9 ng/mL (300–900 ng/L)
Methylmalonic acid, serum—150–370 nmol/L
Osmolality, plasma—275–295 mosm/kg H_2O

Osmolality, serum

275–295 mOsmol/kg

Parathyroid hormone, serum, N-terminal

230–630 pg/mL

Phosphatase, acid, serum—0.5–5.5 U/L
Phosphatase, alkaline, serum—36–92 U/L

Phosphate (alkaline), serum (p-NPP at 30 C)

20–70 U/L

Phosphorus, inorganic, serum—3.0–4.5 mg/dL (0.97–1.45 mmol/L)
Potassium, serum—3.5–5.0 mEq/L (3.5–5.0 mmol/L)

Prolactin, serum (hPRL)

<20 ng/mL

Protein

5.7–8 g/dL

Protein, serum
   Total—6.0–7.8 g/dL (60–78 g/L)
   Albumin—3.5–5.5 g/dL (35–55 g/L)
   Globulins—2.5–3.5 g/dL (25–35 g/L)

Alpha$_1$—0.2–0.4 g/dL (2–4 g/L)
Alpha$_2$—0.5–0.9 g/dL (5–9 g/L)
Beta—0.6–1.1 g/dL (6–11 g/L)
Gamma—0.7–1.7 g/dL (7–17 g/L)

Rheumatoid factor (RF) (Pediatrics)	<1:20
Rheumatoid factor (Medicine)	<40 U/mL (<40 kU/L)
Sodium, serum—136–145 mEq/L (136–145 mmol/L)	
Thyroid-stimulating hormone, serum or plasma	0.5–5.0 µU/mL
Thyroidal iodine (^{123}I) uptake	8–30% of administered dose/24 h
Thyroxine (T$_4$), serum	5–12 µg/dL
Triglyceride	<150 mg/dL
Triglycerides—<250 mg/dL (2.82 mmol/L), desirable	
Urea nitrogen, blood (BUN)	8–25 mg/dL
Urea nitrogen, serum (BUN) (Ob/Gyn)	7–18 mg/dL
Urea nitrogen, serum (Medicine)	8–20 mg/dL (2.9–7.1 mmol/L)
Uric acid, serum (Medicine)	2.5–8.0 mg/dL (0.15–0.47 mmol/L)
Uric acid, serum (Ob/Gyn)	3.0–8.2 mg/dL
Vitamin B$_{12}$, serum—200–800 pg/mL (148–590 pmol/L)	

Cerebrospinal Fluid
Cell count—0–5 cells/µL (0–5 × 10^6 cells/L)
Glucose—40–80 mg/dL (2.5–4.4 mmol/L); <40% of simultaneous plasma concentration is abnormal
Protein—15–60 mg/dL (150–600 mg/L)
Pressure (opening)—70–200 cm H$_2$O

Chemistry

Alanine aminotransferase (ALT)	Male: 13–72 U/L, Female: 9-52 U/L
Alkaline phosphatase	38–126 U/L
Amylase	30–110 U/L
Aspartate aminotransferase (AST)	Male: 15–59 U/L, Female: 14–50 U/L
Bicarbonate (HCO$_3^-$)	19–25 mmol/L
Bilirubin total	0.2–1.3 mg/dL
Bilirubin direct	0.0–0.3 mg/dL
Calcium	8.4–10.2 mg/dL
Carbon dioxide	22–29 mmol/L
Chloride (Cl$^-$)	98–107 mmol/L
Creatinine	Male: 0.8–1.5 mg/dL, Female: 0.7–1.2 mg/dL
Glucose	64–128 mg/dL
Lactate	0.7–2.1 mmol/L
Lactate dehydrogenase (LDH)	300–600 U/L
Magnesium (Mg^{2+})	1.6–2.3 mg/dL
Osmolality	280–303 mOsm/kg
Potassium (K$^+$)	3.3–5.0 mmol/L
Phosphorus (inorganic)	2.4–4.3 mg/dL
Sodium (Na$^+$)	136–144 mmol/L
Urea nitrogen (BUN)	Male: 9–22 mg/dL, Female: 6–22 mg/dL

Endocrine

Adrenocorticotropin (ACTH)—9–52 pg/mL (2–11 pmol/L)

Aldosterone, serum
   Supine—2–5 ng/dL (55–138 pmol/L)
   Standing—7–20 ng/dL (194–554 pmol/L)

Aldosterone, urine—5–19 μg/24 h (13.9–52.6 nmol/24 h)

Catecholamines—epinephrine (supine): <75 ng/L (410 pmol/L);
   norepinephrine (supine): 50–440 ng/L (296–2600 pmol/L)

Catecholamines, 24-hour, urine—<100 μg/m^2 per 24 h
   (591 nmol/m^2 per 24 h)

Cortisol
   Serum—8 A.M.: 8–20 μg/dL (221–552 nmol/L);
   5 P.M.: 3–13 μg/dL (83–359 nmol/L)

1 h after cosyntropin: >18 μg/dL (498 nmol/L);
   usually 8 μg/dL (221 nmol/L) or more above baseline

Overnight suppression test: <5 μg/dL (138 nmol/24 h)

Dehydroepiandrosterone sulfate, plasma—Male: 1.3–5.5 mg/mL
   (3.5–14.9 μmol/L); female: 0.6–3.3 mg/mL (1.6–8.9 μmol/L)

11-deoxycortisol, plasma—Basal: <5 μg/dL (145 nmol/L);
   after metyrapone: >7 μg/dL (203 nmol/L)

Estradiol, serum—Male: 10–30 pg/mL (37–110 pmol/L);
   female: day 1–10, 50–100 pmol/L; day 11–20, 50–200 pmol/L;
   day 21–30, 70–150 pmol/L

Estriol, urine—>12 mg/24 h (42 μmol/day)

Follicle-stimulating hormone, serum—Male (adult): 5–15 mU/mL
   (5–15 U/L); female: follicular or luteal phase, 5–20 mU/mL
   (5–20 U/L); midcycle peak, 30–50 mU/mL (30–50 U/L);
   postmenopausal, >35 mU/mL (35 U/L)

Growth hormone, plasma—After oral glucose, <2 ng/mL (2 μg/L);
   response to provocative stimuli: >7 ng/mL (7 μg/L)

17-hydroxycorticosteroids, urine (Porter-Silber)—Male: 3–10 mg/24 h
   (8.3–28 μmol/24 h); female: 2–8 mg/24 h (5.5–22.1 μmol/24 h)

Insulin, serum (fasting)—5–20 mU/L (35–139 pmol/L)

17-ketosteroids, urine—Male: 8–22 mg/24 h (28–77 μmol/24 h);
   female: up to 15 μg/24 h (52 mmol/24 h)

Luteinizing hormone, serum—Male: 3–15 mU/mL (3–15 U/L);
   female: follicular or luteal phase, 5–22 mU/mL (3–15 U/L);
   midcycle peak, 30–250 mU/mL (30-250 U/L);
   postmenopausal, >30 mU/mL (30 U/L)

Metanephrine, urine—<1.2 mg/24 h (6.1 mmol/24 h)

Parathyroid hormone, serum—10–65 pg/mL (10–65 ng/L)

Progesterone
   Luteal—3–30 ng/mL (0.10–0.95 nmol/L)
   Follicular—<1 ng/mL (0.03 nmol/L)

Prolactin, serum—Male: <15 ng/mL (15 mg/L); female: <20 ng/mL (20 mg/L)

Renin activity (angiotensin-I radioimmunoassay), plasma
   Normal diet: supine, 0.3–1.9 ng/mL per h (0.3–1.9 μg/L per h);
   upright, 0.2–3.6 ng/mL per h (0.2–3.6 μg/L per h)

Sperm concentration—20–150 million/mL (20–50 × 10^9/L)

Sweat test for sodium and chloride—<60 mEq/L (60 mmol/L)

Testosterone, serum—Adult male: 300–1200 ng/dL (10–42 nmol/L);
   female: 20–75 ng/dL (0.7–2.6 nmol/L)

Thyroid function tests (normal ranges vary)
   Thyroid iodine (^{131}I) uptake—10%–30% of administered dose at 24 h
   Thyroid-stimulating hormone (TSH)—0.5–5.0 μU/mL (0.5–5.0 mU/mL)
   Thyroxine (T_4), serum
      Total—5–12 μg/dL (64–155 nmol/L)
      Free—0.9–2.4 ng/dL (12–31 pmol/L)
      Free T_4 index—4–11
   Triiodothyronine, resin (T_3)—25%–35%
   Triiodothyronine, serum (T_3)—70–195 ng/dL (1.1–3.0 nmol/L)
Vanillylmandelic acid, urine—<8 mg/24 h (40.4 μmol/24 h)
Vitamin D
   1,25-dihydroxy, serum—25–65 pg/mL (60–156 pmol/L)
   25-hydroxy, serum—15–80 ng/mL (37–200 nmol/L)

Gastrointestinal
D-xylose absorption (after ingestion of 25 g of D-xylose)—
  Urine excretion: 5–8 g at 5 h (33–53 mmol); serum D-xylose:
  >20 mg/dL at 2 h (1.3 nmol/L)
Fecal urobilinogen—40–280 mg/24 h (68–473 μmol/24 h)
Gastric secretion—Basal secretion: male: 4.0 ± 0.2 mEq of HCl/h
  (4.0 ± 0.2 mmol/h); female: 2.1 ± 0.2 mEq of HCl/h
  (2.1 ± 0.2 mmol/h); peak acid secretion: male: 37.4
  ± 0.8 mEq/h (37.4 ± 0.8 mmol/h); female: 24.9 ± 1.0 mEq/h
  (24.9 ± 1.0 mmol/h)
Gastrin, serum—0–180 pg/mL (0–180 ng/L)
Lactose tolerance test—Increase in plasma glucose:
  >15 mg/dL (0.83 mmol/L)
Lipase, ascitic fluid—<200 U/L
Secretin-cholecystokinin pancreatic function—>80 mEq/L
  (80 mmol/L) of HCO_3 in at least one specimen collected over 1 h
Stool fat—<5 g/day on a 100-g fat diet
Stool nitrogen—<2 g/day
Stool weight—<200 g/day

Hematology
Activated partial thromboplastin time—25–35 sec
Bleeding time—<10 min
Coagulation factors, plasma
   Factor I—150–350 mg/dL (1.5–3.5 g/L)
   Factor II—60%–150% of normal
   Factor V—60%–150% of normal
   Factor VII—60%–150% of normal
   Factor VIII—60%–150% of normal
   Factor IX—60%–150% of normal
   Factor X—60%–150% of normal
   Factor XI—60%–150% of normal
   Factor XII—60%–150% of normal

Erythrocyte count (Ob/Gyn)	Female: 3.5–5.5 million/ mm^3
Erythrocyte count (Medicine)	4.2–5.9 million cells/μL (4.2–5.9 × 10^{12} cells/L)
Erythrocyte sedimentation rate, child (ESR)	0–10 mm/hr
Erythrocyte sedimentation rate (Westergren)	Female: 0–20 mm/h

Erythrocyte survival rate (^{51}Cr)—T$^1/_2$ = 28 days
Erythropoietin—<30 mU/mL (30 U/L)
D-dimer—<15–200 ng/mL (15–200 mg/L)
Ferritin, serum—15–200 ng/mL (15–200 mg/L)
Glucose-6-phosphate dehydrogenase, blood—5–15 U/g
  Hgb (0.32–0.97 mU/mol Hgb)
Haptoglobin, serum—50–150 mg/dL (500–1500 mg/L)

Hematocrit, child	12.5–16.1 mg/dL
Hematocrit (Surgery)	Male: 40.8–51.9%, Female: 34.3–46.6%
Hematocrit (Medicine)	Male: 41%–51; female: 36%–47%
Hemoglobin A$_{1C}$	≤6%
Hemoglobin	Male: 14.6–17.8 g/dL (140–170 g/L); Female: 12.1–15.9 g/dL (120–160 g/L)
Hemoglobin, child	36%–47%

Hemoglobin, plasma—0.5–5.0 mg/dL (0.08–0.80 µmol/L)
Leukocyte alkaline phosphatase—15–40 mg of phosphorus
  liberated/h per 10^{10} cells; score = 13–130/100 polymorphonuclear
  neutrophils and band forms

Leukocyte count	3200–10,600/mm^3

Leukocyte count—Nonblacks: 4000–10,000/µL (4.0–10 × 10^9/L);
  blacks: 3500–10,000/µL (3.5–10 × 10^9/L)
Leukocyte count and differential

Leukocyte count	4500–11,000/mm^3
Segmented neutrophils	54–62%
Bands	3–5%
Eosinophils	1–3%
Basophils	0–0.75%
Lymphocytes	25–33%
Monocytes	3–7%

Lymphocytes
  CD4$^+$ cell count—640–1175/µL (0.64–1.18 × 10^9/L)
  CD4$^+$ cell count—335–875/µL (0.34–0.88 × 10^9/L)
  CD4:CD8 ratio—1.0–4.0
Mean corpuscular hemoglobin (MCH)—28–32 pg

Mean corpuscular hemoglobin concentration (MCHC)	31–37 g/dL Mean corpuscular hemoglobin concentration (MCHC)—32–36 g/dL (320–360 g/L)
Mean corpuscular volume (MCV) (Pediatrics)	75–95 µm^3
Mean corpuscular volume (MCV) (Ob/Gyn, Medicine)	80–100 fL

Osmotic fragility of erythrocytes—Increased if hemolysis occurs
  in >0.5% NaCl, decreased if hemolysis is incomplete in 0.3% NaCl

Partial thromboplastin time (activated) (Ob/Gyn)	25–40 seconds
Partial thromboplastin time (PTT) (Pediatrics)	25–40 sec
Partial thromboplastin time (Surgery)	26–37 s
Platelet count (Peds, Ob/Gyn)	150,000–400,000/mm^3
Platelet count (Medicine)	150,000–350,000/µL (150–350 × 10^9/L)
Platelet count (Surgery)	177,000–406,000 K/µL

Platelet life span (^{51}Cr)—8–12 days
Protein C activity, plasma—67%–131%
Protein C resistance—2.2–2.6
Protein S activity, plasma—82%–144%
Prothrombin time (PT) (Ob/Gyn, Pediatrics)   11–15 sec
Prothrombin time (Medicine)   11–13 sec
Prothrombin time (Surgery)   12–15.5 s
Red cell distribution width (RDW)   11.5%–14.5%
Reticulocyte count—0.5%–1.5% of erythrocytes; absolute:
  23,000–90,000 cells/μL (23–90 × 10^9/L)
Schilling test (oral administration of radioactive cobalamin-labeled
  vitamin B$_{12}$)—8.5%–28.0% excreted in urine per 24–48 h
Sedimentation rate, erythrocyte (Westergren)—Male: 0–15 mm/h;
  female: 0–20 mm/h
Volume, blood
    Plasma—Male: 25–44 mL/kg (0.025–0.044 L/kg) body weight;
    female: 28–43 mL/kg (0.028–0.043 L/kg) body weight
      Erythrocyte—Male: 25–35 mL/kg (0.025–0.044 L/kg) body
      weight; female: 20–30 mL/kg (0.020–0.030 L/kg) body weight

Pulmonary

Forced expiratory volume in 1 second (FEV$_1$)—>80% predicted
Forced vital capacity (FVC)—>80% predicted
FEV$_1$/FVC—>75% (0.75)

Urine

Amino acids—200–400 mg/24 h (14–29 nmol/24 h)
Amylase—6.5–48.1 U/h
Calcium—100–300 mg/day (2.5–7.5 mmol/day) on unrestricted diet
Chloride—80–250 mEq/day (80–250 mmol/day) (varies with intake)
Copper—0–100 μg/24 h (0–1.6 μmol/day)
Coproporphyrin—50–250 μg/24 h (76–382 nmol/day)
Creatine—Male: 4–40 mg/24 h (30–305 mmol/24 h);
  female: 0–100 mg/24 h (0–763 mmol/h)
Creatine clearance   Male: 97–137 mL/min
                                        Female: 88–128 mL/min

Creatinine—15–25 mg/kg per 24 h (133–221 mmol/kg per 24 h)
Creatinine clearance—90–140 mL/min (0.09–0.14 L/min)
5-hydroxyindoleacetic acid (5-HIAA)—2–9 mg/24 h
  (10.4–46.8 μmol/day)
Osmolality (Medicine)   38–1400 mosm/kg H$_2$O
Osmolality (Ob/Gyn)   50–1400 mOsmol/kg
Phosphate, tubular resorption—79%–94% (0.79–0.94) of filtered load
Potassium—25–100 mEq/24 h (25–100 mmol/24 h) (varies with intake)
Protein (Medicine)   <100 mg/24 h
Proteins, total (Ob/Gyn)   <150 mg/24 h
Sodium (Ob/Gyn)   Varies with diet
Sodium (Medicine)   100–260 mEq/24 h (100–260
                                          mmol/24 h) (varies with intake)

Uric acid—250–270 mg/24 h (1.48–4.43 mmol/24 h) (varies with diet)
Urobilinogen—0.05–2.50 mg/24 h (0.08–4.22 μmol/24 h)

BLOCK 1

1. A 44-year-old Hispanic man presents to your office for a routine yearly physical exam. His only concern is that his blood pressure was 153/88 at the local health fair 2 months ago. Past medical history is significant for moderate persistent asthma, for which he takes daily fluticasone and albuterol as needed. He has been hospitalized twice in the last year for asthma exacerbations. On exam today his blood pressure is 155/90. The remainder of his cardiovascular and pulmonary exam is unremarkable. The best initial therapy for this patient's hypertension would be:

   A. Propranolol
   B. Diltiazem
   C. Hydrochlorothiazide
   D. Dietary modification and weight loss only
   E. Clonidine

2. A 29-year-old white woman presents with hypertension found during a pre-employment physical. She is otherwise asymptomatic. She has no prior medical history and takes no medications or herbal supplements. Blood pressure is 170/91. Funduscopic exam shows grade II hypertensive changes without hemorrhages. Cardiovascular and pulmonary exam is normal. Abdominal exam is remarkable for a bruit heard in the left upper quadrant. This patient's hypertension is most likely due to:

   A. Coronary artery disease
   B. Fibromuscular dysplasia of the renal artery
   C. Cushing's syndrome
   D. Benign essential hypertension
   E. Pheochromocytoma

End of Set

The next two questions (items 3 and 4) correspond to the following vignette.

A 41-year-old white man presents with 3 weeks of progressive weight gain and pedal and periorbital edema. He has no prior medical history and takes no medications. Exam is notable for blood pressure of 151/92 with normal cardiovascular and pulmonary exam. 3+ Pedal edema is present. Lab studies are as follows: Creatinine 1.0 mg/dL; sodium 135 mEq/L; BUN 15 mg/dL; potassium 4.2 mEq/L; albumin 2.5 g/dL; urinalysis 4+ protein; no blood.

3. Which of the following additional studies should be ordered next to confirm the diagnosis?

   A. 24-hour urine protein
   B. Liver function tests
   C. Serum cholesterol
   D. Renal ultrasound
   E. Renal biopsy

4. What is the most common primary renal disease that causes this patient's syndrome in adult Americans?

   A. Minimal change disease
   B. Focal segmental glomerulosclerosis
   C. Membranoproliferative glomerulonephritis
   D. Membranous glomerulonephritis
   E. Amyloidosis

End of Set

5. An 18-year-old man presents to your office with a complaint of hematuria. He also complains of an upper respiratory illness that began 2 days ago and consists of clear rhinorrhea, a nonproductive cough, and general myalgias. Blood pressure is

1

SIADH

121/70 and he is afebrile. His nasal mucous membranes are mildly inflamed with clear rhinorrhea noted. His throat is mildly erythematous without tonsillar exudates. His heart is regular without murmurs and his lungs are clear to auscultation. There are no skin rashes. A routine urinalysis shows 2+ blood and 1+ protein. Which of the following statements is true concerning this patient's disease process?

A. Findings on renal biopsy would include mesangial proliferation and glomerular IgA deposits by immunofluorescence
B. Serum IgA levels correlate with course of the disease
C. The use of immunosuppressive treatment is well established
D. 10% to 25% of patients have normal renal function 10 years after diagnosis
E. The natural course of this disease is well known and predictable

6. A 34-year-old man presents with complaints of severe right flank pain that began 4 hours ago. The pain is sharp, severe, and radiates to the right groin. He denies fever and finds it difficult to urinate. On exam, he appears to be in distress secondary to pain. His pulse is 105 and his blood pressure is 148/90. He is afebrile. On physical exam, he has costovertebral angle tenderness over the right flank. The exam is otherwise normal. A urinalysis reveals a urine pH of 6.5, is positive for blood, and is negative for WBCs, leukocyte esterase, and nitrites. An abdominal plain film shows a small 3-mm radio-opaque density over the right flank. A stone is collected and sent for study. The composition of this patient's stone is most likely to be:

A. Uric acid
B. Struvite
C. Cystine
D. Calcium oxalate
E. Calcium hydroxyapatite (HA)

7. A 76-year-old male nursing home patient with small cell lung cancer is brought into the ER for confusion worsening over the last 24 hours. He has no history of fever or recent medication changes. Vital signs reveal that the patient's blood pressure is 118/70, his pulse is 70, and he is afebrile. The exam is notable for a cachectic-appearing elderly man who is disoriented and

unable to answer questions appropriately. Initial lab results are as follows: Sodium 113 mEq/L; glucose 95 mg/dL; calcium 9.0 mg/dL; magnesium 1.8 mEq/L. The patient begins to have a generalized tonic clonic seizure. Which of the following is the most appropriate initial management?

A. Fluid restriction
B. Infuse 3% hypertonic saline
C. Start IV demeclocycline
D. Give 1 ampule of dextrose 50 IV
E. CT of the head

8. You are in the clinic and have ordered a urine dip on a patient with diabetes to evaluate for proteinuria. If this dip is negative for macroscopic protein, you plan on sending the urine for microalbumin levels. Which of the following statements regarding detecting proteinuria on urine dipstick testing is true?

A. A urine dipstick can detect protein in a concentrated urine specimen with the same accuracy as a dilute urine specimen
B. False-positive reactions may occur as a result of some antiseptics and other iodinated agents
C. Normal amounts of protein do not cause a positive reaction in a concentrated specimen
D. Highly acidic urine may cause false-positive reactions
E. Immunoglobulins or light chains in the urine can be reliably detected by urine dipstick

9. A 40-year-old man is admitted after a suicide attempt. He states that he drank a liquid substance found in his garage. He is unable to give more specific details. He is complaining of blurred vision. He is awake and alert with normal vital signs and normal physical exam. Labs are as follows: Glucose 90 mg/dL; sodium 140 mEq/L; potassium 4.9 mEq/L; chloride 95 mEq/L; bicarbonate 15 mEq/L; BUN 17 mg/dL; creatinine 1.3 mg/dL; osmolality 320; pH on arterial blood gas 7.28. No crystals are noted on urinalysis. What substance did this patient most likely ingest?

A. Mannitol
B. Ethylene glycol
C. Methanol
D. Gasoline
E. Isopropyl alcohol

10. A 65-year-old man with chronic renal insufficiency secondary to polycystic kidney disease presents with impaired mental status, nausea, and vomiting. He is disoriented to time and place on exam. Excoriated areas of skin and asterixis are also noted on physical exam. The patient's symptoms are most likely due to elevated:

    A. Phosphorus
    B. Potassium
    C. BUN
    D. Sodium
    E. Bicarbonate

11. A 74-year-old man with congestive heart failure (CHF) presents with generalized weakness. He reports running out of his furosemide 4 days ago, but continuing all other medications including his angiotensin-converting enzyme (ACE) inhibitor, β-blocker, spironolactone, and potassium chloride supplement. Blood pressure is 125/85, and jugular venous distension is present. His cardiovascular exam is notable for a S_3 gallop, his lungs are clear to auscultation bilaterally, and he has 1+ pedal edema. An ECG is obtained (Figure 1-11). What is the most likely diagnosis?

    A. Hypercalcemia
    B. Acute myocardial infarction
    C. Uncontrolled congestive heart failure
    D. Hypokalemia
    E. Hyperkalemia

of 2.0 mg/dL, which was up from his baseline of 1.0 mg/dL. Which of the following urine sediments is most suggestive of acute tubular necrosis?

    A. Red blood cell casts
    B. White blood cell casts
    C. Muddy brown granular casts
    D. Hyaline casts
    E. Eosinophils

The response options for items 13 through 16 are the same. You will be required to select one answer for each item in the set.

    A. pH 7.27; pCO_2 14 mmHg; bicarbonate 7 mEq/L; sodium 134 mEq/L; potassium 2.7 mEq/L; chloride 116 mEq/L
    B. pH 7.0; pCO_2 72 mmHg; bicarbonate 15 mEq/L; sodium 138 mEq/L; potassium 5.7 mEq/L; chloride 90 mEq/L
    C. pH 7.15; pCO_2 18 mmHg; bicarbonate 7 mEq/L; sodium 128 mEq/L; potassium 4.1 mEq/L; chloride 100 mEq/L
    D. pH 7.52; pCO_2 23 mmHg; bicarbonate 20 mEq/L; sodium 135 mEq/L; potassium 4.2 mEq/L; chloride 108 mEq/L
    E. E. pH 7.32; pCO_2 50 mmHg; bicarbonate 19 mEq/L; sodium 138 mEq/L; potassium 5.0 mEq/L; chloride 108 mEq/L

For each clinical scenario, select the most appropriate arterial blood gas and electrolyte values.

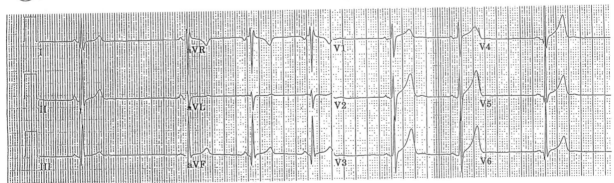

Figure 1-11 • Image Courtesy of Dr. Brenda Shinar, Banner Good Samaritan Medical Center, Phoenix, Arizona.

12. A 54-year-old man was admitted for abdominal pain, nausea, vomiting, and diarrhea for the past 2 days. He has been unable to tolerate any oral intake of food or water for the past 2 days. His blood pressure on admit was 90/50 with a pulse of 140, and his labs were significant for a creatinine

13. A 61-year-old man with diabetes presents with nausea, vomiting, and polyuria.

14. A 23-year-old woman presents with palpitations, chest pain, and an "impending sense of doom."

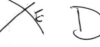

15. A 34-year-old woman presents with watery diarrhea for the last 3 days.

16. A 28-year-old man with a history of asthma presents with tachypnea, wheezing, chest tightness and severe shortness of breath.

End of Set

17. A 55-year-old man is admitted to the hospital with hematemesis. He had no prior abdominal pain and has a significant history of alcohol abuse. You are concerned that the patient may have unrecognized severe liver disease and that his upper GI bleed may be due to esophageal varices. Which of the following is a physical exam finding in a patient with liver cirrhosis that may clue you to the correct etiology of his bleeding?

A. Buffalo hump
B. Palmar erythema
C. Palpable purpura
D. Proptosis
E. Acanthosis nigricans

18. An 18-year-old woman comes to your office with complaints of nausea, vomiting, fever, and right upper quadrant discomfort for the past 4 days. She noticed that the whites of her eyes began to turn yellow yesterday. She has no prior medical history; does not drink alcohol, smoke, or use drugs; and has never had sexual intercourse. She works in a day-care facility. On physical exam, her vital signs are the following: Blood pressure 105/70, heart rate 100, respiratory rate 14, and temperature 99.0°F (37.2°C). She has mild scleral icterus and her mucous membranes are dry. She has a normal cardiac and pulmonary exam, and abdominal exam reveals mild hepatomegaly with tenderness to moderate palpation in the right upper quadrant. There is no splenomegaly. Her laboratories reveal an AST of 1500 U/L, an ALT of 1700 U/L, and total bilirubin of 2.5 mg/dL. Her alkaline phosphase is normal at 80 U/L. You suspect a viral hepatitis. Which of the following is a risk factor for transmission of hepatitis A?

A. IV drug use
B. Tattoos
C. Blood transfusions
D. Work in a health care profession
E. Ingestion of fecally contaminated water

19. A 65-year-old white woman presents to your office with complaints of dysphagia for solids but not for liquids that seems to be getting worse for the past year. She has had to eliminate bread from her diet because of its tendency to get stuck, and to cut up her food in small pieces. She has also noted weight loss of 10 pounds in the last month. She has been taking an over-the-counter H2 blocker and other antacids for symptom relief of her heartburn, which she has had for over 10 years. Past medical history and family history are otherwise negative. The next step in this patient's care is:

A. 24-hour pH esophageal monitor
B. Endoscopy
C. Chest X-ray
D. CT scan of chest
E. Trial a proton pump inhibitor

20. A 46-year-old white woman presents to your office for routine checkup. Past medical history is significant for asthma diagnosed 2 years ago. She states she has an asthma attack two to three times per month, and the episodes usually occur at night. She has not noted any improvement with her current regimen of an albuterol metered dose inhaler. Further review of systems is otherwise negative with the exception of heartburn she has had for the past 3 years. Exam is essentially normal with no evidence of tachypnea or hypoxia. Lung fields are clear bilaterally without wheezes. There is no prolonged respiratory phase and no accessory muscle use. The next step in the treatment of this patient's bronchospasm is:

A. Add a long-acting β-agonist
B. Start an inhaled steroid
C. Add a leukotriene receptor antagonist
D. Trial a proton pump inhibitor
E. No change in therapy at this time

21. A 69-year-old white man presents to the ED with sudden onset of left lower quadrant pain, fever, nausea, and vomiting. He states the pain started 2 days ago. He denies any history of diarrhea, melena, or hematochezia and states that he has not had a bowel movement in 2 days, since the pain started. He says that his only medical problem is constipation. He denies any sick contacts. On exam he has a low-grade temperature of 100.3°F (37.9°C) with otherwise normal vital signs. Abdominal exam is significant for left lower

quadrant tenderness to palpation with some fullness. Bowel sounds are hypoactive and there is no rebound. This patient most likely has:

A. Inflammatory bowel disease
B. Diverticulitis
C. Colon cancer
D. Diverticulosis
E. Appendicitis

22. A 76-year-old man comes to the ER with complaints of bright red blood per rectum (BRBPR). He says that it has occurred a couple of times in the past month and he has noticed some blood surrounding the stool or on the toilet paper. This morning there appeared to be quite a bit of blood in the toilet and the patient said he got a little light-headed. He denies abdominal pain, fever, weight loss, or bleeding at any other site. On physical exam, he is not orthostatic. His abdominal exam is normal, and his rectal exam reveals a small amount of bright red blood. What is the most common cause of lower GI bleeding and therefore his most likely diagnosis?

A. Diverticulosis
B. Hemorrhoids
C. Infectious diarrhea
D. Inflammatory bowel disease
E. Upper GI bleed

23. A 35-year-old white man presents with a 2 to 3 week history of odynophagia. Past medical history is significant for AIDS diagnosed 5 years ago. The patient notes pain with swallowing of both liquids and solids. He denies any sensation of food getting stuck. He has lost approximately 5 pounds secondary to inability to eat. The most likely cause of this person's odynophagia is:

A. Gastroesophageal reflux disease (GERD)
B. Achalasia
C. Barrett's esophagus
D. Infectious esophagitis
E. Diffuse esophageal spasms

24. An 82-year-old woman comes to your clinic with complaints of fatigue and shortness of breath for the past couple of months. She has also noticed that she is not as hungry as usual and when she does eat, she gets full quickly. She denies abdominal pain, chest pain, or cough. She has lost approximately 15 pounds over the past 6 months without intention, but she attributes it to not eating as much. On physical exam, she is thin and in no acute distress. She has normal vital signs. Her exam is unremarkable, including her abdominal exam, although her rectal exam reveals brown, guaiac-positive stool. Her laboratories reveal a microcytic, microchromic anemia with a hemoglobin of 9.2. She is referred for upper and lower endoscopies, and the upper endoscopy reveals a 4-cm ulcerated mass in the antrum of the stomach. Which of the following is an independent risk factor for gastric adenocarcinoma?

A. Alcohol abuse
B. Nonsteroidal anti-inflammatory drug (NSAID)-induced ulcers
C. Tobacco abuse
D. Long-standing GERD
E. *Helicobacter pylori*

25. A 45-year-old obese white woman presents with severe epigastric pain radiating to her back. She states the symptoms started yesterday and are also associated with vomiting. She denies any fever or chills. She also denies any change in bowel habits. On review of systems she states that intermittently she has right-sided abdominal pain after eating out at her favorite Mexican restaurant. She denies any history of alcohol abuse. Physical exam is essentially within normal limits with the exception of her abdomen, which is tender to palpation in the epigastric region. There is no rebound or hepatosplenomegaly. Bowel sounds are normoactive. You order basic labs that reveal normal liver function tests; however, the patient does have an elevated amylase and lipase. The most likely cause of her pancreatitis is:

A. Gallstones
B. Alcohol use
C. Trauma
D. Drugs
E. Tobacco use

26. An 18-year-old white man presents with 2 to 3 days of diarrhea. He denies any recent travel but recently dined at a new restaurant with his family. No other sick contacts are noted. He states the diarrhea is blood-tinged and loose in nature. He complains of crampy abdominal pain. On physical exam the patient is afebrile, heart rate is 96, respiratory rate is 18, and blood pressure is 120/72. In general he is alert, pale appearing, and in no acute distress. HEENT exam is significant

for pale conjunctivae. Chest is clear, and cardio-vascular exam reveals a regular rate and rhythm with a II/VI systolic ejection murmur at the left sternal border. Abdomen is soft with diffuse tenderness and skin exam reveals multiple petechiae on his lower extremities. Labs are as follows: WBCs 15,000/μl; hemoglobin 8.0 g/dL; hematocrit 23.0; platelets 40,000; BUN 100; creatinine 7.8. The infectious organism that would best explain the patient's syndrome is:

A. *Cryptosporidium*
B. *Giardia*
C. Rotavirus
D. *E. coli* O157:H7
E. *Vibrio cholerae*

27. A 24-year-old white woman presents to your office with intermittent, cramping abdominal pain with alternating diarrhea, constipation, and bloating. These symptoms have occurred for the past 3 years and she notes that the symptoms get worse when she is stressed. She denies any family history of colon problems. You suspect irritable bowel syndrome. Which of the following is included in the Rome Diagnostic Criteria for irritable bowel syndrome?

A. Abdominal pain causing nighttime awakening
B. Passage of mucus
C. Steatorrhea
D. Bloody stool
E. Weight loss

28. A 65-year-old white man presents to your ED with sudden-onset severe periumbilical pain. He denies any fevers, diarrhea, or constipation. Past medical history is significant for atrial fibrillation, for which he is on aspirin. On physical exam patient is in severe, distressing pain. He is afebrile, with an irregular tachycardia at 160, and a blood pressure of 120/90. In general he is ill-appearing and his abdominal exam is significant for hypoactive bowel sounds, with mild tenderness to palpation. His rectal exam reveals brown, guaiac-positive stool. The most likely cause of this man's abdominal pain is:

A. Diffuse atherosclerosis
B. Arterial embolism
C. Venous thrombosis
D. Ischemic colitis
E. Small bowel obstruction

29. A 68-year-old white woman presents with a 6-month history of weight loss and hematochezia. She states her last colonoscopy was approximately 5 years ago and a hyperplastic polyp was seen at that time. You refer her for colonoscopy and a 4-cm mass is seen in the proximal sigmoid colon. The pathology of the biopsy specimens is confirmed as adenocarcinoma of the colon. A CT scan of the chest, abdomen, and pelvis is performed and shows no evidence of metastatic disease. The next step for this patient includes:

A. Surveillance colonoscopy every 6 months
B. Surgery for staging and excision
C. Chemotherapy
D. Radiation therapy
E. MRI of the brain to rule out metastases

30. A 40-year-old white woman comes to your office for a preventative care visit. In general she is doing well without any complaints. She takes no medications. She is active, playing tennis three times weekly. She is trying to cut down on red meats, but finds this difficult when cooking for her husband. She does not smoke, but does enjoy 3 to 4 glasses of wine weekly. Her father was diagnosed with colon cancer at age 60. What is (or would have been) the appropriate colon cancer screening recommendations for her?

A. Colonoscopy every 3 to 5 years, starting at age 30
B. Fecal occult blood testing (FOBT) annually, sigmoidoscopy every 3 to 5 years, or colonoscopy every 10 years, starting at age 40
C. FOBT and sigmoidoscopy every 3 to 5 years, colonoscopy every 10 years, starting at age 50
D. Sigmoidoscopy every 1 to 2 years, starting at age 12
E. FOBT every year, no need for sigmoidoscopy or colonoscopy

31. A 30-year-old woman comes to your office with complaints of a skin rash on her lower legs that she has noticed for the past 3 weeks while shaving. She has also noted a few nosebleeds that have occurred spontaneously and have been difficult to stop, over the same time period. She has no other complaints of fever or fatigue. On physical exam, her vital signs are normal. She has petechiae on her soft palate and conjunctiva are pink. Her heart, lungs, and abdominal exams are normal. Her lower extremities reveal a nonblanching petechial rash.

You suspect idiopathic thrombocytopenic purpura (ITP). Which of the follow statements is true regarding ITP?

A. Peak age of occurrence is in the third decade
B. First-line therapy is splenectomy
C. IV immunoglobulin (IVIG) has been shown to increase platelet counts in 60% to 70% of patients
D. It is caused by a membrane defect of the platelets
E. Persistence of thrombocytopenia for more 3 months is considered chronic autoimmune thrombocytopenia

The response options for items 32 through 42 are the same. You will be required to select one answer for each item in the set.

A. HIV infection
B. Cryoglobulinemia
C. Sarcoidosis
D. Diabetes mellitus
E. Hepatitis B
F. Hepatitis C
G. Herpes simplex virus
H. *Pseudomonas aeruginosa*
I. Celiac sprue
J. Systemic lupus erythematosus (SLE)
K. Reiter's syndrome
L. Inflammatory bowel disease
M. Syphilis
N. Lyme disease

For each skin lesion, select the systemic disorder with which it is associated.

32. Pyoderma gangrenosum

33. Acanthosis nigricans

34. Erythema nodosum

35. Erythema multiforme

36. Seborrheic dermatitis

37. Ecthyma gangrenosum

38. Erythema migrans

39. Condyloma lata

40. Dermatitis herpetiformis

41. Keratoderma blenorrhagicum

42. Porphyria cutanea tarda

End of Set

43. A 70-year-old man with no significant past medical history is brought to your office by his wife for complaints of "forgetfulness." His wife tells you that for the past year she has noticed a decline in his short-term memory and cognitive abilities. He has been unable to balance the checkbook as he used to do and is easily frustrated and often irritable, which is not his usual personality. His occupation was real estate sales until he retired approximately 5 years ago. On physical exam, his blood pressure is 150/85, heart rate is 80, and respiratory rate is 14. He is afebrile. He scores a 24/30 on the Mini-Mental Status exam (MMSE). His neurologic exam reveals a pleasant affect and he is alert and oriented to person, place, and time. His cranial nerves are intact and there are no tremors or cogwheel rigidity. His gait is slow, slightly broad-based, and he seems to have difficulty coordinating his foot movements. Reflexes are within normal limits and the rest of the physical exam is within normal limits. Laboratories reveal a normal TSH, B12 level, BUN, creatinine, AST, ALT, bilirubin, and CBC. Which of the following diagnoses is most likely, and what test is the best test to evaluate for it?

A. Normal pressure hydrocephalus (NPH); CT scan of the brain
B. Multi-infarct dementia; MRI of the brain
C. Diffuse Lewy-body disease; brain biopsy
D. Pick's disease; CT of the brain
E. Supranuclear palsy; MRI of the brain

44. A 63-year-old man is admitted to the hospital with fever, malaise, and abdominal pain. His past medical history is significant for hyperlipidemia, for which he takes pravastatin. He was in his usual state of health until several months ago, when he noted unintentional, gradual weight loss; fatigue; and night sweats. These symptoms began to worsen 1 week before admission. He developed abdominal pain the day of admission that prompted him to seek medical attention. On

evaluation of the patient you find the following: Temperature 101.1°F (38.4°C); pulse 94; respirations 16; blood pressure 138/72. Head and neck examination reveals several conjunctival petechiae. His heart examination reveals a III/VI systolic murmur at the right upper sternal border. The patient does not recall being told of a heart murmur in the past. Lung examination is normal. Extremity examination reveals erythematous, macular lesions on several of his fingers that are not tender. Abdominal examination reveals tenderness in the left upper quadrant but normal bowel sounds and no rebound or guarding. You suspect infective endocarditis. You order blood cultures and a transthoracic echocardiogram. Blood cultures are positive for *Streptococcus bovis* in all bottles. Echocardiogram reveals a 4-mm vegetation on the aortic valve. What is the next step in the care of this patient?

A. Transesophageal echocardiogram
B. Computed tomography of the abdomen and pelvis
C. Colonoscopy
D. Evaluation by a cardiothoracic surgeon
E. Skin biopsy of lesions on fingers

paO_2 58 mmHg; $paCO_2$ 30 mmHg; pH 7.48 on room air. What is her alveolar-arterial (A-a) oxygen gradient?

A. 68
B. 48
C. There is not enough information to calculate the A-a gradient
D. 130
E. 55

46. A 62-year-old woman presents to the ED with complaints of sudden onset of dizziness and shortness of breath. Her past medical history is significant for hypertension and diabetes mellitus. On exam, she is afebrile and has a blood pressure of 74/42 with a heart rate of 138. On exam, her lungs have bibasilar crackles and her heart rate is irregularly irregular with no murmurs noted. You obtain an electrocardiogram (Figure 1-46). The most important initial step in her management is:

A. Initiation of warfarin therapy
B. Rate control with IV calcium-channel blockers
C. Initiation of aspirin therapy
D. Cardioversion of her rhythm with amiodarone
E. Synchronized electrical cardioversion

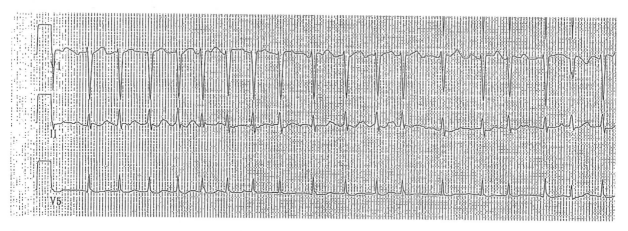

Figure 1-46 • Image Courtesy of Dr. Brenda Shinar, Banner Good Samaritan Medical Center, Phoenix, Arizona.

45. A 45-year-old woman presents to the ED with a 2-day history of left lower extremity pain and swelling and pleuritic chest pain and shortness of breath. She has no past medical history. Oral contraceptives are her only medication. She smokes one pack of cigarettes per day. You suspect a deep venous thrombosis with pulmonary embolism and order a ventilation perfusion scan. While waiting for the scan to be done you receive her arterial blood gas results and they show the following:

47. A 21-year-old previously healthy man collapses while playing basketball with his friends. Paramedics are called and he is found to be in pulseless ventricular tachycardia and is defibrillated with success. He is intubated and transferred to the ED, where he is found to have a blood pressure of 118/80 with a heart rate of 94. His exam reveals a tall, thin man with a harsh midsystolic murmur over the middle upper right sternal area. An ECG reveals evidence for mild

left ventricular hypertrophy (LVH) with no evidence of ischemia. A chest X-ray is normal. His mother arrives and tells you that he had an older sibling who suffered sudden cardiac death. What is the most likely cause of his clinical picture?

A. Ventricular septal defect (VSD)
B. Pulmonary embolus
C. Tension pneumothorax
D. Hypertrophic obstructive cardiomyopathy (HCM)
E. Dissecting aortic aneurysm

48. A 19-year-old woman presents to your office with complaints of progressive dyspnea on exertion and fatigue. Her symptoms started approximately 3 weeks earlier. On examination, you find that she has a blood pressure of 176/98 measured in her right arm. Upon auscultation, you notice a midsystolic murmur that is also heard in her upper back area. A repeat blood pressure measurement in her left arm confirms your earlier findings. You obtain an ECG that shows criteria for LVH. A chest X-ray obtained in the office shows absence of the aortic notch with notching of the ribs. What is the likely diagnosis?

A. Atrial septal defect (ASD)
B. Coarctation of the aorta
C. Aortic stenosis (AS)
D. Patent ductus arteriosis (PDA)
E. HCM

49. You have volunteered to do sports physicals on the athletes at your son's high school to clear them for participation in the competitive events. One of the varsity basketball players is a 16-year-old man without any significant past medical history. You hear a 2/6 systolic murmur in the right upper sternal border. The patient thinks that he was told that he had a heart murmur, but he is unsure. You are worried that there may be a contraindication to him playing basketball. You must have the patient do several maneuvers and be able to interpret them to know the etiology of his murmur. The Valsalva maneuver will make which of the following murmurs louder?

A. HCM
B. AS
C. Aortic insufficiency (AI)
D. Mitral stenosis
E. Tricuspid stenosis

50. A 65-year-old woman with a history of diabetes and hypertension developed chest pain while shoveling her snowy front walk in the early morning. The pain is 8/10 in severity with a "pressure-like" quality and is radiating a little to the jaw. It has persisted for 2 hours. The patient finally called 911 and paramedics brought her to the ER. An ECG reveals normal sinus rhythm without any acute ST-T wave changes. You appropriately treat the patient empirically for an acute coronary syndrome and she is admitted to telemetry to "rule out" a myocardial infarction. In which order, from first to last, would you expect the following markers to peak after an acute myocardial infarction?

A. Troponin-I, LDH, myoglobin, CPK-MB
B. Troponin-I, myoglobin, CPK-MB, LDH
C. Myoglobin, CPK-MB, troponin-I, LDH
D. Myoglobin, troponin-I, CPK-MB, LDH
E. Myoglobin, LDH, troponin-I, CPK-MB

A

Answers and Explanations

1. C	18. E	35. G
2. B	19. B	36. A
3. A	20. D	37. H
4. D	21. B	38. N
5. A	22. A	39. M
6. D	23. D	40. I
7. B	24. E	41. K
8. B	25. A	42. F
9. C	26. D	43. A
10. C	27. B	44. C
11. E	28. B	45. E
12. C	29. B	46. E
13. C	30. B	47. D
14. D	31. C	48. B
15. A	32. L	49. A
16. E	33. D	50. C
17. B	34. C	

1. **C. This patient has hypertension confirmed by two measurements, warranting pharmacologic therapy. First-line medications for hypertension include β-blockers and thiazide diuretics. With this patient's history of asthma, the diuretic would be a better choice for first-line therapy.**

   A. A β-blocker, especially a nonselective β-blocker, would be contraindicated in this patient with asthma.
   B. Calcium channel blockers are not first-line therapy for hypertension. Long-acting calcium-channel blockers may be added to the medication regimen if first-line therapy does not control the blood pressure or if the patient is unable to tolerate first-line medications.
   D. According to the JNC VII guidelines, drug therapy is indicated for stage I hypertension. Stage I hypertension is defined as a systolic blood pressure of 140–159 or diastolic blood pressure of 90–99. Lifestyle modifications should also be encouraged, but not used alone.
   E. A centrally acting adrenergic drug is not considered first-line therapy for hypertension.

2. **B. This patient has features suggestive of a secondary cause for her hypertension including age of onset less than 30, abrupt onset, findings on funduscopic exam, and an abdominal bruit. The abdominal bruit suggests a narrowing of the renal artery. The most common cause of hypertension secondary to renal artery stenosis in young women is fibromuscular dysplasia of the renal artery. (The most common cause of renal artery stenosis in an older population is atherosclerotic disease.)**

   A. Hypertension is a cause of coronary artery disease, not the reverse.
   C. Although Cushing's syndrome is a cause of secondary hypertension, there are no findings on physical exam such as abdominal striae, buffalo hump, or moon facies to suggest Cushing's syndrome as a cause of this patient's hypertension.
   D. This patient has features suggestive of a secondary cause for her hypertension. Further workup should be done to exclude secondary causes of hypertension before a diagnosis of essential hypertension is made.
   E. There are no other features, including headaches, palpitations, or anxiety, to suggest a pheochromocytoma.

3. **A. This patient has significant proteinuria on urinalysis and other findings consistent with nephrotic syndrome. Nephrotic syndrome is defined as urinary protein concentration of greater than 3.0 to 3.5 g over 24 hours. Additional features include hypoalbuminemia, edema, and hyperlipidemia.**

   B. Although abnormal liver function can cause hypoalbuminemia, the urinalysis suggests a renal cause for this patient's low albumin.
   C. Elevated cholesterol is one of the findings in nephrotic syndrome. In nephrotic syndrome, proteinuria leads to hypoalbuminemia and decreased plasma oncotic pressure. This drop in oncotic pressure then stimulates liver lipoprotein synthesis, resulting in hyperlipidemia. However, there are other causes of elevated cholesterol, and serum cholesterol alone cannot confirm the diagnosis of nephrotic syndrome.
   D. Imaging will not aid in establishing the diagnosis.
   E. Biopsy can be used to establish the etiology of the nephrotic syndrome, but is not the initial study of choice to confirm the diagnosis.

4. **D. Membranous glomerulonephritis accounts for 30% to 40% of adult nephrotic syndrome. Biopsy is characterized by thickened glomerular capillary loops. Appropriate renal function is retained at 10 years in 70% of patients with this diagnosis.**

   A. Minimal change disease is the most common cause of nephrotic syndrome in children. Biopsy shows no abnormalities on light microscopy, but effacement of foot processes along capillary loops can be seen on electron microscopy.
   B. Focal segmental glomerulosclerosis is the most common cause of nephrotic syndrome in black adults. Renal biopsy shows glomerulosclerosis. Many patients with this diagnosis progress to renal failure.
   C. Membranoproliferative glomerulonephritis is a less common cause of nephrotic syndrome. Biopsy will show proliferation of the mesangial cells.
   E. Amyloidosis causes renal disease by deposition of immunoglobulin light chains in the kidneys. This can lead to nephrotic syndrome and renal failure. Congo red stain can be used on renal biopsy to show amyloid deposition. Amyloidosis is a *secondary* cause of renal disease leading to nephrotic syndrome, and not a *primary* renal disorder. The most common secondary cause of nephrotic syndrome is diabetes mellitus.

5. **A.** This patient has history and findings consistent with IgA nephropathy. IgA nephropathy can present as asymptomatic hematuria with or without proteinuria *immediately* after, or concomitant with, an upper respiratory tract infection. (This helps distinguish it from poststreptococcal glomerulonephritis, which usually occurs a couple of weeks *after* the pharyngitis). IgA nephropathy also may present in young adults as hematuria that follows vigorous exercise. Biopsy is usually not necessary. However, if a biopsy were to be done, findings would be consistent with those listed in answer choice A.

B. Serum IgA levels do not correlate with the progression of disease.
C. The role of immunosuppressive treatment in IgA nephropathy is not well defined, but is currently under investigation.
D. It is estimated that 80% of patients have normal renal function 10 years after diagnosis.
E. The course of IgA nephropathy is not constant and can include progression to renal failure, slow decline of renal function over years, or little to no change in renal function.

6. **D.** This patient has a typical presentation of nephrolithiasis. 75% of all kidney stones are composed of calcium oxalate or calcium phosphate. Calcium oxalate stones are radio-opaque and are more common in males. Other risk factors for calcium oxalate stones include hypercalciuria, low urine output, hyperuricosuria, hyperoxaluria, and low urine citrate concentrations. In some cases, a cause of the stone is not known.

A. Uric acid stones occur because of the presence of elevated uric acid in the urine. Findings with uric acid stones include an acidic urine pH and radiolucent stone. Uric acid stones account for approximately 5% to 10% of stones in the United States.
B. Struvite stones occur with infections of the urinary tract due to urease-producing bacteria (such as *Proteus* species). This patient does not have indices on the urinalysis that would suggest an infection. Urine pH is usually alkaline. Stones are radio-opaque and can progress to form staghorn calculus. Struvite stones are responsible for 10% to 15% of stones and occur more commonly in women.
C. Cystine stones occur rarely, causing 1% of all kidney stones. It is unlikely that the patient has this type of stone. They occur in patients with defects in renal tubular absorption of cystine, ornithine, arginine, or lysine, and they usually present earlier in life.
E. Calcium HA is the primary mineral of bone and teeth. Abnormal deposition of calcium HA is seen in areas of tissue damage (large muscle hematomas) or in joints of elderly patients. It usually causes a destructive arthropathy, especially in the knees, shoulders, hips, and fingers. Diagnosis is made by electron microscopy of synovial fluid or tissue that identifies the small, nonbirefringent crystals. There is not an association with nephrolithiasis.

7. **B.** This patient has symptomatic hyponatremia. Symptoms of hyponatremia include nausea, vomiting, irritability, mental confusion, and seizures. Hypertonic saline should be given to increase the serum sodium above 120 mEq/L or until asymptomatic. The total mEq of sodium required to increase plasma sodium concentration can be calculated by using the following formula:

Sodium required (mEq) 5 total body water (L) × desired change in sodium (mEq/L)

Total body water averages 60% of body weight. (To calculate total body water, multiply this patient's weight in kilograms by 0.6.) If this patients weighs 70 kg, to raise the serum sodium from 113 to 120 mEq/L (a change of 7 meq), the mEq sodium required = 70 (0.6) × 7, or 294 mEq of sodium. Hypertonic (3%) saline contains 513 mEq of sodium per liter. This patient only requires 294 mEq of sodium to increase his serum sodium to 120 mEq/L. To calculate how much hypertonic saline, in liters, he requires, divide 294 mEq by 513 mEq/liter. Thus, approximately 570 mL of hypertonic saline can be infused to correct this patient's sodium. In symptomatic patients, sodium should be corrected at a rate of 1.5 to 2 mEq/hour for the first 3 to 4 hours or until the patient is asymptomatic.

A. Fluid restriction would be appropriate management for an asymptomatic patient with SIADH. However, this patient is symptomatic and requires immediate intervention to raise his serum sodium.
C. Demeclocycline can be used in the treatment of SIADH refractory to fluid restriction. This drug acts on the collecting tubule by decreasing the response to antidiuretic hormone, causing increased free-water excretion.

D. This patient's glucose level is normal. Therefore, the seizure is not secondary to hypoglycemia and giving glucose is of no benefit.

E. A CT of the head would not be indicated at this time because the low sodium appears to be the cause of the patient's seizure.

8. **B. Some antiseptic washes that contain iodine can cause a false-positive reaction for protein on urine dip. Additionally, false positives can occur when iodinated radiocontrast agents have been given in the last 24 hours.**

A. Highly concentrated urine can cause a false-positive reaction for protein on urine dip. Highly dilute urine will underestimate the amount of proteinuria.

C. Urine dip can detect protein as low as 15 mg/dL. If the urine is concentrated, urine dip may be positive with normal levels of protein in the urine.

D. Highly alkaline urine can cause false-positive reactions.

E. Urine dipstick detects urine albumin. It may not react with immunoglobulins or light chains in the urine. These must be detected by the use of sulfosalicylic acid, which will cause the urine to become turbid and cloudy if protein is present. An alternative that identifies other proteins in the urine besides albumin is urine protein electrophoresis (UPEP).

9. **C. Mannitol, ethylene glycol, methanol, and isopropyl alcohol all produce a serum osmolal gap. Methanol and ethylene glycol also produce an anion gap metabolic acidosis. The absence of urine crystals and complaint of blurred vision points to methanol as the substance that was ingested. The anion gap is calculated by the following equation:**

$$\text{Anion gap} = [\text{sodium (mEq/L)}] - ([\text{chloride (mEq/L)}] + [\text{bicarbonate (mEq/L)}])$$

The anion gap in this patient is 30. Osmolality can be calculated by the following equation:

$$\text{Plasma Osm (mOsm/kg)} = 2 \times [\text{Na+ (mOsm/L)}] + [\text{BUN (mg/dL)}/2.8] + [\text{glucose (mg/dL)}/18]$$

The osmolal gap is equal to the measured serum osmolality minus the calculated osmolality. This patient's osmolal gap = 320 mOsm/kg (measured)

– 292 mOsm/kg (calculated), which equals 38 mOsm/kg. Any value over 10 is abnormal.

A. Mannitol can produce an osmolal gap, but does not produce an anion gap metabolic acidosis.

B. Ethylene glycol ingestion does produce an anion gap acidosis with an osmolal gap. However, calcium oxalate crystals can be found on urinalysis with ethylene glycol ingestion, and patients do not typically complain of visual changes. Other manifestations include changes in mental status and renal failure.

D. Gasoline is usually inhaled if used as a substance of abuse. It may produce nausea, vomiting, and cardiovascular and respiratory effects. The associated metabolic disturbances are not well documented.

E. Isopropyl alcohol produces an osmolal gap, but without an anion gap metabolic acidosis.

10. **C. This patient is uremic and in symptomatic renal failure. Symptoms of uremia include anorexia, nausea, emesis, an unpleasant "metallic" taste in the mouth (known as "dysgusia"), asterixis, encephalopathy, seizures, pruritis, sleepiness, and impaired mental status. Uremic frost may be seen on the skin secondary to urea crystallization of sweat. Note that *uremia* is different from *azotemia*. Azotemia is an elevation of the BUN alone. Uremia is an elevation of the BUN along with the mentioned symptoms of nausea, pruritis, etc.**

A. Hyperphosphatemia does not present with these symptoms. It is usually associated with an underlying disease process such as renal failure.

B. Hyperkalemia presents with neuromuscular weakness, cardiac arrhythmias, and tall peaked T waves on an ECG.

D. Hypernatremia presents with mental status changes that can progress to seizures, coma, and death. Pruritis and asterixis are not present.

E. Elevated bicarbonate does not produce the symptoms noted in this patient.

11. **E. This patient has history and ECG findings consistent with hyperkalemia. Symptoms include muscles weakness and fatigue. More severe hyperkalemia can lead to cardiac manifestations. The ECG will show peaked T waves that progress to a widened QRS, and ventricular fibrillation. Each of the medicines that he was using for heart failure can predispose to hyperkalemia, with the exception of the furosemide, which he stopped.**

A. Symptoms of hypercalcemia include abdominal pain, constipation, nausea, and muscle weakness. A shortened QT interval can be found on the ECG.

B. This patient does not complain of chest pain, shortness of breath, or diaphoresis. The electrocardiograph does not show any ST elevation or depression that would suggest cardiac ischemia.

C. Symptoms of uncontrolled CHF include peripheral edema and shortness of breath. Physical exam findings would include an elevated jugular venous pressure, S_3 gallop, crackles on pulmonary exam, and peripheral edema. The ECG may show evidence of left ventricular hypertrophy. This patient has findings consistent with CHF, but appears to be stable and without evidence of acute worsening.

D. Symptoms of hypokalemia can include muscle cramps, slow bowel motility, and respiratory muscle paralysis. On ECG, T waves can be flat or inverted, and U waves may be present. Severe hypokalemia can lead to ventricular arrhythmias.

12. C. Muddy brown granular casts are most suggestive of acute tubular necrosis. These casts are made of renal tubular cells that have suffered an acute injury, formed casts, and have now become part of the urine sediment. Muddy brown casts do not change the color of the urine but are seen on microscopy. Grossly muddy brown urine may be seen in rhabdomyolysis.

A. Red cell casts indicate glomerulonephritis.

B. White blood cell casts suggest acute interstitial nephritis or pyelonephritis.

D. Hyaline casts are nonspecific and not indicative of renal disease. These casts can be seen in concentrated urine, after exercise, or during diuretic therapy.

E. Urine eosinophils are seen in acute interstitial nephritis, although they are only 70% sensitive for this disorder and 83% specific. Other causes of eosinophiluria are renal atheroembolic disease, rapidly progressive glomerulonephritis, and acute prostatitis.

13. C. This patient is presenting with diabetic ketoacidosis. The labs show an elevated anion gap metabolic acidosis with appropriate respiratory compensation. The anion gap is calculated by the following equation:

Anion gap = [sodium (mEq/L)] − ([chloride (mEq/L)] + [bicarbonate (mEq/L)])

Normal anion gap is 8 to 12. Our patient's anion gap is 21. Respiratory compensation for metabolic acidosis can be calculated by using Winter's formula:

Change in pCO_2 = 1.5 × [bicarbonate (mEq/L)] + 8 (+/− 2)

Our patient's predicted pCO_2 equals 1.5 × 7 + 8 = 18.5. Our patient has appropriate compensation.

14. D. This patient is having an anxiety attack, causing her to hyperventilate. The blood gas reveals an acute respiratory alkalosis and no other electrolyte abnormalities.

15. A. This patient has metabolic acidosis without an elevated anion gap. This can be secondary to GI bicarbonate losses with diarrhea, such as in this patient. It can also be secondary to renal bicarbonate losses such as in a renal tubular acidosis.

16. E. This patient has an acute respiratory acidosis secondary to status asthmaticus. There are no other electrolyte abnormalities and no metabolic compensation because this is acute.

B. This blood gas and electrolyte panel reflects a patient with a combined anion gap metabolic acidosis and a respiratory acidosis.

17. B. Palmar erythema and spider telangiectasias are found in patients with liver disease due to the hyperestrogenic state. This also accounts for the testicular atrophy in men and loss of axillary hair. Findings of portal hypertension in liver disease include ascites, esophageal varices, caput medusa, and hemorrhoids (nonspecific).

A. A buffalo hump is commonly seen on physical exam in a patient with cortisol excess or Cushing's syndrome. Other clinical manifestations include obesity, striae, and easy bruising.

C. Palpable purpura are characteristic of vasculitic processes including Henoch-Schönlein purpura and hypersensitivity vasculitis.

D. Proptosis is a physical exam finding seen with thyroid hormone excess and patients with Graves' disease.

E. Acanthosis nigricans is a clinical exam finding seen with insulin resistance or diabetes mellitus type II. Typically it is a velvety darkening of the skin at the nape of the neck and in the axilla.

18. **E. Hepatitis A is transmitted by fecal-oral route through ingestion of fecally contaminated water or foodstuffs. Those at risk include travelers, children and workers at daycare, and military personnel.**

    A, B, C, D. IV drug use, the presence of a tattoo, history of blood transfusions, and work in the health care profession are all risk factors for Hepatitis B and Hepatitis C transmission.

19. **B. This patient may have an esophageal cancer given the history of dysphagia, weight loss, and heartburn. Endoscopy is the first step in a patient with dysphagia and other warning symptoms for cancer. A biopsy can be performed at the time of endoscopy to confirm diagnosis.**

    A. Twenty-four hour pH esophageal monitoring is the gold standard test for the diagnosis of gastroesophageal reflux disease; however, it would not be the appropriate next step in this patient because of the concern for cancer.
    C. A chest X-ray may help if there is a large mass lesion in the patient's chest, but it would not provide direct visualization or tissue for diagnosis.
    D. Similar to a chest X-ray, a CT scan of the chest would help determine if there was a mass lesion causing compression and extraesophageal dysphagia. A CT would help delineate between anatomic structures better than plain films, but CT is not the gold standard in the evaluation of dysphagia.
    E. This patient has had gastroesophageal reflux disease (GERD) for more than 5 years. Her symptoms are certainly worrisome for cancer. The patient may benefit from a proton pump inhibitor, but evaluation of her dysphagia is most important at this time.

20. **D. This patient may have GERD that is manifesting itself as bronchospasm. Specifically, the patient's nighttime symptoms, normal exam, and inability to improve with a metered dose inhaler suggest an extrapulmonary cause for her bronchospasm. GERD may also present with aspiration syndromes, chronic cough, and dental erosions.**

    A. Long-acting β-agonists are used for treatment in mild-persistent to moderate asthma and may be used in conjunction with inhaled steroids.
    B. Inhaled steroids are indicated for patients with mild-persistent to moderate asthma, where symptoms occur more than once a week, but less than once a day.
    C. Leukotriene receptor antagonists have been shown to improve baseline function and decrease the need for rescue medications in those with moderate asthma.
    E. This patient is obviously symptomatic. Additional etiologies for her bronchospasm, such as GERD, should be sought.

21. **B. This patient most likely has diverticulitis. Patients with a history of constipation are more likely to have diverticuli that may become inflamed secondary to obstruction of the outpouching and microperforation leading to local infection. The presentation of diverticulitis includes left lower quadrant pain, fever, nausea, vomiting, and constipation or diarrhea. Plain films should be obtained to rule out free air, ileus, or obstruction. Sigmoidoscopy should not be performed, because this increases the risk of perforation. The patient should be placed on antibiotics and IV fluids and made NPO.**

    A. Inflammatory bowel disease can present with abdominal pain, fever, and stool changes. Often the patient will give you a history of gross blood in the stool and associated weight loss. The onset of inflammatory bowel disease has a bimodal age distribution, with the first peak occurring in the teens and twenties and the second peak occurring around the fifties and sixties.
    C. Colon cancer can also present with abdominal pain and change in stool habits. Like inflammatory bowel disease, colon cancer is also associated with weight loss and bloody stool.
    D. Diverticulosis is asymptomatic and it describes the herniation of colonic mucosa and submucosa through the colonic wall. A low-fiber diet is thought to contribute to the presence of diverticuli. Diverticulosis can be complicated by bleeding and infection.
    E. Appendicitis usually presents with periumbilical pain that then migrates to the right lower quadrant. It is associated with anorexia and usually does not involve pain in the left lower quadrant.

22. **A.** Diverticulosis and angiodysplasia are the most common causes of lower GI bleeding. The bleeding is thought to occur in the right colon and is secondary to erosion of a diverticular vessel by a fecalith. Patients usually present with sudden onset of cramping with large amounts of hematochezia. Over 90% will stop spontaneously.

    B, C, D, E. Hemorrhoids, infectious diarrhea, and inflammatory bowel disease are all causes of lower GI bleeding. Upper GI bleeding accounts for approximately 10% of those episodes initially thought to be considered lower GI bleeds.

23. **D.** Infectious esophagitis is the most common cause of odynophagia. Candida, cytomegalovirus (CMV), and herpes simplex virus (HSV) are all frequent causes, especially in the immunocompromised patient. Diagnosis is made by biopsy, which shows mucosal inflammation, tissue necrosis, and vascular endothelial involvement. Cytomegalic cells are commonly seen in CMV esophagitis.

    A. GERD causes symptoms of heartburn, atypical angina-like pain, and dysphagia. It does not usually cause odynophagia.
    B. Achalasia typically presents with a dysphagia for solids *and* liquids. Anatomically, it is secondary to failure of lower esophageal sphincter relaxation. Unlike esophagitis, it does not cause odynophagia. Achalasia can also present with symptoms of GERD.
    C. Barrett's esophagus is a precancerous histologic condition in which intestinal columnar epithelium replaces the normal squamous cells in the distal esophagus in response to chronic acid reflux. Barrett's esophagus itself is not symptomatic. Patients will often be symptomatic with heartburn or dysphagia as a result of long-standing GERD.
    E. Diffuse esophageal spasm is a motility disorder in which there are simultaneous and repetitive contractions of the esophagus that can present with symptoms of GERD or chest pain. Patients with diffuse esophageal spasm do not normally present with odynophagia.

24. **E.** Eighty percent of gastric carcinomas are attributable to *H. pylori* and seropositivity confers a three- to six-fold risk of gastric cancer. Gastric lymphomas or mucosa-associated lymphoid tissue (MALT) tumors are also thought to be connected to *H. pylori.* Seventy to 80% of gastric lymphomas or MALT tumors will show regression with eradication of *H. pylori*, though it is unknown whether eradication will prevent gastric cancer.

    A. Alcohol can promote acid secretion and damage the mucosal barrier, but no evidence suggests that it causes chronic peptic ulcer disease and subsequently gastric adenocarcinoma.
    B. NSAID-induced ulcers have no relationship to gastric adenocarcinoma.
    C. Tobacco use is most closely associated with lung cancer.
    D. Long-standing GERD places a patient at risk for Barrett's esophagus and adenocarcinoma of the esophagus.

25. **A.** Gallstones are the most common cause of acute pancreatitis. This patient is also at risk because of her gender, her age, and her obesity. Other causes of pancreatitis include infections (viral and bacterial), hypertriglyceridemia, and hypercalcemia.

    B. Alcohol use is the second most common cause of acute pancreatitis and the most common cause of chronic pancreatitis.
    C. Trauma can also cause pancreatitis and is seen frequently in children who suffer from blunt abdominal trauma. Pancreatitis after endoscopic retrograde cholangiopancreatography (ERCP) is also a well-known entity. This patient gives no history of trauma.
    D. Drugs such as L-asparaginase, Lasix, and didanosine have been known to cause pancreatitis.
    E. Tobacco use has no association with pancreatitis.

26. **D.** This patient has hemolytic-uremic syndrome (HUS), and the likely causative agent is *E. coli* O157:H7. HUS is characterized by a microangiopathic hemolytic anemia, thrombocytopenia, and acute renal failure, and it has a direct correlation to *E. coli* O157:H7. This particular enterohemorrhagic *E. coli* usually causes a bloody diarrhea that may precede the onset of HUS. Renal failure secondary to *E. coli* O157:H7 usually occurs in children aged 5 to 10 years. The organism may be ingested in undercooked beef.

    A. *Cryptosporidium* is an intracellular protozoan parasite. Transmission is typically water-borne, but it can also be person-to-person. It is particularly devastating in the immunocompromised. *Cryptosporidium* is not associated with HUS.

B. *Giardia* is similar to *Cryptosporidium* in that it is a protozoan parasite. Transmission is person-to-person, water-borne, or food-borne. It can present with diarrhea (nonbloody), steatorrhea, malaise, and fatigue, but it is not associated with HUS.

C. Rotavirus is a very common cause of watery, profuse diarrhea in children. It has been associated with intussusception and necrotizing enterocolitis.

E. *Vibrio cholerae* is an enterotoxin-producing, gram-negative bacteria that is water-borne and food-borne. It is very prevalent in Asia and Africa and is known for causing severe dehydration. It is not associated with HUS.

27. **B. In order to meet the Rome Criteria for irritable bowel syndrome, a patient must have abdominal pain that has been present for 12 weeks or more (not necessarily consecutive) in the preceding 12 months. In addition, the pain must have two out of three of the following features: 1) It must be relieved with defecation 2) Its onset must be associated with a change in the frequency of stooling 3) Its onset must be associated with a change in appearance (form) of the stool. These symptoms must be in the absence of any structural or metabolic abnormalities that could explain the symptoms; therefore, it is a diagnosis of exclusion.**

A. Abdominal pain causing nighttime wakening should be taken more seriously to include problems such as malignancy and vascular disease.

C. Steatorrhea is seen in patients with malabsorption. Causes of malabsorption include pancreatic insufficiency or mucosal abnormalities such as celiac disease.

D. Bloody stool with abdominal pain are symptoms often seen in patients with inflammatory bowel disease, such as Crohn's disease or ulcerative colitis.

E. Weight loss in a patient with abdominal pain and changes in stool habits of concern for malignancy. This patient has had no weight loss and also has no family history of colon cancer.

28. **B. This man is suffering from acute mesenteric ischemia. The most common cause of acute mesenteric ischemia is arterial embolism. His risk factor is atrial fibrillation that is not appropriately anticoagulated. Presentation is usually acute in nature and the pain is usually out of proportion to the physical exam.**

A. Patients with diffuse atherosclerosis will often present with postprandial abdominal pain and early satiety. These changes are more chronic in nature and are sometimes called "intestinal angina."

C. Venous thromboses occur secondary to hypercoagulable states, malignancy, or after trauma or surgery. Patients may present with abdominal pain, and significant bowel edema may be present due to compromised venous drainage. Eventually the arterial circulation may also be compromised, resulting in ischemia. The presentation of mesenteric vein thrombosis is usually not as acute as arterial obstruction from an embolus.

D. Ischemic colitis is secondary to a low-flow state, often a decreased cardiac output. Ischemic colitis can present with abdominal pain, hematochezia, or diarrhea.

E. Small bowel obstruction presents with abdominal pain, nausea, and vomiting. A physical exam is usually significant for abdominal distension and hyperactive bowel sounds, often referred to as "rushing" in nature.

29. **B. Surgery is the first step in the treatment of colon cancer, and it is used not only for excision of the tumor but also for staging when there is not already evidence of metastatic disease on imaging (Dukes class D or stage IV disease). Surgery and pathology can determine the depth of tumor penetration of the mucosa (mucosa and submucosa: Dukes class A; muscularis: Dukes class B1; serosa: Dukes class B2) and whether there is any lymph node involvement (Dukes class C).**

A. Surveillance colonoscopy is not enough, because this patient has pathologic evidence of colon cancer. In a patient with stage I (Dukes class A) colon cancer, or cancer confined to the mucosa, 5-year survival is greater than 90%.

C. Chemotherapy in general is adjunctive therapy and used for palliation. Chemotherapy is given in stage III (Dukes class C) and stage IV (Dukes class D). With chemotherapy and surgery, 5-year survival for stage III is 30% to 60%; for stage IV disease it is less than 5%.

D. Radiation therapy is useful in certain types of rectal cancer but is not indicated in colon cancer.

E. Large-bowel cancers usually spread to the regional lymph nodes or to the liver via the portal circulation first. It rarely spreads to other more distant sites without first being seen in these places, and an MRI of the brain is not indicated at this time for staging because the patient does not have neurologic symptoms and there is no evidence of metastases to the liver or lymph nodes.

30. **B. This patient has a first-degree relative with colorectal cancer, so annual fecal occult blood testing is recommended, with a sigmoidoscopy every 3 to 5 years or a colonoscopy every 10 years, to begin at age 40.**

A. There are no recommendations for the general population to begin colonoscopy at age 30.

C. The screening recommendation for the average patient without any risk factors is FOBT annually and a sigmoidoscopy every 3 to 5 years or a colonoscopy every 10 years, starting at age 50.

D. Patients with a risk of familial adenomatous polyposis should have a sigmoidoscopy every 1 to 2 years, starting at age 12.

E. There are no recommendations for FOBT only, without sigmoidoscopy or colonoscopy.

31. **C. IVIG has been shown to play a role in the treatment of ITP. First-line therapy is high-dose steroids. Over 50% of patients will respond to this treatment with increased platelet counts. Patients who do not respond to high-dose steroids can receive IVIG. Another 60% to 70% of patients respond to this treatment with increased platelet counts. The exact mechanism of IVIG is uncertain, but it appears to inhibit the removal of antibody-bound platelets.**

A. The peak age of onset for ITP is during childhood, between ages 2 and 6; it is usually acute and follows a viral illness. Most children recover spontaneously or require a short course of steroids. Adults with ITP are more likely to experience a chronic and refractory course than children.

B. First-line therapy for ITP is high-dose steroids. Splenectomy is indicated for patients who have been refractory to other treatments and suffer bleeding complications from low platelet counts. All patients should be immunized against *Streptococcus pneumoniae*, *Haemophilus influenzae* Type b, and *Neisseria meningitidis* before splenectomy.

D. ITP is caused by IgG and IgM antiplatelet antibodies that attack platelet membrane glycoproteins, leading to platelet destruction.

E. Chronic ITP is defined as persistence of thrombocytopenia for longer than 6 months.

32. **L. Pyoderma gangrenosum is a skin condition that may be idiopathic or may be associated with systemic disorders such as inflammatory bowel disease. It begins as a nodule or hemorrhagic pustule that then breaks down to an ulcer with irregular and raised borders. The ulcer is noninfectious. It is usually treated by treating the underlying disease, but corticosteroids may also be used. The lesion may last months to years.**

33. **D. Acanthosis nigricans is a hyperpigmentation of the skin, occasionally with a velvety appearance. The lesions occur mainly in the axillae, but also other body folds. It is seen in diabetes mellitus and other endocrine disorders; it may also be a paraneoplastic syndrome, primarily associated with adenocarcinoma. The diagnosis is made clinically.**

34. **C. Erythema nodosum is associated with many systemic illnesses, particularly granulomatous diseases. The lesions consist of painful, tender nodules usually on the lower legs but sometimes on the arms. It is frequently seen in sarcoidosis. The diagnosis is clinical and treatment is symptomatic.**

35. **G. Erythema multiforme may be associated with multiple systemic illnesses and may be a reaction to a medication. It is especially common after a herpes simplex viral infection. The lesions consist of target lesions that may be seen on the palms of the hands and soles of the feet. Mucosal involvement may occur. The appearance of the lesions is so characteristic that the diagnosis is usually clinical; the treatment is symptomatic, but corticosteroids may be necessary in severe cases.**

36. **A. Seborrheic dermatitis is a common skin condition characterized by redness of the skin and scaling. The lesions are often greasy. It may involve the scalp and face as well as body folds.**

The incidence of seborrheic dermatitis is significantly increased in patients with HIV infection. It may be difficult to distinguish from psoriasis. Treatments vary from shampoos containing selenium sulfide to oral ketoconazole. Treatment of the condition when it involves the face can be quite difficult.

37. H. Ecthyma gangrenosum results in hemorrhagic bullae that evolve into gangrenous ulcers. It usually occurs in association with *Pseudomonas aeruginosa* bacteremia, primarily in neutropenic or otherwise immunocompromised patients. Diagnosis may be clinical but should be confirmed with biopsy. Treatment is targeted at the underlying bacteremia.

38. N. Erythema migrans is a rash associated with Lyme disease. The lesion is pathognomonic of Lyme disease and consists of a macular, erythematous lesion with central clearing that develops from a macule or papule at the site of the insect bite. The border of the lesion is distinct and red. The lesion may become as large as 15 cm. Most patients have only a solitary lesion, but in a small percentage of patients multiple annular lesions may develop. Treatment targets the underlying Lyme disease.

39. M. Condyloma lata are soft, flat-topped, pale papules and nodules that occur on the genital and perineal skin and are due to secondary syphilis. They are extremely infectious and are similar in appearance to genital warts. Diagnosis is by VDRL, and FTA-ABS may also be positive. Treatment targets the underlying syphilis infection.

40. I. Dermatitis herpetiformis is an intensely pruritic rash that consists of vesicles, papules, and wheals. It usually occurs on the extensor areas of the extremities such as the knees and elbows; it may also occur on the buttocks. It is associated with celiac sprue and/or gluten sensitivity. It may be diagnosed with biopsy. It may be treated with dapsone but is usually completely suppressed by a gluten-free diet.

41. K. Keratoderma blennorhagicum is a lesion that usually occurs on the feet and consists of papules, vesicles, and pustules. The lesions are usually red to brown, and may have a central erosion and become hyperkeratotic. Under the microscope, it looks like psoriasis. The diagnosis of the lesion is mainly clinical. Reactive arthritis and seronegative spondylarthropathy should be ruled out. Treatment is by NSAIDs.

42. F. Porphyria cutanea tarda is associated with hepatitis C, but it may also be idiopathic or secondary to drugs. It consists of vesicles and bullae usually present on the dorsa of the hands. The lesions may occur after minor trauma. Diagnosis is made by biopsy.

B. Cryoglobulins are immunoglobulins and complement that precipitate out of patients' sera and may cause blood vessel damage and inflammation to medium and small vessels. Cryoglobulins are produced in response to infections such as hepatitis C, or they may be a result of hematologic malignancies. They present with palpable purpura of the feet and hands and sometimes ears and tip of the nose.

E. Acute hepatitis B is associated with arthralgia and arthritis due to a serum sickness-type immune complex disease. Patients also can have an associated polyarteritis nodosa-type vasculitis.

J. SLE classically presents with a malar rash and photosensitivity as keratinized skin manifestations and as oral aphthous-like ulcers on oral mucous membranes.

43. A. This patient presents with a decline in cognitive function for the past year or so by history of his wife. His past medical history is unremarkable, and he is on no medications, which makes this case relatively simple. He scores an abnormal 24/30 on the screening Mini-Mental Status exam, which alerts you to the fact that there is truly a cognitive decline. You need to evaluate for any possible reversible causes of dementia in this patient. The laboratories are normal, and therefore, reassuring in some ways; however, because he has an abnormal "broad-based" gait, you should also be worried about NPH as a diagnosis. This requires a CT scan to evaluate the size of the ventricles in comparison to the cortex. If there is suggestion of NPH, then a removal of a large amount of CSF is done to evaluate for improvement in the balance and cognitive dysfunction. This may help to indicate whether shunting surgery will be beneficial. Our patient

had two of the findings in the classic triad for NPH: not every patient will have all three. The triad is: wacky (dementia), wobbly (gait disturbance), and wet (urinary incontinence.)

B. Patients with multi-infarct dementia, also known as vascular dementia, usually have a history of hypertension, hyperlipidemia, and other risk factors for stroke. Often the history will be of sudden, step-like cognitive decline instead of slow, gradual decline that is seen in Alzheimer's and other dementias. Their physical exams usually reveal focal neurologic deficits that are a result of multiple ischemic insults. An MRI scan of the brain reveals one or more cerebral infarcts of varying size, or severe diffuse white matter abnormalities. This patient did not present with vascular dementia.

C. Diffuse Lewy-body dementia is now considered the second most common cause of dementia after Alzheimer's disease, accounting for 20% to 25% of dementias. Initial features include impaired attention, concentration, and visuospatial orientation, but often with preserved short-term memory at onset. Patients may have Parkinsonian features of rigidity and cogwheeling, and, interestingly, may have sleep disturbances in which they lose the normal REM sleep paralysis and physically act out their dreams while they are asleep.

D. Pick's disease is a type of frontotemporal dementia. The initial most prominent features include personality and behavioral changes with apathy. The Mini-Mental Status exam may be normal early in the disease process. CT or MRI of the brain reveals frontal and/or temporal lobe atrophy. Biopsy reveals "Pick bodies," which are cytoplasmic inclusions that stain with silver stain. Clinically, patients may develop hyper-oral behavior, emotional lability, and language disturbance in addition to the dementia.

E. Supranuclear palsy is a degenerative disorder characterized by gliosis; neurofibrillary tangles (different from those in Alzheimer's disease); and neuronal loss in the midbrain, pons, basal ganglia, and cerebellum. Clinically, patients have paresis of voluntary eye movements, specifically downward gaze. Limb rigidity and bradykinesia mimic Parkinson's disease, but there is usually not a tremor. Patients may have frequent falls because of their rigidity and supranuclear ophthalmoplegia. Patients respond poorly to anti-Parkinsonian drugs, and the course is usually progressive, with death occurring within 10 years of diagnosis.

44. **C. Colonoscopy. Patients who are found to be bacteremic with either *Streptococcus bovis* or *Clostridium septicum* must undergo a colonoscopy, because many of them have colon cancer.**

A. A transesophageal echocardiogram is more sensitive for detecting infective endocarditis than a transthoracic echocardiogram. If the suspicion for infective endocarditis is high and the transthoracic echocardiogram is negative, a transesophageal echocardiogram should be performed. However, in this patient, the transthoracic echocardiogram was positive and provided the necessary confirmation of the diagnosis; therefore, a transesophageal echocardiogram is not necessary.

B. A CT of the abdomen may be helpful in evaluation of the patient's abdominal pain, which may be due to splenic infarction from embolization from his infected heart valve. However, at this time he does not have an acute abdomen, and a colonoscopy would be more important to rule out cancer.

D. A cardiothoracic surgeon is probably not necessary for this patient at this point. Cardiothoracic surgery evaluation is recommended for patients with infective endocarditis and the following: acute CHF, valve ring abscess, vegetations larger than 1 cm, persistent embolization despite appropriate antibiotic treatment, positive blood cultures despite antibiotic treatment, and first- or second degree heart block.

E. These skin lesions are most likely Janeway lesions in this patient with a high suspicion of infective endocarditis. Therefore, a skin biopsy is not necessary. Osler's nodes, also seen in the fingers and toes of patients with infective endocarditis, are nodular and painful, as opposed to Janeway lesions, which are macular and painless.

45. **E. 55. This patient has probably had a pulmonary embolism. She is a smoker over the age of 35 and takes oral contraceptives, putting her at risk for**

venous thromboembolism. The A-a oxygen gradient is the difference between the partial pressure of oxygen in the alveoli and that in the blood. It is often elevated in lung disease that results in ventilation/perfusion mismatch such as pulmonary embolism. The equation for the A-a gradient is as follows:

$$A-a = pAO_2 - paO_2$$

pAO_2 is the partial pressure of oxygen in the alveoli, and paO_2 is the partial pressure of oxygen in the artery. The value for paO_2 is obtained from the arterial blood gas measurement. The value for pAO_2 is obtained by the following equation:

$$pAO_2 = (FiO_2[\text{barometric pressure} - \text{water vapor pressure}]) - (paCO_2/0.8)$$

FiO_2 is the percent of oxygen in inspired air. In the case of room air it is 21% or 0.21. Barometric pressure is 760 mmHg, and water vapor pressure is 47 mmHg at standard conditions. The barometric pressure varies, but for calculations, usually the barometric and water vapor pressures at standard conditions are used. The $paCO_2$ is obtained from the arterial blood gas measurement. The term 0.8 is a respiratory quotient. Under standard conditions, therefore, the equation may be reduced to the following formula:

$$paCO_2 = (0.21)(760 - 47) - (paCO_2/0.8) -$$
$$paO_2 = 150 - [paO_2 + (1.25 \times paCO_2)]$$

The normal value for the A-a gradient is 5 to 15 in young patients. The value for the A-a gradient increases with age. This patient's very elevated value of 55 was obtained with the following calculation.

$$paCO_2 = 0.21(760 - 47) - (30/0.8) - 58$$
$$= 150 - [58 + (1.25 \times 30)]$$

A,B,C,D. See explanation for E.

46. E. The patient presented is clinically unstable, as demonstrated by her symptoms (dizziness, shortness of breath and hypotension). She requires immediate intervention to try to restore her to sinus rhythm. This can be accomplished with medications such as amiodarone, but synchronized cardioversion is faster and the preferred method in an unstable patient requiring immediate intervention.

A, C, D. Whether or not to anticoagulate a patient with atrial fibrillation is an important clinical decision to make. However, this intervention is done to prevent long-term complications of atrial fibrillation, specifically to reduce the incidence of thromboembolic events such as cerebrovascular accidents. It is not the first line of therapy in a patient with unstable atrial fibrillation. Whether to use aspirin or warfarin for long-term prophylaxis depends on various risk factors that must be assessed in each patient, as well on the underlying cause of the atrial fibrillation.

B. Although rate control is the most important initial therapeutic goal in a *stable* patient with atrial fibrillation with rapid ventricular response, the patient described above is *unstable*. Both calcium-channel blockers and β-blockers can be used to suppress AV nodal conduction and subsequently control the rate.

47. D. This is a classic presentation of HCM in a young patient. Patients with HCM who are older often present just like patients with valvular aortic stenosis: with angina, syncope (or presyncope) with exertion, or CHF. Fifty percent of patients who present at a younger age have a family history of sudden cardiac death. As the heart rate increases, the filling time of the left ventricle decreases, which decreases the load-dependent cardiac output, resulting in syncope or presyncope.

A. VSDs typically present with dyspnea or are asymptomatic. They rarely present with sudden cardiac death. The murmur associated with VSD is usually holosystolic and located at the left lower sternal border. In addition, although the chest X-ray may be normal, one would expect to see some ventricular enlargement if the VSD were significant enough to cause his symptoms.

B. Pulmonary embolus may present as sudden cardiac death, but not usually in healthy, younger patients (unless there is an underlying hypercoagulable state present). In addition, a pulmonary embolus does not produce the murmur noted on his exam. There are a variety of chest X-ray findings that can be seen with a pulmonary embolus, one of which is a normal chest X-ray.

C. Tension pneumothorax is certainly a consideration for sudden collapse in a tall, thin, otherwise healthy patient. However, his chest X-ray would have revealed evidence of this, and it did not.

E. An aortic dissection is uncommon in healthy young people. Also, the murmur heard on his exam was not consistent with an aortic aneurysm. Again, one would expect to see changes on his chest X-ray such as widening of the mediastinum, which was not noted.

48. **B. This case illustrates classic findings of coarctation of the aorta. Patients who have coarctation often present with progressive symptoms of fatigue and dyspnea. Although the diagnosis is usually made in childhood, it is occasionally not made until early adulthood. Due to the location of the narrowing, or coarctation, in the descending aorta, the arteries supplying the upper extremities and chest experience a high back pressure, whereas the arterial supply to the lower extremities remains relatively normal or diminished. This explains the typical finding of isolated upper extremity hypertension and often diminished pulses in the lower extremities. The elevated blood pressure within the intercostal arteries account for the rib notching seen on the chest X-ray.**

A. ASDs often result in a left-to-right shunt, which lead to increased pressures within the right side of the heart. This ultimately leads to right ventricular enlargement that can sometimes be seen on a chest X-ray in addition to "shunt vascularity." The ECG finding with ASD is usually right-axis deviation with or without right-bundle branch block, not usually LVH. In addition, the ASD does not usually result in hypertension.

C. AS occurs proximal to the arteries supplying the upper extremities and chest, and subsequently does not result in upper extremity hypertension and rib notching on a chest X-ray. Although the murmur of AS is often midsystolic, it is usually best heard at the right upper sternal border with radiation into the carotid arteries, not the back.

D. PDA produces a continuous murmur that is heard throughout systole and diastole. In addition, PDA does not cause rib notching and hypertension. Calcification of the ductus arteriosis is the classic finding of PDA on a chest X-ray.

E. HCM involves the intraventricular septum and does not cause isolated upper extremity hypertension. Although it can cause LVH, it does not account for the rib notching seen on the chest X-ray.

49. **A. The murmur of HCM is the result of turbulent flow through the narrowing of the left ventricular outflow tract. This narrowing is caused by hypertrophy of the intraventricular septum and the anterior motion of the mitral valve leaflets that occur during systole. As blood flow through this area decreases, the intraventricular septum is allowed to move closer to the mitral leaflets, making the outlet narrower. This in turn makes the murmur louder. Conversely, as flow across this narrowing increases, the septum is pushed further away from the mitral leaflets resulting in a wider outlet, decreased turbulence and a softer murmur. The Valsalva maneuver increases intrathoracic pressure and subsequently decreases venous return to the heart. As a result, there is less blood to fill the ventricle, allowing the obstruction to worsen and the murmur to become louder.**

B. AS results in a valve that has a relatively fixed obstruction. The Valsalva maneuver decreases venous return to the heart. Subsequently, as blood flow across this tight, stenotic valve decreases, so does the amount of turbulence; the murmur of AS thus becomes softer.

C. The murmur of AI is the result of retrograde blood flow across the aortic valve that occurs during diastole. Because the Valsalva increases intrathoracic pressure and decreases venous return to the heart, it causes less blood to flow back across the aortic valve into the heart, making the murmur softer.

D. The relationship between blood flow and turbulence across a stenotic mitral valve is similar to that of AS. As flow across the valve decreases, so does the murmur. Therefore, the murmur of mitral stenosis is made softer with the Valsalva maneuver.

E. Again, the relationship between the murmur and the flow across a stenotic tricuspid valve is no different than that outlined for the stenotic aortic or mitral valves. Therefore, by decreasing venous return to the heart and ultimately decreasing flow across the valve, the Valsalva maneuver makes the murmur of tricuspid stenosis softer.

50. C. The above markers are released from the myocyte during injury or death, which is often the result of an acute myocardial infarction. The rates at which they rise, peak, and return to normal are all different. Myoglobin is the first to become elevated at 1 to 4 hours and the first to peak at 6 to 7 hours. Myoglobin peak is followed, in order, by CPK-MB, troponin-I, and LDH. The order in which they return to baseline differs, however. Myoglobin is the first to return to baseline, followed by CPK-MB, and then LDH. Troponin-I remains elevated for up to 10 to 12 days after an acute myocardial infarction.

A, B, D, E. See explanation for C.

BLOCK 2

The next two questions (items 51 and 52) correspond to the following vignette.

An otherwise healthy 31-year-old woman presents with complaints of new-onset substernal chest pain. She states the pain is persistent, worse with inspiration, and improved by leaning forward. She states she has had subjective fevers for the past 2 days. On exam, she has normal vitals signs and is afebrile. She appears uncomfortable, but is in no acute distress. Her lungs are clear to auscultation and you think you hear a faint friction rub. Chest X-ray is normal. You obtain the following ECG (Figure 1-51). *Pericarditis*

A. Aortic stenosis (AS)
B. Aortic regurgitation
C. Mitral stenosis
D. Mitral regurgitation
E. Tricuspid stenosis
F. Tricuspid regurgitation
G. Patent ductus arteriosis (PDA)
H. Coarctation of the aorta

For each description, select the appropriate murmur.

53. Diastolic rumbling murmur with opening snap heard best in the area of the apex. *C*

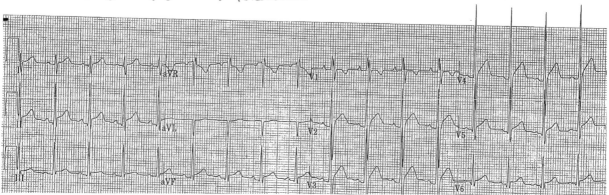

Figure 1-51•Image Courtesy of Dr. Brenda Shinar, Banner Good Samaritan Medical Center, Phoenix, Arizona.

51. What is the diagnosis?
    A. Pulmonary embolus
    B. Acute myocardial infarction
    C. Pericarditis
    D. Tension pneumothorax
    E. Cardiac tamponade

52. What is the initial treatment of choice for this patient?
    A. Anticoagulation with IV heparin
    B. Treatment with β-blockers
    C. Initiation of anti-inflammatory medication
    D. Thoracostomy with placement of chest tube
    E. Pericardiocentesis with placement of pericardial window

End of Set

The response options for items 53 through 58 are the same. You will be required to select one answer for each item in the set.

54. High-pitched, decrescendo mid- to holodiastolic murmur heard at the third and fourth intercostal space at the left sternal border *E*
    AR B

55. Diastolic murmur heard best at the left lower sternal border. *TS* *E*

56. Diamond-shaped <u>systolic</u> ejection murmur heard at the right upper sternal border. *A*

57. Pansystolic decrescendo murmur heard best at the apex with radiation into the axilla. *D*

58. Systolic murmur heard best at the left lower sternal border that increases with inspiration. *G*

End of Set

The next two questions (items 59 and 60) correspond to the following vignette.

A 70-year-old man with long-standing hypertension presents to the ED with complaints of acute onset of substernal chest pain. He describes the pain as "tearing" in nature with radiation into his back. On exam, his blood pressure is 172/102 with a pulse of 118. He appears uncomfortable and diaphoretic. His cardiac exam reveals tachycardia with a normal S_1 and S_2. There are no murmurs noted. You suspect an aortic dissection.

59. Which of the following would be the test of choice to confirm your diagnosis?

    A. ECG
    B. Chest X-ray
    C. Transesophageal echocardiogram (TEE)
    D. Transthoracic echocardiogram (TTE)
    E. CT scan of the chest

60. The above test confirms the presence of a 7-cm ascending thoracic aortic dissection. Your first step in the initial therapeutic management of this patient is to:

    A. Transfuse platelets and fresh-frozen plasma.
    B. Treat with IV β-blockers and nitroprusside
    C. Obtain a cardiothoracic surgery consult
    D. Observe the patient and perform serial echocardiograms
    E. Treat with oral angiotensin-converting enzyme (ACE) inhibitors

End of Set

61. You have just started your hematology-oncology rotation and you are seeing a patient in the clinic for follow-up of breast cancer treatment. She is frightened about her diagnosis, and asks you questions regarding mortality from breast cancer and other kinds of cancers. You counsel her that which of the following cancers is responsible for the most cancer-related deaths in women in the United States per year?

    A. Colorectal cancer
    B. Lung cancer
    C. Breast cancer
    D. Leukemia
    E. Ovarian cancer

The next two questions (items 62 and 63) correspond to the following vignette.

A 25-year-old Hispanic woman presents to your office after finding a lump in her left breast. She found the lump when taking a shower 3 months ago and has not noticed any change in the size or consistency of the lump with her menstrual cycles. She has no significant medical history and takes no medications. She began menses at age 10 and gave birth to a son at age 21. Family history is significant for a paternal aunt with breast cancer. On physical exam there is a palpable mass in the left upper outer quadrant of the left breast. It is approximately 3 cm in diameter, smooth, and well circumscribed. No axillary nodes are palpable.

62. The next step in evaluating this patient should be:

    A. Excisional biopsy
    B. Mammogram
    C. Ultrasound
    D. Mastectomy
    E. Reassurance and follow up in 6 months

63. Which of the following is a risk factor for breast cancer in this patient?

    A. Personal history of breast cancer
    B. First-degree relative with breast cancer
    C. Race
    D. Age at menarche
    E. Age at first live birth

End of Set

The next two questions (items 64 and 65) correspond to the following vignette.

A 34-year-old white man presents with a complaint of blood in his bowel movements for the last 2 weeks. He also has noted some symptoms of constipation and change in stool caliber. He does not report any weight loss, fatigue, or emesis. He has noted a mild decrease in appetite. His family history is positive for a father with colon cancer diagnosed at age 50, a female sibling with colon cancer diagnosed at age 45, and an aunt with colon cancer diagnosed at age 54. A colonoscopy is performed with biopsy of a single ulcerative mass in the descending colon. The pathology shows adenocarcinoma.

64. Which genetic condition do you suspect in this patient?

A. Familial adenomatous polyposis (FAP)

B. BRCA-1 mutation

C. Gardner's syndrome

D. Hereditary nonpolyposis colorectal cancer (HNPCC)

E. Peutz-Jeghers syndrome

65. What recommendations do you have for screening this patient's other family members?

A. One stool guaiac card per day for three consecutive days done annually starting at age 15 for all family members

B. Colonoscopy for all family members starting at age 20 or 10 years younger than the age at which the youngest family member was diagnosed with colon cancer, whichever comes first

C. Female family members should abide by the usual screening rules for gynecologic cancers

D. Colonoscopy for all family members at age 30, and if it is normal, repeat every 10 years

E. Flexible sigmoidoscopy for all family members when they are 10 years younger than the age at which the youngest family member was diagnosed with colon cancer

End of Set

66. A 76-year-old man presents to your office with a complaint of hemoptysis for 1 week. He states that he coughs up about a teaspoon of blood a couple of times a day. He denies fever or purulent sputum. He also reports a weight loss of 10 pounds over the last month and increasing dyspnea. He has a cigarette smoking history of 60 packs/year. Physical exam does not reveal any abnormalities on cardiovascular or pulmonary examination. The chest X-ray shows mediastinal enlargement, and the CT shows a perihilar mass and significant lymphadenopathy. A bronchoscopy is performed, and biopsies of the mass are taken. The pathology reveals islands of small, round, deeply basophilic-staining epithelial cells that look like lymphocytes, but are about twice the size of normal lymphocytes. Which of the following statements is true regarding his disease?

A. Untreated patients with his disease have median survival rates of 12 to 14 months

B. Surgery is a mainstay of treatment

C. Subacute cortical cerebellar degeneration is a paraneoplastic syndrome associated with his disease

D. His disease is not associated with his tobacco use

E. The tumor arises from type II pneumocytes in the alveolar wall

The response options for items 67 through 69 are the same. You will be required to select one answer for each item in the set.

A. Human T-lymphotrophic virus 1 (HTLV-1)

B. Epstein-Barr virus (EBV)

C. *Helicobacter pylori*

D. Cytomegalovirus (CMV)

E. Human herpesvirus 8 (HHV-8)

For each lymphoma, select the associated infection.

67. Burkitt's lymphoma

68. Mucosa-associated lymphoid tissue (MALT) lymphoma

69. Adult T-cell lymphoma

End of Set

70. A 60-year-old man with an 80 packs/year history of smoking presents with a complaint of "turning yellow" over the last 2 weeks. He reports nausea, but no vomiting or abdominal pain. He has no other significant medical history and no history of alcohol abuse. He notes a decrease in his appetite over the last month, a 5-pound weight loss, and a slight increase in abdominal girth. On physical exam, the vitals signs are within normal limits. His skin is visibly jaundiced, and his sclera are icteric. The exam otherwise reveals a minimally distended, nontender abdomen. Labs reveal the following: WBC 6000/μL with normal differential; hemoglobin 11.8 g/dL; blood smear normal; total bilirubin 13.0 mg/dL; direct bilirubin 11.5 mg/dL; indirect bilirubin 1.5 mg/dL; AST 45 U/L; ALT 55 U/L; alkaline phosphatase 200 U/L. What is the most likely diagnosis?

A. Cholecystitis

B. Pancreatic cancer

C. Ascending cholangitis

D. Gilbert's syndrome

E. Autoimmune hemolytic anemia

71. A 70-year-old man presents with bone pain in his lower back and pelvis bilaterally for the past 2 weeks. He has been increasingly fatigued over the last 2 months. He denies weight loss, night sweats, easy bruising, or bleeding. He has been to an urgent care for upper respiratory infections twice in the last 3 months. On physical examination you note spinous process tenderness to palpation over the lumbar vertebrae and tenderness of the pelvis and long bones of the thighs. Otherwise the examination is unremarkable. Labs are as follows: Hemoglobin 8.9 g/dL; WBCs 5000/μL; platelets 300,000/μL; creatinine 1.9 mg/dL; calcium 11.2 mg/dL; total protein 9.1 g/dL. The remainder of electrolytes and liver function tests are normal. What is the most likely diagnosis?

    A. Acute lymphocytic leukemia
    B. Monoclonal gammopathy of uncertain significance (MGUS)
    C. Waldenström's macroglobulinemia
    D. Chronic myelogenous leukemia
    E. Multiple myeloma

72. A 20-year-old man presents with shortness of breath for the last 6 weeks. He complains of dyspnea on exertion, palpitations, weight loss of 15 pounds, fever, and night sweats. On examination his pulse is 120, respiratory rate 18, and oxygen saturations are 98% on room air. A fixed, firm, 3-cm left anterior cervical lymph node is palpable. Lungs are clear to auscultation bilaterally, and the patient has no enlargement of the liver or spleen. The remainder of the exam is

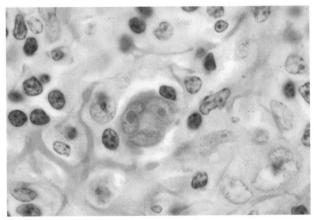

Figure 1-72 • Image Courtesy of Dr. Brenda Shinar, Banner Good Samaritan Medical Center, Phoenix, Arizona.

normal. A chest X-ray shows mediastinal lymphadenopathy. Excisional biopsy of the cervical lymph node reveals cells seen in Figure 1-72. What is his most likely diagnosis?

    A. CMV
    B. Hodgkin's lymphoma
    C. Non-Hodgkin's lymphoma
    D. Scrofula
    E. Sarcoidosis

73. A 75-year-old man with small-cell carcinoma presents with shortness of breath, facial swelling, and headache. On physical exam, his respiratory rate is 18, his oxygen saturation is 94% on room air and he is not in any acute distress. There is cervical venous distension, plethora of the face, and facial edema. You suspect superior vena cava (SVC) syndrome. Which of the following statements is true regarding this diagnosis?

    A. Lymphoma is the most common cause of SVC syndrome
    B. Stridor due to tracheal obstruction is a medical emergency and should be treated immediately with radiation
    C. The most common physical finding is facial edema
    D. Symptoms can be decreased by elevating the head of the bed, providing oxygen, and gentle diuresis
    E. Radiation therapy has no effect on the prognosis

74. You are asked to design a screening test for disease "X." Knowing that approximately 20% of the general population has disease "X," you develop a screening test, which you use on 1000 randomly selected patients. The following numbers are obtained: People *with* the disease and a positive screening test, 180; people *without* the disease and *with* a positive screening test, 160; people *with* the disease and a negative screening test, 20; people *without* the disease and *with* a negative screening test, 640.

Which of the following statements regarding the screening test is true?

    A. The specificity is 90%
    B. The specificity is 60%
    C. The sensitivity is 40%
    D. The sensitivity is 66%
    E. The sensitivity is 90%

The next two questions (items 75 and 76) correspond to the following vignette.

A 28-year-old man presents to the ED with complaints of abdominal pain, nausea, and vomiting. He has had three episodes of emesis over the past 24 hours. His abdominal pain is localized to the epigastric and right upper quadrant areas. He has had no diarrhea. He reports increasing jaundice, but denies dark urine or light-colored stools. He has had no recent travel. On examination, he is afebrile and has normal vital signs. He is in no acute distress, but obviously does not feel well. He has mild scleral and mucosal icterus, but the remainder of his head and neck exam is unremarkable. His lungs are clear and his heart examination is normal. He has diffuse abdominal tenderness that is worse in the right upper quadrant area. His abdomen is not distended. He has no rebound, guarding, or rigidity. His genitourinary (GU) examination is normal and his stool is negative for occult blood. You obtain the following laboratory results: AST 4800 U/L; ALT 3900 U/L; total bilirubin 2.1 mg/dL; alkaline phosphatase 152 U/L; PT 12.6 seconds.

75. What is the most likely cause of this patient's clinical presentation?

    A. Viral hepatitis
    B. Cholelithiasis
    C. Alcoholic hepatitis
    D. Hemochromatosis
    E. Hepatocellular carcinoma

76. What is the next appropriate test to obtain on this patient?

    A. Abdominal ultrasound
    B. Ethanol level
    C. Percutaneous liver biopsy
    D. Serum ferritin level
    E. Acute hepatitis panel

End of Set

77. A 54-year-old man presents to your office for a pre-employment physical. He is currently treated for allergic rhinitis with a steroid preparation nasal spray, but is otherwise healthy and takes no other medications. He offers no specific complaints during his visit. He drinks infrequently and smokes approximately two packs of cigarettes per day for the past 10 years. His physical examination is normal, including

his vital signs. He gives you some papers from his employer to complete regarding his physical exam and health status. The forms include a request for an ECG, a chest X-ray, and some routine labs. You order these as requested. His ECG is normal, as are his routine labs. You receive a report that his chest X-ray reveals a single, round lesion near the periphery of his right upper lobe. It is approximately 2 cm in diameter and is surrounded by normal lung parenchyma. There is no evidence of lymphadenopathy on the chest X-ray. There are no old chest X-rays available for comparison. You obtain a CT scan of his chest, which confirms the presence of an eccentric 2-cm lesion in the right upper lobe near the chest wall. Which of the following is the most appropriate next step in the management of this patient?

    A. Have him follow up in 3 months for a repeat chest X-ray
    B. Have him follow up in 6 months for a repeat chest X-ray
    C. Make arrangements for him to have a CT-guided needle biopsy of the lesion
    D. Make arrangements for him to have a bronchoscopy with transbronchial biopsies of the lesion
    E. Apply a PPD and start empiric therapy for tuberculosis

78. A 72-year-old woman presents to the ED with a severe exacerbation of her chronic obstructive pulmonary disease (COPD). She is in respiratory distress and requires immediate intubation and placement on a mechanical ventilator. Once she is stabilized, she is admitted to the intensive care unit where you are working. A nurse asks you about the possibility of her developing a deep venous thrombosis (DVT) and possible pulmonary embolus (PE). Which of the following statements is correct regarding the prevention of venous thromboembolism (VTE) in this patient?

    A. She is at low risk for VTE and does not need prophylaxis
    B. 5000 U of subcutaneous heparin should be given every 8 to 12 hours
    C. Sequential compression devices (SCDs) should be applied to her lower extremities
    D. Full-dose IV heparin should be initiated
    E. She should be evaluated for a hypercoagulable state before beginning DVT prophylaxis

79. You are rotating in the intensive care unit and taking care of several patients. On rounds, your attending asks you to choose which one out of five of your patients is at the highest risk for the development of a stress ulcer complication. Your choice is:

    A. A 62-year-old woman on a mechanical ventilator because of severe COPD exacerbation
    B. A 58-year-old man who is on IV heparin therapy for an acute myocardial infarction
    C. A 60-year-old woman with acute pancreatitis with a prior history of upper GI bleed
    D. A 55-year-old man with COPD and a large pulmonary embolus who developed respiratory failure requiring ventilation and is on IV heparin therapy
    E. A woman with rheumatoid arthritis with a septic knee and hypotension

80. A 62-year-old woman presents to your office complaining of a cough that has been present for the past 8 weeks. She says the cough is nonproductive and is not associated with fevers or shortness of breath. There is no history of tobacco use. She has not noticed the cough being worse at night, but does report it seems worse when she lies flat. She has hypertension that is well controlled with a β-blocker, but has been healthy otherwise. She has no history of asthma and denies wheezing with this cough or any recent respiratory tract infections. There is no history of seasonal allergy symptoms. There are no identifiable risk factors for tuberculosis. She states that she has fairly frequent heartburn but denies weight loss or dysphagia. Her vital signs are normal and she is afebrile. Her physical examination is completely normal. What is the most likely cause of her chronic cough?

    A. Seasonal allergies
    B. Postnasal drip
    C. Gastroesophageal reflux
    D. Asthma variant
    E. Bronchogenic carcinoma

81. A 58-year-old man, accompanied by his wife, presents to your office with complaints of progressive difficulty swallowing. He has a sensation of the food getting "stuck" in his chest. He says that the difficulty swallowing first started with breads and meats a few months ago and

now occurs with most foods. He has no trouble swallowing liquids. He denies any nausea or vomiting. He does not choke on his food or have any difficulty chewing or initiating a swallow. His wife confirms this and states she believes he has lost approximately 15 pounds over the past 4 months. His past medical history is significant only for hypertension, which is well controlled. He reports chronic reflux-type symptoms that he treats with over-the-counter antacids. He is not a smoker. His vital signs are normal and his physical examination is unremarkable. An ECG and chest X-ray are obtained, both of which are normal. What is the most likely diagnosis and the best test to evaluate for it?

    A. Achalasia; upper GI barium study
    B. Diverticulum; CT scan
    C. Adenocarcinoma: esophagogastroduodenoscopy (EGD)
    D. Squamous cell carcinoma: EGD
    E. Candidiasis; candida skin testing

The next two questions (items 82 and 83) correspond to the following vignette.

A 26-year-old white woman comes to your office after noticing a lump in her breast approximately 1 week ago. She states that she had never noticed it before. She is fearful because her grandmother had breast cancer diagnosed at age 75. She notes that the lump is tender and moveable. She does not recall any trauma to the area. She is due for her period in 2 weeks. On exam you note a smooth, round, 1.5-cm mass that is fluctuant and minimally tender.

82. What is the most likely diagnosis?

    A. Breast adenocarcinoma
    B. Fibrous adenoma
    C. Breast abscess
    D. Fat necrosis
    E. Breast cyst

83. You have advised her to observe the mass throughout her menses and return if it does not go away. She returns 2 weeks later and is concerned that the mass is still present and is, in fact, larger. On exam it has grown to 2 cm in size but still remains smooth, round, and fluctuant. The next diagnostic step is:

A. BRCA1 and BRCA 2 gene testing
B. Ultrasound
C. Mammogram
D. Surgical referral for excision
E. Wait and re-examine in 3 months

End of Set

84. A 19-year-old white woman presents to your office with complaints of irregular periods. She states she has had irregular periods since menarche at age 14. Her periods occur every 28 to 40 days and last 4 to 5 days. It has been approximately 60 days since her last period. She is very athletic and plays basketball on her college team. Her weight has been stable without any recent extreme losses or gains. She states she is currently sexually active but states she and her boyfriend always use condoms. Her BMI is 25, and her physical exam, including pelvic exam, is within normal limits. What should you do next to evaluate the cause of her irregular periods?

A. Start a low estrogen/progestin oral contraceptive pill to regulate her cycle
B. Get a urine β-HCG to rule out pregnancy
C. Recommend that she check daily basal body temperatures to evaluate for ovulation
D. Order a TSH
E. Refer for an endometrial biopsy

85. A 55-year-old white woman with a history of hypertension presents to your office with complaints of a red right eye. She states that she noticed it approximately 2 days ago. She denies any recent viral illness or eye discharge. She is very uncomfortable with a deep, severe aching pain behind her right eye that she has never felt before. She had associated nausea and vomiting today secondary to the severe pain. On physical exam, the eye is diffusely erythematous without discharge. The cornea appears cloudy. The pupil is moderately dilated and fixed, without a response to light. The vision in the affected eye is markedly blurred. What is the most likely diagnosis?

A. Viral conjunctivitis
B. Herpes simplex keratitis
C. Corneal abrasion
D. Acute angle-closure glaucoma
E. Allergic conjunctivitis

86. A 28-year-old Hispanic woman comes to your office for a routine health exam. She states she has not had a Pap and pelvic exam in 6 years. She is currently sexually active, and has been in a monogamous relationship for 4 years. She has had a total of two sexual partners starting at age 20. She denies alcohol, tobacco, or IV drug abuse (IVDA). Her exam, including pelvic, is within normal limits. You obtain her Pap results and it reveals atypical squamous cells of uncertain significance (ASCUS). What do you do next in the management of this patient?

A. Repeat Pap and pelvic in 1 year and repeat yearly until three are consecutively negative.
B. Refer for colposcopy with biopsy
C. Human papilloma virus (HPV) gene typing
D. Refer for colposcopy with cryotherapy
E. Repeat Pap and pelvic every 4 to 6 months until three are consecutively negative.

87. A 60-year-old white man presents to your office for a new patient visit. He states that in general he is fairly healthy with the exception of hypertension for which he is taking hydrochlorothiazide. On review of systems, his only concern is that his last doctor told him that he had blood in his stool when checked in the office and that he would need follow-up. He was unable to do this at that time because he lost his insurance. He denies any weight loss or change in appetite. He also denies any change in stools. He denies any family history of colorectal cancer. Exam reveals internal hemorrhoids. Repeat fecal occult blood test is positive. The next step in his evaluation is:

A. Single contrast barium enema
B. Anoscopy, to evaluate the hemorrhoids for bleeding
C. Flexible sigmoidoscopy
D. Colonoscopy
E. CT scan of abdomen and pelvis

The response options for items 88 through 91 are the same. You will be required to select one answer for each item in the set.

A. Intrauterine device (IUD)
B. Progestin only, injection form
C. Combination oral contraceptive (OCP) (estrogen/progesterone)
D. Condom

For each description, select the appropriate form of contraceptive.

88. Inhibits ovulation by suppressing follicle stimulating hormone (FSH) and luteinizing hormone (LH). Success is determined by taking this medication consistently.

89. Long-term suppression of ovulation, often used in adolescents. Side effects include irregular uterine bleeding, headache, breast tenderness, weight gain, and acne.

90. Progesterone-containing device associated with an increased risk of pelvic inflammatory disease (PID) in high-risk patients, such as those with multiple sex partners or with a history of sexually transmitted diseases (STDs). Side effects include increased uterine cramping and bleeding.

91. When used with spermicide it is associated with increased effectiveness. Is also associated with a decreased transmission of STDs.

End of Set

The next two questions (items 92 and 93) correspond to the following vignette.

A 20-year-old white woman presents to your office with a 3- to 4-day history of dysuria and increased frequency of urination. She denies fever, chills, or flank pain. She is currently sexually active with her boyfriend. She states they use condoms all of the time. She has recently noted a vaginal discharge that has an unusual odor. Urine dip in the office is negative. On pelvic exam you note a thin, white vaginal discharge adhering to the vaginal wall. The cervix is otherwise within normal limits. There is no cervical motion tenderness. The pH of the vaginal discharge is 6. A wet mount preparation reveals epithelial cells that are covered with coccobacillary bacteria, which makes the cells appear stippled.

92. What is the most likely diagnosis?
    A. Urinary tract infection with *E. coli*
    B. Bacterial vaginosis
    C. *Trichomonas* infection
    D. *Chlamydia trachomatis* infection
    E. Vulvovaginal candidiasis

93. The most appropriate therapy for bacterial vaginosis is:

A. Trimethoprim-sulfamethoxazole
B. Ciprofloxacin
C. Metronidazole
D. Diflucan
E. Ceftriaxone

End of Set

---

94. A 55-year-old obese man comes to your office with concerns regarding diabetes. His mother and father both suffer from type II diabetes, diagnosed in their adult years. He denies any history of polyuria or polydipsia. His past medical history is significant only for hypertension, for which he is trying diet and exercise with little success. His body mass index (BMI) is 40, heart rate 90, respiratory rate 18, and blood pressure 149/79. Exam is significant for an obese man with noted acanthosis nigricans. You suspect he has type II diabetes mellitus and you order laboratories. Which of the following would be consistent with a diagnosis of diabetes?
    A. Random glucose >180
    B. Postprandial 2-hour plasma glucose >120
    C. HgbA1C of 7.0
    D. Fasting glucose >126
    E. + glucose on urine dipstick

95. A 56-year-old white woman presents to you with complaints of urinary incontinence. She notes that she senses an intense need to use the bathroom but often does not make it to the bathroom on time. She is not incontinent with coughing or sneezing. She denies any dysuria, fevers, or abdominal pain. She is not currently taking any medications. She is incontinent two or three times per week. Physical exam is essentially within normal limits. Urinalysis is within normal limits and postvoid residual is
    A. Overflow and urge incontinence
    B. Overflow and stress incontinence
    C. Urge incontinence
    D. Stress incontinence
    E. Overflow incontinence

The next three questions (items 96 through 98) correspond to the following vignette.

A 41-year-old man with diabetes mellitus presents with a cough associated with pleuritic chest pain, which began yesterday. His cough is productive of thick, rust-colored sputum. He has been having fevers up to

103.0°F (39.4°C) and shaking chills. On examination, you find a well-developed man with temperature 102.6°F (39.2°C), blood pressure 118/68, heart rate 98, and respiratory rate 24. Room air pulse-oximetry reveals an oxygen saturation of 86% that increases to 94% on 2 L/min nasal cannula. His lung exam reveals bronchial breath sounds in his right lower lung base with egophany. His heart rate is mildly tachycardic without murmur or ectopy noted. Abdominal and GU exams are normal. A CBC reveals a WBC count of 18,400 with a left shift. His chest X-ray demonstrates a focal, consolidative infiltrate in the right lower lobe area with an associated pleural effusion.

96. Which of the following organisms has most likely caused his presentation?

    A. *Mycoplasma pneumoniae*
    B. *Pneumocystis carinii*
    C. *Bacteroides fragilis*
    D. *Streptococcus pneumoniae*
    E. *Bacillus anthracis*

97. Which of the following antibiotics would be the best choice for initial therapy of his infection?

    A. Clindamycin
    B. Ceftriaxone
    C. Sulfamethoxazole-trimethoprim
    D. Ampicillin
    E. Amantadine

98. You perform a thoracentesis to obtain fluid to evaluate this patient's new pleural effusion. A simultaneous serum sample is drawn and shows a total protein (TP) level of 6.5 and an LDH level of 220. Which of the following are you most likely to find on his pleural fluid analysis (Table 1-98)?

■ TABLE 1-98

Answer	Effusion Total Protein (TP)	Effusion LDH
A	4.0	180
B	3.0	60
C	2.5	80
D	2.0	100
E	1.0	120

End of Set

The next two questions (items 99 and 100) correspond to the following vignette.

A 31-year-old man presents to the ED with complaints of a painful, swollen right finger. He states that the onset of swelling and pain started the day before. Other than a subjective fever and malaise, he has no other complaints. On review of systems, he reports some mild dysuria which began approximately 2 weeks ago. He denies penile discharge. He has had several female sexual partners over the past few months. He denies any GI complaints or skin rashes. On examination, he is afebrile and his vital signs are normal. He has mild erythema of the conjunctiva of the right eye without photophobia. The remainder of his examination is unremarkable with the exception of his right index finger (Figure 1-99).

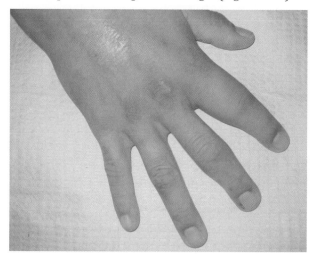

Figure 1-99 • Image Courtesy of Dr. Brenda Shinar, Banner Good Samaritan Medical Center, Phoenix, Arizona.

99. What is the most likely cause of this patient's symptoms?

    A. Psoriatic arthritis
    B. Rheumatoid arthritis
    C. Reiter's syndrome
    D. Gonococcal arthritis
    E. Osteoarthritis

100. Which of the following is most likely to be positive in this patient?

    A. Culture of joint aspirate
    B. Rheumatoid factor
    C. Urethral DNA probe for gonorrhea
    D. HLA-B27
    E. Plain film periosteal elevation and thickening

End of Set

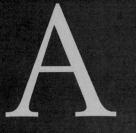

Answers and Explanations

51. C	68. C	85. D
52. C	69. A	86. C
53. C	70. B	87. D
54. B	71. B	88. C
55. E	72. E	89. B
56. A	73. D	90. A
57. D	74. E	91. D
58. F	75. A	92. B
59. E	76. E	93. C
60. B	77. C	94. D
61. B	78. B	95. C
62. C	79. D	96. D
63. D	80. C	97. B
64. D	81. C	98. A
65. B	82. E	99. C
66. C	83. B	100. D
67. B	84. B	

51. **C. This patient has classic findings of pericarditis. These include pleuritic chest pain that is affected by positioning, fevers, and a friction rub. The ECG shows diffuse ST segment elevation that is suggestive of a global process, and PR depression.**

    A. Although a pulmonary embolus can cause substernal chest pain and fever in a young woman, the pain is usually not affected by positioning. In addition, the ECG findings most often show sinus tachycardia with or without evidence of right-sided heart strain.

    B. Acute myocardial infarction would be an unusual cause of chest pain in a young patient. Pain resulting from myocardial ischemia does not usually have a pleuritic component to it. In addition, one would not expect to see diffuse ST segment changes on the ECG, but rather a specific pattern of injury (for example, leads II, III, and AVF would be affected in an inferior wall myocardial infarction).

    D. Tension pneumothorax could also cause pleuritic chest pain in a young patient, but it is not usually affected by positioning. Additionally, it would not account for the ECG changes shown, and one would not expect to see a normal chest X-ray.

    E. Cardiac tamponade does not usually present with chest pain, but rather with dyspnea and symptoms similar to those of congestive heart failure, such as orthopnea and lower extremity edema. However, patients in tamponade should have clear lung fields on auscultation, which distinguishes them from patients in left heart failure. In addition, tamponade does not usually cause diffuse ST segment elevation on ECG, but rather low voltage throughout all the leads. This is due to the dampening of the electrical impulse as it traverses the fluid surrounding the heart.

52. **C. The patient with pericarditis should be started initially on anti-inflammatory medications such as aspirin or NSAIDs. For refractory cases of pericarditis, other medications such as colchicine or steroids may be indicated.**

    A. The treatment of choice for a pulmonary embolus would be to initiate anticoagulation with IV heparin. However, this is contraindicated in a patient with pericarditis because of the increased risk of bleeding from the inflamed pericardium, which could lead to a hemorrhagic effusion and tamponade.

    B. Although β-blockers would be indicated if she were having an acute myocardial infarction, they are of no benefit in the treatment of pericarditis.

    D. Thoracostomy with placement of chest tube would be helpful in a patient with a pneumothorax. However, it will be of no benefit to our patient.

    E. Pericardiocentesis with placement of pericardial window may be indicated in some cases of cardiac tamponade; however, it is of no benefit in the treatment of pericarditis without pericardial effusion. An echocardiogram will help you determine whether or not a pericardial effusion is present.

53. **C. The murmur of mitral stenosis is best heard in the area of the mitral valve (the apex) and occurs during diastole. The murmur is the result of turbulent blood flow across the stenotic valve, which occurs during the filling of the left ventricle.**

54. **B. Aortic regurgitation results in the backflow of blood across the valve into the left ventricle during diastole. This murmur is best heard at the third and fourth intercostal space at the *left* sternal border when it is due to aortic *valve* disease, and at the *right* sternal border when it is due to aortic *root* disease (Right = Root). In severe cases, a second diastolic murmur can be heard in the area of the left lower sternal border. This murmur, known as the Austin-Flint murmur, is the result of the regurgitant stream of blood striking the mitral leaflets and making a "relative" mitral stenosis.**

55. **E. Similar to mitral stenosis, tricuspid stenosis results in turbulent blood flow across the valve during filling of the right ventricle (diastole). This murmur, however, is best heard in the area of the tricuspid valve (left lower sternal border).**

56. **A. AS results in turbulence of blood flow across the valve during ejection of the blood from the left ventricle (systole). It is best heard in the right upper sternal border area and often radiates into the carotids.**

57. **D. The murmur of mitral regurgitation, which is best heard in the apical area, results from retrograde blood flow across the insufficient valve into the left atrium during systole.**

58. **F.** Tricuspid regurgitation is similar to mitral regurgitation, in that the murmur is the result of retrograde blood flow across the valve during systole. It can be distinguished from mitral regurgitation, tricuspid regurgitation, and right-sided murmurs, because as a general rule, they increase in intensity with inspiration. This is because blood is "sucked" into the right atrium with the negative intrathoracic pressure that occurs during inspiration and increases the volume of blood that travels across the stenotic or regurgitant valve. Tricuspid regurgitation is also heard best in the area of the tricuspid valve (along the left lower sternal border) as opposed to the apical area where mitral regurgitation is best heard.

G. Although a PDA can result in a murmur along the left sternal border, it is usually closer to the clavicular area and is a continuous "machine gun" type of murmur (i.e., it is heard throughout systole and diastole).

H. The murmur of coarctation of the aorta sounds similar to AS, but it is often heard in the upper back area. Checking the peripheral pulses also helps distinguish between AS and coarctation of the aorta. In coarctation of the aorta, the pulses in the lower extremities are diminished when compared with the pulses in the upper extremities. AS should not result in a discrepancy in the peripheral pulses.

59. **E.** A CT scan of the chest is the test of choice to evaluate for a possible thoracic dissection. It is the most rapid and precise test that is readily available. The classic finding of a dissection on CT is widening of the aorta with extravasation of blood into the wall of the aorta causing the "double barrel" sign.

A. The ECG may show evidence of ischemia if the coronary arteries are involved, but otherwise is not useful in the diagnosis of thoracic aortic dissection.

B. A chest X-ray may show widening of the mediastinum, which should raise concern for dissection, but it does not confirm the diagnosis or identify the exact portion of the aorta that is involved. It also cannot be used to estimate the size of the dissection.

C. TEE will give a better assessment of the descending portion of the aorta, and is also a good way to assess the ascending aorta, next to the aortic valve. However, TEE is not as readily available as a CT scan. In addition, if there is any concern or evidence of an acute myocardial infarction, then a TEE is contraindicated. However, if the patient is in the ICU and is too unstable to go to a CT scan, an emergent TEE is a good option to diagnose a dissection of the aorta.

D. TTE is a relatively rapid, noninvasive way of assessing cardiac function and valvular abnormalities. However, the aortic root and ascending aorta are not always well visualized on an echocardiogram. In addition, the descending aorta is difficult to thoroughly assess with the transthoracic approach, thereby increasing your chances of missing the diagnosis.

60. **B.** This patient's condition is a medical emergency and the first step in the treatment of the dissection is to rapidly decrease his blood pressure. This is best accomplished by using IV medications such as nitroprusside and β-blockers. Nitroprusside should be used with a β-blocker, not alone. If nitroprusside is used alone, the arterial vasodilatory properties will cause a reflex tachycardia that can worsen "shearing forces" in the dissection. Therefore, it is important to use arterial vasodilators at the same time as β-blockers to avoid this phenomenon.

A. Transfusing platelets and fresh-frozen plasma may be necessary during his operative procedure or postoperatively; however, it will do nothing acutely to stop the advancement of his dissection.

C. Dissections of the ascending aorta almost always require surgical intervention, so a cardiothoracic surgery consult should be obtained expeditiously. However, attempts at reduction in blood pressure should be initiated while you are awaiting the arrival of the surgical team.

D. Observing the patient with serial echocardiograms is not acceptable management. This patient has a medical emergency requiring prompt and rapid treatment (including surgical intervention). Simply observing this patient is putting him at significant risk of death.

E. Although blood pressure may be treated with oral ACE-inhibitors, this is not appropriate given the longer onset of action of the oral medications and the need for immediate reduction of blood pressure.

61. **B.** Although lung cancer is second to breast cancer in incidence for women in the United States, it is the most common cause of cancer *death*. Lung cancer accounts for 12% of cancers in this population, but accounts for 25% of cancer deaths.

   A. Colorectal cancer accounts for 11% of cancer incidences in this population and 11% of cancer deaths. This makes it the third most common cancer and the third leading cause of cancer death for women in the United States.
   C. Breast cancer has the highest incidence of cancers among women in the United States, accounting for 30% of cancers. However, it falls behind lung cancer as a cause of cancer death at 15%.
   D. Leukemia accounts for only 4% of cancer deaths among women in the United States. Leukemia makes up less than 2% of cancer types for this population.
   E. Ovarian cancer accounts for 4% of cancers among women in the United States, making it the fifth most common cancer in women. Additionally, it is the fifth leading cause of cancer death in this population, accounting for 5% of all cancer deaths.

62. **C.** When evaluating breast masses, the clinical suspicion for cancer and the age of the patient help to guide the work-up. Mammograms are less diagnostic in premenopausal women because of the generally higher density of the breast tissue. Therefore, a palpable mass in a 70-year-old woman should trigger a mammogram evaluation. A palpable mass in a woman who is age 35 or younger is better evaluated by an initial ultrasound to determine whether the mass is cystic or solid. *It is important to remember that a patient with a persistent palpable breast mass who has a normal mammogram still requires further work-up.*

   A. Ultrasound can determine whether the lesion is a simple cyst or if it has septations and/or solid components. An excisional biopsy may be indicated *after* the ultrasound, if the ultrasound determines that the lesion is not a simple cyst.
   B. See explanation for C.
   D. Mastectomy should be undertaken only after a tissue diagnosis of cancer is obtained and treatment options are discussed with the patient.

   E. Occasionally, it may be reasonable in a woman who is considered very low risk for cancer to be observed through one menstrual cycle to determine if the mass lesion goes away with normal hormone fluctuations. However, this patient had observed the lesion through three menstrual cycles without any change in the lesion, and therefore it warrants further evaluation.

63. **D.** A younger age at menarche is a known risk factor for breast cancer. The longer time of menses increases exposure to hormones, thereby increasing the risk of breast cancer. The average age of menarche in the United States is 12.2 years, so this patient has undergone menarche relatively early at age 10.

   A. A personal history of breast cancer increases the risk of new or recurrent cancer in either breast. Our patient did not have a personal history of breast cancer.
   B. The number of first-degree relatives with breast cancer increases the risk. First-degree relatives include mother, sisters, and daughters. One first-degree relative affected increases the risk by almost two-fold. However, this patient had an aunt with breast cancer.
   C. Whites have the highest rate of breast cancer after age 40. Black women have the second-highest rate, but the highest mortality. Hispanic women have the third-highest rate of breast cancer.
   E. Older age at first live birth increases the risk of breast cancer. Women who give birth at age 35 or more have 1.5 times the risk of breast cancer than those who give birth before age 25.

64. **D.** This patient meets the Amsterdam Criteria for diagnosis of HNPCC (also known as Lynch syndrome). It is inherited in an autosomal dominant pattern. The Amsterdam Criteria are: three or more relatives with colorectal cancer, one affected relative is a first-degree relative, two generations of family with colorectal cancer, and one case is diagnosed in a family member younger than 50 years of age. Although it is often difficult to distinguish HNPCC from FAP, the findings on colonoscopy should rule out FAP in this case (see explanation for A).

A. FAP typically presents in the second to third decade of life. FAP is caused by a mutation in the adenomatous polyposis coli gene (APC) and is transmitted in an autosomal dominant manner. Multiple polyps, typically 500 to 2500 polyps "carpeting" the mucosal surface, can be found on colonoscopy. There is a tremendous risk that these polyps will transform into adenocarcinoma of the colon over time.

B. BRCA-1 mutation is associated with breast cancer, ovarian cancer, and prostate cancer.

C. Gardner's syndrome is a subset of familial APC. In addition to the colonic polyps, patients also have soft tissue and bony tumors and ampullary cancers.

E. Peutz-Jeghers syndrome is a rare autosomal dominant syndrome characterized by multiple hamartomatous polyps scattered throughout the gastrointestinal tract. Patients have small macular "freckle" appearing areas of pigmentation on the oral mucosa, lips, face, and palmar surface of the hands. Although the hamartomatous polyps carry no risk of malignancy, the patients are at risk of pancreatic, lung, breast, ovarian, and uterine cancers.

65. **B. Screening recommendations for family members include a colonoscopy at age 20 to 25 years OR 10 years younger than the age of diagnosis for the youngest person in the family, whichever comes first. This should be repeated every 1 to 2 years because of the rapid progression of malignancy in these patients, even if the first colonoscopy is normal.**

A. Fecal occult blood testing, a screening test used in the general population, is not adequate in this patient population.

C. Female family members are at increased risk for endometrial and ovarian cancer. Annual screening for these malignancies should begin at age 25. Screening includes pelvic examination with endometrial aspirate or transvaginal ultrasound.

D. Colonoscopy should be repeated more frequently than is recommended for the general population. Current recommendations are to repeat the exam every 1 to 2 years.

E. Flexible sigmoidoscopy is not adequate to screen for colon cancer in this patient population. The entire colon must be examined.

66. **C. This patient has small cell carcinoma (also called "oat cell" carcinoma) of the lung. The cancer is highly malignant and is in the family of small, round, blue (basophilic-staining) tumors of neuroendocrine origin. Small cell carcinomas often produce paraneoplastic syndromes because of their production of ectopic hormones such as ACTH (resulting in Cushing's syndrome). Other, less well-known paraneoplastic syndromes include subacute cortical cerebellar degeneration, which presents as vertigo, dysarthria, diplopia, and nystagmus. It is thought to be due to antibody-mediated destruction of the cerebellar Purkinje cells and their axons.**

A. The prognosis for small cell carcinoma is poor, both with and without treatment. Without treatment, life expectancy is 2 to 4 months. Staging is simple: Limited-stage disease (30% of patients) means that the disease is confined to one hemithorax and its regional lymph nodes. Extensive-stage disease is that which is not confined to the above "limits."

B. Treatment with chemotherapy with or without radiation can prolong the duration and quality of life for those with small cell lung cancer, but overall the prognosis is not very good. There is no role for surgery in the treatment of small cell lung cancer.

D. Small cell lung cancer is highly related to smoking. Only 1% of patients with the disease are nonsmokers.

E. The tumor arises from neuroendocrine cells of the lining of bronchial epithelium.

67. **B. Burkitt's lymphoma is a type of non-Hodgkin's lymphoma. Patients with this type of lymphoma can present with a rapidly enlarging mass on the head or neck. African Burkitt's lymphoma cells express the Epstein-Barr virus receptor and have the EBV virus genome in the tumor cells.**

68. **C. *H. pylori* infection has a known association with gastric MALT lymphoma. MALT lymphoma can progress to large B-cell lymphoma.**

69. **A. Adult T-cell lymphoma is associated with HTLV-1 infection. Adult T-cell lymphoma presents with diffuse adenopathy, hepatosplenomegaly, cutaneous lesions, hypercalcemia, lytic bone lesions, and interstitial pulmonary infiltrates. The WBC count is high and peripheral smear shows highly convoluted, abnormal nuclei.**

D. CMV is not associated with a lymphoma.

E. HHV-8 has been linked to Kaposi's sarcoma, but not to lymphoma.

70. **B. This man is presenting with painless jaundice, anorexia, and weight loss over a time period of several weeks. He has a significant smoking history that is a risk factor for pancreatic cancer. Obstruction of the biliary tree by the mass leads to jaundice. Obstruction of the duodenum leads to nausea and vomiting. Often patients will also have dull epigastric and back pain which they may describe as "gnawing" or "boring" in quality.**

A. Cholecystitis is caused by obstruction of the cystic duct by a gallstone. This patient does not present with a history of right upper quadrant pain, fever, or vomiting after meals. There is no tenderness to palpation over the right upper quadrant on exam, and his WBC count is normal. These findings go against a diagnosis of cholecystitis. In addition, cholecystitis by itself should not cause jaundice, unless a stone is obstructing the bile duct; in this case, the more likely diagnosis is ascending cholangitis.

C. The classic presentation for ascending cholangitis is fever, jaundice, and right upper quadrant pain. Cholangitis is an infection proximal to obstruction of the common bile duct.

D. Gilbert's syndrome is a mild, persistent, unconjugated (indirect) hyperbilirubinemia caused by a decrease in glucuronosyltransferase activity. This is the enzyme that conjugates bilirubin from the indirect portion to the direct portion. It is a common syndrome, thought to be present in 3% to 10% of the general population. The total bilirubin usually runs from 1.5 to 3.0 mg/dL, and rarely exceeds 5.0 mg/dL, and it will be mostly indirect. A feature of Gilbert's that can be diagnostically useful is that the indirect bilirubin increases after fasting. Our patient does not display any of these features.

E. Autoimmune hemolytic anemia would not cause a direct hyperbilirubinemia as in our patient. The hemoglobin is usually low and the mean corpuscular volume (MCV) is usually elevated because of the larger size of the reticulocytes that are being pumped out of the bone marrow to make up for the decreased life span of the hemolyzed red cells.

71. **B. This presentation is consistent with Hodgkin's lymphoma. There is a bimodal distribution of disease at ages 15 to 35 and again over 50. Patients usually present with lymphadenopathy including mediastinal adenopathy. "B" symptoms include fever, night sweats, and weight loss. When Reed-Sternberg cells are found on lymph node biopsy, the diagnosis of Hodgkin's disease can be made with certainty. The malignant cells are frequently binucleate and more closely resemble macrophages than lymphocytes.**

A. CMV is a virus in the herpes family. It has a number of clinical presentations including neonatal infection, primary infection in late childhood or adulthood (which resembles a mononucleosis-type illness), and infection of immunocompromised patients. Cytomegalic cells are infected epithelial cells that are two to four times the size of the surrounding cells. They have an 8- to 10-μm intranuclear inclusion that is eccentrically placed and surrounded by a clear halo that looks like an "owl's eye." This patient does not have hepatosplenomegaly, which is common with primary CMV in an adult. Also, the lymph node biopsy reveals a Reed-Sternberg cell.

C. Non-Hodgkin's lymphoma typically presents with painless lymphadenopathy and may also have "B" symptoms. Reed-Sternberg cells are diagnostic for Hodgkin's lymphoma, however, not non-Hodgkin's lymphoma.

D. Scrofula (or tuberculous lymphadenitis) is in the differential of a firm lymph node often in the cervical region. Patients may or may not have evidence of prior tuberculosis on chest X-ray. The biopsy should show acid-fast bacillus (AFB) organisms, however, not Reed-Sternberg cells.

E. Sarcoidosis may manifest with mediastinal adenopathy and the malaise and dyspnea that our patient feels. However, the biopsy of the nodes would reveal noncaseating granulomas consistent with sarcoidosis.

72. **E. One of the symptoms of multiple myeloma is bone pain. Radiographs of the bones affected will show "punched out" lesions due to activation of osteoclasts by the cytokines released by the malignant cells. Multiple myeloma occurs as a result of a monoclonal malignant proliferation of plasma cells. The malignant plasma cells secrete immunoglobulins, which are reflected**

in the elevated serum total protein, and should make you think of the diagnosis. Additional findings of this disease include anemia, hypercalcemia, and renal failure. Anemia occurs secondary to the decreased RBC production by the bone marrow. Bone pain, lytic lesions, and hypercalcemia are due to increased osteoclastic activity. Renal failure occurs as a result of the toxic effects of the light chains on the renal tubules. Recurrent infections are due to hypogammaglobulinemia of all other immunoglobulins except the monoclonal (M) chain. Diagnosis can be made by serum protein electrophoresis (SPEP) or urine protein electrophoresis (UPEP). SPEP detects the M component and UPEP detects a light chain predominance.

A. Acute lymphocytic leukemia typically presents in children, but can occur in adults. Patients present with fatigue and bone pain. Hepatosplenomegaly, lymphadenopathy, and an anterior mediastinal mass are often present. Punched-out lesions and hypercalcemia are not present.
B. MGUS occurs when there is only an elevation of total serum protein with a predominance of M component. The other findings that are seen with multiple myeloma, including renal failure, anemia, punched-out bone lesions, and hypercalcemia, are not present with MGUS. Approximately 25% of patients with MGUS progress to multiple myeloma.
C. Waldenström's macroglobulinemia is a low-grade proliferation of plasmacytoid lymphocyte cells that secrete IgM. There are no bone lesions. Patients can have symptoms related to hyperviscosity.
D. Chronic myelogenous leukemia presents in the chronic phase with fevers, night sweats, fatigue, and splenomegaly. They do not have bone lesions.

73. D. Simple measures such as elevation of the head of the bed, providing oxygen, and gentle diuresis can improve the patient's symptoms while a diagnosis is pursued.

A. Lung cancer is the leading cause of SVC syndrome. Lymphoma is the second leading cause. Other causes include infection and clot formation from catheters or pacer wires.
B. Glucocorticoids and acute airway management should be the first step in the management of a patient with tracheal obstruction due to SVC syndrome. Radiation may be used later in treatment if appropriate for diagnosis.
C. The most common physical finding is cervical venous distension. Other physical findings include facial edema, facial plethora, cyanosis, and conjunctival edema.
E. Radiation can affect the prognosis if the underlying tumor is radiation responsive.

74. E. Sensitivity and specificity are two statistical formulas that are used to help evaluate clinical tests. The sensitivity is the ratio of patients *with* a disease who have a positive test divided by all the patients with the disease. A test with high sensitivity will result in very few patients with false negative results. In other words, it will not miss many patients who have the disease. Therefore, if a test with high sensitivity is negative, the patient most likely does not have the disease, making it a good test for "ruling out" the disease. Specificity is the ratio of all the patients *without* a disease who have a negative test result divided by all the patients who do not have the disease. A test with high specificity will have very few false positives. Therefore, if you use a test with high specificity to screen for a disease, a patient with a positive result most likely has the disease, making it a good test to "rule in" the disease. To calculate the sensitivity and specificity of a particular test, you need to know the total number of people tested, the prevalence of the disease and the results of the test. In our example, 1000 people were tested and the disease prevalence was high (20%). Table 1-74 is an example of a "two by two table" that illustrates this concept applied to our results. Of the 1000 patients tested, 200 actually have the disease that we are screening for (20%) and 800 do not. Of the 200 that do have the disease, 180 have a positive test result, making the sensitivity 90%. The specificity of this test would then be 80%.

A, B, C, D. See explanation for E.

75. A. The term "liver function tests" can be somewhat misleading, so one must be careful when analyzing them. The tests that are often included in the hepatic function panel include

TABLE 1-74   Two by Two Table

	Patients *with* the Disease	Patients *without* the Disease
+ test results	180 (True Positive)	160 (False Positive)
− test results	20 (False Negative)	640 (True Negative)

Sensitivity = True Positives/(True Positives + False Negatives)
Specificity = True Negatives/(True Negatives + False Positives)

the AST, ALT, bilirubin, alkaline phosphatase, albumin, and total protein. Of these tests, the albumin is the only test that truly reflects the synthetic function of the liver (as does the PT, which is not included above). The levels of AST, ALT, alkaline phosphatase, and bilirubin do not necessarily correlate with the functional status of the liver. In other words, the AST (or other labs listed above) can be elevated, but the function of the liver may not be compromised. These tests give the clinician insight into the type of process occurring when these laboratory values are abnormal. Typically, these abnormalities can be categorized as either "obstructive" or "hepatocellular injury." With hepatocellular injury (without obstruction), one would expect to see increased AST and ALT levels, because these are dumped into the bloodstream from the injured cells. However, you would not expect to see a significant increase in the bilirubin or alkaline phosphatase levels. In an obstructive process, such as cholelithiasis or choledocholithiasis, the biliary tree is unable to drain normally. As biliary fluid accumulates behind the obstruction, one would expect to see increases in the bilirubin and alkaline phosphatase levels. When this blockage occurs, some mild hepatocellular injury can be revealed by an increase in the AST and ALT levels, but not to the same extent as with other processes. Processes which cause hepatocellular injury can have varying degrees of injury. For example, in alcohol-induced hepatitis, one typically sees an increase in the AST and ALT into the low hundreds range. Classically, AST to ALT is at a ratio of 2:1 to 3:1. However, in viral hepatitis (most commonly type A or B), one sees a significantly higher degree of cellular injury with higher transaminase values (in the thousands). There are only a handful of conditions that can cause a person's AST and ALT to reach the thousands. Other conditions include viral hepatitis, acetaminophen (or other drug) toxicity, ischemia (shock liver), and sometimes autoimmune disease.

B. Cholelithiasis would show more of an obstructive picture. One would expect to see the bilirubin and alkaline phosphatase higher, with only mild increases in AST and ALT.

C. See explanation for A.

D. Hemochromatosis is an infiltrative disease in which excess iron is deposited into the tissue of the liver. The liver function tests can be normal or show mild evidence of hepatocellular injury, but should not reveal this presentation or degree of injury.

E. Changes due to hepatocellular carcinoma should give a picture of hepatocellular injury. However, if the tumor is encroaching on or compressing an intrahepatic duct or the biliary tree, an obstructive picture may also be present. Hepatocellular carcinoma is most commonly seen in patients who are already cirrhotic, usually from chronic viral hepatitis.

76. E. As in the explanation to question 75, there are only a few conditions that can cause ALT and AST levels to reach into the thousands: viral hepatitis, acetaminophen toxicity, liver ischemia, and sometimes autoimmune disease. In this scenario, it would be advisable to check an acute hepatitis panel and an acetaminophen level (this was not a choice, however).

A. Abdominal ultrasound is the recommended radiologic study to evaluate for cholelithiasis, but it is not necessarily useful in the diagnosis of viral hepatitis.

B. It would be reasonable to check an ethanol level in a patient if you felt the liver injury pattern was consistent with alcoholic hepatitis. However, alcohol should not increase transaminases to these levels, and should give an AST:ALT ratio of 2:1 to 3:1.

C. Percutaneous liver biopsy would be indicated if there were concern for hepatocellular carcinoma or if the underlying diagnosis was not clear. However, in this case, the changes in the liver function tests would not be typically seen in a patient with hepatocellular carcinoma.

D. A serum ferritin level would be useful in helping assess a patient for hemochromatosis, but this disease would not result in the degree of transaminase elevation seen in this patient.

77. **C. This patient has a new lesion present in his lung and has risk factors for cancer (age and smoking). Therefore, a tissue specimen should be obtained to make certain this is not cancer. If the lesion had been present on a previous chest X-ray and had not changed for 2 years, then one could conceivably follow it clinically with follow-up chest X-rays. However, we do not have the luxury of previous chest X-rays on this patient. To wait and follow this lesion may allow a possibly malignant tumor to grow and metastasize. The location of the lesion is helpful in determining the best approach to obtaining a biopsy. Central lesions are usually accessible by bronchoscopy with biopsy. However, peripheral lesions, such as the one in our patient, are not as easily accessible with the bronchoscope, so a CT-guided needle biopsy is the method of choice.**

A, B. New or suspicious pulmonary lesions should be evaluated promptly to exclude the presence of a malignant lesion. Having him follow up in 3 or 6 months for a repeat chest X-ray is not an acceptable way of managing this patient.

D. See explanation for C.

E. The presence of an upper lobe lesion should raise your concern about the possibility of mycobacterial disease (e.g., tuberculosis). Although there is a small possibility this could be the cause of this patient's lesion, it is unlikely. Placing a PPD skin test is never a bad idea in this clinical setting, but it is not the most appropriate next step in working up this patient.

78. **B. This patient is at high risk for the development of DVT and subsequent PE, and should therefore be started on prophylactic therapy. There are several possible treatments that can prevent VTE. These include subcutaneous administration of unfractionated heparin at 5000 U every 8 to 12 hours or low-molecular-weight heparins on a reduced dosing schedule (e.g., enoxaparin 40 U subcutaneously once a day).**

A. See explanation for B.

C, E. If the patient has a risk of bleeding that would make you want to avoid such anticoagulation medications as low-dose heparin, you may use sequential compression devices on the lower extremities. However, the graduated compression stockings and sequential compression devices are not appropriate to use alone in patients who are at high risk of DVT. Only moderate- to low-risk patients, or patients at high risk of significant bleeding, should be given SCDs alone.

D. Full-dose anticoagulation with IV heparin or full-dose anticoagulation with low-molecular-weight heparin is indicated for the treatment of VTE, but not prevention of VTE, as in this patient.

79. **D. Patients who are admitted to the hospital have altered physiologic and metabolic processes due to their illnesses. Some of these patients have a higher risk of stress-related gastric ulcers and subsequent upper GI bleeding events. Hospital patients who should be placed on stress ulcer prophylaxis are those who are intubated, are coagulopathic (i.e., at risk for bleeding), or have prior histories of upper GI bleeding. The man described in example D has two of the three risk factors and is therefore at the highest risk.**

A, B, C, E. See explanation for B.

80. **C. The four most common causes of chronic cough include asthma, gastroesophageal reflux, postnasal drip, and allergies. Of these, her history is most suggestive of reflux-type symptoms, because the cough is worse with being supine and she has frequent heartburn.**

A, B, D. She does not have classic symptoms of cough secondary to asthma (wheezing, worse at night, identifiable triggers) or postnasal drip (worse in the morning, nasal congestion, etc.).

E. Although bronchogenic carcinoma can cause a persistent cough, it is usually seen in patients with a history of tobacco abuse, which she denies. It is also usually associated with other symptoms such as weight loss and hemoptysis, neither of which she reports.

81. **C. When assessing a patient with dysphagia, it is helpful to assess whether their symptoms are caused only by solids or if they also occur when drinking liquids. This helps to distinguish between a motility disorder and an underlying obstructive lesion. With a motility disorder, the patient should have symptoms with both solids and liquids. With an obstructive lesion in the esophagus (e.g., a tumor), you would expect solids to stick but liquids to pass without difficulty. Determining whether symptoms are intermittent or progressive also helps the diagnosis. Problems such as diffuse esophageal spasm and esophageal rings are usually intermittent, whereas achalasia and tumors are progressive. This patient reports progressive dysphagia with solids only, which is concerning for possible malignancy. The two main types of esophageal cancer are adenocarcinoma and squamous cell carcinoma. Patients at increased risk for adenocarcinoma are those with long-standing untreated gastroesophageal reflux and Barrett's esophagus. Adenocarcinoma usually affects the distal portion of the esophagus near the gastroesophageal junction. Squamous cell carcinoma typically affects the midportion of the esophagus, and is more prevalent in patients who abuse tobacco and alcohol. Therefore, given this patient's history, he is at risk of esophageal adenocarcinoma. The appropriate diagnostic test is an EGD with biopsy.**

A. Achalasia typically presents with progressive dysphagia with solids and liquids, which this patient does not report. An upper GI can be done to evaluate for achalasia, but this is not the most likely diagnosis.

B, D, E. See explanation for C.

82. **E. This patient likely has a breast cyst, given the physical exam findings of smoothness, fluctuance, and mild tenderness. The timing of the breast mass with her period is also suggestive of a breast cyst. Fibrocystic disease is the most common cause of a breast mass in premenopausal women.**

A. Breast adenocarcinoma on physical exam is often firm, irregular, nontender, and fixed.

B. Fibrous adenomas are common in this age group but tend to persist throughout several menstrual cycles.

C. Breast abscesses are seen in lactating women, and the bacterial etiology is usually *Staphylococcus aureus* or *Streptococcus*. This patient is not lactating and does not give any history of fevers or chills, so a breast abscess is less likely.

D. Fat necrosis occurs with trauma and presents as a firm, tender mass.

83. **B. Since this mass has not disappeared, it is likely that it is a fibroadenoma. The next step in evaluation of the mass is to perform an ultrasound. Doctors who are trained in the procedure of fine needle aspiration will sometimes put a needle in the part of the breast that is suspicious for a cyst to see if it is possible to aspirate fluid before ordering the ultrasound. If the fluid that is aspirated is clear and the lump goes away, then it is reasonable to follow the patient to see if the fluid reaccumulates. If the lump returns, then it must be evaluated further with ultrasound. If the aspirated fluid is bloody, it must be sent for cytology, and further evaluation with ultrasound should be done. If the mass on ultrasound appears solid, then the patient *must* have a tissue diagnosis made, either by excisional biopsy, fine needle, or core biopsy.**

A. BRCA 1 and BRCA 2 gene mutations are associated with malignant disease. There are many questions that must be asked when deciding to test for such genes, such as, "What is the sensitivity and specificity of the test?" and "Is there a proven intervention available?" Testing for BRCA 1 and 2 is not recommended for people at average risk for breast cancer because of the incidence of false positives in that population. It is appropriate for a patient with a strong family history of breast cancer to consider gene testing; however, it is not currently recommended to test for the gene in other patients except in research protocols. Given our patient's history, physical exam, and family history, she would not be a candidate for gene testing.

C. A mammogram is not as sensitive or specific in a woman younger than age 35 than it is in older women, because of the relatively higher density of premenopausal breast tissue. It is recommended that the evaluation of a palpable lump in a woman who is 35 or younger be initiated with an ultrasound as opposed to a mammogram. In a woman older than 35, it is reasonable to start the evaluation of a lump with a mammogram. However, if the mammogram is normal, further imaging needs to be done and, eventually, perhaps a biopsy.

D. See explanation for B.

E. It would be negligent to wait on this patient's breast mass, especially because it did not disappear after her period.

84. **B. Any woman who presents with secondary amenorrhea (meaning that she has had periods in the past that have now ceased) needs evaluation for possible pregnancy as the cause. Even though this patient states that she could not be pregnant because of her use of condoms with her boyfriend, you need to check a pregnancy test. If she is not pregnant, then she is probably having intermittent anovulatory cycles that account for her irregular periods. Anovulatory cycles are common in adolescents in the first 2 to 3 years after menarche secondary to an immature hypothalamic-pituitary-ovarian axis.**

A. Oral contraceptive pills have many uses; they are used for contraception, in patients with dysfunctional uterine bleeding to decrease the amount of endometrium shed, and in patients with polycystic ovarian syndrome. They can also be used to regulate the cycles of women with irregular cycles, such as this patient. An oral contraceptive pill may be used in her future, but is not the next step in her evaluation.

C. Basal body temperatures are often used in the fertility process to determine if a woman is ovulating, noted by a rise in temperature after ovulation secondary to increased progesterone. It is not something to recommend to our patient at this point.

D. A TSH could be measured if there were a concern that hypothyroidism was causing her irregular cycles. Hypothyroidism, if it effects the menstrual cycle, usually manifests as heavy flow, or menorrhagia.

E. Endometrial biopsy is indicated in all women over the age of 35 with abnormal uterine bleeding to rule out cancer or premalignant lesions. This does not apply to our patient.

85. **D. Acute angle-closure glaucoma usually presents with a deep aching pain, nausea, and vomiting. Other clues to the diagnosis include a mid-dilated fixed pupil that is unresponsive to light and clouding of the cornea. It is considered an emergency and needs to be evaluated right away by measuring the intraocular pressures and consulting an ophthalmologist.**

A. Viral conjunctivitis is usually preceded by an upper respiratory infection and is usually bilateral. Often, there is discharge. There is no effect on vision or pupillary response to light.

B. Keratitis results in inflammation of the corneal limbus and may result in ulceration of the cornea. It may be caused by bacteria, fungi, or viruses, and can present with irritation, photophobia, and tearing. When it is due to herpes simplex, which is the most common cause of keratitis in the United States, it is minimally painful, which can be very helpful diagnostically. If the center of the cornea is affected, there may be reduction in vision.

C. Allergic conjunctivitis is usually associated with itchy, watery eyes and other atopic symptoms such as clear rhinorrhea and sneezing. It is usually bilateral and nonpainful, and the pupils react normally. There is no vision loss.

E. Corneal abrasions usually present as excruciating eye pain with the sensation of a foreign body present in the eye. The patient will often give you a history that "something got in my eye" and the initial foreign body sensation progressed to severe pain. Photophobia is the result of painful contraction of the hyperemic iris. Often, the use of anesthetic drops can help in the examination of the eye. The pupil should be normally reactive.

86. **C. According to the guidelines of the American Society for Colposcopy and Cervical Pathology (ASCCP) that were based on the ALTS trial (Atypical Squamous Cells of Undetermined Significance/Low-Grade Squamous Intraepithelial Lesions Triage stufy), patients who present with ASCUS on Pap should undergo HPV serotyping**

to check whether they are at high or low risk for malignancy. If the serotype is low risk, then it is reasonable to put them back into the normal cervical cancer screening group, and repeat the Pap smear in 1 year. If the serotype is high risk, then the next step would be colposcopy with biopsy, and possible cryotherapy if needed.

A. You cannot continue to keep a patient in the normal screening population category once they have had an abnormal Pap smear. You cannot wait for a year to re-evaluate the abnormal Pap.

B, D, E. See explanation for C.

87. **D. Colon cancer is the second leading cause of cancer death in the United States. Once someone has a positive fecal occult blood test, the next step is to perform a colonoscopy to evaluate for cancer.**

A. Single contrast barium enemas are used in older patients or patients who are unable to tolerate the air injected in a double contrast enema. It is not as sensitive as colonoscopy to look for polyps or small cancers, and is not recommended.

B. Anoscopy can be done to look for bleeding of the hemorrhoids, but the evaluation should *not* stop there. A patient with guaiac-positive stool needs to have evaluation of the *entire* colon to look for cancerous or precancerous lesions.

C. Flexible sigmoidoscopy is not recommended, because the patient needs to have the entire colon examined.

E. A CT scan of the abdomen and pelvis can aid in looking for metastatic lesions, but does not give direct visualization of the mucosal surface of the colon, and small polyps or cancers can be missed.

88. **C. The combination OCP is a good choice for birth control for women who are able to take a pill consistently every day. Other advantages include decreased menstrual flow and dysmenorrheic symptoms, improvement of acne with certain formulations, and decreased risk of ovarian cancer over time. It is not a good choice for birth control for women who are not able to take pills consistently. It also does not protect against STDs, including those with no cure such as herpes, HPV, or HIV.**

89. **B. Injectable progesterone in a depo form (Depo-Provera) is a birth control option for women who do not want to have to take a pill every day. It is given every 3 months in an intramuscular injection. Side effects include irregular bleeding and eventual amenorrhea in most women, acne, and minimal weight gain. Like OCPs, it does not protect against STDs.**

90. **A. Progesterone-containing IUDs are birth control options for women who do not want to take a pill every day and do not want intramuscular injections. It is an object that must be inserted by a gynecologist, and there is a low possibility of mechanical complications such as uterine perforation. Patients who are in monogamous relationships are better candidates for the device, because there is an increased risk of PID in patients with IUDs who are having sex with multiple partners.**

91. **D. Condoms and diaphragms are forms of barrier contraception. They have a better chance of preventing pregnancy when they are used in combination with a spermicide-containing product. Condoms can help to prevent the spread of HIV and other STDs, but they are not perfect and do not protect well against HPV, which is the virus that causes cervical cancer.**

92. **B. This patient has bacterial vaginosis caused by *Gardnerella vaginalis*. Risk factors for vaginosis include early age of onset of intercourse, multiple sex partners, cigarette smoking, and douching. Other diagnostic criteria include a pH >4.5 and a positive whiff test (fishy odor upon application of KOH to vaginal discharge samples). The cells on the wet mount fit the description of "clue cells," which are epithelial cells coated with the *G. vaginalis* bacteria.**

A. This patient's urinalysis is normal, so urinary tract infection is unlikely.

C. Patients with trichomoniasis often present with dysuria, pruritis, and discharge, and may have punctate "strawberry spot" lesions on the cervix. Patients may also have intense pruritis and a frothy, watery, greenish-gray discharge.

D. Chlamydia, like trichomoniasis, is sexually transmitted and presents with vaginal discharge, burning, and itching. It can also be asymptomatic. It is diagnosed by antigen detection of cervical swab specimens, by genetic probe methods of cervical swab methods, or, most recently, by nucleic acid amplification techniques to detect the organism in urine specimens. The nucleic acid amplification techniques are extremely sensitive for Chlamydia detection, and are convenient because they don't require a pelvic exam and can be done on urine specimens, which are less invasive.

E. Vaginal candidiasis presents with dysuria, irritation, dyspareunia, and a thick, white clumpy discharge. The yeasts (spores and/or pseudohyphae) can be seen on a KOH wet mount.

93. **C. Metronidazole is the first-line treatment for patients with bacterial vaginosis. It is also used in the treatment of trichomoniasis.**

A, B. Trimethoprim-sulfamethoxazole and ciprofloxacin are used for treatment of the uncomplicated urinary tract infection.

D. Diflucan, in a one-time dose, is used for treatment of candidiasis. Other topical antifungal agents can be used as well.

E. Ceftriaxone is used to treat *Neisseria gonorrhoeae* infection.

94. **D. The definitive criteria for the diagnosis of diabetes includes a fasting glucose >126, a random glucose >200 with symptoms of polyuria and polydipsia, or a 2-hour postprandial glucose greater than 200. HgbA1C measurements are not considered diagnostic criteria for diabetes.**

E. Glucose on urine dip can be present from hyperglycemia or an inability of the kidneys to reabsorb glucose, as seen in Fanconi's syndrome.

A, B, C. See explanation for D.

95. **C. Urge incontinence is caused by an overactive urinary bladder detrusor muscle. The patient describes an intense, sudden urge to urinate that may be difficult to control. Patients may avoid social situations because of the fear of accidents. Often, the etiology of detrusor muscle spasm is idiopathic, but bacterial cystitis must be ruled out.**

D. Stress incontinence is seen in patients with weak pelvic floor muscles and presents with incontinence during coughing, sneezing, or

laughing. These actions cause increased intra-abdominal pressure, which allows the hypermobile urethra to move and allows urine to leak. Ten percent of patients may have intrinsic sphincter deficiency as a cause of their stress incontinence. Risk factors for stress incontinence include aging, estrogen deficiency, a prior traumatic vaginal delivery, or pelvic surgery. Stress incontinence is the most common cause of urinary incontinence in younger women, and the second most common cause of urinary incontinence in older women.

E. Overflow incontinence is secondary to weakened detrusor activity and/or bladder outlet obstruction. Postvoid residual is usually elevated in overflow incontinence (>100 mL) and the stream is often hesitant.

A, B. See explanations for C, D, and E.

96. **D. This patient has the classic presentation of community-acquired pneumonia (CAP) caused by *Streptococcus pneumoniae*, which includes abrupt onset of high fevers with rigors, productive cough with rust-colored sputum, pleuritic chest pain, and a lobar consolidation on chest X-ray. Although any of the organisms listed above may cause pneumonia, they typically have a different natural history and affect different hosts.**

A. *M. pneumoniae* is one of the organisms responsible for causing an "atypical" form of CAP. Patients with *M. pneumoniae* generally have a more indolent course with low-grade fevers, cough, and usually do not appear so abruptly ill. On chest X-ray, they can have focal consolidative changes, but chest X-rays can range from normal to those with patchy bilateral infiltrates.

B. *P. carinii* is most often seen in patients who are immunocompromised. *P. carinii* typically presents with a more indolent onset of several days to weeks time. The fevers are usually low-grade, and the sputum is usually not purulent. Chest X-ray is often normal, but can show patchy bilateral interstitial infiltrates.

C. *B. fragilis* is responsible for a significant number of anaerobic pulmonary infections. These infections are most often seen in patients who have aspirated, such as those with seizures or alcoholism. Aspiration pneumonia can involve any portion of the lung, but notoriously affects the right lower and middle lobes.

E. Pulmonary *B. anthracis* typically presents with a prodromal viral-like illness with myalgias, fatigue, and upper-respiratory infection-like symptoms that are then followed by rapid respiratory collapse. Chest X-ray classically shows widening of the mediastinum because of the associated lymphadenopathy.

97. **B.** There is much debate about the appropriate empiric antibiotic therapy for *Streptococcus pneumoniae*; however, of the choices listed, a third-generation cephalosporin would be best initially. Most practitioners would also start this patient on empiric macrolide therapy to treat for any possible "atypical" organism such as *Mycoplasma* or *Chlamydia*. However, this patient does not present with signs of infection by "atypical" organisms.

A. Clindamycin would be a good choice if you were treating an aspiration or anaerobic pneumonia, but that is not the case here.

C. Sulfamethoxazole-trimethoprim is the drug of choice for the treatment of pneumonia caused by *P. carinii*; however, it is not appropriate for first-line therapy against pneumococcal disease in a sick patient.

D. Penicillin should not be used as first-line therapy against pneumococcal pneumonia because of the high resistance patterns that are present within some communities.

E. Amantadine can decrease the time course of some viral forms of pneumonia such as that caused by influenza A if it is initiated early in the course. However, it has no efficacy against pneumococcal disease.

98. **A.** Pleural effusions are divided into two major categories: exudative and transudative. *Transudative* effusions are the result of a pressure difference between the vasculature space and the surrounding tissue and pleural spaces. This pressure difference is from either a low oncotic pressure in the vasculature (such as a hypoalbuminemic state, which allows fluid to shift out of the vascular space and into the extravascular space), or high hydrostatic pressure (such as in congestive heart failure, which pushes the fluid out of the vascular space and into the extravascular space). In a transudative effusion, the vascular membrane remains intact, figuratively speaking. *Exudates* are the result of inflammation, usually from infection or malignancy, which weakens the vascular membrane and allows fluid and associated proteins to leak into the pleural space. Understanding this, one would expect to see *lower* levels of protein and LDH in the fluid if it were caused by pressure changes (i.e., transudative) and *higher* levels if it were caused by inflammatory changes (i.e., exudative). Light's criteria, which are based on these principles, are used to determine whether a pleural effusion is exudative or not. To be classified as an exudative effusion, *only one of the following three criteria must be met*:

- $TP_{effusion}/TP_{serum} > 0.5$
- $LDH_{effusion}/LDH_{serum} > 0.6$
- $LDH_{effusion} > 2/3$ the upper limit of normal LDH_{serum}

In this clinical case, one would expect that the patient has an inflammatory effusion as the result of his pneumonia (i.e., exudative). Of the choices listed, A is the only answer in which the above criteria are met.

B, C, D, E. See explanation for A.

99. **C.** This patient has the classic triad of Reiter's syndrome: conjunctivitis (or uveitis), urethritis, and arthritis. Reiter's syndrome is a type of reactive arthritis, which is a type of seronegative (rheumatoid factor-negative) spondylarthropathy. Other seronegative spondylarthropathies include ankylosing spondylitis, psoriatic arthritis, and inflammatory bowel disease–associated arthritis. To be diagnosed with Reiter's, the patient must have all three portions of the triad. Patients with Reiter's syndrome are usually young men who present with an abrupt onset of monoarticular or asymmetric oligoarticular arthritis with a history of a preceding urethritis (often from *Chlamydia* infection) or diarrheal illness (often from *Shigella*, *Salmonella*, *Campylobacter*, or *Yersinia*). They have ocular disease ranging from a mild conjunctivitis to a severe uveitis. The arthritis usually involves the knee, ankle, or foot, but also may involve the wrist and fingers. This patient had a finding on his examination of

dactylitis, or "sausage digit," which is seen in Figure 1-99. Dactylitis is seen most often in psoriatic arthritis and Reiter's syndrome. Our patient had no evidence of psoriasis. There are other clinical features that can help distinguish between the other types of arthritis given as possible answers.

A. Psoriatic arthritis is the other arthritis in the differential when a patient presents with a "sausage digit." It is important to look for evidence of subclinical skin disease, especially in places such as the scalp, umbilicus, and gluteal cleft. Most patients with psoriatic arthritis have obvious skin disease. Our patient did not have psoriasis, but did have many of the findings of Reiter's syndrome.

B. Rheumatoid arthritis presents with symmetrical polyarthritis and is more common in women in this age group. Rheumatoid arthritis does not cause dactylitis as seen in our patient.

D. Gonococcal arthritis is more common in women than in men. It is abrupt in onset, and patients may have urethritis, although usually associated with a discharge in men. Gonococci are found on culture of the penile discharge. There is usually not a dactylitis, although tenosynovitis may be present. Patients also do not usually have conjunctivitis with gonococcal arthritis.

E. Osteoarthritis is a noninflammatory arthritis and is due to wear and tear of the cartilage of joints. It is mostly seen in the elderly and affects the distal phalangeal joints (with classic Heberden's and Bouchard's nodes) as well as the weight-bearing joints of the knees and hips. It is a gradual process and is not likely to be the cause of this patient's symptoms.

100. D. To date, only two clear predisposing factors have been identified for the development of a reactive arthritis or other seronegative (rheumatoid factor-negative) spondylarthropathy: a preceding infection (enteric or GU) with a pathogen such as *Chlamydia, Shigella, Salmonella, Campylobacter,* or *Yersinia,* and the presence of HLA-B27. The presence of the HLA-B27 major histocompatibility complex (MHC) is the *most* important factor in determining the predisposition for developing a seronegative spondylarthropathy.

A. A culture of fluid aspirated from the joint may be positive in a patient who has septic arthritis, but it will be negative in patients who have reactive arthritis or Reiter's. The arthritis that develops in these latter conditions is the result of an autoimmune process, not an infectious one.

B. Rheumatoid factor can be positive in a host of autoimmune processes that can cause arthritis; however, one would not expect it to be positive in this case.

C. It is unusual for gonorrhea to cause urethritis without urethral discharge. In addition, reactive arthritis from gonococcal infection does not present with "sausage digits" as described in Table 1-99. Although he is at risk for contracting gonorrhea and should be tested, one would not expect this to be the cause of his symptoms.

E. Periosteal thickening and elevation along with bone erosion and soft tissue swelling are radiographic findings of osteomyelitis. Acute dactylitis usually presents radiographically with soft-tissue swelling alone.

BLOCK 3

101. A 24-year-old man presents with a history of increasing left knee pain and swelling for the past 3 days. He has had subjective fevers and is now unable to bear weight on his left knee. He denies any recent trauma and has never had an episode like this before. His past medical history is significant for hepatitis C, which he contracted by using IV drugs. On examination, he has a temperature of 101.6°F (38.7°C), a heart rate of 92, respiratory rate of 16, and blood pressure of 126/82. He is nontoxic in appearance, but is in a significant amount of pain. His examination is unremarkable with the exception of his left knee. There is marked swelling noted as depicted in Figure 1-101. He has no specific joint line tenderness or crepitus, but does have pain with passive flexion in the middle range of motion of his knee. You perform a diagnostic arthrocentesis at the bedside and obtain approximately 20 mL of yellow fluid that you send to the laboratory for immediate analysis. The following results are obtained: Color yellow and opaque; viscosity low; WBCs 108,800; PMNs 78%. Culture is pending and crystal analysis is negative. Which of the following statements is most accurate?

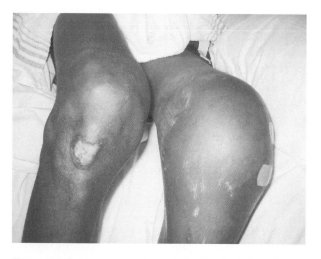

Figure 1-101 • Image Courtesy of Dr. Brenda Shinar, Banner Good Samaritan Medical Center, Phoenix, Arizona.

A. The patient likely has a septic arthritis and should be started on empiric IV antibiotic therapy while awaiting culture results
B. The patient likely has a septic arthritis and culture results should be obtained before starting IV antibiotics
C. The patient likely has an effusion secondary to trauma and should be observed until culture results are available
D. The patient likely has an inflammatory arthritis secondary to hepatitis C and should be started on intra-articular corticosteroid injections
E. The patient likely has a meniscal tear with an effusion. He should be given nonsteroidal anti-inflammatory drugs (NSAIDs) and an orthopedic referral

102. A 17-year-old woman presents with shortness of breath and a nonproductive cough that started approximately 12 hours before her arrival in the ED. In addition to shortness of breath, she complains of wheezing and chest tightness. She denies fever or chest pain. She was diagnosed with asthma when she was 10 years old and has had numerous exacerbations since that time. She has previously been admitted to the ICU for observation, but has never been intubated. Her home medication regimen includes inhaled albuterol, inhaled fluticasone, and oral montelukast. She also takes loratidine for seasonal allergy symptoms. On examination, you find her sitting in a tripod position on the bed speaking in short sentences. She is anxious with a respiratory rate of 26. Room-air oxygen saturation is 91%. She is afebrile with a heart rate of 88 and blood pressure of 116/74. Pulmonary examination reveals diffuse expiratory wheezes in all of her lung fields with diminished air exchange. The remainder of her examination is unremarkable. You obtain baseline labs, a chest X-ray and a room air arterial blood gas (ABG). Chest X-ray reveals mild flattening of the diaphragms bilaterally, but no focal infiltrates or abnormalities. She is started on continuous inhaled β-agonist therapy, oxygen supplementation, and IV corticosteroids. The results of the ABG drawn on room air show: pH 7.40; $paCO_2$ 42; paO_2 88; HCO_3^- = 22; oxygen saturation 92%. Which of the following statements is most accurate?

A. Her ABG is reassuring and she should be continued on her current medications and monitored
B. Her ABG shows an oxygenation problem and the focus of her care should be on improving her paO_2
C. Her ABG reveals a respiratory acidosis, which is expected in an acute exacerbation of asthma
D. Her ABG is worrisome and endotracheal intubation should be considered
E. Her ABG is normal and she can be discharged after she is given IV corticosteroids

The response options for items 103 through 108 are the same. You will be required to select one answer for each item in the set.

A. Transudative effusion in a patient with congestive heart failure (CHF)
B. Chylous effusion in a patient with lymphoma
C. Rheumatoid effusion in a patient with severe rheumatoid arthritis (RA)
D. Tuberculous effusion in a patient with primary tuberculosis (TB) and HIV
E. Empyema in a patient with *Streptococcal pneumoniae* pneumonia
F. Malignant effusion in a patient with metastatic squamous cell carcinoma
G. Pleural effusion secondary to pulmonary infarction resulting from a pulmonary embolism

For each of the pleural fluid findings, select the appropriate disease state (in each case the patient has a serum total protein of 7.0 g/dL and an LDH of 150 U/L).

103. Appearance thick, grayish-white; pH 6.9; LDH 2000 U/L; glucose 25 mg/dL; Gram stain reveals numerous neutrophils with Gram-positive cocci in pairs

104. Appearance clear, yellow; pH 7.40; LDH 50 U/L; glucose 70 mg/dL; total protein 2.0 g/dL; Gram stain reveals no organisms

105. Appearance milky green; pH 7.0; LDH 1500 U/L; glucose 5 mg/dL; WBCs 500; 85% lymphocytes; triglycerides 30 mg/dL

106. Appearance straw-colored; pH 7.30; LDH 600 U/L; protein 5.5 g/dL; glucose 70 mg/dL; WBCs 4000; 60% lymphocytes

107. Appearance milky; pH 7.60; LDH 450; total protein 5.0 g/dL; WBCs 1000; 60% lymphocytes; triglycerides 120 mg/dL

108. Appearance bloody; pH 7.40; LDH 1000; total protein 4.5 g/dL; glucose 70 mg/dL; RBCs 10,000; WBCs 2,000; eosinophils 15%

End of Set

109. Light's criteria has been modified by Heffner et al to allow clinicians to determine whether a patient has an exudative or a transudative pleural effusion without the need to get serum values simultaneously. Which of the following are the correct values used in the modified criteria?

A. Pleural fluid LDH >66% of serum upper limit of normal; pleural fluid cholesterol >45 mg/dL; or pleural fluid protein >2.9 g/dL
B. Pleural fluid LDH >45% of serum upper limit of normal; pleural fluid cholesterol >45 mg/dL; or pleural fluid protein >2.9 g/dL
C. Pleural fluid albumin >45% of serum upper limit of normal; pleural fluid cholesterol >100 mg/dL; or pleural fluid ANA >1:80 titer
D. Pleural fluid LDH >66% of serum upper limit of normal; pleural fluid triglyceride >110 mg/dL; or pleural fluid protein >5.0 g/dL
E. Pleural fluid LDH >45% of serum upper limit of normal; pleural fluid cholesterol >45 mg/dL; or pleural fluid albumin >4.0 g/dL

110. A 55-year-old man comes to your clinic with complaints of hemoptysis. He states that for the past month he has occasionally coughed up some sputum that is streaked with blood. This has never happened to him before. His past medical history is significant for 50 pack-years of tobacco abuse, high blood pressure, and diabetes type II. He denies fever, chest pain, and weight loss. Physical exam is normal. You order a chest X-ray and some baseline labs. His CBC reveals a normal WBC with a hemoglobin of 16 g/dL and a hematocrit of 48%. His chest X-ray reveals some hyperinflation and flattening of the diaphragm without any sign of infiltrate or mass. What is the most appropriate next step in the evaluation of his hemoptysis?

A. Order a sputum for cytology
B. Give the patient reassurance and advise him to stop smoking
C. Treat the patient empirically for acute bronchitis and have him follow up in 1 month
D. Order a CT scan of the chest
E. Send the patient to a pulmonologist for a bronchoscopy

111. A 30-year-old woman comes to your office complaining of chronic coughing for the past month. She has never had problems with her lungs or smoked, but approximately 1 month ago she was working as a house cleaner and became acutely ill while cleaning a bathroom with a mixture of ammonia and bleach. The fumes made her very short of breath and wheezy and she was hospitalized for treatment and observation of her pulmonary status. Since that incident, she complains of recurrent cough and shortness of breath when she exercises and when she is exposed to cold air. On physical exam, her vital signs are normal. Her lung exam is clear with good air movement and she does not wheeze on forced expiration. You send her for a chest X-ray and pulmonary function tests, which are normal. The patient insists that she has significant damage to her lungs, and that she has been harmed by this event. What is the next step in evaluation of her complaints?

A. Refer her to psychiatry for evaluation of post-traumatic stress disorder and anxiety
B. Reassure her that her pulmonary function tests and chest X-ray are normal and she does not need further testing
C. Obtain a room air arterial blood gas to look for an A-a gradient
D. Obtain pulmonary function tests with methacholine challenge to diagnose reversible reactive airway disease
E. Do pulse oximetry at rest and with exercise to determine whether she desaturates

The response options for items 112 through 116 are the same. You will be required to select one answer for each item in the set.

A. Right lower lobe consolidation due to streptococcal pneumonia
B. Right-sided pneumothorax
C. Left-sided pneumothorax
D. Right-sided pleural effusion
E. Left-sided pleural effusion
F. Severe obstructive lung disease due to emphysema
G. Impending respiratory failure
H. Acute asthma exacerbation

For each of the following physical exam findings, select the appropriate diagnosis.

112. Right lower lobe bronchial breath sounds, egophony, and increased tactile fremitus

113. Right lower lobe decreased breath sounds, decreased tactile fremitus, and dullness to percussion

114. Bilateral decreased breath sounds, increased anteroposterior (AP) diameter of the chest, and prolonged expiration to inspiration ratio

115. Right lower lobe decreased breath sounds, hyperresonance to percussion, and trachea deviated to the left

116. Abdominal wall retraction during inspiration

End of Set

The response options for items 117 through 120 are the same. You will be required to select one answer for each item in the set.

A. Spherocytes
B. Target cells
C. Tear drop cells
D. Schistocytes
E. Howell-Jolly bodies
F. Heinz bodies
G. Rouleaux formation

For each clinical scenario, select the appropriate finding on blood smear.

117. A 60-year-old man on quinine for leg cramps is brought to the ER for fever, headache, and visual changes, and is found to be thrombocytopenic and anemic on his CBC.

118. A 60-year-old woman with a history of chronic lymphocytic leukemia has a hemoglobin of 8.0 g/dL and an LDH of 1000.

119. A 35-year-old woman with a history of sickle cell disease comes to the ER with a pain crisis.

120. A 45-year-old man with cirrhosis due to hepatitis C and a hemoglobin of 10 g/dL.

End of Set

The next two questions (items 121 and 122) correspond to the following vignette.

A 38-year-old white man presents to your office with complaints of nasal congestion for 6 months. He states it started with a cold and the symptoms have not gotten better. He notes congestion with intermittent rhinorrhea. He denies any fevers, headache, or itchy and watery eyes. Past medical history is significant for hypertension, for which he takes a thiazide diuretic and over-the-counter nasal medication that he takes three to four times a day as needed for his congestion. On exam he is afebrile and his vital signs are normal. In general, he is alert and in no acute distress. HEENT is significant for edematous nasal mucosa with clear rhinorrhea. The tympanic membranes are within normal limits and the oropharynx is without erythema or exudates. Chest is clear and heart exam is regular without murmur rub or gallop. Skin exam is normal.

121. What is the likely etiology of this man's congestion?

    A. Allergic rhinitis
    B. Foreign body
    C. Nasal polyp
    D. Vasomotor rhinitis
    E. Rhinitis medicamentosa

122. What is the treatment for this patient's disorder?

    A. Inhaled nasal corticosteroids
    B. ENT evaluation
    C. Change hypertension medication to propanolol
    D. Discontinue inhaled nasal decongestant
    E. Nasal smear to check for eosinophils

End of Set

123. A 35-year-old white man comes to your office with complaints of headache, congestion, and fever accompanied by purulent nasal drainage for 2 weeks. He states a history of recurrent sinus infections since he was young. He has a past medical history of allergic rhinitis, for which he takes an inhaled nasal corticosteroid. On review of systems he notes generalized fatigue. He denies any weight loss or gain. He tells you that he has frequent episodes of diarrhea that is watery and associated with bloating and flatulence. On exam, the patient's vital signs are within normal limits. In general he is alert and in no acute distress. His body mass index (BMI) is 17, and he is pale appearing. HEENT is significant for pink edematous nasal mucosa with purulent discharge. He has maxillary tenderness, right greater than left. His conjunctivae are pale. The rest of his exam is essentially normal except that is labs reveal iron-deficiency anemia. What immunodeficiency does this patient likely have?

    A. C5–C9 membrane attack complex (MAC) deficiency
    B. X-linked congenital agammaglobulinemia
    C. IgG deficiency
    D. IgA deficiency
    E. IgM deficiency

124. A 20-year-old Hispanic man presents to your office with swelling and induration on his left shoulder. He states that he received a tetanus booster yesterday. This hypersensitivity reaction is best described as:

    A. Immediate hypersensitivity
    B. Arthus type III reaction
    C. Delayed type IV reaction
    D. Late phase IgE-mediated reaction
    E. Anaphylaxis

The next two questions (items 125 and 126) correspond to the following vignette.

A 23-year-old black woman with a history of asthma presents with a 3-day history of increased shortness of breath and audible wheezing. She states she has been using her β-agonist inhaler every 2 hours without improvement. She notes that before this flare her allergies had been worsening. She states she has never been hospitalized for her asthma but has made many ER visits (about three times per year). She has had many steroid bursts. In an average week she uses her β-agonist inhaler three to four times. She regularly has nighttime cough. Triggers include pets, colds, and allergies. She has never used any other medication.

125. This patient's asthma could be best described as:

    A. Mild intermittent
    B. Mild persistent
    C. Moderate persistent
    D. Severe
    E. Exercise-induced

126. What is the best daily medical management for patients with this type of asthma?

    A. Inhaled β-agonist only as needed
    B. Inhaled β-agonist as needed and daily inhaled corticosteroid
    C. No therapy needed
    D. Long-acting β-agonist
    E. Leukotriene receptor antagonist

End of Set

127. A 24-year-old woman with a history of asthma since childhood presents to the ER with shortness of breath, which has been worsening over the past 3 days. On exam she is afebrile and tachypneic at 30 respirations per minute. Oxygen saturations are 99% on room air. She can converse with you in short phrases but appears to be in some respiratory distress. Her lung exam is significant for poor air movement and bilateral inspiratory and expiratory wheezes. There is also accessory muscle use noted. She is becoming drowsy and is able to interact less as your exam progresses. Your next step is to:

    A. Draw an ABG, then intubate
    B. Admit to the floor for observation
    C. Inhaled corticosteroid therapy
    D. One dose IV corticosteroid, then home on a steroid burst
    E. Continuous inhaled β-agonist therapy and admit to ICU

The next two questions (items 128 and 129) correspond to the following vignette.

A 45-year-old white man presents to your office with episodes of dry cough, malaise, and chills. He states this has been happening for the last few months. He recently moved with his family from the city to a farm to fulfill his lifelong dream of becoming a farmer. He denies any recent foreign travel or any known occupational or tuberculosis exposures. He denies hemoptysis, chest pain, or shortness of breath.

He has noted some weight loss with a decrease in appetite. He recently visited his sister back in the city and noted that was the last time he felt well.

128. What is the likely antigen responsible for his symptoms?

    A. Actinomycetes
    B. Animal proteins
    C. Fungi
    D. Work-related chemicals
    E. Arthropods

129. What is the optimal treatment for patients with hypersensitivity pneumonitis?

    A. Inhaled β-agonist therapy before known exposure
    B. High-dose IV steroids
    C. Antibiotic therapy
    D. Avoidance of antigen
    E. Short oral steroid bursts

End of Set

130. An 18-year-old black woman presents to your office with recurrent episodes of leg and tongue swelling. She states these have been occurring for the last few years. She states that she will suddenly swell up without provocation. She denies any itching. She states her sister suffers from the same symptoms. Her immunodeficiency is best described as:

    A. C5–C9 MAC deficiency
    B. C3 deficiency
    C. C2 deficiency
    D. C1-esterase inhibitor deficiency
    E. IgA deficiency

131. A 36-year-old white woman in respiratory distress is brought to your ED by her friend, who states that they were at a picnic when the patient developed hives and difficulty breathing. They raced her to your ED. Your patient cannot communicate secondary to respiratory distress. Her friend thinks she has an allergy to bees. On physical exam she is afebrile, tachycardic at 130, blood pressure is 80/50, and saturations are 92% on room air. In general she is in moderate respiratory distress and she is diffusely erythematous with angioedema of her face and hands. Lungs are tight with wheezes throughout. Your next course in treatment is:

A. IV epinephrine
B. IV steroids
C. Antihistamines
D. Subcutaneous epinephrine
E. Inhaled β-agonists

132. A 25-year-old white woman presents to your office for a new-patient visit. She denies any current complaints. On review of her past medical history she says that she had been hospitalized frequently as a child secondary to recurrent infections, in particular pneumonia. She was recently diagnosed with lupus. What laboratory test would be helpful in diagnosing her immunodeficiency?

A. Serum immunoglobulins
B. Nitroblue tetrazolium (NBT) dye reduction test
C. Total hemolytic complement activity
D. Anti-nuclear antibodies
E. X chromosome inactivation analysis

The next two questions (items 133 and 134) correspond to the following vignette.

A 71-year-old woman presents with a complaint of bilateral hand pain that has been getting progressively worse over the past 6 months. She has also noticed increasing pain in her knees, with the right being worse than the left. She states she has approximately 10 minutes of morning stiffness each day and the pain seems worse after excessive activity. She denies any history of trauma or fevers. The joints in her hands and knees have not been red or swollen. The pain is most severe in her distal (DIP) and proximal (PIP) interphalangeal joints and her right knee. She has had no numbness or parasthesias. On examination, she is an obese woman in no acute distress. Her vital signs are normal and she is afebrile. Her heart and lung examinations are normal. Her abdomen is benign and her neurologic examination is nonfocal. Her hands reveal a full range of motion without evidence of effusions or erythema. There are nodules involving the DIP joints bilaterally. Her knee examination reveals full range of motion with a bony enlargements over the medial aspect of both knees. In addition, there is significant crepitus noted with motion. She has no joint-line tenderness or effusions. You obtain X-rays of her hands and knees, which show osteophyte formations in both knees and in her DIP joints.

133. What is the most likely diagnosis?

A. RA
B. Systemic lupus erythematosus (SLE)
C. Osteoarthritis (OA)
D. Calcium pyrophosphate dihydrate (CPPD) deposition disease
E. Reactive arthritis

134. Which of the following is the best initial treatment for this patient?

A. Methotrexate
B. Prednisone
C. Allopurinol
D. Ibuprofen
E. Colchicine

End of Set

The next three questions (items 135 through 137) correspond to the following vignette.

A 48-year-old man presents to your clinic with complaints of severe right toe pain that began 36 hours ago. The pain is accompanied by redness and swelling in the toe. He does not recall any trauma to his toe and there have been no prior occurrences. The patient reports subjective fevers, but has not objectively documented them. He states that the pain is so severe he cannot bear weight on his foot. He has no other medical problems. The only medication he takes is one aspirin a day. He does report ongoing IV drug use and drinks alcohol daily. On examination, he is afebrile with normal vital signs. His examination is essentially unremarkable with the exception of his right toe. There is marked swelling and redness over the first metatarsophalangeal joint, and exquisite tenderness with minimal movement of the joint. His other joints appear normal on examination. You obtain labs and an X-ray of his right foot. The lab results show a normal WBC count and a uric acid level of 9.4 mg/dL. The X-rays of his right foot reveal soft-tissue swelling, but no bony changes. You then aspirate a small amount of fluid from the joint and send the specimen to the laboratory. The lab reports needle-like structures in the fluid that have strong negative birefringence.

135. What is the most likely cause of this patient's pain?

A. Septic arthritis
B. Gout
C. CPPD
D. Traumatic fracture
E. SLE

136. Which of the following statements regarding the patient's uric acid level is true?

    A. It is normal, so gout can reliably be excluded
    B. It is normal, but gout cannot be excluded
    C. It is normal, making the diagnosis of CPPD more likely
    D. It is elevated, confirming the diagnosis of gout
    E. It is elevated, but cannot be used to make the diagnosis of gout

137. Which of the following would be the best choice for the initial treatment of this patient?

    A. Allopurinol
    B. Nafcillin
    C. Prednisone
    D. Indomethacin
    E. Immobilization with splints

End of Set

The next three questions (items 138 through 140) correspond to the following vignette.

A 40-year-old man presents with complaints of worsening low back pain over the past several weeks. The pain is mostly in his low back and gluteal areas. He states the pain is usually worse when he wakes up or after he has been resting for a while. As he becomes more active, the pain seems to diminish. He denies any trauma or heavy lifting. He has had no fevers, rashes, or pain in other joints. He says his diet is unchanged and he has had no weight loss. Bowel habits are normal. He has no significant medical history and takes no regular medications. He is not sexually active but does use IV drugs occasionally. There has been no recent travel. On examination, his vital signs are normal and he is in no acute distress. His cardiovascular and lung exams are normal. His abdomen examination is benign and his skin reveals no abnormal findings. Upon standing, he has noticeable stiffness and discomfort in his lower back area. He has no focal tenderness over his spinous processes. He has slightly limited range of motion in his lumbar spine. There is tenderness over his sacroiliac region. His straight-leg raise test is negative. His muscle strength, deep-tendon reflex, and sensory testing are all normal. You obtain blood work and X-rays of his lumbosacral spine. The X-rays show squaring and increased density anteriorly of the vertebral bodies. The sacroiliac joint margins are blurred with evidence of erosions.

138. What is the most likely diagnosis?

    A. Vertebral osteomyelitis
    B. Ankylosing spondylitis (AS)
    C. Reactive arthritis
    D. RA
    E. Inflammatory bowel disease (IBD)

139. Testing for which of the following will most likely yield a positive result in this patient?

    A. HLA-B27
    B. Blood culture
    C. Rheumatoid factor
    D. Anti-nuclear antibody
    E. Stool guaiac

140. In addition to spinal cord injuries, patients with this disease are at increased risk for the development of which complication?

    A. Nephritis
    B. Serositis
    C. Cerebritis
    D. Cutaneous lesions
    E. Uveitis

End of Set

The next two questions (items 141 and 142) correspond to the following vignette.

A 74-year-old woman presents to the ED complaining of a headache and fatigue that started approximately 24 hours ago. She has no prior history of migraines and states the pain is worse over the right side of her head. She denies focal weakness or slurred speech, but does report that her jaw becomes painful when eating. She also has noticed visual changes that she describes as "a black curtain starting to cover my vision." She also reports progressive pain in her shoulders and hips with morning stiffness, but denies chest pain or claudication of the arm. On examination, you find a pleasant, elderly woman in no acute distress. She has marked visual field defects in her right eye, but her left eye is normal. Funduscopic examination of the left eye is normal and the right eye reveals a swollen, pale disc with blurred margins. The remainder of her neurologic examination is normal with the exception of pain in her shoulders and hips bilaterally. Her cardiovascular examination is normal and she has strong peripheral pulses bilaterally. The lungs are clear to auscultation and the abdomen is benign. Laboratory studies reveal normal CBC, renal function, and electrolytes.

141. Which of the following is the most likely cause of her symptoms?

    A. Takayasu's arteritis
    B. Cerebrovascular accident (CVA)
    C. Temporal arteritis
    D. SLE
    E. Acute aortitis

142. Which of the following is the most appropriate next step in the management of this patient?

    A. Obtain arteriography and initiate steroid therapy
    B. Obtain anti-nuclear antibodies and initiate prednisone therapy
    C. Obtain a CT scan of the brain and initiate antiplatelet therapy
    D. Obtain a biopsy of the temporal artery and initiate prednisone
    E. Obtain rapid plasma reagin (RPR) results and initiate intramuscular penicillin therapy

End of Set

The next three questions (items 143 through 145) correspond to the following vignette.

A 45-year-old woman with RA presents to your clinic for a routine follow-up. She was diagnosed approximately 9 years ago and has had a rapidly progressive disease course. She has morning stiffness for approximately 1 hour every morning and she has suboptimal pain control. Most of her pain involves the bilateral proximal interphalangeal (PIP) and metacarpophalangeal (MCP) joints. She is known to have high titers of rheumatoid factor (RF). Her treatment regimen consists of oral prednisone 20 mg daily and methotrexate 7.5 mg weekly. Entanercept was recently initiated at a dose of 25 mg subcutaneously twice weekly. On examination, she is afebrile and has normal vital signs. Head and neck exams are normal. Heart and lung examinations are unremarkable. Her spleen is enlarged, nontender, and easily palpated when examining her abdomen. Her skin exam reveals rheumatoid nodules on the extensor surface of her forearms. Joint exam reveals moderate synovitis in the PIP and MCP joints diffusely. You are concerned that she has developed Felty's syndrome, so you order appropriate laboratory studies.

143. Which of the following abnormalities would support the diagnosis of Felty's syndrome?

    A. Uremia
    B. Prolonged partial thromboplastin time (aPTT)
    C. Elevated aspartate aminotransferase (AST)
    D. Neutropenia
    E. Direct hyperbilirubinemia

144. Which of the following is a common extra-articular manifestation of RA?

    A. Peptic ulcer disease
    B. Pericardial effusion
    C. Autoimmune hemolytic anemia
    D. Nephrotic syndrome
    E. Spontaneous pneumothorax

145. Methotrexate has many side effects. Patients are given folate to help to prevent some of these side effects. Which of the following side effects of methotrexate may be ameliorated by the addition of folate to the patient's medication regimen?

    A. Rash
    B. Stomatitis
    C. Pneumonitis
    D. Liver transaminitis
    E. Teratogenicity

End of Set

146. A 32-year-old Hispanic woman presents with 5 weeks of fatigue, generalized weakness, and pallor. She denies fever, chills, or weight loss, but has had two urinary tract infections in the last month. She works in a factory that makes tires, but is unsure what chemicals are used at her workplace. Physical examination reveals pale conjunctiva and mucous membranes, heart rate of 95, but otherwise normal cardiovascular and pulmonary examinations. There is no palpable lymphadenopathy. Abdominal examination is benign with no evidence of hepatosplenomegaly. A CBC is obtained with the following results: WBC 2000/μL; differential: 60% neutrophils, 30% lymphocytes, 6% monocytes, remainder eosinophils and basophils. Hemoglobin level is 9.2 g/dL; hematocrit 29%; mean corpuscular volume (MCV) 85 fL; platelet count 45,000/μL,

reticulocytes 0.5%. A bone marrow aspirate is obtained showing all cell lines to be hypocellular with an increase in fat cells. The diagnosis most consistent with this patient's presentation is:

A. Myelodysplastic syndrome
B. Aplastic anemia
C. Paroxysmal nocturnal hemoglobinuria
D. Chronic myelogenous leukemia
E. Folate deficiency

147. A 60-year-old woman presents with a new deep venous thrombosis (DVT). She denies any trauma, recent travel, or family history of hyper-coagulable states. She is not a smoker and has no other significant medical history. Additional history is notable only for pruritus in the morning, noted after her showers. Vital signs include pulse 82, respiratory rate 18, oxygen saturation 98% on room air, and blood pressure 121/83. Physical examination is remarkable for facial plethora, spleen tip palpable 4 cm below the left costal margin, and normal cardiovascular and pulmonary examinations. Labs show the following results: Hemoglobin is 18 g/dL; hematocrit 52%. Which of the following statements is true concerning polycythemia vera?

A. A serum erythropoetin level of greater than 30 U/L is diagnostic of polycythemia vera
B. RBC mass studies are not useful in confirming the diagnosis of polycythemia vera
C. Phlebotomy is the treatment of choice and should be done until the patient develops an iron-deficiency anemia
D. Splenomegaly is not a common physical exam finding in polycythemia vera and should alert the physician to investigate for an underlying leukemia
E. WBC and platelet counts are typically normal in polycythemia vera

148. A 24-year-old man with Crohn's disease presents with 1 month of progressive fatigue and weakness. He currently takes sulfasalazine and recently completed a course of oral steroids. Vital signs include a pulse of 90, respiratory rate of 16, blood pressure of 110/75, and oxygen saturation of 98% on room air. Physical examination reveals pale mucous membranes, tachycardia with an otherwise normal cardiovascular examination, diffuse

tenderness to palpation on abdominal examination without palpable hepatosplenomegaly. A CBC with peripheral smear is obtained. The peripheral smear is shown in Figure 1-148. This patient's anemia is most likely due to:

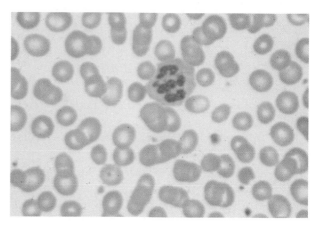

Figure 1-148 • Image Courtesy of Dr. Brenda Shinar, Banner Good Samaritan Medical Center, Phoenix, Arizona.

A. Iron deficiency
B. Blood loss
C. Chronic disease
D. B12 deficiency
E. Folate deficiency

149. You are in the clinic and seeing a patient with the diagnosis of "anemia" who has been placed on iron therapy empirically. You are unsure if the patient truly has iron deficiency or whether the problem is really anemia of chronic disease when you look through the chart. Which of the following statements is true regarding iron-deficiency anemia?

A. Iron studies will show a low iron, low total iron-binding capacity, and high ferritin
B. The most common cause of iron-deficiency anemia is decreased iron intake
C. An increase in hemoglobin by 2 g/dL over 4 weeks of treatment is considered an acceptable response to iron therapy
D. Pica is an uncommon symptom of untreated iron-deficiency anemia
E. Ferritin levels are not affected by acute illness

150. A 17-year-old previously healthy woman presents to your office after being told she has anemia at a sports preparticipation screening.

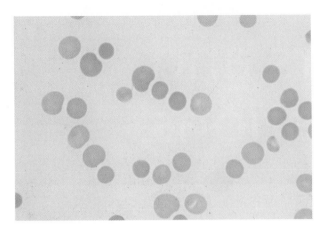

Figure 1-150 • Image Courtesy of Dr. Brenda Shinar, Banner Good Samaritan Medical Center, Phoenix, Arizona.

She reports occasional right upper quadrant pain after large meals, but is otherwise asymptomatic. Family history is remarkable for a mother with anemia. Physical examination is notable for splenomegaly, but otherwise is normal. Laboratory studies include: Hemoglobin 9.2 g/dL; MCV 85 fL; reticulocytes 7%; total bilirubin 3.4 mg/dL. The peripheral smear is shown in Figure 1-150. The next most appropriate step in management would be:

A. Bone marrow biopsy
B. Osmotic fragility test
C. Quantitative G6PD levels
D. Splenectomy
E. Obtain IgG and IgM autoantibody levels

A Answers and Explanations

101. A	118. A	135. B
102. D	119. E	136. E
103. E	120. B	137. D
104. A	121. E	138. B
105. C	122. D	139. A
106. D	123. D	140. E
107. B	124. B	141. C
108. G	125. B	142. D
109. B	126. B	143. D
110. E	127. E	144. B
111. D	128. A	145. B
112. A	129. D	146. B
113. D	130. D	147. C
114. F	131. A	148. D
115. B	132. C	149. C
116. G	133. C	150. B
117. D	134. D	

101. A. This patient has clinical findings concerning for septic arthritis: fever, arthralgia, and pain with passive motion of the joint. In addition, the results of his arthrocentesis suggest an infectious process (Table 1–101). Once a bacterial infection has developed in a joint space, treatment must be initiated rapidly to prevent destruction of the joint. Given that he likely has a septic arthritis, he should be started on empiric IV antibiotic therapy as soon as possible and before culture results are available.

B. As in the explanation for A, antibiotic therapy should not be withheld in a case of suspected septic arthritis because of the increased risk of joint destruction. You should start empiric therapy and modify this once culture results are available.

C. Traumatic effusions are usually not inflammatory (immune mediated). Occasionally, they are hemorrhagic, which will be evident by gross visualization of the fluid.

D. Although hepatitis C can cause arthralgias, it is not common to see large effusions associated with it. In addition, the synovial fluid would have a more inflammatory than septic appearance (Table 1-101).

E. The patient gives no history of trauma, and the fluid that was aspirated is significantly inflamed, which suggests infection. Patients with meniscal tears typically can state the time and place of their injury, and should not have fever or the other indicators of an infected joint.

102. D. This patient is in the midst of a serious asthma exacerbation. She is anxious, dyspneic, and tachypneic. She is sitting in a tripod position trying to breath easier and she is becoming hypoxemic. All are warning signs for impending respiratory failure. In the initial phase of an acute exacerbation of asthma, the minute ventilation (respiratory rate × tidal volume) increases. As the minute ventilation increases, more CO_2 is exhaled and the $paCO_2$ should decrease. Therefore, you should not expect to see a normal $paCO_2$ in a patient who is compensating well for their acute attack. As our patient's exacerbation persisted, she has became more fatigued and, as a result, the tidal volumes she was able to generate became progressively smaller. As the tidal volumes decreased, she was unable to increase her respiratory rate any further and her minute ventilation began to decrease and $paCO_2$ to rise. Therefore, the "normal" $paCO_2$ obtained during her acute attack of asthma is worrisome because it suggests that the $paCO_2$ is on an upward trend. This patient is becoming fatigued and is on the verge of respiratory failure. She should be considered for endotracheal intubation before a complete respiratory collapse occurs.

A, E. Her ABG appears normal, but it is not reassuring. Recognizing this subtlety can help you intervene more rapidly before the patient becomes unstable.

B. Although her oxygenation status is suboptimal, it is not the primary problem. It is a result of her ventilation problem. Although supplemental oxygen should be provided, further correction of her paO_2 is not our primary concern.

C. Although she is likely to develop respiratory acidosis if her condition continues to deteriorate, she has not yet become acidemic, as indicated by her neutral pH.

TABLE 1-101 Arthrocentesis Results

	Normal	Inflammatory	Septic	Hemorrhagic
Volume (mL)	<3.5	>3.5	>3.5	>3.5
Color	Clear	Yellow	Yellow/green	Red
Clarity	Clear	Clear to opaque	Opaque	Bloody
Viscosity	High	Low	Low to high	Low to high
WBCs	<200	2000–10,000	>100,000	200–2000
PMNs	<25%	>50%	>75%	50–75%

103. **E.** Light's criteria helps to diagnose pleural fluid as transudative or exudative. If any one of the three criteria is positive, then the fluid is an exudate. These criteria are: (1) A pleural fluid protein to serum protein ratio of >0.5, (2) a pleural fluid LDH to serum LDH ratio of >0.6, or (3) a pleural fluid LDH >2/3 the upper limit of normal serum LDH. This effusion is thick and grayish-white in color, which is probably pus. The pH is acidic, and the glucose is low along with a high LDH. Most importantly, the Gram stain is positive for organisms, which makes this an empyema. This effusion will need to be drained with a chest tube, and the patient may need to go to decortication to treat the infection.

104. **A.** This effusion is a transudate, because the pH is normal, the pleural fluid protein to serum protein ratio is 0.28, and the pleural fluid LDH to serum LDH ratio is 0.33.

105. **C.** This effusion is due to RA. First, by analysis of the protein and LDH ratios, it is an exudate. It is milky green, which might confuse you into thinking that this is a chylous effusion; however, the triglycerides are <50 mg/dL, which virtually excludes a chylous effusion. Also, the glucose is extremely low, at 5 mg/dL, which is most commonly seen with rheumatoid effusions. The WBC count is not very high, but is mostly lymphocytic, which also goes along with a rheumatoid-related effusion.

106. **D.** This effusion is consistent with a tuberculous effusion (which needs to be distinguished from a tuberculous empyema). Tuberculous effusions are caused by a delayed hypersensitivity reaction to the AFB antigen, which may leak into the pleural space. They are usually straw-colored and exudative. The pH may be low (around 7.30) and the glucose may be low, but not as low as in a tuberculous empyema or a rheumatic effusion. The white cells are predominantly lymphocytic, and there is usually a paucity (<5%) of mesothelial cells in TB effusions.

107. **B.** Chylous effusions are turbid or milky-appearing because of their high lipid content, and are usually a result of a thoracic duct disruption. Causes of this disruption can be traumatic or nontraumatic. The most common nontraumatic cause is a lymphoma in the chest.

Other nontraumatic causes include sarcoidosis or tuberculosis. Traumatic causes are most often related to surgeries of the chest. A triglyceride content in the effusion of >110 mg/dL strongly suggests a chylous effusion, whereas a triglyceride content of <30 mg/dL virtually rules out the diagnosis. It the content falls between these two numbers, then a lipoprotein analysis should be done on the fluid. If chylomicrons are found, then the diagnosis of a chylous effusion can be made.

108. **G.** An eosinophilic pleural effusion can have many causes. It may be associated with a pneumothorax, a hemothorax, a pulmonary infarction, on a parasitic or tuberculous infection; it can also be drug-induced. This pleural effusion was bloody, and it was exudative, making the best choice of answers "G."

F. An effusion related to metastatic cancer lung cancer will most likely be exudative and is often grossly bloody. The cytology may be helpful if it is positive, but if negative, the sensitivity of cytology is not good enough to rule out cancer.

109. **B.** The values as given by Heffner et al (*Chest*, 1997;111:970–980) are convenient to use because they eliminate the need for drawing a patient's serum the same time (or as close as possible to the same time) as performing a thoracentesis. Remember, just as in Light's criteria, if just *one* of the criteria are met, the pleural effusion is considered an exudate. The criteria are: Pleural fluid LDH >45% of the serum upper limit of normal; pleural fluid cholesterol >45 mg/dL; or pleural fluid total protein >2.9 gm/dL. There is no albumin, ANA, or triglyceride in the Heffner criteria of transudate vs. exudative pleural effusion.

A, C, D, E. These values are incorrect. See explanation for B.

110. **E.** Studies have shown that small endobronchial cancerous lesions may be found as a cause for hemoptysis in patients with clear chest X-rays between 0% and 20% of the time. Factors that increase the risk for occult malignancy in patients with hemoptysis and a clear chest X-ray include cigarette smoking, age >40 years, and hemoptysis that continues for longer than 1 week.

Because lung cancer may be resectable in its early stages, it is important to look for it. In this patient, who is 55 years old with a significant smoking history and the hemoptysis lasting a month, the most appropriate next step is to refer him to a pulmonologist for a bronchoscopy.

A. Sputum for cytology would be helpful if it were positive, because the next step would be to go to bronchoscopy to look for the source of malignant cells. However, sputum cytology is not sufficiently sensitive, and many small cancers can be missed. Therefore, it is not the appropriate next step for this patient.

B. It is always important to advise patients who smoke of the risks to their health, and to encourage them to quit; however, it is not appropriate to give this patient reassurance regarding his hemoptysis.

C. In a patient who is low risk for occult malignancy, such as a younger patient, one who does not smoke, or one who presents with upper respiratory symptoms and a cough with minimal streaks of hemoptysis, it may be appropriate to treat for empiric bronchitis to see if the hemoptysis resolves. However, that is not the correct choice for management in this patient scenario.

D. A *high-resolution* CT scan of the chest may be an alternative to a fiberoptic bronchoscopy in a patient for whom bronchoscopy is contraindicated (such as patients with bleeding disorders). However, a plain CT scan is not appropriate. A high-resolution CT scan takes coronal slices through the chest at smaller intervals than a normal CT scan and is more sensitive for smaller lesions. Bronchoscopy, however, is preferred for both diagnosis and cost-effectiveness.

111. D. Asthma is a combination of bronchial hyperreactivity, constriction, and chronic inflammation. There are many causes of occupational asthma, including metal salts, wood and vegetable dusts, industrial chemicals and plastics, and others. There are probably three separate mechanisms for this type of asthma: 1) The agent may trigger an IgE antibody resulting in immunologic sensitization; 2) The substance itself can release factors that cause bronchoconstriction; and 3) The substance can cause a direct or a reflex stimulation of the airways in latent (or already diagnosed) asthmatics. The

methacholine challenge is the appropriate test to evaluate this patient, to see whether she develops signs of airway bronchoconstriction and obstruction on pulmonary function tests when exposed to methacholine. A negative challenge (the FEV_1 remains 80% or greater than predicted) in a patient not on anti-asthma medications excludes the diagnosis of asthma with 95% certainty.

A. This patient should not be referred to psychiatry, because you have not eliminated reactive airway disease as a diagnosis based on the tests that you have performed.

B. Patients with asthma may have completely normal chest X-rays and pulmonary function tests when they are not in an acute attack. This patient needs a methacholine challenge before asthma can be ruled out.

C. A room-air arterial blood gas would not help make the diagnosis of asthma in this patient who is currently asymptomatic.

E. Oxygen desaturation with exercise is a sensitive indicator of gas exchange abnormalities, but is not specific. It will not help make the diagnosis of asthma in this patient. Oxygen desaturation with exercise may be pronounced in patients with HIV and *Pneumocystis carinii* pneumonia (PCP), patients with early interstitial lung disease, and patients with pulmonary vascular disease, such as primary pulmonary hypertension.

112. A. This patient has bronchial breath sounds in the right lower lobe. (Bronchial breath sounds are synonymous with "tubular" and "tracheal" breath sounds.) These sounds are different from the usual alveolar sounds that are heard in the periphery of the lung. If you listen to a normal chest at either lower lobe, you will hear a fine noise on inspiration and nothing on expiration. If you listen over the trachea, you will hear a loud noise during inspiration *and* expiration. The noise that you hear over the trachea is *abnormal* to hear in the lung periphery, and it means that large airway noises are being transmitted to the periphery. This is usually because the alveoli are full of a material (fluid, pus) and are consolidating the lobe. (Bronchial breath sounds can also be heard when large effusions "squish" the lung parenchyma and allow the large airway noise to be heard in the periphery, but usually effusions cause decreased breath

sounds.) Egophony is also heard with consolidation. With your stethoscope over the area of consolidation, ask the patient to say "eeeeee"; the sound will change to "aayyyy." Increased tactile fremitus is seen in consolidation as well. To test for this, you should place your hands *firmly* against the patient's back or chest wall (or you can alternate the same hand back and forth, like your stethoscope) and have the patient say "ninety-nine" over and over again. You will sense an increased vibration over the area of consolidated lung, meaning that there is a direct, solid communication from the bronchus, through the lung, and out to the chest wall—a sign of consolidation.

113. D. This patient has decreased breath sounds over the right lower lobe. The next step in evaluating the pathology is palpation to determine whether it is dull or hyperresonant. The dullness signifies either an effusion or consolidation of the lobe. The decreased tactile fremitus indicates a probable effusion between the lung tissue and the chest wall, as opposed to a consolidation, which would cause *increased* tactile fremitus.

114. F. This patient has decreased breath sounds bilaterally. The increased AP diameter of the chest (also known as a "barrel chest") implies chronic air trapping. The long expiration to inspiration ratio suggests obstruction to air flow, which is seen in patients with chronic obstructive lung disease or asthma. However, the barrel shape of the chest makes you think that this is something more chronic and long-standing than an asthma exacerbation, and severe obstructive lung disease due to emphysema is the correct answer.

115. B. This patient has decreased breath sounds over the right lung; however, he is hyperresonant to percussion, which should make you think of a pneumothorax. The trachea is deviated *away* from the pneumothorax, because the large volume of air in the pleural space is pushing it away. A large right-sided pleural effusion also may deviate the trachea to the left (as would anything with high volume), but there would be dullness, and not hyperresonance, to percussion.

116. G. The abdominal wall usually expands with inspiration. This patient's abdomen is retracting with inspiration, which is called respiratory paradox. The most common reason for this is a patient who is becoming severely tired from respiratory effort, and the diaphragm is being pulled upward as the intercostal muscles do all the work of breathing. Respiratory alternans is seen when a patient has normal abdominal wall expansion with breathing that alternates with paradoxical abdominal wall movement. Both of these scenarios are serious and indicate impending respiratory failure.

C. The left-sided pneumothorax would have the same findings as "B," but on the left side.

E. The left-sided effusion would have the same findings as in "D," but on the left side.

117. D. This patient is presenting with four of the five classic signs of thrombotic thrombocytopenic purpura (TTP): fever, neurologic changes, anemia, and thrombocytopenia. In addition, he takes a medication known to have a rare side effect of TTP. TTP is a disorder of endothelial injury that causes the activation of platelets (and thrombocytopenia) and the formation of fibrin strands within blood vessels. The fibrin strands shear the RBCs, resulting in a microangiopathic hemolytic anemia. Schistocytes are fragmented RBCs seen on the blood smears of patients with microangiopathic hemolytic anemias such as TTP, hemolytic uremic syndrome (HUS), and the hemolysis, elevated liver enzymes, low platelets (HELLP) syndrome of pregnancy.

118. A. Spherocytes are seen in the peripheral smears of patients with autoimmune hemolytic anemias (AIHAs). In this anemia, the patient forms antibodies to the RBC membrane; in the spleen, a "bite" of the membrane is taken out, effectively giving the cell a "facelift" and changing its shape from a biconcave disk to a sphere. Patients with chronic lymphocytic leukemia are prone to the development of AIHA.

119. E. Howell-Jolly bodies are nuclear remnants that are left in the circulating RBCs of patients who have had their spleen removed or have functional asplenia. The spleens of patients with sickle cell disease have usually infarcted by late childhood; these patients will be functionally asplenic.

120. **B.** **Target cells are formed when the RBC has an increased surface area (membrane) to volume (cytoplasm) ratio. Any process that increases the amount of cell membrane or decreases the amount of cytoplasm will cause a target cell. Chronic liver disease causes target cells by increasing the amount of phospholipids deposited in the cell membrane (thereby increasing the ratio), and thalassemia and severe iron deficiency cause target cells by decreasing the cytoplasmic volume (which also increases the ratio).**

    C. Tear drop cells are seen in myelofibrosis.
    F. Heinz bodies are aggregates of denatured hemoglobin and are most often seen in glucose 6-phosphate dehydrogenase (G6PD) deficiency and in thalassemias.
    G. Rouleaux formation is seen on the peripheral smear in approximately 50% of patients with multiple myeloma. It consists of RBCs that appear in stacks, like coins.

121. **E.** **Rhinitis medicamentosa can occur with many drugs, but the most common precipitant is over-the-counter sympathomimetic nasal sprays used to treat congestion. When used for several days, one can develop rebound congestion when the medication wears off. The patient often starts to use more of the nasal spray at higher doses, which then begins a vicious cycle.**

    A. Allergic rhinitis is usually seasonal and accompanied by other symptoms such as watery, itchy eyes and sneezing. Patients give a history of worsening symptoms at different times of the year. Common allergens include dust mites and animal proteins. People typically give a personal or family history of rhinitis, eczema, or asthma. Exam is significant for turbinate edema with pallor or a bluish hue. This patient does not give any temporal relationship to symptoms and his exam is more consistent with nonallergic rhinitis.
    B. This patient does not give any history of placing or inserting foreign objects in his nose, a very common occurrence in children. Physical exam is often significant for unilateral congestion (where foreign object is located) and purulent discharge.

    C. Nasal polyps are associated with chronic allergic rhinitis. On exam they are pale, polypoid masses that are insensitive to pain. Treatment begins with nasal steroids, but if the patient is still symptomatic, surgery can be performed.
    D. Vasomotor rhinitis is chronic nasal congestion worsened by changes in temperature and humidity and with new odors. Physical exam is significant for pink, boggy nasal mucosa. Nasal itching is very rare, as is the presence of eosinophils, which are common in allergic rhinitis. Avoidance of triggers and inhaled nasal steroids aid in treatment.

122. **D.** **This man has rhinitis medicamentosa caused by continual use of a sympathomimetic nasal spray. His symptoms worsen when the medication wears off and thus begins the vicious cycle. Treatment is removal of the offending agent. Nasal corticosteroids have been used with some improvement. Symptoms can remain for up to 1 year.**

    A. Inhaled nasal corticosteroids are used primarily in the treatment of allergic rhinitis. They can also be used with rhinitis medicamentosa, but studies have shown only some improvement in symptoms.
    B. ENT evaluation at this point is unnecessary, given the patient history and physical exam. It is unlikely that he is suffering from a nasal tumor or foreign body.
    C. Antihypertensives are known to cause rhinitis. The main offending agent is propanolol. Thiazides are less likely to cause rhinitis.
    E. A nasal smear to check for eosinophils would help differentiate allergic rhinitis from nonallergic rhinitis. Because this patient does not have allergy-type symptoms, this is not necessary.

123. **D.** **IgA deficiency is the most common immunoglobulin deficiency with an incidence reaching 1/600 in white populations. This patient gives a history of recurrent sinopulmonary infections and intermittent diarrhea, which are consistent with IgA deficiency. There is a concordance with IgA deficiency and celiac sprue, and this patient has diarrhea and iron-deficiency anemia, which should make you think of celiac disease. Another manifestation**

of IgA deficiency includes anaphylactic reactions to blood transfusions. The diagnosis is made by measuring quantitative IgA levels. Treatment includes prophylactic antibiotics to lessen the number of infections. If this does not help, IV immune globulin (IVIG) has been tried with some success.

A. C5–C9 MAC deficiency is also called terminal complement deficiency. Complement proteins C5 through C9 are responsible for the membrane attacking complex after initiation of the immune response by antibodies in both the classic and alternative activation cascades. Deficiency of these proteins leads to increased infections with *Neisseria* species including both meningococcal and gonococcal infections. This patient does not give this type of history.

B. X-linked agammglobulinemia presents in males, usually ages 6 to 18 months, with recurrent sinopulmonary infections secondary to *Staphylococcus*, *Streptococcus*, and meningococcus. There are no B cells present in serum. These patients have normal resistance to viral illnesses, fungi, and gram-negative organisms. If caught early, the prognosis is good with IVIG treatment.

C. IgG deficiency is also known as common variable hypogammaglobulinemia. Patients have decreased resistance to encapsulated organisms such as *Streptococcus pneumoniae* and *Haemophilus influenzae*. Peak incidence occurs between 25 and 40 years of age. Clinical manifestations include recurrent sinopulmonary infections, recurrent enteroviral infections, and an association with autoimmune disorders and rheumatologic disorders. Treatment is IVIG over 2 to 4 weeks.

E. IgM deficiency is also known as Wiskott-Aldrich syndrome. Patients often present in infancy with thrombocytopenia, recurrent sinopulmonary infections, eczema, and other autoimmune disorders. IgM levels are generally low on diagnosis. Treatment includes bone marrow transplant, IVIG, splenectomy, and prophylactic antibiotics.

124. B. Arthus (hypersensitivity type III) reactions are mediated by IgG antibodies, which form complexes with antigens. These hypersensitivity reactions are less common than IgE-mediated hypersensitivity reactions. Arthus reactions are described as deposition of immune complexes that cause a localized inflammatory reaction. They occur about 8 to 24 hours after inoculation. An antigen that has been injected (in this case the tetanus vaccine) stimulates this patient's localized immune response. This will not progress on to anaphylaxis.

A. Immediate hypersensitivity occurs within 1 hour of exposure to an allergen. Typically allergens include stings, drugs, and foods. Urticaria and hives are initial presenting signs that can advance to anaphylaxis. This reaction is IgE mediated.

C. Delayed type IV reactions are mediated by T cells, not antibodies. They typically occur 24 to 48 hours after exposure. Exposure to mycobacterial proteins or poison ivy are examples of type IV reactions. Reactions are typically local, with erythema, induration, and dermatitis present.

D. Late-phase IgE-mediated reactions present as local erythema, burning, and induration typically seen with reactions to local skin testing. The reaction is secondary to mast cell release.

E. Anaphylaxis is an extreme form of immediate hypersensitivity reaction that is usually IgE mediated. There are non-IgE-mediated forms of anaphylaxis secondary to release of cytoplasmic granules. These are called "anaphylactoid" reactions. An example of an anaphylactoid reaction is the usual reaction to radiocontrast dye.

125. B. This patient's asthma can best be described as mild persistent. Mild persistent asthma is defined as having symptoms more than once per week that require bronchodilators, nighttime awakening once every 2 weeks, and fluctuations in peak flows of 20% or more.

A. Mild intermittent asthma criteria include symptoms two times or fewer in a week, fewer than two nighttime awakenings per month, and peak flows consistently above 80%.

C. Moderate persistent asthma is defined as daily symptoms with bronchodilator use, at least one nighttime awakening per week, and peak flows ranging from 60% to 80% of predicted values.

D. Severe asthma is defined as symptoms with any trigger, usually occurring daily and requiring the use of a bronchodilator. Awakening four to seven times nightly and peak flows less than 60% of predicted normal values are also criteria for severe asthma.

E. Exercise-induced asthma usually falls into the mild intermittent category, because symptoms are usually only related to exercise and peak flows remain greater than 80% of predicted values.

126. **B. The initiation of an anti-inflammatory agent is indicated in cases of mild persistent asthma. In this case, the patient would most likely benefit from an inhaled corticosteroid. She should use an inhaled β-agonist as needed for rescue purposes. This therapy should lower the number of symptomatic episodes she has per week.**

A. An inhaled β-agonist would not be adequate therapy for this patient. This would treat only the acute symptoms, which she is having quite frequently. There would be no therapy for the underlying inflammation in her bronchioles.

C. This patient requires medical therapy on an outpatient basis. Not treating her would be a medical liability.

D. A long-acting β-agonist is often added to therapy of patients with moderate persistent and severe asthma. It cuts down on the number of short-acting β-agonists needed. It does not treat the inflammatory component of asthma.

E. Leukotriene receptor antagonists inhibit leukotrienes, which are released during asthma exacerbations. Leukotrienes are responsible for airway edema, mucus secretion, and bronchoconstriction that especially awaken the patient at night, because they are the late-phase mediators of inflammation. These antagonists can be started in patients with mild persistent asthma after initiation of β-agonist and corticosteroid therapy, but are more frequently used in patients with moderate to severe asthma.

127. **E. This patient is very ill, as witnessed on her physical exam (in particular, her worsening ability to converse, poor air movement, and new-onset lethargy). Sending her home would not be an option. This patient should be started on continuous nebulizer therapy and transferred** to the ICU for close monitoring as soon as possible. Other treatment additions would include IV steroid and IV β-agonist therapies.

A. An ABG would help you determine if this patient was unable to oxygenate or ventilate (showing signs of tiring). This would be manifested even if the CO_2 level was normal, because it should NOT be normal in a patient that is breathing 30 times a minute and ventilating appropriately. The CO_2 would be a late sign that the patient was tiring and should worry you that this patient will need to be intubated soon.

B. This patient does need to be admitted, but observation on the floor would be inadequate. This patient has exhibited signs of impending respiratory decline with her lung exam, her decreasing ability to speak, and her worsening neurologic status.

C. Inhaled corticosteroid therapy is used in the treatment of mild persistent and moderate asthma. Use in the acute setting of status asthmaticus has not been shown to affect outcome.

D. In a patient with status asthmaticus, IV steroids should be started immediately and continued until the asthma improves.

128. **A. This patient likely has farmer's lung, the most common hypersensitivity pneumonitis. Symptoms are generally vague, presenting as malaise, fevers, and chills with an associated cough. There may be some shortness of breath and even hemoptysis. Farmer's lung is caused by thermophilic actinomycetes that are present in moldy compost or hay.**

B. Animal proteins can also be responsible for hypersensitivity pneumonitis. The most common form is bird-breeder's lung; bird droppings are responsible for the antigenic response. Other animal proteins that can cause this condition include rodent urine and shell dust.

C. Fungi can also cause hypersensitivity pneumonitis. Cheese worker's lung (*Penicillium* spp) and woodworker's lung (*Alternaria* spp) are other examples. Our patient gives no history of working with cheese or wood.

D. Work-related chemicals that can cause hypersensitivity pneumonitis include epoxy resin and trimellitic anhydride (plastic worker's lung). This patient gives no history of these exposures.

E. Arthropods, in particular the wheat weevil, *Sitophilus grainarius*, can cause hypersensitivity pneumonitis (miller's lung).

129. **D.** Avoidance of antigen exposure is difficult and can cause a financial burden on farmers with hypersensitivity pneumonitis. Reduction of antigenic burden can be difficult also; if compost or hay is wetted down before handling, the number of mobile actinomycetes is reduced. Avoidance of the antigen is the primary treatment in hypersensitivity pneumonitis.

A. Inhaled β-agonist therapy has not been shown to help with farmer's lung. The major etiology of symptoms is diffuse inflammation of the lung parenchyma secondary to antigen exposure. A bronchodilator is not the first-line therapy.

B. High-dose IV steroids are not part of the initial treatment regiment for farmer's lung. Oral steroids have been studied and are used in patients with moderate symptoms.

C. Antibiotic therapy is not indicated as the mechanism for a patient's symptoms is inflammation of lung parenchyma secondary to antigen exposure and sensitization. Avoidance of the antigen and treatment of inflammation are necessary therapies.

E. Oral steroids have been shown to result in some improvement in patients with moderate acute symptoms. In studies comparing steroids to antigen exposure removal, at 6 months patient symptoms were similar, suggesting that steroids can help in the acute phase.

130. **D.** The complement cascade is initiated when antibodies or immunoglobulins bind to an antigen. The cascade is composed of two parts, classical and alternative. The alternative differs from the classical in that it can be indirectly initiated by cell wall proteins. Hereditary angioedema is an autosomal dominant disorder. It is caused by a decrease in the C1-esterase inhibitory protein. This protein is responsible for the breakdown of the first part of the complement cascade to prevent excessive complement activation. With excessive complement activation, patients have increased bradykinin release, which increases vasopermeability. Patients are subject to asymmetric swelling of extremities, tongue, and larynx, and do not have associated urticaria. Treatment is with androgens, which help increase levels of C1-esterase inhibitor. Fresh frozen plasma can be given to acutely replete the C1 inhibitor. C1 inhibitor deficiency is different from mast cell-mediated forms of angioedema that respond to antihistamines. Itching is often a component of these forms of angioedema.

A. A deficiency of C5 through C9 results in increased infections with the *Neisseria* spp (meningococcal and gonococcal). Patients with recurrent disseminated gonococcal infections should be screened for terminal complement deficiency.

B. C3 deficiency leads to recurrent bacterial infections with encapsulated organisms. Patients present soon after birth.

C. C2 deficiency results in the development of lupus. It can also present in childhood with recurrence of pyogenic infections. It is the most common complement deficiency.

E. IgA deficiency is associated with recurrent sinopulmonary infections and celiac disease. It is not associated with intermittent edema of the extremities, tongue, or larynx.

131. **A.** This patient is having an anaphylactic reaction, as evidenced by her respiratory distress, hives, and hypotension. IV epinephrine is first-line therapy in patients with anaphylaxis who present with hypotension and bronchospasm. It has been shown that delay of epinephrine therapy increases mortality.

B. IV steroids are used to prevent late-phase reactions in patients with IgE-mediated reactions. They do not work in the acute phase.

C. Antihistamines, including both H1 and H2 blockers, are used to prevent symptoms secondary to histamine release, such as hives and itching. It has been shown that it is more effective to use H1 and H2 blockers together. However, these will not help this patient's hypotension and respiratory distress.

D. Subcutaneous epinephrine is given if a patient has mild to moderate symptoms including urticaria and hives. It may be repeated every 15 to 20 minutes. If a patient develops respiratory distress or hypotension, IV epinephrine should be administered.

E. Inhaled β-agonists can be used in concert with IV epinephrine in patients suffering from respiratory distress due to anaphylaxis to help ease the bronchospasm. It will not help with the hypotension.

132. **C. This patient likely has C2 deficiency, which is the most common complement deficiency in whites. It may present with lupus, or patients may have a history of recurrent pyogenic infections as children. The appropriate test is the total hemolytic complement activity test (CH50). This is an initial screen to determine whether there is a problem in the function of the complement cascade. Individual complement components can be measured after a positive test.**

A. Serum immunoglobulins should be ordered in a person suspected to have a humoral immunity deficiency. Typically, these patients present with recurrent sinopulmonary infections with encapsulated organisms. Quantitative immunoglobulins can also be measured.

B. The NBT dye test measures the ability of phagocytes to generate oxygen radicals used in the killing of microbes. Tests of phagocytosis are ordered when a patient gives a history of recurrent skin and respiratory infections with bacteria and fungi.

D. Anti-nuclear antibodies are checked when an autoimmune disorder is suspected, not an immunodeficiency. It is important to remember, however, that some cases of lupus are due to complement deficiencies.

E. X-chromosome inactivation analysis is performed when Wiscott-Aldrich (recurrent infections, eczema, and diarrhea), severe X-linked combined immunodeficiency, or hyper-IgM syndromes is suspected.

133. **C. This patient has classic findings of OA. It typically has a slow, progressive onset and is the result of chronic trauma. The joints that are typically affected are the weight-bearing joints (hip, knee, and spine) and the small joints in the hand (specifically the DIP and PIP joints). Patients with OA typically have less than 30 minutes of morning stiffness, whereas patients with RA have longer periods of stiffness. They also typically do not have other evidence of systemic illness (fevers, malaise, etc.). Changes seen on physical exam include bony deformities (nodules) at the DIP (Heberden's nodes) and PIP (Bouchard's nodes) joints. Crepitus is commonly felt on examination of the effected joint (especially the knee). Classic X-ray findings are osteophytes and narrowing of the joint space.**

A. RA typically presents more acutely and has more systemic signs and symptoms associated with it. These include fevers, malaise, morning stiffness (lasting between 45 minutes and several hours), anorexia, and weight loss, to name a few. The joints that are typically affected in RA include the PIP joints and the metacarpophalangeal joints—the DIP joints are spared. Although the knee is the most common single joint involved in RA, it tends to affect mostly the smaller joints in the body.

B. Although the majority of patients with SLE have joint involvement, it is rarely the only part of the body involved. Similarly to RA, patients with SLE typically have more systemic signs of illness (fever, malaise, etc.). In addition, they do not typically develop the bony changes or crepitus seen in patients with OA.

D. CPPD deposition disease is a crystalline arthropathy that can mimic many disease processes. It can present as pseudo-RA, pseudo-OA, or pseudo-ankylosing spondylitis, or can even be asymptomatic. It is most often referred to as pseudo-gout because of its acute presentation (fairly abrupt onset as a monoarticular arthritis with an exquisitely painful joint). CPPD disease usually involves the knee and spares the smaller joints. The onset of disease is not usually as rapid as gout. The joint examination during an acute attack of CPPD disease is similar to that of gout (single joint, very painful, may or may not have overlying redness and swelling). The radiologic feature that identifies CPPD disease is the presence of chondrocalcinosis (calcium deposition in the cartilage) seen on plain X-rays (usually of the knee).

E. Reactive arthritis, or acute gout attacks, typically present as an abrupt monoarticular arthritis often with overlying redness and swelling (can easily mimic a septic joint). The smaller joints are usually spared with the exception of the large toe (first metatarsophalangeal joint). Physical findings are discussed above. X-rays taken during an acute gout attack may well be normal. Patients with chronic gouty arthritis can develop tophi (uric acid deposits) and joint erosions on X-ray.

134. **D.** Weight reduction, aerobic exercise (e.g., swimming), and NSAIDs are the mainstay for initial treatment of osteoarthritis. Orthotics, braces, canes, and other assistive devices may be beneficial for some patients. Patients who fail more conservative medical treatment may benefit from intra-articular injections with glucocorticoids. However, oral steroid therapy is not indicated for the treatment of OA (remember, it's the result of trauma; it is not a systemic autoimmune process). Patients with more advanced disease affecting the hips or knees may be referred for consideration for arthroplasty.

A. Methotrexate is commonly used in the treatment of RA but has no indication for the treatment of OA.
B. Prednisone is commonly used in the treatment of autoimmune processes such as RA and SLE, but not for OA.
C. Allopurinol, a xanthine oxidase inhibitor, is used for the chronic treatment of gout to decrease the production of uric acid. It is of no benefit in the treatment of OA.
E. Colchicine is used in select patients for the treatment of an acute flare of gout.

135. **B.** This patient has a classic presentation of gout. Gout is a crystalline arthropathy that can present acutely and is often exquisitely painful. Although the joint that is most commonly affected is the first metatarsal-phalangeal (MTP) joint (referred to as podagra), the knee is often involved as well. The inflammation in the joint can be quite intense and resemble that of an infected joint (redness, warmth, swelling, pain with motion, etc.). During an initial attack, X-rays of the affected joint may appear normal. It is only after recurrent attacks or a long-standing history of gout do you see the bony changes (tophi, joint erosions). Synovial fluid analysis reveals clear fluid with monosodium urate crystals which have strong negative birefringence (i.e., they look like yellow needles when lined up with the polarizing light of the microscope). The remainder of the synovial fluid studies can mimic those of an infected joint (leukocytosis, etc.).

A. Septic arthritis needs to be excluded in any patient with the presentation of a monoarticular arthritis and a history of IV drug use. The presence of crystals in the synovial fluid helps us make the diagnosis of gout in this case. However, one has to maintain a high index of suspicion, because patients with underlying joint disease (gout, RA, etc.) are at higher risk for the development of septic arthritis (actually, both processes can be present at the same time).
C. CPPD deposition disease—also known as pseudogout—can have a very similar presentation. The joint distribution, onset of disease, and physical examination findings are very similar, but the joint aspirate and X-ray findings are different. Synovial fluid from a patient with CPPD disease reveals rhomboid crystals that are weakly positively birefringent. X-rays of the affected joint reveals chondrocalcinosis as discussed above.
D. Traumatic fracture is less likely given there was no history of trauma. Also, fractures often result in hemorrhagic effusions, which the patient did not have.
E. SLE is often accompanied by joint involvement, but it usually is not monoarticular. The joint involvement in SLE is more diffuse and symmetric (it can often mimic RA). In addition, if synovial fluid were obtained from a joint affected by SLE, it should not contain monosodium urate crystals.

136. **E.** Gouty arthritis results from the deposition of monosodium urate crystals in the joint space. Although patients with high serum uric acid levels are at increased risk of developing gout, it cannot be used to make the diagnosis of gout. Many patients have elevated serum uric acid levels but never develop gout. Even in patients who develop gout, it is not the degree of elevation of uric acid in the serum that precipitates deposition of the crystals into the joint space, but rather how fast the level of uric acid changes. That is why many patients with gout will have an acute flare of their disease when they are admitted to the hospital (where they receive IV fluids or diuretics that alter their uric acid levels). In addition, if a high uric acid level is abruptly lowered (e.g., with IV fluids), an acute gout flare may result even though the uric acid level may be measured as normal at that point.

A, B, C, D. See explanation for E.

137. **D.** Patients with gout develop hyperuricemia by two potential mechanisms. They either overproduce uric acid (idiopathic, leukemia, hemolytic anemia, G6PD, etc.) or undersecrete it (idiopathic, chronic renal disease, lead nephropathy, alcohol, diabetic ketoacidosis [DKA], drugs, etc.). The treatment of *acute* gout flares and *chronic* gout is different. For acute gout, indomethacin is the preferred treatment. Colchicine can also be used for acute gout, but it has more side effects, such as diarrhea, nausea, and abdominal pain. Both indomethacin and colchicine are contraindicated in renal insufficiency, in which case intra-articular or oral steroids may be used, or even narcotics alone, just to control pain. Notice that the treatment focus of the acute attack is to decrease inflammation, not to alter the uric acid level.

   A. Drugs that are used to treat chronic gout focus on decreasing production (allopurinol) or increasing renal excretion (probenecid). These drugs may precipitate an acute flare, because they change the uric acid level; therefore, they should *not* be initiated during an acute attack. Doing so may prolong the initial attack, which the patient will not be happy about.

   B. IV nafcillin may be considered if septic arthritis were possible; however, this patient has gout.

   C. Prednisone may be given during an acute attack of gout, but this should be considered only if the patient is unable to take oral NSAIDs or colchicine. Intra-articular steroids can also be given if the patient cannot be given other forms of treatment.

   E. You would consider immobilizing an extremity if you were concerned about a fracture until you could further evaluate it. However, this patient's findings are not consistent with a fracture. Immobilization may offer comfort to the patient with an acute gout flare, but it will not halt the disease process.

138. **B.** This patient has AS. AS is one type of the seronegative spondylarthropathies that are immune mediated, usually involve the spine, and have asymmetric joint involvement. Reactive arthritis and psoriatic arthritis are other types of seronegative spondylarthropathies. Patients with AS, all of whom have symptomatic sacroiliitis, usually develop the disease during young adulthood. Men are more commonly afflicted with the disease (some argue that there is equal prevalence, but that women have a milder disease process and often miss detection). The pain associated with AS is always decreased with exercise. Common physical findings include decreased range of motion in the affected spine and tenderness over the sacroiliac joint. Patients with AS can also develop "sausage digits" (as can those with reactive and psoriatic arthritis). Classic radiographic findings include the formation of new bone on vertebral bodies near the annulus fibrosis (which gives the vertebral bodies the classic "shiny corner" or "window pane" appearance). In addition, syndesmophytes are commonly seen. These collections of bone growth between the vertebral bodies eventually cause the vertebrae to fuse and have the bamboo appearance. Sacroiliitis is commonly seen on plain X-rays, with occasional fusion of the sacroiliac joints.

   A. Vertebral osteomyelitis should be considered in any patient with low back pain and a history of IV drug use. Patients with vertebral osteomyelitis may or may not have systemic signs of illness (fevers, malaise, etc.). Bacterial causes of osteomyelitis tend to produce a more abrupt and systemic illness. However, infections such as mycobacterium (tuberculosis) or coccidioidomycosis can cause vertebral osteomyelitis with a more indolent course. One of the most reliable clinical signs of vertebral osteomyelitis is pain with palpation over the affected spinous process (which the patient does not have).

   C. Reactive arthritis is another type of seronegative spondylarthropathy. However, patients with reactive arthritis do not develop the X-ray findings like those seen in AS. Reactive arthritis is an acute arthritis that occurs as the result of an infection elsewhere in the body (e.g., *Chlamydia, Ureaplasma, Salmonella, Shigella, Yersinia, Klebsiella*, and *Campylobacter*). Reiter's syndrome is a term often used interchangeably with reactive arthritis. Although both terms refer to a similar process, Reiter's syndrome should be used only when there is the triad of conjunctivitis, arthritis, and nongonococcal urethritis.

   D. Although RA shares some of the features of AS (morning stiffness, improvement in symptoms with activity, etc.), it should be noted that RA typically does *not* affect the spine or sacroiliac joints.

E. IBD can result in enteropathic arthropathy, which are joint attacks related to flares of IBD, but not associated with sacroiliitis. These attacks typically involve only a few of the joints of the lower extremities and are followed by complete remission. Occasionally, these patients may develop erythema nodosum or pyoderma gangrenosum.

139. **A.** HLA-B27 is very common among patients with seronegative spondylarthropathies. Approximately 90% of patients with AS will be positive for HLA-B27. Sixty percent to 80% of patients with Reiter's syndrome, 60% of patients with spondylitis with psoriasis or IBD, and 10% of the healthy population are HLA-B27 positive.

   B. Blood culture is not likely to be positive, because this is not caused by an infectious process. Even in the presence of vertebral osteomyelitis, fewer than 50% of patients will have a positive blood culture.
   C. Rheumatoid factor can be present in a variety of conditions, with the most obvious one being RA. Again, our patient has spinal involvement, which rarely happens in RA.
   D. Anti-nuclear antibodies are present in approximately 10% of the normal population and are not useful in the diagnosis of AS. They are a very sensitive test for SLE (i.e., their absence makes SLE very unlikely), but not very specific (i.e., if they are positive, it doesn't confirm your diagnosis of SLE).
   E. Stool guaiac positivity along with clinical features of IBD may support a diagnosis of enteropathic arthropathy; however, our patient had none of these. This type of arthropathy does not give the X-ray findings typically seen in AS.

140. **E.** The incidence of spinal cord injuries in patients with AS is ten times that of the normal population. Other important associated findings/complications include uveitis and aortitis. Approximately 30% of patients with AS will develop uveitis, which presents as unilateral pain, photophobia, and lacrimation. Fortunately, only approximately 3% of patients with AS will develop aortitis, which causes aortic insufficiency and CHF.

   A, B, C, D. Nephritis, serositis, cerebritis, and cutaneous lesions are all complications of SLE, but are not associated with AS.

141. **C.** This patient has temporal headaches, jaw claudication, and amaurosis fugax, which are consistent with temporal arteritis. These patients often have scalp tenderness as well. Temporal arteritis, or giant cell arteritis, is one of the large vessel vasculitides. It is the result of the infiltration of the blood vessels arising from the aortic arch by multinucleated giant cells. This usually occurs in a patchy or segmental fashion along the artery. Patients with temporal arteritis are more often female, usually over 50 years of age, and with sedimentation rates >60. There is a strong association with polymylagia rheumatica (30% to 50% of patients). Without treatment, approximately half of the patients with temporal arteritis will progress to develop ischemic optic neuropathy with blindness (unilateral).

   A, E. The other two major types of large vessel vasculitis are Takayasu's arteritis and aortitis. Takayasu's arteritis typically affects younger women of Asian descent and results in "pulseless disease" (i.e., upper extremity claudication with arterial obstruction). They may or may not have associated Raynaud's syndrome. Aortitis is seen primarily in two conditions, ankylosing spondylitis and syphilis. Aortitis usually results in aortic insufficiency and CHF.
   B. An embolic CVA could result in ischemic optic neuritis; however, it would not account for her jaw claudication. In addition, embolic CVAs are not usually accompanied by headaches.
   D. SLE can be complicated by the development of cerebritis, which can result in a headache. However, there are often changes in mental status with cerebritis, and normally it is not accompanied by visual changes or jaw claudication.

142. **D.** This situation should be treated as a medical emergency, because the patient has started having visual involvement from her temporal arteritis. The patient should be immediately started on prednisone 60 mg per day. She should also have a biopsy of her temporal artery to confirm the diagnosis. The biopsy should be taken from a tender area of the artery, and a substantial piece should be obtained, because the disease can be patchy or segmental. Ideally, the biopsy is obtained before starting treatment; however, with visual field involvement, treatment should

not be delayed to get a biopsy. The histologic changes seen in temporal arteritis take several weeks to resolve, so the biopsy can be delayed for a short time if necessary.

A. Initiating steroid therapy and obtaining arteriography may be reasonable if you were concerned about aortitis; however, this is not the typical presentation of aortitis.

B. Anti-nuclear antibodies are not helpful in the diagnosis of temporal arteritis.

C. Obtaining a CT scan of the brain and initiating anti-platelet therapy would be reasonable if there were concern for an embolic CVA.

E. The RPR can be useful in the diagnosis of syphilis, which can cause aortitis. However, this patient doesn't have findings consistent with aortitis. Penicillin is the treatment of choice for syphilis.

143. D. Felty's syndrome is composed of the triad of RA, splenomegaly, and neutropenia. It may also be associated with anemia and thrombocytopenia. It is most often seen in patients with high rheumatoid factor titers and subcutaneous rheumatoid nodules. Patients with significant neutropenia with Felty's syndrome may develop opportunistic infections. The treatment for Felty's syndrome is basically getting control of the RA with immunosuppressant medications such as methotrexate, glucocorticoids, and sometimes, gold therapy. Methotrexate may cause neutropenia as a side effect, and it may be hard to tell if the neutropenia is due to methotrexate treatment or Felty's syndrome. Granulocyte colony stimulating factor (G-CSF) may be used to boost the white count in patients with recurrent infections. Splenectomy is reserved for patients with refractory disease.

A. It is important to understand the difference between uremia and azotemia. Azotemia is the elevation of the blood urea nitrogen, usually seen in patients with renal insufficiency. Uremia is a constellation of symptoms experienced by a patient who is severely azotemic. The symptoms of uremia are nausea, vomiting, dysgusia (which patients describe as a "metallic" taste in their mouths), encephalopathy, pericarditis, and pruritis. Neither uremia or azotemia is part of Felty's syndrome.

B. A prolonged partial thromboplastin time (aPTT) may indicate a lupus anticoagulant, a factor deficiency, or an inhibitor of the clotting cascade. It is not associated with Felty's syndrome.

C. Aspartate aminotransferase (AST) is an enzyme that may be released from hepatocytes or muscle cells when either of these tissues is injured. It is not elevated in Felty's syndrome.

E. Hyperbilirubinemia is considered either directly or indirectly, meaning that the predominant portion of the elevated bilirubin is either conjugated or unconjugated, respectively. Direct hyperbilirubinemia can be a result of obstruction of bile anywhere along the outflow tract, either intrahepatically or extrahepatically. Direct hyperbilirubinemia is not a part of Felty's syndrome.

144. B. Besides Felty's syndrome, there are numerous other extra-articular manifestations of RA. These include pericarditis, myocarditis, amyloid renal disease, keratoconjunctivitis sicca (eye dryness), scleritis, episcleritis, pleuritis, severe bronchiolitis, pulmonary interstitial fibrosis, anemia of chronic disease, vasculitis (resembles polyarteritis nodosa), and rheumatoid nodules. Of these, the nodules, severe anemia, and Felty's syndrome occur more commonly in rheumatoid factor-positive patients. Echocardiographic evidence of pericardial effusion is seen in almost 50% of RA patients who have no clinical symptoms.

A. Peptic ulcer disease is not a complication of RA itself, but may be a complication of therapy with NSAIDs. The only GI symptoms seen in RA are xerostomia in patients with associated Sjögren's disease, and intestinal ischemia in patients with associated vasculitis.

C. The anemia associated with RA is common and is a result of inflammatory cytokine-induced suppression of normal erythropoiesis resulting in anemia of chronic disease.

D. Glomerular disease resulting in proteinuria is uncommon in RA (whereas it is very common in SLE). Proteinuria may rarely occur in RA secondary to amyloid-induced renal disease, or it may more commonly occur secondary to drug therapy such as penicillamine or gold.

E. Pulmonary extra-articular manifestations of RA are common and include pleuritis with pleural effusion and interstitial fibrosis. Autopsy findings confirm histologic evidence of interstitial lung disease in most patients with RA, most of whom were never symptomatic. Spontaneous pneumothorax is an extremely rare complication.

145. **B. Methotrexate works by interfering with the cellular use of folic acid. The depletion of folic acid in rapidly dividing cells is thought to be responsible for the symptoms of stomatitis, alopecia, diarrhea, and bone marrow suppression. Patients with low baseline levels of folic acid before initiation of treatment with methotrexate may experience more of the toxicities of therapy. Furthermore, many studies have found that these side effects may be ameliorated by adding folate to the patient's medication regimen without significantly affecting the efficacy of therapy.**

A. A rash may occur within days of each weekly dose of methotrexate and may clear before the next week's dose. Some patients may develop photosensitivity on the drug. These skin reactions are not significantly changed by the addition of folate therapy.
C. Interstitial lung disease from pneumonitis (that may progress to fibrosis) occurs in 3% to 5% of RA patients who are on methotrexate therapy, and is unrelated to folic acid depletion. A new cough in patients on methotrexate therapy needs to be completely evaluated for the possibility of lung-related toxicity. It can be confusing to know whether the patient's interstitial lung disease is related to the methotrexate or to the underlying RA. An open lung biopsy may be required to determine the etiology of the patient's disease.
D. Liver injury also may be seen with methotrexate therapy and is unrelated to folic acid depletion. Patients on methotrexate should have their liver enzymes followed regularly, and some advocate periodic liver biopsies to assess for possible liver damage.
E. Folate supplementation does not reverse or lessen the teratogenic effects of methotrexate therapy. Women of child-bearing age should not be given methotrexate therapy unless they completely understand the risks to an unborn fetus and comply with contraception. It is recommended that both men and women be off of methotrexate therapy for at least 3 months before conception to decrease the risks of teratogenicity.

146. **B. The clinical presentation of aplastic anemia can include fatigue and pallor due to anemia, mucosal bleeding due to thrombocytopenia, and recurrent infections due to neutropenia. Peripheral blood counts will reveal pancytopenia with a normocytic anemia and poor reticulocyte count. Bone marrow aspirate shows all cell lines to be hypocellular with increased bone marrow fat cells. The causes of aplastic anemia include chemicals such as benzene and arsenic; drugs such as chloramphenicol and carbonic anhydrase inhibitors; and viral infections including cytomegalovirus, Epstein-Barr virus, and parvovirus. In many cases of aplastic anemia, a cause is never established. The ultimate cure is a bone marrow transplant.**

A. Myelodysplastic syndromes have a clinical presentation that is similar to that of aplastic anemia, because both cause pancytopenia. However, myelodysplastic syndromes cause abnormal features of the cells that can be seen on the peripheral smear. In addition, bone marrow aspirate usually reveals hypercellularity with dysplasia of marrow precursor cells. Myelodysplastic syndromes are more common in elderly patients. The only definitive cure is chemotherapy followed by bone marrow transplant.
C. Paroxysmal nocturnal hemoglobinuria is also included in the differential of pancytopenia. It is an uncommon disease that includes chronic hemolytic anemia, pancytopenia, and thrombophilia. Cells are predisposed to lysis because of a defective membrane protein.
D. Chronic myelogenous leukemia can cause anemia; however, leukocyte count is typically elevated. Acute leukemias are more likely to cause pancytopenia.
E. Severe folate deficiency can cause pancytopenia. The anemia caused by folate deficiency is megaloblastic with MCV values above 100 fL. Hypersegmented neutrophils should also be seen on peripheral blood smear with folate deficiency.

147. **C. Phlebotomy is the treatment of choice for polycythemia vera. The treatment consists of phlebotomy once or twice weekly until the patient is iron deficient and hemoglobin is <14 g/dL. Hydroxyurea can also be used in conjunction with phlebotomy to control blood counts.**

    A. A low-to-normal serum erythropoetin level is consistent with polycythemia vera. An elevated level can be seen in secondary erthyrocytosis due to pulmonary disease, smoking, or sleep apnea.

    B. RBC mass studies can be useful in confirming the diagnosis of polycythemia vera. RBC mass is elevated in polycythemia vera, but not in other myeloproliferative disorders. It cannot distinguish polycythemia vera from secondary erythrocytosis, because RBC mass can be elevated in both.

    D. Splenomegaly is a common physical exam finding in polycythemia vera occurring in nearly 70% of patients. It does not necessarily indicate an underlying leukemia. Patients with polycythemia vera do have a 2% to 5% lifetime risk of leukemic transformation, but splenomegaly is not a specific physical finding to indicate this transformation.

    E. Fifty percent to 60% of patients have an elevated platelet count. Forty percent to 50% of patients have an elevated WBC count.

148. **D. The smear in Figure 1-148 shows a macrocytic anemia. Patients with Crohn's disease often have inflammation of the distal ileum where B12 is absorbed, leading to the deficiency. A B12 level can be obtained to confirm the diagnosis.**

    A. Patients with Crohn's disease can have iron-deficiency anemia due to iron malabsorption with duodenal involvement, or due to chronic GI bleeding. However, iron deficiency causes a microcytic anemia, and Figure 1-148 shows a macrocytic anemia.

    B. Anemia secondary to blood loss, if acute, is typically normocytic. If the blood loss is chronic, a microcytic anemia can be seen due to iron deficiency. This patient has a macrocytic anemia.

    C. Anemia of chronic disease can be seen in Crohn's disease, but it will be a microcytic or normocytic anemia.

    E. Folate deficiency is a macrocytic anemia. However, folate deficiency is not typically seen in patients with Crohn's disease.

149. **C. Iron-deficiency anemia is treated most commonly with ferrous sulfate. The reticulocyte count can be expected to increase within 7 to 10 days after starting iron therapy. Hemoglobin levels increase over the first month of treatment with an increase of 2 g/dL being considered an adequate response to treatment. It is important, however, to determine whether a patient has iron deficiency before putting them on iron supplements.**

    A. In iron-deficiency anemia, iron studies show low iron, high total iron binding capacity, and low ferritin. The profile shown of low iron, low total iron binding capacity, and high ferritin is consistent with anemia of chronic disease.

    B. The most common cause of iron-deficiency anemia is blood loss either from the GI tract or from menstrual bleeding. Intake of iron is adequate for most people, with the exception of pregnant women and toddlers.

    D. Pica (which means eating "non-nutritive" substances) occurs in over 50% of patients with untreated iron-deficiency anemia. The word specific for ice craving is "pagophagia."

    E. Ferritin is an acute phase reactant and is affected by acute illness, infectious processes, and chronic diseases. Therefore, if the other iron studies indicate the presence of an iron-deficiency anemia, an elevated ferritin should not be used to eliminate the diagnosis.

150. **B. This patient has a history and peripheral smear that indicate hereditary spherocytosis. This is the most common hemolytic anemia due to an RBC membrane defect. Inheritance is autosomal dominant. Patients with a milder form can present into early adulthood with anemia and cholelithiasis. Typical laboratory findings include anemia with elevated reticulocyte count. MCV is usually not helpful, but the mean corpuscular hemoglobin concentration (MCHC) and red cell distribution width (RDW) can be elevated. Peripheral smear will show spherocytes with hemolytic cell fragments as depicted in Figure 1-150. Diagnosis should be confirmed with the osmotic fragility test. In this test, RBCs are placed**

in progressively more dilute saline solutions. Spherocytes hemolyze at hypotonic concentrations at which normal cells survive.

A. Bone marrow biopsy is not necessary. The diagnosis can be obtained through clinical history, peripheral smear, and osmotic fragility testing.

C. History and peripheral smear are not consistent with G6PD deficiency. There is no history of a new medication, infection, or other offending agent in this patient.

D. Splenectomy may be indicated in this patient for future treatment, but should not be done before the diagnosis is confirmed. It is indicated in patients with moderate to severe anemia who require multiple transfusion therapies. The risk of splenectomy is later development of infection and sepsis with encapsulated organisms. All patients who receive a splenectomy should receive pneumococcal, haemophilus, and meningococcal vaccines a few weeks before surgery.

E. IgG and IgM autoantibody levels could be obtained if immune-mediated hemolytic anemia were suspected. History and peripheral smear do not suggest this diagnosis.

BLOCK 4

151. You are seeing a new patient in your clinic who comes to establish care. He is a 24-year-old man from the Mediterranean region with a history of anemia since childhood. You consider the possibility of a hemolytic anemia. Which of the following statements is true regarding hemolytic anemia?

    A. Hemolytic anemia occurs only when there is destruction of the erythrocyte by an antibody
    B. Direct bilirubin and haptoglobin levels are elevated
    C. Pyruvate kinase deficiency is the most common cause of enzyme deficiency hemolysis in RBCs
    D. IgG antibodies are associated with cold autoimmune hemolytic anemia
    E. Glucose 6-phosphate dehydrogenase (G6PD) deficiency is an X-linked disorder that induces hemolysis after exposure to oxidant drugs

152. A 25-year-old black man with sickle cell anemia presents with 1 day of chest pain, cough, and fever. Physical examination is remarkable for tachypnea with oxygen saturations of 88% on room air, tachycardia, and diminished breath sounds in the right lower lobe. A chest X-ray reveals a new infiltrate in the right lower lobe. Which of the following is the most appropriate next step in the management of acute chest syndrome?

    A. Start IV heparin protocol
    B. Begin ceftriaxone and azithromycin
    C. Exchange transfusion
    D. Limited supplemental oxygen to keep paO_2 at 70
    E. Aggressive IV fluid hydration

153. A 28-year-old previously healthy woman presents with petechiae and epistaxis for the last 2 weeks. She denies fatigue, fever, weight loss, or any other associated symptoms. She takes no medications and has no significant past medical history. Physical examination is notable for scattered petechiae over the lower and upper extremities. No hepatosplenomegaly or mucous membrane lesions are noted. Labs are as follows: WBCs 8200/μL; differential normal; hemoglobin 15.4 g/dL; hematocrit 36%; platelets 14,000/μL; PT 12.1 seconds; PTT 21 seconds; bleeding time 2 minutes. The most likely diagnosis is:

    A. Drug-induced thrombocytopenia
    B. Acute immune thrombocytopenia
    C. Von Willebrand's disease
    D. Hemophilia A
    E. Hypersplenism

The response options for items 154 through 157 are the same. You will be required to select one answer for each item in the set.

    A. Von Willebrand's disease
    B. Hemophilia A
    C. Vitamin K deficiency
    D. Disseminated intravascular coagulation (DIC)
    E. Hemophilia B

For each of the laboratory results, select the most likely clinical syndrome.

154. Prolonged prothrombin time (PT) that corrects when mixed with normal plasma; decreased factor VII; and prolonged PTT if severe

155. Slightly elevated activated partial thromboplastin time (aPTT); prolonged bleeding time; low factor VIII

156. Prolonged PTT; prolonged PT; low fibrinogen

157. Prolonged PTT; normal bleeding time; low factor VII

End of Set

158. A 28-year-old woman with a history of SLE presents with shortness of breath and pleuritic chest pain that was acute in onset 4 hours ago. She has had two pregnancies complicated by spontaneous abortions in the first trimester. On physical examination she is tachypneic and tachycardic, and oxygen saturations are 85% on room air. Pulmonary examination reveals no focal crackles, wheezes, or other abnormalities. Arterial blood gas shows a respiratory alkalosis with hypoxia. Which of the following would be the most likely laboratory finding in this patient?

A. No correction of prolonged aPTT with addition of normal patient plasma serum
B. Normal aPTT time
C. Elevated platelet count
D. Elevated PT
E. Negative anti-cardiolipin antibody

159. A 32-year-old white man with no significant past medical history presents with a 3-day history of right calf swelling and warmth. He completed a cross-country car trip 2 days ago. He denies shortness of breath, chest pain, or any other symptoms. The patient's father has a history of recurrent deep venous thrombosis (DVT) with pulmonary embolism. Physical examination is normal except for significant swelling of the right calf with a palpable cord. The patient is admitted and an evaluation for hypercoagulable state is begun. The most likely underlying disorder in this patient would be:

A. Protein C deficiency
B. Antithrombin deficiency
C. Anti-phospholipid syndrome
D. Malignancy
E. Factor V Leiden defect

160. A 63-year-old woman presents to your office for preoperative evaluation for a total knee replacement. Her past medical history is significant only for osteoarthritis for which she takes non-steroidal anti-inflammatory drugs (NSAIDs). She is concerned about the possibility of a blood transfusion either during the surgery or during the postoperative period. She asks about the risks of transfusion therapy. Which of the following is a true statement regarding transfusion therapy?

A. The patient should be transfused for a hemoglobin of 10 g/dL
B. Acute hemolytic transfusion reactions occur primarily in patients who have had many transfusions
C. HIV is the most common viral infection that can be acquired from a transfusion
D. The risk of acquiring hepatitis C from a blood transfusion is approximately 1:100,000 units of blood transfused
E. Delayed transfusion reaction is usually due to ABO incompatibility

The next two questions (items 161 and 162) correspond to the following vignette.

A 45-year-old white woman comes to your office for a new-patient visit. She denies any current concerns or complaints. She has no past medical history except for obesity. She has a family history of type II diabetes. She denies tobacco use and IV drug use. She drinks socially once or twice per month. She is interested in starting an exercise regimen and diet. On exam the patient is afebrile, pulse is 90, respiratory rate 18, blood pressure 125/76, and BMI 31. In general she is obese, in no acute distress. Exam is essentially within normal limits with the exception of the following skin findings seen in Figure 1-161.

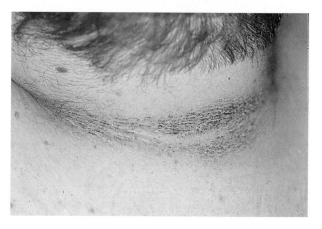

Figure 1-161 • Image Courtesy of Dr. Robert Raschke, Banner Good Samaritan Medical Center, Phoenix, Arizona.

161. This skin finding is called:

A. Acanthosis nigricans
B. Necrobiosis lipoidica
C. Granuloma annulare
D. Tinea corporis
E. Carotenodermia

162. You are concerned that this patient may have type II diabetes. Which of the following values confirms the diagnosis of diabetes?

A. A random plasma glucose >190 mg/dL
B. A fasting plasma glucose >126 mg/dL
C. A 2-hour plasma glucose concentration >140 mg/dL during an oral glucose tolerance test
D. A hemoglobin A1C >7.0
E. Ketosis and an anion gap acidosis

End of Set

163. A 32-year-old white woman presents to your office with amenorrhea. She states she is not sexually active. She has had regular periods for

most of her life until recently. She also notes the recent onset of headaches that are frontal and constant in nature. She does not note any visual changes. Physical exam is essentially normal with the exception of galactorrhea. A pregnancy test is negative and prolactin level is 500 ng/mL. The next diagnostic step in this patient is:

A. CT of the brain
B. MRI of the brain
C. Skull films
D. Review of the patient's medication list
E. A bromocriptine trial

164. A 24-year-old white woman presents to your office with symptoms of weight loss and diarrhea, and complaints of sweating. These symptoms have progressed for approximately 1 month. She denies any past medical history. She also denies any tobacco, alcohol, or drug use. She currently takes no medications or herbs and family history is noncontributory. On physical exam the patient is afebrile, thin appearing with stable vital signs. HEENT is notable for lid lag bilaterally, and neck exam is notable for thyromegaly without bruit or obvious nodule. Heart and lung exams are within normal limits. Neurologic exam is significant for hyperreflexia throughout. Skin is noted to be warm with fine hair throughout. The most likely cause of this patient's symptoms is:

A. Subacute thyroiditis
B. Toxic adenoma
C. Addison's disease
D. Hashimoto's thyroiditis
E. Graves' disease

165. A 19-year-old white man is brought to your office by his parents. They are concerned that he has become more distant. He has lost 20 pounds in the last 4 months and has intermittent abdominal pain and nausea. He has also complained of increasing fatigue. He denies any past medical problems, tobacco, alcohol, or drug use. On physical exam, his heart rate is 110, respiratory rate 18, blood pressure 90/60, and oxygen saturations are 99 percent on room air. On exam he appears thin and withdrawn. His lungs are clear and his heart is tachycardic without murmurs. His abdomen is soft without hepatosplenomegaly. He appears slightly tanned, especially in his palmar creases. You order basic labs that reveal the following: WBC

6000/µL; eosinophils 5%; hemoglobin 14 g/dL; sodium 130 mEq/dL; potassium 5.8 mEq/dL; chloride 107 mEq/dL; bicarbonate 24 mEq/L; BUN 18 mg/dL; creatinine 0.8 mg/dL; glucose 68 mg/dL. What is the most likely diagnosis?

A. Hyperthyroidism
B. Hypothyroidism
C. Primary hypoadrenalism
D. Secondary hypoadrenalism
E. Hyperaldosteronism

166. A 35-year-old white woman presents to your office with complaints of irregular menses. She started menstruating at age 15. Her periods have always been irregular, occurring every 28 to 50 days. She is currently trying to get pregnant and has been trying for more than 3 years. She is on phenobarbital for a seizure disorder. She denies any illicit drug, alcohol, or tobacco use. Her vital signs are within normal limits. Her BMI is 28. Physical exam is notable for dark hair on her upper lips, arms, and abdomen. She has mild acne on her face and her upper back. Initial CBC and pregnancy tests are both within normal limits. TSH is 3.5 mU/L and free T4 is normal. The most likely cause of her hirsutism is:

A. Idiopathic hirsutism
B. Polycystic ovarian syndrome
C. Pituitary neoplasm
D. Phenobarbital
E. Hypothyroidism

167. A 75-year-old Hispanic man was recently seen in the ED for complaints of fatigue, weight loss of 15 pounds in 6 months, and cough. He has brought the results of basic labs taken at that time to your office and wants you to interpret the results. The patient has a past medical history significant for hypertension on a β-blocker and a smoking history of one pack per day for 40 years. Vitals are within normal limits with the exception of a respiratory rate of 24 and saturations of 90% on room air. Exam is significant for a thin man in no acute distress. Lung exam is significant for decreased breath sounds at the left lung base. The rest of his exam is essentially normal. The labs values are: Sodium 140 mEq/dL; potassium 4.6 mEq/dL; chloride 105 mEq/dL; bicarbonate 23 mEq/L; BUN 27 mg/dL; creatinine 1.1 mg/dL; glucose 80 mg/dL; calcium 12.5 mg/dL. The most likely etiology for this man's laboratory abnormality is:

A. Parathyroid adenoma
B. Sarcoidosis
C. Squamous cell lung carcinoma
D. β-blocker
E. Thyrotoxicosis

A. Glucocorticoid
B. Furosemide
C. Bisphosphonate
D. Calcitonin
E. Normal saline bolus

168. A 24-year-old white woman presents to your office with complaints of palpitations, shaking hands, and sweatiness. She states the symptoms started about 1 hour ago. You quickly review her chart and see that she has a medical history significant for depression and one suicide attempt 5 years ago. She denies any ingestions, drug, alcohol, or tobacco use. Her family history is significant for depression and type I diabetes in a 14-year-old sister. Her vital signs are within normal limits, but she is pale and diaphoretic. You check a glucose level and it is 30 mg/dL. As you replete her glucose stores, you order some lab tests. Which would be the most helpful in determining the etiology of her hypoglycemia?

A. Insulin level
B. C-peptide level
C. Sulfonylurea level
D. Liver enzyme tests (AST and ALT)
E. Thyroid function tests

169. A 36-year-old white woman comes to your office with her husband. He states that for the last few days she has been complaining of diffuse abdominal pain and bone pain. Today he noted that she was acting a bit confused. She has a past medical history significant for hypertension for which she takes a thiazide diuretic. This has never happened before and he denies any alcohol, drug, or tobacco use. She has not had any fevers or chills, nausea, vomiting, or diarrhea. He thinks she has been constipated lately. On exam, temperature is 98.8°F (37.1°C), heart rate 80, respiratory rate 16, blood pressure 140/80, and oxygen saturations 99% on room air. Abdominal exam is significant for mild left lower quadrant pain to deep palpation. On neurologic exam, cranial nerves II through XII are intact, and muscle strength and sensorium are intact. Deep tendon reflexes are diminished throughout. You order basic labs, which reveal the following: CBC normal; sodium 140 mEq/L; potassium 4.6 mEq/L; chloride 108 mEq/L; bicarbonate 24 mEq/L; BUN 28 mg/dL; creatinine 0.8 mg/dL; glucose 90 mg/dL; calcium 13.0 mg/dL. The next step in the treatment of this patient is:

170. A 55-year-old white man comes to your office for a routine check-up. He currently has no complaints. He has well-controlled hypertension on a β-blocker and a history of gout controlled with NSAIDs. His exam is essentially within normal limits. You note that he has not had his cholesterol level checked in the last 5 years. The fasting lipid panel reveals: LDL 116 mg/dL; HDL 50 mg/dL; triglycerides 600 mg/dL. You decide to start him on a fibrate. The mechanism by which this medication works is:

A. Reduces secretion of very low-density lipoprotein (VLDL), increased stimulation of lipoprotein lipase
B. Reduces intrahepatic cholesterol, leading to increases in LDL receptor turnover
C. Inhibits production of VLDL, reduces transfer of HDL to VLDL
D. Binds bile acids in the intestine, thus lowering the cholesterol pool
E. Impairs dietary cholesterol absorption at the intestinal brush border

The response options for items 171 through 175 are the same. You will be required to select one answer for each item in the set.

A. Elevated calcium, low phosphate, elevated parathyroid hormone (PTH)
B. Elevated calcium, variable phosphate, low PTH
C. Low calcium, elevated phosphate, low PTH
D. Low calcium, elevated phosphate, elevated PTH
E. Low or normal calcium, low phosphate, elevated PTH

For each disease state, select the most appropriate laboratory findings.

171. Vitamin D deficiency

172. Malignancy

173. Hypoparathyroidism

174. Pseudohypoparathyroidism

175. Hyperparathyroidism

End of Set

176. A 65-year-old Hispanic man comes to your office with concerns regarding his sexual function. He states that he has had no difficulty obtaining erections until the last couple of months. He denies any recent psychosocial stressors and tells you that he has occasionally awakened with an erection during this time period. He has a past medical history significant for hypertension and is taking a thiazide diuretic. His physical exam is essentially within normal limits, including normal testicular size and firmness and a positive cremasteric reflex. What is the most likely cause of his erectile dysfunction?

   A. Neurogenic
   B. Vascular
   C. Medication induced
   D. Depression
   E. Hypogonadism

The response options for items 177 through 180 are the same. You will be required to select one answer for each item in the set.

   A. Anti-phospholipid antibody syndrome
   B. DIC
   C. Von Willebrand's disease
   D. Hemophilia A
   E. Hemophilia B

For each clinical scenario, select the most appropriate laboratory results.

177. A 36-year-old gravida 2 para 0 woman presents with new DVT. Laboratories show thrombocytopenia and an elevated PTT that does not correct when mixed with normal plasma. PT is normal.

178. A 17-year-old man presents with right knee hemarthrosis. Laboratories show prolonged PTT, normal PT, normal bleeding time, and low factor IX.

179. A 28-year-old woman presents with menorrhagia and easy bruising. Laboratories show slightly elevated aPTT, prolonged bleeding time, and low factor VIII.

180. A 76-year-old man is admitted to the intensive care unit for urosepsis. Laboratories show prolonged PTT, prolonged PT, decreased platelets, and low fibrinogen.

End of Set

The response options for items 181 through 185 are the same. You will be required to select one answer for each item in the set.

   A. Multiple myeloma
   B. Primary hyperparathyroidism
   C. Familial hypocalciuric hypercalcemia
   D. Sarcoidosis
   E. Squamous cell carcinoma

For each disease, select the associated mechanism of hypercalcemia.

181. Excessive secretion of PTH by a parathyroid adenoma or by parathyroid hyperplasia

182. Excessive renal tubular absorption of calcium and magnesium

183. Parathyroid hormone-related protein (PTH-rP) production

184. Elevated concentrations of 1,25-dihydroxyvitamin D secondary to the excessive conversion of 25-hydroxyvitamin D to 1,25-dihydroxyvitamin D (the active metabolite)

185. Cytokine-mediated activation of osteoclasts, which resorb bone

End of Set

The response options for items 186 through 190 are the same. You will be required to select one answer for each item in the set.

   A. Ginkgo biloba
   B. Echinacea
   C. Ginseng
   D. Saw palmetto
   E. St. John's Wort

For each disorder, select the most commonly used herbal medication.

186. Benign prostatic hypertrophy (BPH)

187. Depression

188. Dementia

189. Respiratory infections

190. Fatigue

End of Set

The response options for items 191 through 193 are the same. You will be required to select one answer for each item in the set.

    A. Initiate drug therapy
    B. Initiate diet therapy
    C. No therapy

For each clinical scenario, select the appropriate management. Each answer may be used more than once.

191. A 56-year-old white man with a past medical history significant for hypertension comes to your office for a routine follow-up. His blood pressure is fairly well controlled. Exam is essentially within normal limits. You order basic labs and note an LDL of 176 mg/dL.

192. A 45-year-old Hispanic woman comes to your office for a well woman exam. She has no significant past medical history. She is active and denies any tobacco, alcohol, or drug use. Her mother has been told she has elevated cholesterol, and the patient would like to be checked. Her LDL is 170 mg/dL.

193. A 65-year-old white woman with a recent myocardial infarction comes to your office for a post-hospitalization checkup. Her current medications include a β-blocker, an angiotensin-converting enzyme (ACE) inhibitor, and aspirin. A check of her cholesterol reveals an LDL of 130 mg/dL.

End of Set

The response options for items 194 through 199 are the same. You will be required to select one answer for each item in the set.

    A. Perifollicular purpura
    B. Perifollicular hyperkeratosis
    C. Hypopigmented macules and patches on flexural skin areas
    D. Alopecia
    E. Erythema, edema, blisters, and bullae of the dorsa of the hands
    F. Angular stomatitis
    G. Seborrhea

For each vitamin deficiency, select the most likely skin finding.

194. Vitamin A

195. Vitamin B3 (niacin)

196. Vitamin B2 (riboflavin)

197. Vitamin B12 (cyanocobalamin)

198. Vitamin C

199. Vitamin B6 (pyridoxine)

End of Set

---

200. A 50-year-old Hispanic man with a history of hypertension comes to your office as a new patient. He has no complaints, but his family history is significant for several members with type II diabetes mellitus, and he is concerned that he also might develop the disease. On physical exam, his blood pressure is 140/90 and other vital signs are within normal limits. His BMI is 32 and you note a velvety dark pigment on the back of his neck and his axillary regions. His fasting glucose is 149 and 151 on two separate evaluations. What is the appropriate management for this patient with newly diagnosed diabetes?

A. Diet and exercise therapy alone
B. Diet and exercise, begin metformin as monotherapy
C. Diet and exercise, begin a sulfonylurea as monotherapy
D. Diet and exercise, begin long-acting lantus insulin as monotherapy
E. Confirm the diagnosis with an elevated hemoglobin A1C

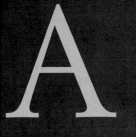

A Answers and Explanations

151. E	168. B	185. A
152. A	169. E	186. D
153. B	170. A	187. E
154. C	171. E	188. A
155. A	172. B	189. B
156. D	173. C	190. C
157. B	174. D	191. A
158. A	175. A	192. B
159. E	176. C	193. A
160. D	177. A	194. B
161. A	178. E	195. E
162. B	179. C	196. F
163. B	180. B	197. C
164. E	181. B	198. A
165. C	182. C	199. G
166. B	183. E	200. B
167. C	184. D	

151. **E.** G6PD deficiency is the most common enzymatic deficiency in RBCs. It can induce a hemolytic anemia after exposure to oxidant drugs such as sulfa, dapsone, and primaquine. Hemolysis can also be induced by infection and other agents, including fava beans.

    A. Hemolytic anemia can be caused by membrane defects, enzyme abnormalities, hemoglobinopathies, immune or autoimmune processes, or drugs.

    B. Laboratory findings in hemolytic anemia include an elevated reticulocyte count, an elevated indirect bilirubin, an elevated lactate dehydrogenase level, and a decreased haptoglobin.

    C. G6PD deficiency is the most common RBC enzymatic defect.

    D. IgM antibodies are associated with cold autoimmune hemolytic anemia. IgG antibodies are associated with warm autoimmune hemolytic anemia. You can remember this as follows: When I am *warm*, I want a *glass* of iced tea (Warm: IgG); when I am *cold*, I want a *mug* of hot cocoa (Cold: IgM). In both disorders, 50% of the patients have an underlying disorder such as AIDS, systemic lupus erythematosus (SLE), or inflammatory bowel disease.

152. **B.** The cause of acute chest syndrome is not fully known. Both infection and infarction have been indicated as possible causes. Therefore, it is appropriate to treat the patient for both community-acquired organisms and atypical pneumonias.

    A. Anticoagulation therapy should be started only if there is a documented thromboembolic event.

    C. Exchange transfusion is indicated in acute chest syndrome if there are progressive infiltrates on the chest X-ray or progressive hypoxia.

    D. Supplemental oxygen is necessary to prevent further sickling. PaO_2 should be maintained above 70, and brought to 100 if possible.

    E. IV fluid hydration is important in the management of acute chest syndrome, but should be monitored closely. Fluid hydration that is too aggressive can lead to pulmonary edema.

153. **B.** This patient has a low platelet count with no other associated cytopenias. There is no history of medications or other underlying illnesses. Immune thrombocytopenia is a diagnosis of exclusion. It is due to anti-platelet antibodies directed against membrane proteins. The process can be self-limited, or it can reoccur and become chronic. Treatment includes steroids, IV immune globulin (IVIG), and possible splenectomy if other treatments fail.

    A. Drug-induced thrombocytopenia is due to a medication that causes destruction of platelets. Heparin is the most well-known offending drug. It causes platelet destruction by heparin-dependent antibodies that act against platelets.

    C. Von Willebrand's disease is an autosomal-dominant inherited disorder of hemostasis. It affects platelet function, but does not affect platelet count.

    D. Hemophilia A is an X-linked inherited bleeding disorder. It does not affect platelet count. Partial thromboplastin time is prolonged. Patients usually present with prolonged bleeding, hematomas, or hemarthrosis.

    E. Hypersplenism can cause decreased platelet count, leading to petechiae. This patient does not have a palpable spleen on exam and has no underlying diagnosis that would account for an enlarged spleen.

154. **C.** Vitamin K deficiency initially prolongs PT with decreased factor VII levels. As other factors begin to decrease, the PTT will also prolong. Vitamin K-dependent factors include factors II, VII, IX, and X; protein C; and protein S. Replacement with vitamin K will correct the coagulopathy.

155. **A.** Von Willebrand's disease is the most common inherited bleeding disorder. Patients usually have easy bruising, nosebleeds, menorrhagia, or prolonged bleeding with trauma. Von Willebrand factor plays a critical role in platelet function and is also a carrier protein for factor VIII. Defective von Willebrand factor can therefore decrease factor VIII and prolong PTT.

156. **D.** DIC is triggered by systemic illness and can be a catastrophic hematologic event. Possible associations with DIC include sepsis, trauma,

malignancy, and burns. Initially, fibrinogen and platelets are consumed in clot formation. This is later followed by hemorrhage as the clots are degraded by fibrinolysis.

157. **B. Hemophilia A is an X-linked inherited bleeding disorder. Patients usually present with prolonged bleeding, hematomas, or hemarthrosis. In hemophilia A, factor VIII is deficient.**

    E. Hemophilia B is due to a factor IX deficiency. (It is also called "Christmas disease.") Patients present with varying degrees of bleeding secondary to the deficient factor IX. This is also an X-linked recessive disease like hemophilia A.

158. **A. This patient has anti-phospholipid antibody syndrome. Patients with this syndrome have antibodies directed toward certain phospholipid-bound plasma proteins that are involved in the coagulation pathway. Patients are predisposed to recurrent arterial and venous clot formation as well as fetal loss. This syndrome is more commonly seen in patients with autoimmune syndromes, but can also be associated with malignancies, infections, and some drugs. Laboratory testing includes lupus anticoagulant. The patient's serum is mixed with normal patient serum to see if the aPTT corrects. If no correction is seen, the test is positive for lupus anticoagulant, indicating that the patient has the syndrome.**

    B. Activated PTT can be normal in anti-phospholipid antibody syndrome, but typically is elevated.
    C. Thrombocytopenia is associated with this syndrome.
    D. PT is not affected by the lupus anticoagulant.
    E. Anti-cardiolipin is one of the anti-phospholipid antibodies and can be positive in this syndrome. It is detected by enzyme-linked immunosorbent assay (ELISA).

159. **E. Factor V Leiden defect is the most common inherited hypercoagulable state accounting for nearly 50% of inherited thrombophilic disorders. Estimated prevalence of the defect is 2% to 5%, with whites having the highest prevalence. The risk of venous thrombosis in patients who are heterozygous for this defect is approx-** imately seven times that of persons without the defect. Several factors should alert the clinician to an underlying defect, including family history of thrombosis, age of first thrombotic event <50, and recurrent thrombotic events.

    A. Protein C deficiency is less common, with a prevalence of less than 1%. Protein C, once activated, breaks down factors V and VIII. This deficiency is associated with a high incidence of thrombosis, even among patients who are heterozygous. Most patients present in their 20s or 30s with a venous thromboembolism.
    B. Antithrombin inactivates procoagulant factors including factors II, IX, and X. Initial presentation with thrombosis typically occurs before age 50. This defect also has a prevalence of less than 1%.
    C. Anti-phospholipid antibodies occur in 2% to 5% of otherwise healthy people, but are most frequent in patients with autoimmune disorders such as SLE. Patients with this syndrome are at risk for both venous and arterial thromboembolisms.
    D. Malignancy is a risk factor for hypercoagulable state; however, this patient has no history to suggest this as an underlying diagnosis.

160. **D. Hepatitis C is the second most common viral infection that can be acquired from blood transfusion. Hepatitis B is the most common with a risk of 1:60,000 units transfused. Although all blood is screened for infection, current screening methods do not detect early stages or some subclinical infections.**

    A. There is no evidence to support transfusion of an asymptomatic patient with no underlying cardiovascular disease based solely on the hemoglobin level.
    B. Acute hemolytic transfusion reactions are serious and life-threatening, and can occur in any patient receiving a blood transfusion. Acute hemolytic transfusion reactions are due to ABO incompatibility. Symptoms include fever and back pain with development of renal failure.
    C. Hepatitis B and C have a higher transmission rate than HIV. The risk of acquiring HIV from a blood transfusion is 1:500,000 units transfused.

E. Delayed transfusion reactions are seen in patients who have developed autoantibodies due to prior transfusion or pregnancy. Rh, Kidd, Duffy, and Kell are the typical antigens to which the antibodies are directed. Onset of delayed transfusion reaction can occur by 5 to 10 days after transfusion and manifests with fever, jaundice, and anemia due to extravascular hemolysis.

161. **A. Acanthosis nigricans is a common manifestation of insulin resistance, often seen in patients with type II diabetes. It is a nonspecific skin reaction that presents with symmetric brown thickening of the skin. Acanthosis can develop a warty-like appearance and is typically found in the axilla, neck flexures, and groin. It is also seen in syndromes of excess steroid, in obesity, and in other endocrine disorders.**

B. Necrobiosis lipoidica is unknown in its origin, but approximately 50% of patients with this condition have diabetes. It usually appears before the onset of diabetes in the third or fourth decade in women. Lesions are oval, violaceous patches that have a red, slowly expanding border. The central portion of the lesion is brown with telangiectasias.

C. Granuloma annulare is a ring-shaped, firm, flesh-colored papule. It is usually found on the lateral and dorsal portions of the hands and feet. Isolated lesions have no association with diabetes, but disseminated lesions do. These lesions usually spontaneously involute.

D. Tinea corporis is a fungal infection of the skin. Diabetics do have a predisposition to fungal infections, but more often in the form of thrush.

E. Carotenodermia is the yellowing of skin seen in diabetes.

162. **B. Diagnostic criteria for diabetes include any one of the following: 1) a fasting blood sugar ≥126 mg/dl on two separate occasions; 2) a random blood sugar ≥200 mg/dl in a patient with symptoms of diabetes such as polyuria, polydipsia, and weight loss; and 3) a 2-hour plasma glucose concentration of >200 mg/dL during a glucose tolerance test.**

A. This value is incorrect. See explanation for B.

C. A 2-hour plasma glucose tolerance test may be used when a patient does not have a fasting blood sugar >126 mg/dL, but there is still concern for diabetes. An oral glucose load of 75 g is given to the patient, and blood sugar is measured at 1 and 2 hours. A blood sugar >140 mg/dL and <200 mg/dL at the 2-hour mark constitutes "glucose intolerance," but not frank diabetes. These patients are at risk for the development of overt diabetes and should be monitored carefully.

D. Hemoglobin A1C, or glycosylated hemoglobin, is currently not used as a diagnostic criterion for diabetes, because standardization of these tests is lacking between laboratories. Variation in A1C numbers can also be seen in various states of anemia (iron deficiency, hemolysis) and in end-stage renal disease.

E. Ketosis and an anion gap acidosis does not diagnose diabetes. It may be due to alcoholism or starvation as well as insulin deficiency states, and is differentiated from diabetic ketoacidosis by the normal or low blood sugar seen in this entity. There is also a higher ratio of acetoacetate to beta-hydroxybutyrate seen in alcoholic or starvation ketoacidosis versus diabetic ketoacidosis.

163. **B. MRI is the preferred imaging test to evaluate a patient for a prolactinoma. Prolactinomas are the most common pituitary tumor, and present in women with symptoms of oligomenorrhea, amenorrhea, and galactorrhea. Microadenomas are lesions <1 cm, and macroadenomas are >1 cm.**

A. CT of the head is not the first-line choice in patients with elevated prolactin levels and symptoms of hyperprolactinemia; MRI can better evaluate the hypothalamic/pituitary stalk for masses.

C. Plain skull films cannot help in the evaluation of a hypothalamic/pituitary mass.

D. It is always essential to search for other causes of high prolactin levels, such as hypothyroidism, dopamine-antagonist drugs such as antiemetics and antipsychotics, and pregnancy. Usually, however, a patient with a prolactin level >300 ng/mL will have a prolactin-secreting tumor.

E. Dopamine agonists such as bromocriptine decrease the prolactin level whether the cause of elevated prolactin is a prolactin-secreting tumor or there is a secondary cause. Therefore, it is not helpful to use bromocriptine to diagnose a prolactinoma. Bromocriptine is the primary therapy for prolactinomas. Side effects include nausea, vomiting, and orthostatic hypotension, which can make it hard to tolerate. Some patients who cannot tolerate the GI side effects can use an intravaginal preparation, which is better tolerated.

164. **E. Symptoms of hyperthyroidism include palpitations, diarrhea, tremulousness, unintentional weight loss, heat intolerance, and hair thinning. Graves' disease is the most common cause of hyperthyroidism and typically occurs in women between the ages of 20 and 40 years old. Clinical findings of Graves' disease include hyperthyroidism with a diffuse, nontender goiter; opthalmopathy (to include lid lag, lid retraction, proptosis, extraocular muscle weakness), and pretibial myxedema. Patients do not need all three components to have Graves'. The diagnosis is made by finding a decreased thyroid stimulating hormone, an elevated thyroxine level and an increased radioactive iodide uptake value. Multiple options are available for treatment of Graves' disease: Surgical removal or radioactive iodine ablation of the gland will permanently alter the gland, and many patients become hypothyroid either immediately or over time. Medical therapies to block hormone synthesis with methimazole or propylthiouracil are other alternatives.**

    A. Subacute thyroiditis, also called de Quervain's thyroiditis, is probably virally mediated. Other forms of thyroiditis include chronic and postpartum forms. In thyroiditis, a transient thyrotoxicosis exists secondary to leakage of hormone from the gland, then transient hypothyroidism, then a return of thyroid function to normal. Radioactive iodide uptake scan, which is ordered to evaluate the cause of the clinical hyperthyroidism, usually shows a low uptake due to injury or inflammation of the gland.

    C. Addison's disease is the name for primary adrenal insufficiency. Symptoms include weakness, anorexia, vomiting, diffuse abdominal pain, and hypotension. The diagnosis is made by doing a corticotropin stimulation test. This involves obtaining a baseline cortisol level and then giving the patient a dose of adrenal corticotropin hormone (ACTH) to try to stimulate the adrenal glands. A cortisol level is obtained at 30, 60, and 90 minutes after the ACTH is given. The cortisol level should rise appropriately to indicate that the adrenals are able to function appropriately when stimulated. This patient does not have Addison's disease.

    D. Hashimoto's thyroiditis is a clinical state of hypothyroidism. It is usually seen in women aged 20 to 60 years and may be secondary to autoimmune destruction with lymphocytic infiltration of the thyroid gland. Thyroid-stimulating hormone is usually elevated and patients present with symptoms of hypothyroidism including fatigue, depression, cold intolerance, and weight gain. Treatment is with thyroid hormone replacement.

165. **C. This patient likely has primary adrenal insufficiency, or Addison's disease. Symptoms include weakness, lethargy, and fatigue as well as nausea, vomiting, abdominal pain, headaches, and weight loss. The adrenal glands produce cortisol, mineralocorticoids, and sex hormones. Deficiency of mineralocorticoids such as aldosterone causes the hyponatremia and hyperkalemia that are the hallmark electrolyte disturbances of primary adrenal insufficiency. Patients may be somewhat hypoglycemic due to cortisol deficiency. The patient's skin pigmentation is due to overproduction of ACTH-pro-opiate melanocorticotropin (POMC) from the hypothalamus/pituitary that is an attempt to stimulate the failing glands. The precursor hormone of ACTH is ACTH-POMC. POMC is cleaved from ACTH and stimulates melanocytes to produce melanin. Lastly, eosinophilia is sometimes seen in primary adrenal insufficiency. In the United States, primary adrenal insufficiency is most often due to an autoimmune destruction of the gland.**

    A. Patients with hyperthyroidism also experience weight loss, anxiety, and tremulousness, but they should not have the hyperpigmentation or the electrolyte disturbances that are seen in primary adrenal insufficiency.

    B. Hypothyroidism gives a clinical picture of fatigue, sluggishness, and lethargy. Patients will also complain of weight gain, constipation, and cold intolerance. They will not have skin color changes or electrolyte abnormalities.

D. Secondary hypoadrenalism is a lesion of the pituitary and presents with symptoms similar to primary hypoadrenalism, with the exception of hyperkalemia and increased pigmentation. In these patients, ACTH levels are low. Remember that aldosterone is released from the adrenal gland because of the stimulation of the renin-angiotensin system and *not* because of the stimulation of ACTH. This is why, in secondary adrenal insufficiency, the potassium is usually normal. (Glucocorticoids affect water/sodium balance, allowing patients with secondary hypoadrenalism to have some degree of hyponatremia.)

E. Hyperaldosteronism usually manifests itself as hypertension and hypokalemia. This patient is hypotensive and hyperkalemic, which is more suggestive of someone with relative hypoaldosteronism, effects of which can be seen with primary adrenal insufficiency.

166. **B. Polycystic ovarian syndrome is a constellation of oligo-ovulation, hyperandrogenism, and ovarian cysts. Hirsutism is secondary to increased levels of androgens.**

A. Idiopathic hirsutism is associated with regular ovulatory cycles and no other medical problems. It may be related to ethnicity, and some people from Mediterranean populations are especially hairy. The most important question to ask a woman who presents with complaints of hirsutism is whether her menses are regular or not. If she says that her menses are extremely regular, then there is no further work-up to do. Patients may be referred to dermatologists or cosmetologists for hair removal.

C. Pituitary neoplasms, such as prolactinomas, can cause irregular periods but usually cause other symptoms such as headache, visual changes (depending on tumor size), and galactorrhea. Prolactinomas are not associated with hirsutism.

D. Medications can cause hirsutism, but phenobarbital is not one of these medications. Phenytoin, glucocorticoids, and pencillamine are known to cause increased hair growth.

E. Hypothyroidism can cause irregular periods and changes in hair growth (more coarse), but this patient has normal TSH and thyroxine levels.

167. **C. This patient's hypercalcemia is likely secondary to malignancy, especially given his history of weight loss, smoking, and physical exam findings. Malignancy can cause hypercalcemia by many different paraneoplastic syndromes. Solid tumors such as squamous cell carcinoma and renal cell carcinoma often secrete parathyroid hormone-related peptide (PTH-rP) that stimulates the release of calcium from bone into the circulation. Breast cancer and melanoma may cause hypercalcemia because of the direct invasion of bone. Lymphomas often cause an increase in calcium secondary to an increase in the amount of 1,25 hydroxyvitamin D.**

A. Primary hyperparathyroidism causes elevated calcium by secretion of PTH. Parathyroid adenomas account for 80% of these cases, and parathyroid hyperplasia accounts for 15% to 20% of primary hyperparathyroidism. The diagnosis is often made by incidental laboratory findings of mildly elevated calcium levels. When work-up is done to evaluate the cause of the hypercalcemia, the intact PTH is found to be elevated inappropriately for the calcium level. (Normally, hypercalcemia should suppress intact PTH.)

B. Vitamin D excess can cause hypercalcemia. Vitamin D levels may become elevated, resulting in hypercalcemia, secondary to granulomatous disease such as sarcoidosis, coccidioidomycoses, histoplasmosis, and tuberculosis.

D. Various medications can cause hypercalcemia. β-blockers are not common contributors. Thiazides, lithium, vitamin A, and calcium-containing antacids are known to cause hypercalcemia.

E. Hyperthyroidism can cause hypercalcemia secondary to increased bone turnover. Immobilization and Paget's disease also cause hypercalcemia by the same mechanism. This patient's history and physical exam do not suggest elevated thyroid hormone levels.

168. **B. A C-peptide level would help determine the difference between endogenous and exogenous insulin administration. If this patient had surreptitiously injected insulin, her C-peptide level should be low. C-peptide is a portion of the proinsulin produced endogenously.**

A. An elevated insulin level would suggest either an endogenous source of insulin such as an insulinoma or exogenous insulin levels. It cannot distinguish between the two.

C. A sulfonylurea level would help determine if the patient had ingested sulfonylurea. This patient has no contact with anyone taking oral hypoglycemics, so this is unlikely.

D. Elevated liver enzymes can suggest a toxic (e.g., acetaminophen overdose), shock, or viral insult to the liver that causes hypoglycemia. This patient denies any Tylenol use and has no history of chronic alcohol use, which could also cause hypoglycemia.

E. Hypothyroidism may rarely cause hypoglycemia, but this patient has no evidence of hypothyroidism on physical exam.

169. **E. This patient has hypercalcemia manifesting as mental status changes and abdominal and bone pain. A possible etiology is her thiazide diuretic use, but regardless of the etiology, patients with hypercalcemia have undergone an osmotic diuresis due to the high calcium's effect on the kidneys and are significantly volume depleted. A normal saline bolus, even upwards of 4 to 6 liters, is required to lower her serum calcium levels before any other intervention, such as Lasix. Giving fluids is the first step in treating a patient with symptomatic hypercalcemia.**

A. Glucocorticoids are useful in treating hypercalcemia that is related to high levels of vitamin D, such as the hypercalcemia found in sarcoidosis and certain lymphomas. The calcium level improves within days, and the mechanism of action is unknown.

B. Furosemide, along with normal saline, is also one of the first steps in treating symptomatic hypercalcemia. It is only started after a patient is intravascularly repleted. Like normal saline, it promotes natriuresis and therefore increases calcium excretion.

C. Bisphosphonates inhibit osteoclast function. Osteoclasts resorb bone, which releases calcium into the circulation; therefore, bisphosphonates inhibit the release of calcium. They are very useful in treating the hypercalcemia of malignancy. Onset of action is 1 to 2 days, and duration of therapy is up to 2 weeks.

D. Calcitonin simulates the endogenous hormone that is produced by the parathyroid glands and that aid in putting serum calcium into bone. Onset is within hours, and duration of effect is 2 to 3 days. Unfortunately, a major side effect is tachyphylaxis.

170. **A. Fibrates decrease secretion of VLDL and increase stimulation of lipoprotein lipase, which in turn leads to increased clearance of triglycerides. Fibrates are used primarily to reduce elevated triglycerides, but also may increase serum HDL.**

B. Statins are inhibitors of hydroxy-methylglutaryl-coenzyme A (HMG CoA) reductase, which is the rate-limiting step in cholesterol synthesis. Inhibition of this reductase leads to increased LDL receptor turnover, thus leading to decreases in serum LDL. Statins are the most effective medication for reducing LDL levels. Side effects include hepatitis and myopathy, and are more common in patients who are on both statins and fibrates. Therefore, it is very important to educate patients about the side effects.

C. Niacin inhibits production of VLDL and, in turn, LDL. It also reduces the transfer of HDL to VLDL, thereby increasing serum HDL levels. Niacin is used in patients to lower LDL, increase HDL, and decrease triglycerides. Side effects include flushing, pruritis, and insulin resistance.

D. Bile acid sequestrants such as cholestyramine inhibit bile acid reabsorption, which leads to a decreased pool of cholesterol. This in turn increases the number of LDL receptors, which lowers serum LDL levels. These medications primarily work to lower LDL levels. Side effects include abdominal distension and change in bowel habits.

E. Cholesterol absorption inhibitors are a relatively new class of medications that inhibit the absorption of cholesterol at the intestinal brush border without affecting the absorption of fat-soluble vitamins. This treatment is currently thought to be adjunctive therapy to statins in lowering serum LDL levels. Side effects include hepatitis, so liver function tests should be followed.

171. E. Vitamin D deficiency can be caused by decreased intake, inadequate production in the skin, or renal failure. In renal failure there is decreased hydroxylation of calcidiol to calcitriol, the end product of vitamin D. The function of vitamin D is to increase absorption of calcium and phosphate at the level of the intestine. Deficiency causes reduced absorption of both calcium and phosphate, which leads to increased production of PTH (secondary hyperparathyroidism) as an attempt to improve serum calcium levels, which then lowers serum phosphate levels.

172. B. Hypercalcemia of malignancy can be secondary to the production of a PTH-related protein or local osteoclastic activity at the level of bone. Calcium levels are elevated and phosphate levels can vary depending on the etiology of the elevated calcium. Endogenous PTH levels will be low in response to feedback inhibition from the elevated serum calcium.

173. C. Hypoparathyroidism can be isolated, secondary to surgery, or due to decreased magnesium levels. PTH is responsible for increasing serum calcium from bone, increasing serum calcium resorption at the level of the kidney, and decreasing serum phosphate levels by excretion by the kidney. Thus, in hypoparathyroidism, calcium levels should be low and phosphate levels should be elevated.

174. D. Pseudohypoparathyroidism is defined as PTH end-organ resistance. This syndrome is also associated with skeletal abnormalities and retardation. Consequently, serum calcium levels are low, serum phosphate levels are elevated, and serum PTH levels are elevated.

175. A. Hyperparathyroidism is caused by an adenoma 80% of the time. It can also be caused by hyperplasia and carcinoma. With too much PTH, there is increased serum concentration of calcium from bony turnover and increased renal absorption of calcium. Phosphate excretion is increased at the level of the kidney.

176. C. Many medications can lead to impotence. Of the antihypertensive medications, thiazides and β-blockers have potential side effects of impotence. Most antidepressants, some H2 blockers, and antifungal drugs can also cause impotence.

A. People with spinal cord injuries can develop erectile dysfunction. Patients with neurogenic causes of impotence such as spinal cord injury are unable to have erections while sleeping and should not have the cremasteric reflex.
B. Any patient with evidence of peripheral vascular disease can develop impotence. Like patients with neurogenic causes of impotence, however, they do not have erections during REM sleep.
D. Depression and anxiety are major causes of impotence. Sudden loss of an erection, or inability to maintain an erection, is a common sign. These patients can maintain an erection at night while sleeping.
E. Hypogonadism is a common problem plaguing older men. Decreased libido and impotence are common manifestations. Testosterone replacement is the treatment. This patient is unlikely to have this problem, because he does not have testicular atrophy.

177. A. This patient has anti-phospholipid antibody syndrome. Patients with this syndrome have antibodies directed toward certain phospholipid-bound plasma proteins that are involved in the coagulation pathway. Patients are predisposed to recurrent arterial and venous clot formation and fetal loss. Laboratory testing includes lupus anticoagulant. The patient's serum is mixed with normal patient serum to see whether the aPTT corrects. If it does not, the test is positive for lupus anticoagulant, indicating the patient has the syndrome. Thrombocytopenia is also associated with this syndrome. PT is not affected.

178. E. Hemophilia B is an X-linked inherited bleeding disorder. Patients usually present with prolonged bleeding, hematomas, or hemarthrosis. Factor IX is deficient in hemophilia B, and factor VIII is deficient in hemophilia A.

179. C. Von Willebrand's disease is the most common inherited bleeding disorder. Patients usually have easy bruising, nosebleeds, menorrhagia, or prolonged bleeding with trauma. Von Willebrand factor plays a critical role in platelet function and is also a carrier protein for factor VIII. Defective von Willebrand factor can therefore decrease factor VIII and prolong PTT.

180. B. DIC is triggered by systemic illness and can be a catastrophic hematologic event. Possible associations with DIC include sepsis, trauma, malignancy, and burns. Initially, fibrinogen and platelets are consumed in clot formation. This is later followed by hemorrhage as the clots are degraded by fibrinolysis.

181. B. Primary hyperparathyroidism occurs in women three times more often than men, and it is usually seen in the early postmenopausal years. It is most commonly asymptomatic and is diagnosed because a mildly elevated calcium level is seen on blood that is being tested for some other reason. Patients have an elevated PTH, and in 80% of cases it is due to a parathyroid adenoma. Approximately 20% of the time, the elevated PTH is due to diffuse parathyroid gland hyperplasia.

182. C. Familial hypocalciuric hypercalcemia (FHH) is an autosomal dominant trait that consists of moderate hypercalcemia (usually asymptomatic) and a relative hypocalciuria. The renal tubular resorption of calcium and magnesium is abnormally high. The *best* test to determine whether or not a patient has FHH is *not* a 24-hour total calcium excretion level, but rather a ratio of calcium clearance to creatinine clearance. The clearance ratio in FHH is one-third that of primary hyperparathyroidism, with a cutoff value at 0.01. This test helps to distinguish FHH from primary hyperparathyroidism.

183. E. PTH-rP is a protein that is released in excess in certain malignancy states. It mimics PTH and binds its receptor with equal affinity. It causes a humoral hypercalcemia of malignancy, and is most often seen in squamous cancers of the head, neck, and lungs. PTH-rP activates osteoclasts to resorb bone and release calcium. Intact PTH (iPTH) is suppressed in the hypercalcemia that is related to PTH-rP excess.

184. D. Hypercalcemia secondary to granulomatous diseases, such as sarcoidosis, is mediated by an abnormally elevated 1,25-dihydroxyvitamin D level. The conversion of hydroxyvitamin D to dihydroxyvitamin D appears to be unregulated in these patients, and is suppressed by glucocorticoids, which is the appropriate treatment.

185. A. Hypercalcemia occurs in 20% to 40% of patients with multiple myeloma during their disease course. Myeloma cells in the bone marrow produce cytokines that activate the nearby osteoclasts to resorb bone. Interestingly, there is not a close correlation between the amount of bony destruction and bone pain in myeloma and the development of hypercalcemia.

186. D. Often used by men to relieve symptoms of BPH, saw palmetto is thought to inhibit 5-α reductase type I or androgen receptor activity. It is associated with few adverse side effects.

187. E. Used in the treatment of mild to moderate depression, St. John's Wort has ten active ingredients, the effects of which are unclear.

188. A. Ginkgo biloba is used primarily in the treatment of dementia and claudication. Adverse side effects include headache and intestinal discomfort.

189. B. Derived from the purple coneflower, echinacea is used to fight the common cold or respiratory viruses. No significant side effects are noted.

190. C. Although no data are available regarding its safety, ginseng is used by many to combat fatigue.

191. A. LDL cholesterol goals are based on a number of risk factors for coronary artery disease (CAD). Patients with one risk factor initiate diet control at levels >160 mg/dL and drug therapy at levels >190 mg/dL, and the goal is <160 mg/dL. Patients with two risk factors for CAD initiate diet control at levels >130 mg/dL and drug therapy at levels >160 mg/dL, and the goal is >130 mg/dL. Risk factors include age >45 in men and >55 in women; tobacco use, hypertension, diabetes, family history, and HDL <35 mg/dL. This patient has two risk factors (age and medically controlled hypertension), thus it would be recommended to start statins for a goal LDL of <130 mg/dL.

192. B. This patient has one risk factor for CAD: her family history. At this point, her therapy should consist of lifestyle changes, with goal of LDL <160 mg/dL.

193. A. This patient has a history of CAD. Her LDL goal should be <100 mg/dL. Statins are added once LDL reaches 130 mg/dL, and are considered when LDL is between 100 and 130 mg/dL.

194. B. Vitamin A deficiency occurs mainly in the third world and is due to dietary vitamin deficiency. The main manifestations of vitamin A deficiency are related to the eye, and vitamin A deficiency is a leading cause of blindness in the third world. Skin manifestations that may occur consist of hyperkeratosis of the epidermis, especially the follicular area. This results in a perifollicular hyperkeratosis called phrynoderma or "toad skin."

195. E. Deficiency of niacin causes pellagra, the symptoms of which are commonly referred to as the "three Ds": diarrhea, dementia, and dermatitis. The dermatitis may manifest in several ways but usually consists of erythema of the dorsa of the hands (due to the distribution in sun-exposed areas), which progresses to blisters, then bullae. These lesions are pathognomonic for niacin deficiency.

196. F. Riboflavin deficiency may result in several dermal manifestations, such as angular stomatitis, glossitis, and conjunctivitis.

197. C. Vitamin B12 deficiency is known to cause megaloblastic anemia, nail changes, and beefy red tongue. Skin manifestations consist of hypopigmented macules that tend to be distributed on flexural areas of skin.

198. A. Vitamin C deficiency is uncommon in developed countries. It causes scurvy, a syndrome characterized by myalgias, malaise, and weakness; perifollicular purpura follow, primarily on the legs. Hemarthroses may also occur, resulting in significant pain.

199. G. Vitamin B6 deficiency may result from treatment with isoniazid or other medications without supplementation of pyridoxine. It may also result from dietary deficiency. It results in constitutional symptoms and neurologic disturbances. Skin findings in pyridoxine deficiency include seborrhea involving the face, scalp, neck, shoulders, buttocks, and perineum.

    D. Alopecia is defined as an absence of hair from areas where it normally grows. It may be due to hormones, as in male-pattern baldness; to infections, as in tinea capitis; or to autoimmune diseases, as in alopecia areata or alopecia totalis. There are no vitamin deficiencies that cause alopecia.

200. B. This patient has type II diabetes mellitus that is confirmed by two separate fasting glucose measurements >126. He is obese and has significant insulin resistance based on the physical exam finding of acanthosis nigricans. This patient also appears to have the "metabolic syndrome" with his hypertension, diabetes, and obesity, and should have his lipids evaluated. It is reasonable to encourage diet and exercise therapies, but it is unlikely that this approach alone will change the metabolic profile in this patient, unless he is extremely motivated. Therefore, the first choice of pharmacotherapy is metformin. This is the only oral agent used for the treatment of type II diabetes that does not cause weight gain in overweight patients and that does not cause hypoglycemia in patients whose fasting blood sugar is less than 150 mg/dL. Therefore, it is the optimal choice in this patient.

    A. Diet and exercise should be encouraged. The patient should have a thorough cardiac evaluation before beginning an exercise program because of the significant cardiac risks of diabetes and hypertension (and probable hyperlipidemia). Diet and exercise alone, however, are not likely to change the metabolic picture, and it is reasonable to start pharmacologic therapy.

    C. Sulfonylureas are often chosen first-line in diabetes management; however, it is not a good choice in this patient for two reasons. First, it can cause weight gain, and this patient is already obese (BMI >30). Second, sulfonylureas can cause hypoglycemia as a side effect, and should not be used to start therapy in patients whose fasting blood sugar is ≤150 mg/dL. They also should be used with caution in patients who are elderly or who have renal insufficiency.

    D. All type II diabetics who live long enough will eventually require insulin as the β-cell function of the pancreas fails. However, this patient still has good function with a fasting blood sugar of 150 or so, and should not require insulin at this point.

    E. The diagnosis of diabetes is made by the fasting blood sugar measurements. There is no need to "confirm" the diagnosis with a hemoglobin A1C measurement. Even if the A1C were normal, he would still have the diagnosis of diabetes based on the fasting sugars.

BLOCK 1

1. A 29-year-old G_3P_2 personal injury attorney at 30 weeks gestational age (GA) presents after 2 days of fevers, chills, and nausea. She had been attributing her symptoms to the viral gastroenteritis that is keeping her 5-year-old son home from school, but she began to experience right-sided flank pain during a deposition this morning, and decided to come in to the emergency room. She reports no dysuria. Her temperature is 39°C. On physical exam, her lungs are clear and her breathing is not labored. She is very tender at the right costovertebral angle. Her urine dips 2+ leukocyte esterase, 1+ white blood cells, trace protein, and no glucose. Urine and blood cultures are sent to the microbiology laboratory. The most appropriate initial treatment for this patient is:

   A. Wait for culture results
   B. Outpatient therapy with oral Bactrim
   C. Outpatient therapy with oral nitrofurantoin
   D. Admission for IV ampicillin and gentamicin
   E. Admission for IV ciprofloxacin

2. A 33-year-old G_3P_3 woman presents to the emergency department (ED) with shortness of breath that began suddenly 30 minutes ago. She is now 3 days postpartum following an uncomplicated vaginal delivery. She denies any history of trauma. Her vital signs are BP 110/75, T 37.5°C, P 110, RR 30, and O_2 saturation is 88% on room air. Chest X-ray is within normal limits and EKG is notable only for sinus tachycardia. A pulmonary angiogram is shown (Figure 2-2). Supplemental oxygen (10L by face mask) is started, bringing the patient's O_2 saturation to 93%. Which of the following is the most appropriate next intervention?

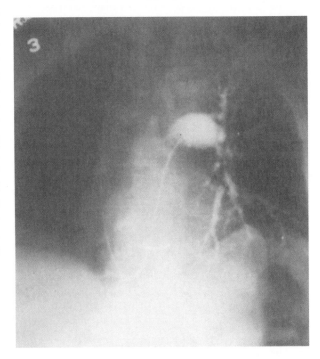

Figure 2-2 • Reproduced with permission from Dildy, G. Critical Care Obstetrics. Blackwell Science, 2004. Fig. 20-7, p. 284.

   A. IV Lasix (furosemide)
   B. Oral Coumadin (warfarin)
   C. IV heparin
   D. Surgical placement of a vena cava filter
   E. IV protamine sulfate

The response options for items 3 to 6 are the same. You will be required to select one or more answers for each item in the set.

A. Ductal carcinoma in situ
B. Fibroadenoma
C. Fibrocystic change
D. Galactocele
E. Infiltrating ductal carcinoma
F. Intraductal papilloma
G. Invasive lobular carcinoma
H. Lobular carcinoma in situ
I. Mammary duct ectasia
J. Paget's disease

For each description, select the appropriate breast lesion(s). Answer choices may be used more than once.

3. The most common breast lesion in women under 30, commonly presenting as a firm, painless, solitary, mobile mass (**SELECT 1**)

4. A benign tumor arising from duct epithelium, often worrisome for malignancy because of its presentation with spontaneous bloody nipple discharge (**SELECT 1**)

5. Subacute inflammation with dilated ducts, commonly presenting with tender nipples, a thick, dark discharge, and subareolar mass without evidence of infection (**SELECT 2**)

6. The most common benign breast condition, frequently presenting as cyclic, bilateral pain or tenderness (**SELECT 1**)

End of Set

7. A 26-year-old woman presents to your clinic after finding a firm breast mass on self-exam. Her last menstrual period was 2 weeks ago, and she has no family history of breast cancer. Physical exam confirms a 2-cm firm mass in the upper outer quadrant of the right breast. No other masses are palpated, her breasts are nontender, and no skin changes or nipple discharge are noted. An ultrasound (US) shows a 2-cm solid mass. A mammogram is normal. The most appropriate next step is:

A. No further work-up required, the mass is likely to be benign
B. Repeat mammogram
C. Fine needle aspiration
D. Radical mastectomy
E. Modified radical mastectomy

8. A 25-year-old woman presents to clinic complaining of dull abdominal pain on the left side. She reports that she has had this pain several times this year, but never this severely. She has normal monthly menses, which do not seem to correlate with the pain, and denies irregular bleeding. Urine pregnancy test is negative. Pelvic US reveals a 3-cm thin-walled left ovarian cyst. What is the most appropriate management of this patient?

A. No further action required
B. Repeat US in one month
C. Exploratory laparotomy
D. Pelvic CT
E. Pelvic MRI

9. A 60-year-old G_2P_2 woman comes to your office for a routine annual exam. Her last menstrual period was 10 years ago. She has not been on hormone replacement therapy but now desires to start due to concerns about osteoporosis. On routine pelvic exam, you palpate a small uterus and cervix along with palpable ovaries bilaterally. Which of the following is the most appropriate next step in the management of this patient?

A. Exploratory laparotomy
B. Start cyclic hormone replacement therapy: Premarin days 1 to 25, Provera days 16 to 25
C. Start continuous hormone replacement therapy: Premarin and Provera once a day
D. Pelvic US
E. Dual photon densitometry for evaluation of bone density

The next three questions (items 10 to 12) correspond to the following vignette.

A 50-year-old G_1P_1 woman presents for an annual exam. Her last menstrual period was 2 years ago. She is without complaints, and her physical exam is unremarkable. Although she has no relevant family history, she is very concerned about her risk of cancer and would like to know what steps she should take to detect malignancy at an early stage.

10. For which of the following malignancies has routine screening of asymptomatic patients been most effective in reducing mortality?

A. Breast cancer
B. Cervical cancer
C. Endometrial cancer
D. Ovarian cancer
E. Vulvar cancer

11. Which of the following malignancies is most likely to be present with advanced disease, and carries the worst overall prognosis for 5-year survival?

A. Breast cancer
B. Cervical cancer
C. Endometrial cancer
D. Ovarian cancer
E. Vulvar cancer

12. For which of the following malignancies is histologic grade the most important prognostic factor?

A. Breast cancer
B. Cervical cancer
C. Endometrial cancer
D. Ovarian cancer
E. Vulvar cancer

End of Set

13. A 21-year-old woman presents to the emergency department at 11 weeks GA with 2 days of painless vaginal bleeding. A US at 7 weeks was interpreted as a normal intrauterine pregnancy. Pelvic exam in the emergency room now reveals only a small amount of blood. A pelvic US reveals a thickened placenta with multiple cysts and a fetus consistent with her dating, but no cardiac activity. Quantitative ß-hCG is 166,000. What is the most likely diagnosis?

A. Incomplete molar pregnancy
B. Complete molar pregnancy
C. Spontaneous abortion of normal intrauterine pregnancy
D. Ectopic pregnancy
E. Normal intrauterine pregnancy complicated by incompetent cervix

14. A 24-year-old G_1P_0 woman arrives to the ED by ambulance after she began having tonic-clonic seizures at home 30 minutes ago. Her husband reports that she is at 33 weeks GA, has no previous history of seizures or other medical problems, and has had no difficulties in this pregnancy. He does report that she had a severe headache for several hours before the seizure began. On arrival to the ED, her blood pressure is 165/115. A brief neurological exam is unremarkable, with no focal findings. What is the most appropriate next intervention?

A. Postpone intervention until a head CT can be obtained
B. Perform immediate cesarean section

C. Administer IV magnesium sulfate and hydralazine
D. Administer IV calcium gluconate
E. Administer SQ terbutaline

15. A 31-year-old G_3P_2 presents for a routine prenatal visit at 28 weeks GA. Her previous pregnancy was notable for delivery of a 4200 gm baby. This pregnancy has been uncomplicated. The results of her third trimester labs are now available, and her blood glucose 1 hour after a 50-g load was elevated at 155. What is the most appropriate next step?

A. Initiate insulin therapy
B. Check a 3-hour glucose tolerance test
C. Check a serum HgbA1c level
D. Check a serum ß-hCG level
E. Induce labor

The next three questions (items 16 to 18) correspond to the following vignette.

A 24-year-old G_3P_1 at 13 weeks GA presents to the ED with 2 days of nausea, vomiting, and vaginal bleeding. Her blood pressure is 110/80, and her urine dipstick shows trace proteinuria. Physical exam reveals a uterus 16 weeks in size, and active bleeding is seen at the cervical os. ß-hCG is 130,000 mIU/ml. Pelvic US shows an enlarged uterus filled with hydropic trophoblastic tissue and no fetal tissue, as depicted in Figure 2-16.

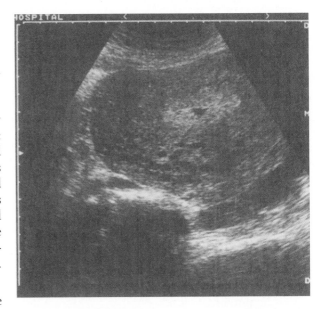

Figure 2-16 • Reproduced with Permission from Impey, L. Obstetrics & Gynecology. Blackwell Science, 1999. Fig. 14.7, p. 100.

16. What is the origin of the chromosomes of the trophoblastic tissue seen on the US ?

    A. Maternal haploid
    B. Paternal haploid
    C. Maternal diploid
    D. Paternal diploid
    E. Maternal triploid

17. What is the most appropriate initial management of this patient?

    A. Suction evacuation and curettage
    B. Methotrexate therapy
    C. Combination oral contraceptives
    D. Hysterectomy
    E. Expectant management, monitoring ß-hCG levels

18. Which of the following is most accurate regarding the differences between incomplete and complete molar pregnancies?

    A. Incomplete moles result from the fertilization of an empty ovum
    B. Incomplete moles are more likely to result in persistent trophoblastic disease
    C. Incomplete moles do not require uterine evacuation
    D. Complete moles are more likely to present with hyperthyroidism, hyperemesis, or preeclampsia
    E. Complete moles are viable

End of Set

The next two questions (items 19 and 20) correspond to the following vignette.

A 19-year-old G$_3$P$_2$ woman at 34 weeks gestation is found to have a blood pressure of 150/100 on a routine prenatal visit. Her urine dips 1+ protein, and repeat blood pressure is 140/95. She is asymptomatic. The patient is admitted for observation and testing for preeclampsia.

19. Which of the following diagnostic tests, when combined with this patient's presentation, would establish this diagnosis?

    A. 24-hour urine protein collection
    B. 24-hour uric acid collection
    C. Serum ß-hCG level
    D. Unconjugated estradiol
    E. Alpha-fetoprotein (AFP)

20. Which of the following features of this patient's history, if true, would be protective against the risk of preeclampsia?

    A. The patient has pregestational diabetes
    B. The patient has had two previous uncomplicated pregnancies
    C. The patient has a history of chronic hypertension
    D. The patient is pregnant with dizygotic twins
    E. The patient is African-American

End of Set

21. A 42-year-old woman presents with complaints of vaginal bleeding, especially after intercourse. She reports that her symptoms have been worsening for the past several months. She has no past medical history, and her sexual history includes first sexual intercourse at the age of 14 and numerous partners since then. Given this history, you are concerned that she may now have a gynecologic cancer. A history of infection of which of the following organisms would be most likely to increase the risk of a reproductive tract cancer?

    A. Herpes simplex virus (HSV) Type 1
    B. Epstein-Barr virus (EBV)
    C. *Trichomonas vaginalis*
    D. Human papilloma virus (HPV) type 18
    E. *Mycoplasma hominis*

22. A 23-year-old sexually active woman returns to your clinic for a follow-up visit following an abnormal Papanicolaou smear consistent with cervical intraepithelial neoplasia grade II (CIN II). On colposcopy, you are able to visualize the entire transformation zone and notice a small, cauliflower-shaped punctate lesion on the cervix. A directed biopsy of the lesion confirms CIN II. Based on these findings, the patient undergoes a therapeutic loop electrosurgical excision procedure (LEEP). Which of the following is accurate regarding LEEP?

    A. Because the instrument uses electric current as it cuts, there is frequently no need for anesthesia during this procedure
    B. Cervical stenosis is an occasional complication of this procedure
    C. LEEP is the only method of conization deemed safe for use during pregnancy
    D. Follow-up Papanicolaou smears are not necessary following LEEP since it is 100% curative
    E. The excised tissue does not provide useful information on pathology study

23. A 45-year-old recent immigrant presents to your office for her very first annual examination. Before performing all parts of the physical examination, you take a detailed history and find that her mother used diethylstilbestrol (DES) during her pregnancy. Which of the following disorders has been linked to in utero exposure to DES?

    A. Ovarian carcinoma
    B. Vaginal prolapse
    C. Squamous cell cervical cancer
    D. Polycystic ovarian syndrome (PCOS)
    E. Clear cell vaginal adenocarcinoma

The response options for items 24 to 27 are the same. You will be required to select one or more answers for each item in the set.

    A. Glucose of 44
    B. Blood pressure 145/92
    C. Blood pressure 166/114
    D. 238 mg of protein on a 24-hour collection
    E. 459 mg of protein on a 24-hour collection
    F. 897 mg of protein on a 24-hour collection
    G. AST of 97, ALT of 119
    H. Pulmonary edema
    I. Schistocytes on peripheral smear
    J. Platelet count of 88,000

For each scenario regarding blood pressure, select the most appropriate finding(s). Answers may be used more than once.

24. Gestational hypertension **(SELECT 1)**

25. Mild preeclampsia **(SELECT 3)**

26. Severe preeclampsia **(SELECT 5)**

27. HELLP syndrome **(SELECT 3)**

End of Set

28. A couple presents to a fertility clinic after trying to conceive unsuccessfully for 2 years. In your evaluation, you ask the man questions regarding his work exposures, history of mumps, hernia repair, testicular trauma, steroid use, and sexual function. Initial evaluation of this couple will include a semen analysis (SA). The couple is instructed to abstain for 2 days and then bring a sample of semen to the clinic within 2 hours of ejaculation. Which of the following are components of a semen analysis?

    A. Sperm count per milliliter, motility, morphology, DNA analysis
    B. Sperm count per milliliter, motility, morphology, DNA analysis, acrosome count
    C. Sperm count per milliliter, pH, volume, motility, acrosome count
    D. Sperm count per milliliter, pH, volume, motility, morphology, WBC
    E. Sperm count per milliliter, pH, volume, motility, WBC

29. You are reading a report about contraceptive trends and find a list of the most used methods in the United States. Of the following, which is considered the most popular method of controlling fertility in the United States?

    A. IUD
    B. Combined oral contraceptive pills
    C. Depo-Provera
    D. Condom
    E. Sterilization

The next two questions (items 30 and 31) correspond to the following vignette.

A 26-year-old healthy G_1P_0 woman at 28 weeks GA by last menstrual period is here for a routine prenatal visit. As part of your standard exam, you perform Leopold measurements on the mother.

30. Assuming the calculated GA of 28 weeks is accurate and the fetus is developing normally, what would be your estimate of the distance between the uterine fundus and the mother's symphysis pubis (i.e., fundal height)?

    A. 28 in
    B. 28 cm
    C. 28 fingerbreadths
    D. 28 mm
    E. Unable to determine from the information given

31. Upon examination, you find that the fundal height is far less than you predicted. Which of the following is a possible cause of size being less than the date in this patient?

    A. Multiple gestations
    B. Polyhydramnios
    C. Gestational diabetes mellitus (GDM)
    D. Intrauterine fetal demise
    E. Fetus in breech presentation

End of Set

32. A 22-year-old G_1P_0 at 22 weeks GA by LMP is undergoing a biophysical profile (BPP) to assess fetal well-being. So far, the information gathered includes: normal fetal breathing movements, normal gross body movements, normal fetal tone, and adequate amniotic fluid volume by qualitative analysis. Which of the following additional information will complete the BPP for this patient?

    A. Lecithin:Sphingomyelin ratio (L:S)
    B. US for fetal anatomy
    C. Fetal heart tracing and tocometry (nonstress test)
    D. Mother is morbidly obese
    E. Fundal height

33. A 29-year-old G_2P_1 is at 16 weeks GA by LMP. Her pregnancy has thus far been normal. Her last pregnancy, however, was significantly more complicated. She developed GDM, and her baby was born with Klinefelter's syndrome (47, XXY). Her past medical history is significant for GERD of 3 years, for which she takes omeprazole regularly. She has no other medical history and no drug allergies. Her father is alive and well; her mother is deceased after suffering an embolic stroke at the age of 61. Based on the above, which piece of history is the biggest indication for her to undergo prenatal testing via amniocentesis?

    A. Advanced age
    B. Previous GDM
    C. Family history of cerebrovascular disease
    D. Medication use
    E. Previous chromosomal abnormality

34. You are working in an inner-city clinic and your next patient is a pregnant woman who was recently diagnosed with HIV. You suggest she start highly active anti-retroviral therapy (HAART) and explain to her that the chances of having an infant affected with HIV if she is not treated are:

    A. 5%
    B. 25%
    C. 50%
    D. 65%
    E. 80%

35. You are seeing a pregnant patient in clinic and she tells you she is going on a vacation. You urge her to get up and walk around occasionally throughout her flight. You explain that pregnancy increases her risk of developing deep vein thrombosis (DVT) secondary to venous stasis. Which of the following pregnancy factors contributes to this hypercoagulable state?

    A. Increased hematocrit
    B. Decreased estrogen
    C. Increased progesterone
    D. Decreased ambulation
    E. Increased right atrial pressures

The next two questions (items 36 and 37) correspond to the following vignette.

A 25-year-old G_1P_0 woman at 8 weeks GA by LMP presents for her first prenatal visit. You do the standard set of prenatal tests for an initial visit and find that she is rubella nonimmune (i.e., she does not have antibodies to the rubella virus). You worry that this puts her at increased risk for such complications as spontaneous abortion or congenital rubella syndrome (CRS), especially if she is infected in the first trimester.

36. Which of the following is a finding associated with CRS?

    A. Mental retardation
    B. Paralysis
    C. Polycystic kidney disease
    D. Cleft lip/palate
    E. Congenital adrenal hyperplasia (CAH)

37. At this point in the patient's pregnancy, what is the most appropriate intervention?

    A. Immediate immunization for rubella
    B. Prophylactic antibiotic treatment for rubella
    C. Therapeutic abortion
    D. Treatment with intravenous immunoglobulin (IVIG)
    E. Rubella vaccination immediately postpartum

End of Set

38. A 26-year-old sexually active obese woman complains of amenorrhea for 6 months. She has no past medical history, achieved menarche at age 14, and has had irregular menses every 1 to 3 months since then. She denies skin or hair changes, takes no medications, and reports a 10-lb weight gain over the last few months. She has experienced no alteration in her exercise or sleeping patterns. What is the first step that should be taken in this patient's work-up?

A. Order an abdominal/pelvic CT
B. Obtain gonadotropin and prolactin levels
C. Start her on a trial of combined oral contraceptive pills
D. Obtain a psychiatry consult to rule out depression
E. Draw a serum β-hCG level

The next two questions (items 39 and 40) correspond to the following vignette.

A 34-year-old G_2P_2 woman complains of amenorrhea for the last 8 months. In contrast to her normal menses of 3 days and moderate flow, her last menstrual period consisted of 2 days of spotting. She achieved menarche at age 16 and had a normal menstrual cycle through her 20s. Her pregnancies were uncomplicated.

39. Which of the following terms most accurately describes the patient's current condition?

    A. Primary amenorrhea
    B. Secondary amenorrhea
    C. Oligomenorrhea
    D. Hypomenorrhea
    E. Menometrorrhagia

40. You perform a physical exam and find that aside from her menstrual changes, the patient is obese and exhibits signs of acne and abnormal body hair growth. You decide to check her gonadotropin levels as part of your work-up and find that her follicle stimulating hormone (FSH) is near normal but her luteinizing hormone (LH) is markedly elevated. Based on this evidence, what is this patient's most likely diagnosis?

    A. Ovarian dysgenesis
    B. Asherman's syndrome
    C. PCOS
    D. Testicular feminization syndrome
    E. Ectopic pregnancy

End of Set

41. A 14-year-old girl comes to your clinic because she has not yet begun menstruating. She has not developed any appreciable pubic hair or breast mass. She has no past medical history and is very active in athletics, having participated in national and international gymnastics competitions continuously since the age of 7. She eats and sleeps regularly, and does not use any tobacco or illicit substances. On exam, you notice that she is normal height and very well-toned even though she weighs a mere 80 lbs. You also determine that her breasts are Tanner stage 3 (early pubescent), and pubic hair is Tanner stage 2 (presexual). Motor, sensory, and mental status exams are all normal. Given this information, what is the most likely cause of this patient's pubertal delay?

    A. Pituitary malignancy
    B. Hypothalamic dysfunction secondary to repeated cranial injury at gymnastics competitions
    C. Decreased weight and body fat stores secondary to intense athletic training
    D. Kallman's syndrome
    E. CAH

42. A 30-year-old G_1P_0 at 32 weeks gestation is complaining of lower abdominal pain but denying dysuria or contractions. She is afebrile and has no costovertebral tenderness. You send her urine for analysis and culture and find it is nitrite and leukocyte esterase positive and eventually grows out >100,000 colonies/ml of *Escherichia coli* bacteria. To best manage this patient you decide to:

    A. Treat her with oral antibiotics
    B. Admit her for IV antibiotics to prevent an ascending infection
    C. Explain to her that it is normal to have bacteriuria during pregnancy and urge her to stay well hydrated
    D. Send another urine sample because it is likely a lab error given the lack of classic urinary tract infection (UTI) symptoms
    E. Put her on antibiotic prophylaxis for the remainder of her pregnancy

43. A 19-year-old primigravida comes into clinic for prenatal care at 36 weeks gestation. You perform a culture to check for colonization by group B *Streptococcus* (GBS). You explain to her that if the test is positive, management will consist of which of the following?

    A. The patient needs to be treated to prevent transmission to the fetus in utero
    B. The neonate should receive antibiotics for 24 hours after delivery
    C. The patient is more likely to have STDs
    D. Penicillin is given when the patient is in labor to prevent fetal transmission
    E. She is more likely to deliver early

44. A 37-year-old G_4P_2 at 28 weeks gestation presents with vaginal tingling and itching. She denies any new sexual contacts and explains that she had similar symptoms about one year ago and was treated at that time for herpes simplex virus (HSV). On examination of her vulva you see multiple, small, vesicular lesions as in Figure 2-44. Which of the following is the best way to manage this patient?

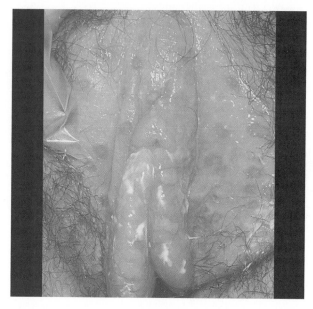

Figure 2-44 • Reproduced with Permission from Callahan TL, Caughey AB. Blueprints Obstetrics & Gynecology, 4th ed. Baltimore: Lippincott Williams & Wilkins, 2007. Fig. 16-2, p. 177.

A. Start her on acyclovir and continue throughout the rest of her pregnancy
B. Treat her infection with acyclovir but explain to her that HSV-1 cannot be transmitted to the baby at delivery
C. Treat her current infection and consider prophylactic therapy at 36 weeks
D. Stress the importance of treatment because secondary lesions have a higher fetal attack rate
E. Plan for scheduled cesarean section because any woman with an outbreak of HSV during pregnancy should not deliver vaginally, even in the absence of active lesions

45. A 35-year-old patient in latent labor complains of sudden onset pleuritic chest pain, shortness of breath, and hemoptysis. Her oxygen saturation acutely drops to 88%. She is given oxygen and an electrocardiogram is done at the bedside. Your clinical suspicion is supported by:

A. A widened QRS complex
B. A prolonged P-R interval
C. Sinus bradycardia
D. Left axis deviation
E. Peaked T waves

46. You are called to see a 24-year-old G_2P_1 at 11 weeks gestation in the emergency room. She came in complaining of unilateral leg pain and foot swelling. Ultrasound examination reveals a DVT. Which of the following is the most appropriate treatment?

A. Coumadin therapy with an INR goal of 2 to 3 throughout the remainder of the pregnancy
B. Low-molecular-weight (LMW) heparin initially, followed by Coumadin therapy for prophylaxis
C. LMW heparin throughout the pregnancy, changing over to unfractionated heparin at 36 weeks
D. Coumadin therapy followed by compression stockings for prophylaxis
E. LMW heparin followed by compression stockings for prophylaxis

The response options for items 47 to 50 are the same. You will be required to select one answer for each item in the set.

A. Normal uterus
B. Arcuate uterus
C. Septate uterus
D. Unicornuate uterus
E. Bicornuate uterus
F. Uterus didelphys

For each diagram, select the appropriate müllerian anomalies.

47. Figure 2-47.

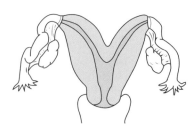

Figure 2-47 • Reproduced with Permission from Callahan TL, Caughey AB. Blueprints Obstetrics & Gynecology, 4th ed. Baltimore: Lippincott Williams & Wilkins, 2007. Fig. 14-1, p. 155.

48. Figure 2-48.

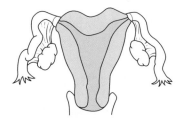

Figure 2-48 • Reproduced with Permission from Callahan TL, Caughey AB. Blueprints Obstetrics & Gynecology, 4th ed. Baltimore: Lippincott Williams & Wilkins, 2007. Fig. 14-1, p. 155.

50. Figure 2-50.

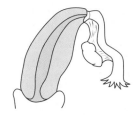

Figure 2-50 • Reproduced with Permission from Callahan TL, Caughey AB. Blueprints Obstetrics & Gynecology, 4th ed. Baltimore: Lippincott Williams & Wilkins, 2007. Fig. 14-1, p. 155.

End of Set

49. Figure 2-49.

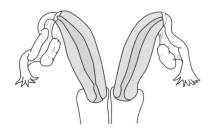

Figure 2-49 • Reproduced with Permission from Callahan TL, Caughey AB. Blueprints Obstetrics & Gynecology, 4th ed. Baltimore: Lippincott Williams & Wilkins, 2007. Fig. 14-1, p. 155.

A Answers and Explanations

1. D
2. C
3. B
4. F
5. D, I
6. C
7. C
8. B
9. D
10. B
11. D
12. C
13. A
14. C
15. B
16. D
17. A

18. D
19. A
20. B
21. D
22. B
23. E
24. B
25. B, E, F
26. C, G, H, I, J
27. G, I, J
28. D
29. E
30. B
31. D
32. C
33. E
34. B

35. C
36. A
37. E
38. E
39. B
40. C
41. C
42. A
43. D
44. C
45. E
46. C
47. E
48. B
49. F
50. D

1. **D.** This patient presents with classic features of pyelonephritis—fever, nausea, flank pain—and should be admitted for empiric IV therapy with a beta-lactam and gentamicin. Pyelonephritis is the most common serious medical complication in pregnancy (seen in 1% to 2% of all pregnancies). Endotoxin-mediated toxicities can include pulmonary edema and ARDS, hemolytic anemia, renal insufficiency, sepsis, and premature labor. It is important to note that not all women with pyelonephritis report a history of UTI symptoms (e.g., dysuria, increase in urinary frequency).

   A. Pyelonephritis poses significant maternal and fetal risks (e.g., it is estimated that 10% to 20% of women with pyelonephritis are bacteremic, and many in this group will develop septic shock). Empiric therapy should be initiated immediately.

   B. Although nonpregnant patients are often treated for pyelonephritis on an outpatient basis, this approach has only been recently described in pregnant patients. If it is used, patients need to be selected based on the acuity of their illness as well as their reliability to return for follow-up. Intramuscular ceftriaxone is begun Q 24 hours and the patient is advised to use oral hydration at home and follow her temperatures. After 24 hours afebrile, the patient can be switched to oral antibiotics to complete a 10-day course. Even for patients selected for this treatment approach, oral Bactrim is inadequate as initial therapy.

   C. Daily low dose oral nitrofurantoin (or cephalexin) is often given after resolution of an episode of pyelonephritis as a prophylaxis to help prevent recurrence for the duration of the pregnancy. It is not considered appropriate therapy for acute illness.

   E. Fluoroquinolones are effective in treating pyelonephritis is nonpregnant patients, but are not used in pregnancy because of concerns of adverse effects on cartilage development.

2. **C.** This patient's presentation and pulmonary angiogram are most consistent with a pulmonary embolus (PE). Intravenous heparin is generally the medical therapy of choice. Pregnancy is considered a "hypercoagulable state," and the risk of DVT and PE is increased. (Pulmonary embolus is now the leading cause of maternal death in pregnancy.) The etiology of this hypercoagulable state is not well understood, but appears to be related to a combination of increased coagulation factors, endothelial damage, and venous stasis. This increased risk does not end with delivery and, in fact, PE is more common postpartum than antepartum. Other therapeutic options to consider are substitution of subcutaneous LMW heparin (which allows patients to be discharged as soon as they are stable) and/or the addition of a thrombolytic (e.g., streptokinase) in the setting of an unstable patient.

   A. A diuretic might be appropriate if this patient's symptoms were secondary to pulmonary effusion, as can occur when preeclampsia or infection complicates pregnancy.

   B. Warfarin therapy is an inappropriate choice for this patient for medical, not obstetric, reasons. Its slow onset of efficacy (days) is unacceptable in the acute setting of pulmonary embolus. When stable, patients are routinely anticoagulated for a minimum of 6 months; conversion from heparin to warfarin is appropriate for long-term anticoagulation. Warfarin is considered to be compatible with breast-feeding by the American Academy of Pediatrics (but is contraindicated during pregnancy due to strong evidence of teratogenicity).

   D. For the majority of patients, a vena cava filter offers no advantage over heparin anticoagulation. It may be considered in patients who develop recurrent emboli despite heparin therapy or in patients at high risk for hemorrhage (e.g., an antepartum patient with known placenta previa).

   E. Protamine sulfate is used to reverse the effect of heparin, and thus is not a treatment for PE.

3. **B.** Fibroadenoma, a benign tumor with epithelial and stromal components, is the most common tumor in younger women. A healthy, young woman with this classic presentation, and without a family history of breast cancer, can usually be followed clinically without further immediate workup. Fine needle aspiration (FNA) is performed in other cases to rule out malignancy or cystosarcoma phyllodes (a rare variant of fibroadenoma with malignant potential).

4. **F.** Intraductal papilloma is a benign solitary lesion involving the epithelium of lactiferous ducts. Malignant transformation is rare, but cytology and/or excisional biopsies are needed to rule out malignant causes of bloody discharge, including papillary carcinoma.

5. **D, I.** Inflammation resulting from a blocked excretory duct is termed galactocele in a lactating woman, and mammary duct ectasia in a non-lactating woman. Mammary duct ectasia is most common at or after menopause; an excisional biopsy is indicated in this population to rule out carcinoma.

6. **C.** Fibrocystic change is the most common benign breast condition. It is not associated with an increased risk of cancer. Of note, malignant disease rarely presents as a painful lesion.

7. **C.** A solid breast mass in a woman this age requires pathological diagnosis, and FNA is generally the first step. Fine needle aspiration is often, but not always, diagnostic, and is usually used first in these cases because it is less invasive. A nondiagnostic result from FNA, however, requires an excisional biopsy. Figure 2-7 depicts common locations for breast masses.

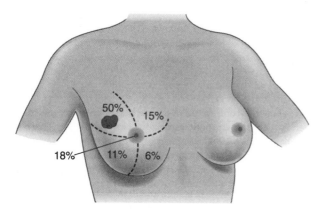

Figure 2-7 • Image Provided by Departments of Radiology and Obstetrics & Gynecology, University of California, San Francisco.

A. If this patient's mass appeared cystic on US, it could be observed with no further immediate workup, as it would be very unlikely to be malignant.
B. Mammograms are often nondiagnostic in younger women, as dense breast parenchyma limits their ability to distinguish lesions.
D, E. Although the solid nature of this mass makes it suspicious for malignancy, mastectomy without a pathologic diagnosis is not appropriate. The mass is still very likely to be benign, and FNA can provide a minimally invasive diagnosis.

8. **B.** The management of ovarian masses is highly dependent not only on the character of the mass, but also on the age of the patient. A thin-walled, noncomplex 3-cm cyst in a woman of reproductive age is almost certain to be a physiologic (functional) cyst, and concern for malignancy should be very low. Although the risk of malignancy is low, a repeat US is needed to be certain that the cyst has regressed. Large cysts carry the additional risk of ovarian torsion, and size must be monitored for this reason as well.

A. See explanation for B.
C. Although a laparotomy is not indicated for this patient, the same presentation in a premenarchal or postmenopausal woman would require surgical exploration, as concern for malignancy would be much higher.
D, E. Although a pelvic CT and MRI can offer useful information in certain cases, they do not play a significant role in the diagnosis of most ovarian cancers, and are certainly not required for the initial evaluation of a cyst so likely to be benign.

9. **D.** In a postmenopausal woman, the ovaries should not be palpable; if they are, it should raise concern for ovarian malignancy. Whereas the large majority of women of reproductive age with this presentation will be found to have functional cysts or other benign processes, an ovarian mass in a woman over 50 is more likely to be malignant than benign. Ultrasound is the initial imaging method of choice for adnexal masses.

A. Before performing an operative evaluation, an initial workup of the adnexal masses should include radiologic assessment by US , along with tumor markers. A CT scan may also be warranted to assess for metastatic disease.
B, C. Although these are accepted regimens for hormone replacement therapy, palpable ovaries need to be evaluated to rule out malignancy.
E. Dual photon densitometry will give a reliable measure of bone density, but this patient's palpable ovaries require a more immediate workup.

10. **B.** The reduction in mortality from cervical cancer is one of the great success stories of modern medicine. Routine screening with the Papanicolaou smear has allowed diagnosis of premalignant lesions and earlier diagnosis of cervical carcinoma. Cervical cancer was the leading cause of death from malignancy in women at the turn of the century, but is now the sixth leading cause.

A. Screening for breast cancer has contributed to a reduction in breast cancer mortality rates, but this effect is not as dramatic as it is for cervical cancer. There is now general agreement that a screening mammography should be offered to women over 50, but there is controversy surrounding the efficacy of self-examination and mammograms for younger women as routine screening tests. The current American Cancer Society guidelines call for baseline screening mammograms at ages 35 to 39, every 1 to 2 years between 40 and 50, and annually after age 50. Monthly self-exams and an annual physician exam are recommended in all women over 20 years of age.

C. There are currently no effective screening tests for endometrial cancer. Endometrial biopsies on asymptomatic patients are not cost effective. Although 30% to 40% of patients with endometrial cancer will have an abnormal Papanicolaou smear, it is not considered a good screening test for endometrial malignancy.

D. Ovarian cancers are often associated with tumor cell markers (e.g., CA-125 in epithelial ovarian cancer). CA-125 is useful in monitoring response to treatment, but its value as a screening tool has not been established, as it is a nonspecific marker that is elevated in pregnancy, endometriosis, fibroids, and many benign (e.g., pancreatitis) and malignant (e.g., lung cancer) nongynecologic diseases. The situation is similar for other types of ovarian cancers.

E. Effective routine screening for vulvar cancer is not available.

11. D. Nearly 75% of patients with ovarian cancer present with Stage III (extension into the abdominal cavity) or more advanced disease. There is no effective screening test, symptoms are often vague, and extension into the peritoneal cavity is facile. As a result, ovarian cancer is responsible for 50% of deaths from cancer of the female genital tract, even though it accounts for only 25% of gynecologic malignancies. Overall 5-year survival is 25% to 30%.

A. Improved diagnosis of earlier-stage breast cancer (combined with improvements in adjuvant therapy) have improved prognosis. The overall 5-year survival rate is now more than 90%.

B. Cervical cancer is often detected at a premalignant stage, or in the early stages of malignancy, because of the efficacy and widespread use of the Papanicolaou smear.

C. Although no good screening test exists, endometrial cancer presents with abnormal vaginal bleeding in 90% of patients (e.g., prolonged heavy periods or intermenstrual spotting in premenopausal women, or postmenopausal vaginal bleeding). Because patients are so often symptomatic, 75% of cases are Stage I (confined to uterus, not extending to cervix) at the time of diagnosis, and the overall 5-year survival is 65%.

E. Vulvar cancer commonly presents with a history of vulvar pruritus (and in some cases vulvar bleeding or a vulvar mass). The overall 5-year survival rate is 75%.

12. C. Endometrial cancer is the only gynecological malignancy for which histology is the most important prognostic factor. High-grade, poorly differentiated tumors are more likely to spread aggressively and are associated with a much poorer prognosis.

A, B, D, and E. Surgical staging of breast, cervical, ovarian, and vulvar cancer is of greater prognostic value than tumor histology.

13. A. The combination of markedly elevated ß-hCG and US findings make molar pregnancy the most likely diagnosis. The presence of fetal tissue is consistent with an *incomplete* mole.

B. Complete molar pregnancy is characterized by the absence of fetal parts.

C. Spontaneous abortion could also present with vaginal bleeding, but the elevated ß-hCG makes molar pregnancy more likely.

D. Ectopic pregnancy could also present with vaginal bleeding, but ß-hCG would be *low* for gestational age and intrauterine fetal tissue would not be seen on US.

E. Incompetent cervix does not explain the ß-hCG value or the US findings, and would generally not manifest until the second trimester.

14. C. This patient's likely diagnosis is eclampsia, which is the occurrence of grand mal seizures in the preeclamptic patient not attributable to other causes. Initial management requires first stabilizing the patient with seizure prophylaxis (magnesium sulfate) and blood pressure control (usually hydralazine or labetolol). Once stable, the patient should be delivered, as this is the only cure for preeclampsia-eclampsia.

A. A head CT would provide useful information to rule out nonobstetric causes of this patient's seizure, but treatment should not be delayed when the diagnosis of eclampsia is as probable as it is in this case. Complications of eclampsia include cerebral hemorrhage, aspiration pneumonia, hypoxic encephalopathy, and thromboembolic events.

B. Although cesarean rates are certainly found to be higher in this population, cesarean section should be reserved for obstetric indications.

D. Calcium gluconate is used to reverse toxicity from magnesium overdose.

E. Terbutaline is used as a tocolytic. It is imperative to induce or augment labor in an eclamptic patient, not delay it.

15. **B. A 1-hour glucose load test is a common *screening* test for diabetes in pregnancy. A value greater than 140 mg/dL is positive, and necessitates the *diagnostic* test: a 3-hour glucose tolerance test (fasting blood glucose levels, then 1 hour, 2 hours, and 3 hours after 100 gm glucose load).**

A. This patient should not be treated for diabetes until a diagnosis is made, and even then, blood sugar control with diet would be the initial management. Insulin therapy, used when diet alone is ineffective, is usually not required in patients with true gestational diabetes.

C. Serum HgbA1c estimates blood glucose levels over the last 6 to 8 weeks. It is not an appropriate diagnostic test.

D. Although serum ß-hCG is somewhat decreased in pregnancies complicated by diabetes, it is not a useful diagnostic test.

E. Patients with diabetes are often induced at 39 to 40 weeks due to concern for shoulder dystocia secondary to macrosomia, as well as fear of intrauterine fetal demise. Induction at 28 weeks, however, would be wholly inappropriate.

16. **D. A complete mole, which does not have associated fetal tissue, results from the fertilization of an empty ovum by a normal sperm. Chromosomes are paternally derived and diploid (95%XX, 5%XY). Due to high levels of ß-hCG, hydatidiform moles can be associated with hyperthyroidism, theca lutein cysts, and hyperemesis gravidarum. They can also be associated with preeclampsia in the first trimester.**

A, B, C, and E. See explanation for D.

17. **A. Treatment of molar pregnancy is immediate evacuation of the uterus, followed by monitoring for persistent disease by serial ß-hCG levels. This follow-up period should be at least 1 year, during which time reliable contraception is essential.**

B. Chemotherapy (most commonly methotrexate) is indicated for persistent malignant disease, which follows 15% to 25% of complete molar pregnancies (and 4% of incomplete molar pregnancies). It is not indicated as initial treatment.

C. While effective contraception is required during the follow-up period to allow monitoring of persistent disease, the first step in management should be uterine evacuation. Oral contraceptives do not treat the underlying disease process.

D. Hysterectomy is an alternate therapy for hydatidiform moles, but is not considered necessary, and can be avoided in this patient who desires future childbearing. Of note, hysterectomy does *not* eliminate the risk of recurrent disease (which remains 3% to 5%).

E. Following ß-hCG levels for persistent disease is an important component of management, but evacuation of the uterus is required on presentation.

18. **D. Complete moles are more likely to lead to preeclampsia than incomplete moles. They are also more likely to lead to medical complications such as hyperthyroidism (due to the structural homology of ß-hCG and TSH) and hyperemesis gravidarum.**

A. An incomplete mole results from the fertilization of a normal ovum by two sperm. Cells are triploid, with two sets of paternal origin and one set of maternal origin (most commonly 69,XXY). In contrast, a complete mole results from the fertilization of an empty ovum.

B. Incomplete moles are less likely to result in persistent trophoblastic disease compared to complete moles (4% vs. 15% to 25%).

C. Uterine evacuation is indicated for both complete and incomplete moles.

E. Neither complete nor incomplete moles are viable pregnancies. Complete moles do not actually result in the development of a fetus. In contrast, triploid incomplete molar pregnancies are complicated by congenital malformations and growth restriction so severe that the fetus survives only several weeks in utero before being spontaneously aborted.

19. **A. The classic triad of preeclampsia is hypertension, proteinuria, and edema. Formal diagnosis requires at least 300 mg protein in a 24-hour collection (or persistent ≥1+ dipstick) and blood pressures greater than 140 mm Hg systolic or 90 mm Hg diastolic on two occasions at least 6 hours apart. A 24-hour urine protein collection should be started while following her blood pressures. The patient should also be carefully monitored for preeclamptic symptoms (e.g., headache, visual changes, RUQ pain).**

    B. Uric acid has been noted to be elevated in patients with preeclampsia, and is being investigated as a screening test, but is not used to make the diagnosis of preeclampsia.

    C, D, E. Alterations in serum ß-hCG (i.e., elevated), unconjugated estradiol (i.e., elevated), and AFP (i.e., decreased or normal) are seen in preeclampsia, but these are poor screening tests, and certainly are not used to make the diagnosis in a patient with a suspicious presentation. It should be noted that ß-hCG would be useful if this patient presented similarly in the first trimester, as preeclampsia is seen in the first trimester only in the setting of molar pregnancy.

20. **B. Preeclampsia is sometimes described as a disease of first pregnancies, and although the reasons remain controversial, it is clear that previous normal pregnancy significantly reduces the risk of preeclampsia in future pregnancies.**

    A. Diabetes is a risk factor for preeclampsia.

    C. Chronic hypertension is a risk factor for the development of "superimposed" preeclampsia.

    D. Multiple gestation is a risk factor for preeclampsia.

    E. African-Americans are at increased risk for preeclampsia.

21. **D. Certain types of HPV have been implicated as probable causative agents of cervical carcinoma. Specifically, types 16, 18, 31, 33, 35, 39, 45, 51, 52, 56, and 58 have been associated with cancer. Other types, especially 6 and 11, can cause condyloma acuminata (venereal warts), but they are not involved in the pathogenesis of carcinoma.**

    A. HSV is the causative agent in multiple disorders, including oral cold sores (usually type 1), genital ulcers (usually type 2), and temporal lobe encephalitis. There is also some evidence that it may be an independent risk factor for cervical carcinoma. However, unlike HPV, it is not a causative agent.

    B. EBV is linked to infectious mononucleosis and certain types of lymphoma. It does not cause reproductive tract cancers.

    C. *Trichomonas* is a flagellated protozoan, and the cause of trichomonal vaginitis. Symptoms include vaginal burning and itching, foul-smelling "frothy" discharge, and dysuria. It generally does not cause vaginal bleeding, and is not associated with reproductive tract cancers.

    E. *Mycoplasma hominis* is part of the natural vaginal flora. It can be a cause of bacterial vaginosis if it overgrows in the vagina due to such factors as nutritional changes, douching, or antibiotic use. It is not, however, a cause of reproductive tract cancers.

22. **B. Cervical stenosis is a rare, albeit serious, complication of cervical conization, whether via LEEP, cold knife, or laser. Other potential complications of conization include heavy bleeding (most common), infection, and cervical incompetence.**

    A. The cervix has a reasonably rich nerve supply, and significant manipulation of any nature can cause pain. While the electrical nature of LEEP minimizes discomfort compared to other conization methods, local anesthesia, usually provided via paracervical block, is absolutely required for this procedure.

    C. No conization methods are considered safe during pregnancy. ALL of them are associated with an increased risk of premature delivery.

    D. Follow up Papanicolaou smears and colposcopies are usually done 3 months after the procedure to ensure that the wound is healing well, that the entire lesion was in fact removed, and that there is no new evidence of dysplasia.

    E. Because the tissue is removed as a single specimen, pathologic study is possible and is frequently undertaken to ensure that the borders of the specimen are free of dysplastic changes. If this is found to be the case, it suggests that the removed tissue contains the entire abnormal region and no dysplasia has been left behind.

23. **E. Any female fetus exposed to DES in utero has an increased likelihood of developing clear cell adenocarcinoma of the vagina and cervix. Prior to 1965, these adenocarcinomas were extremely**

rare. However, a case series of 7 was reported in women whose mothers had been treated with DES for miscarriage prevention. This led to larger epidemiologic studies that showed a strong intergenerational association between DES and these rare adenocarcinomas. DES daughters are also at increased risk for vaginal, cervical, uterine, and renal anomalies. An annual or biennial Papanicolaou smear and colposcopy is recommended for all exposed women.

A. There is no link between DES and ovarian carcinoma.

B. Prolapse of the vaginal vault can sometimes be seen as a result of relaxation of pelvic muscles in aging women. It is especially common in those who have undergone hysterectomy. This phenomenon is not associated with DES exposure. One effect DES does have on the vagina, however, is an increased risk of vaginal clear cell adenocarcinoma, especially if exposure occurred before 18 weeks gestation.

C. While DES is associated with an increased risk of clear cell adenocarcinoma of the cervix, it is not associated with squamous cell carcinoma, the most common type of cervical cancer.

D. PCOS generally presents with enlarged, polycystic ovaries, secondary amenorrhea or oligomenorrhea, hirsutism, obesity, and infertility. Women between 15 and 30 years of age are primarily affected. While the precise etiology has not been determined, it is known that DES is not associated with this disorder.

24. B. Gestational hypertension, also known as pregnancy induced hypertension (PIH), is diagnosed when blood pressures are consistently elevated above 140/90, but not above 160/110.

25. B, E, F. Mild preeclampsia is diagnosed by having mildly elevated blood pressures between 140/90 and 160/110 as well as mild proteinuria, between 300 mg and 5 gm in a 24-hour urine collection. Preeclampsia is also associated with nondependent edema of the face and hands.

26. C, G, H, I, J. Sever preeclampsia is diagnosed in the setting of elevated blood pressures and proteinuria and having any of the following additional signs or symptoms: Severe headache, visual changes—particularly flashing lights in the visual field—blood pressures elevated above 160/110, pulmonary edema, RUQ pain/tenderness, elevated AST/ALT, hemolysis characterized by schistocytes or elevated LDH, thrombocytopenia, oliguria with either <30 mL per hour for 3 hours or more, and severe proteinuria with >5 grams on a 24-hour urine collection.

27. G, I, J. HELLP syndrome is characterized by hemolysis, elevated liver enzymes, and low platelets. Any of these three findings is seen in severe preeclampsia, but the three can be seen together to make the diagnosis of HELLP syndrome, an even more severe variant of preeclampsia. Because of the hemolysis and thrombocytopenia, coagulopathy and disseminated intravascular coagulation (DIC) should be screened for with fibrin split products, fibrinogen, and PT/PTT/INR.

28. D. Sperm count per ml, pH, volume, motility, morphology, and WBC count are all components of a semen analysis. Sperm count should be between 20 and 250 million/mL; pH should be between 7.2 and 7.8; volume should be at least 2 mL of semen that liquefies normally; motility should be at least 50% of sperm with forward progression; morphology should be at least 30% normal forms; and WBC count should be less than 1×10^6 leukocytes/mL.

A, B, C, E. DNA testing is not part of a semen analysis and there is no such thing as an acrosome count. The semen analysis is designed to rule out factors that may prevent sperm from reaching and penetrating the egg.

29. E. Sterilization is employed by 1/3 of all married couples and is the most popular form of birth control if the female partner is over 30 years of age or the couple has been married more than 10 years. Nearly 1 million sterilization procedures are performed in this country every year.

A, B, C, D. See explanation for E. Each of these methods considered separately is not as popular as sterilization as a means of contraception.

30. B. Until about 36 weeks gestational age, the GA in weeks is approximately equal to the fundal height in centimeters. Thus, a 28-week fetus will show a 28-cm fundal height. At some point after 36 weeks, the fetal head can move distally, or "drop," below the pubic symphysis, making fundal height measurements less accurate. All of this, of course, is only

true if GA was correctly calculated, and there is no intrinsic problem in the fetus' development or mother's health.

A, C, D, E. See explanation for B.

31. D. A finding of size less than dates can be attributed to a few known causes, including inaccurate GA calculations, hydatidiform mole, oligohydramnios, fetal growth restriction, and intrauterine fetal demise. Size greater than dates, on the other hand, is caused by polyhydramnios, multiple gestations, and GDM, as well as hydatidiform mole and inaccurate GA calculations.

A. The presence of more than one fetus will create a larger uterus than a singleton pregnancy will due to the sheer volume of the additional fetus and amniotic fluid.
B. Polyhydramnios, or amniotic fluid volume greater than 2000 mL, will cause enlargement of the uterine corpus to greater than normal size. Polyhydramnios is also associated with an increased incidence of placental abruption, preterm labor, and postpartum uterine atony.
C. The classic effect of gestational diabetes is increased fetal growth and size, called macrosomia. Macrosomia is generally defined as a fetal weight greater than 4500 grams at term.
E. Breech presentation is when the fetal breech (buttocks) is the presenting part, as opposed to babies that are cephalic, or "head down." In the absence of fetal malformations, fetal presentation should not contribute to uterine size.

32. C. The biophysical profile consists of the four parameters described in the question stem as well as a nonstress test. Each parameter is scored as normal (worth 2 points) or abnormal/absent (worth 0 points). A total score of 8 to 10 is considered normal, 6 points is equivocal, and 4 or fewer points is distinctly abnormal and likely requires intervention. The results are generally accurate, although maternal use of sedatives or alcohol and spontaneous uterine activity can affect scores.

A. L:S ratio is an important means of assessing fetal lung maturity. A high lecithin level compared to sphingomyelin means the lungs are producing adequate surfactant. This is especially important to assess if there is a threat of premature labor and delivery. However, L:S ratio is not a part of the BPP.

B. Ultrasound is a useful modality to detect any gross structural or position anomalies, but is not part of the BPP.
D. Obesity is not considered in the BPP.
E. Fundal height is measured from the fundus of the uterus to the pubic symphysis and the length in centimeters should correspond to GA in weeks. Any inconsistency between the two must be evaluated. This is a useful part of the examination, but is not a part of the BPP.

33. E. Previous chromosomal abnormality in pregnancy is an indication for testing in subsequent pregnancies. Other indications include maternal age greater than 35 years, a triple screen with a positive result, and a known chromosomal abnormality in one or both parents. This testing can be achieved either via amniocentesis beyond 15 weeks gestation or chorionic villus sampling (CVS) from 10 to 12 weeks gestation.

A. This woman is 29 years old and not considered to be of advanced age.
B. GDM does not cause chromosomal abnormalities and is not an indication for amniocentesis.
C. In the absence of a suspected genetic syndrome, family history of cerebrovascular disease is not an indication for prenatal testing.
D. Omeprazole is not known to be teratogenic or mutagenic in any way. There is no danger to the pregnancy with use of this medication.

34. B. A 25% transmission rate is thought to occur late in pregnancy or at delivery. HIV therapy can help reduce this risk by decreasing viral load. In the largest study of the use of anti-retroviral therapy in pregnancy, zidovudine (AZT) was administered throughout pregnancy, in labor, and postpartum. Transmission was reduced by 2/3 in women who underwent treatment. In more recent studies, patients who are treated aggressively with combination therapy and have undetectable viral loads have even lower vertical transmission rates.

A, C, D, E. See explanation for B.

35. C. High levels of progesterone lead to smooth muscle relaxation and subsequent decreased venous tone and stasis in pregnancy. Additionally, increased levels of estrogen result in increased hepatic production of clotting factors.

A. A *decreased* hematocrit is more common in pregnancy due to an increase in blood volume that exceeds the increase in red blood cells.

B. Estrogen increases rather than decreases in pregnancy.

D. While decreased ambulation is a risk factor for DVTs, it is not specific to the pregnant state. However, there are some complications of pregnancy that require bed rest. These patients should be placed on heparin or other DVT prophylaxis.

E. Right atrial pressures are not affected by pregnancy and therefore do not contribute to venous stasis during pregnancy, although IVC compression does.

36. **A. CRS is a rare occurrence in this country due to intensive screening and vaccination policies as part of standard prenatal care. From 1990 to 1996, only 92 cases were reported to the National Congenital Rubella Syndrome Registry. Typical signs and symptoms of the disease include mental retardation, cataracts/congenital glaucoma, congenital heart disease (most commonly patent ductus arteriosus or peripheral pulmonary artery stenosis), and sensorineural hearing loss. Other findings include retinopathy, splenomegaly, jaundice, microcephaly, meningoencephalitis, and bone disease. Incidence is highest when infection occurs in the first trimester, although symptoms may not present for years after birth.**

B. Paralysis is not a component of CRS.

C. Polycystic kidney disease is an autosomal dominant disorder that usually presents initially with flank pain, hematuria, and hypertension. Kidneys are cystic, enlarged, and frequently palpable on exam. Cyst infection is a common occurrence. Associated conditions include nephrolithiasis, cerebral aneurysms, and cardiac valvular pathology. However, this disease is not associated with CRS.

D. Cleft lip and palate are congenital malformations due to incomplete fusion of lip tissue and palatal bones, respectively. A fairly common anomaly, it occurs in some form in 1 in 700 live births. These can be unilateral or bilateral, but the vast majority of cases are easily corrected and afford no lasting sequelae. These anomalies are not associated with CRS.

E. Congenital adrenal hyperplasia (CAH) is a common cause of premature or abnormal virility. The most common type (deficiency of 21-hydroxylase) leads to inefficient production of cortisol from precursor compounds. These precursors are androgens, and their accumulation in women leads to such symptoms as hirsutism, alopecia, amenorrhea, infertility, and virilization. While this disorder is hereditary, it is not caused by rubella.

37. **E. The rubella vaccine consists of a live virus, and therefore vaccination during or up to 3 months prior to pregnancy is contraindicated because of the theoretical risk of transmission of disease to the fetus. Approximately 15% of the female population in this country is seronegative for rubella and thus susceptible to infection and CRS. The vaccine (as well as prior infection) affords lifelong immunity and induces antibodies in greater than 95% of patients.**

A. See explanation for E.

B. There is no antibiotic treatment for an active rubella infection as it is a self-limited viral illness in most cases.

C. The implementation of abortion based solely on the possibility of infection, without direct evidence of severe deformity, chromosomal abnormality, or other life-threatening complication, is not indicated.

D. IVIG is of no benefit in this situation.

38. **E. The overwhelming majority of secondary amenorrhea is caused by pregnancy. A pregnancy test is the first step that should be taken in the work-up of any woman of child-bearing age, regardless of her sexual status. This is especially true in a case where no other signs or symptoms of endocrine dysfunction exist. Of note, the strict definition of secondary amenorrhea is the absence of menses for three cycles or 6 months in a previously menstruating woman.**

A. Imaging is a bit premature in the absence of a working diagnosis and should not be done on any woman without first knowing her pregnancy status.

B. This would certainly be done to rule out hypothalamic-pituitary-ovarian dysfunction, but only in the setting of a negative pregnancy test.

C. This is a reasonable solution if you suspect ovarian dysfunction, such as premature ovarian failure or PCOS. However, it should not be done without first knowing whether the patient is pregnant.

D. Psychiatric etiologies are always diagnoses of exclusion, and should only be considered after a thorough organic work-up comes up negative. Also, her maintenance of exercise habits and lack of change to her sleeping pattern suggests depression is unlikely.

39. B. Secondary amenorrhea is defined as failure to menstruate for 6 or more months after having had normal menses prior to the current episode. There are a myriad of etiologies for amenorrhea, including pregnancy (the most common etiology), hypothalamic-pituitary abnormalities, ovarian dysfunction, and genital tract outflow obstruction.

A. Primary amenorrhea is defined as the absence of any menses at any time.
C. Oligomenorrhea is amenorrhea of 40 days to 6 months duration.
D. Hypomenorrhea is a reduction in the amount or length of flow, but with normal frequency.
E. Menometrorrhagia is heavy, irregular bleeding.

40. C. PCOS is a functional ovarian problem consisting of bilateral, large, polycystic ovaries, anovulation, oligo- or amenorrhea, infertility, acne, and hirsutism. A hyperestrogenic state results from the increased estrogen and peripheral conversion of androgens into estrogens caused by chronic anovulation. This causes an absence of the LH surge and perpetuates the cycle by inhibiting ovulation leading to infertility and changes in menstruation. LH also stimulates ovarian production of androgens, leading to hirsutism and acne, and further increases in peripheral conversion. Thus, a positive feedback cycle develops, keeping the patient anovulatory and oligo/amenorrheic. Treatment is aimed at breaking the positive cycle hormonally with combined oral contraceptives or clomiphene citrate and with weight reduction.

A. Ovarian dysgenesis is a rare occurrence and is due to abnormal embryologic development in the womb. Considering the patient has had normal menses and pregnancies in the past, there is no question that she has ovaries.
B. Asherman's syndrome is scarring of the uterine cavity leading to obstruction of menstrual flow and amenorrhea. It is generally the result of uterine infection, or iatrogenic causes such as vigorous dilation and curettage. It is a structural problem and does not cause the other symptoms seen in this patient.

D. Testicular feminization syndrome is the result of a genetically XY male having testes, but dysfunctional or absent androgen receptors. People with this disorder have no female reproductive organs (due to müllerian inhibiting hormone secretion by the embryonic testes), but do have a partial vagina due to the lack of formation of male external genitalia (which occurs under the influence of androgens). This patient's history of menses and successful pregnancy rules out this disorder.
E. Ectopic pregnancy does not cause hirsutism or acne.

41. C. Studies have shown that competitors in intense athletic sports such as gymnastics, running, and ballet do not develop sufficient stores of fat or adequate body weight to undergo pubertal changes at appropriate ages. A weight of 85 to 105 pounds is considered necessary before menses can begin, and a body fat proportion of 15% to 25% is needed for a regular ovulatory cycle. Rigorous exercise and sports training regimens usually keep girls from meeting these parameters at normal times in their growth. However, pubertal development will commence once their level of training decreases enough to satisfy these criteria. Thus far, no negative long-term sequelae of delayed puberty have been elucidated.

A. A pituitary malignancy such as a hamartoma of the pituitary stalk is a possible cause of these symptoms. However, this is a relatively rare disorder, and a pituitary stalk disorder would likely present with additional signs such as short stature (due to impaired growth hormone secretion).
B. Similar to the explanation for A, if this patient had sustained enough cranial injury to affect hypothalamic function, many other symptoms and signs would likely be present including motor dysfunction or changes in mental status.
D. Kallman's syndrome is a rare disease involving hypoplastic olfactory tracts and a lack of GnRH secretion by the arcuate nucleus in the hypothalamus. Common findings include absence of breast and hair growth and no sense of smell. The patient's normal sensory exam rules out this disorder.
E. CAH manifests as some form of adrenal insufficiency. In the most common type, a deficiency of 21-hydroxylase leads to inadequate cortisol

production and secretion, which then leads to a build-up of precursor androgen hormones. This accumulation causes higher than normal levels of androgens in the blood and leads to a syndrome of precocious (or early) puberty—the opposite of what this patient is experiencing.

42. **A. A simple UTI can be treated with oral antibiotics in pregnant patients. If a patient has a history of multiple UTIs or bacteriuria persists after treatment, prophylactic therapy can decrease the risks associated with UTIs in pregnancy, such as higher rates of pyelonephritis.**

    B. Hospital admission and IV antibiotics are only indicated in a patient with clinical evidence of pyelonephritis.
    C. Although bacteriuria is not rare in pregnancy (approximately 5% of pregnant women), it is still abnormal and 25% will develop into a more severe infection and should be treated aggressively.
    D. Pregnant women do not always exhibit classic UTI symptoms. A repeat urine is not necessary in order to treat this patient.
    E. This patient's UTI needs to be treated. However, since this is her first infection in this pregnancy and it is uncomplicated, continued prophylaxis is unnecessary.

43. **D. Neonatal transmission occurs at the time of delivery and can lead to severe sepsis. Because of this, women who are known to be colonized with GBS are treated with IV penicillin in labor. Women with unknown GBS status should be started on penicillin if they have rupture of membranes greater than 18 hours.**

    A. Colonization occurs in 10% to 35% of pregnant women and is of little concern in the antepartum period.
    B. Antibiotics are given prior to delivery in order to prevent neonatal infection, and therefore empiric antibiotics are not necessary in the neonatal period.
    C. GBS is not sexually transmitted, and therefore has no bearing on whether or not a patient has likely been exposed to other STDs.
    E. Although infection is associated with preterm labor, GBS is a colonizing, not a pathogenic, bacteria in the mother and should not increase the risk of early labor.

44. **C. Acyclovir is the treatment of choice for this patient. Whether this is a primary or secondary outbreak does not change the management. Once a patient has an outbreak in pregnancy, she is usually placed on suppression with acyclovir at 36 weeks gestation. This approach is taken to decrease the rate of transmission at delivery by decreasing the chance of having another outbreak and by likely decreasing asymptomatic shedding.**

    A. Fetal transmission is most likely to occur at the time of delivery, so acyclovir is not usually used throughout the pregnancy.
    B. Although genital lesions are generally associated with HSV-2, both HSV-1 and HSV-2 can cause severe infection in the neonate including herpetic lesions, sepsis, pneumonia, encephalitis, and even death.
    D. Primary infection with HSV during pregnancy has a higher fetal and neonatal attack rate.
    E. If the patient is asymptomatic and there is no evidence of herpetic lesions at the time of delivery, the risk of neonatal transmission is very low, especially in the setting of prophylactic therapy.

45. **E. Although not a sensitive or specific test, in the setting of PE, an EKG may show peaked T waves, sinus tachycardia, right axis deviation secondary to right heart strain, and nonspecific ST changes. In this patient, PE is of concern because of the constellation of symptoms and pO2 desaturation all in the setting of pregnancy. She will need to be evaluated via spiral CT, or more traditionally with V/Q scan and pulmonary angiogram.**

    A, B, C, D. See explanation for E.

46. **C. Low-molecular-weight heparin is used for treatment and prophylaxis. This is important in a patient who will remain hypercoagulable throughout the remainder of her pregnancy. Because of its longer half-life, LMW heparin is usually converted to unfractionated heparin at 36 weeks of gestation to lower the risk of bleeding at the time of delivery. Postpartum, the patient can be treated with Coumadin, although some patients will prefer to remain on LMW heparin to avoid multiple visits to have their PT/INR checked.**

A, D. Coumadin is teratogenic, causing skeletal abnormalities and nasal hypoplasia when given during the first trimester.

B. Again, Coumadin is generally contraindicated in pregnancy.

E. Medical management is mandatory in a patient who has proven she is at high risk for development of DVT. Compression stockings are more useful for a patient on bed rest with no history of DVT.

47. E. Uterine anomalies arise when errors occur during the fusion of the Müllerian (paramesonephric) ducts. These anomalies can range in severity from an arcuate uterus, which is heart-shaped or mildly indented at the fundus, to uterus didelphys, which is complete lack of fusion of the duct systems, resulting in two separate uterine horns, cervices, and vaginas.

48. B. Uterine anomalies arise when errors occur during the fusion of the Müllerian (paramesonephric) ducts. These anomalies can range in severity from an arcuate uterus, which is heart-shaped or mildly indented at the fundus, to uterus didelphys, which is a complete lack of fusion of the duct systems, resulting in two separate uterine horns, cervices, and vaginas.

49. F. Uterine anomalies arise when errors occur during the fusion of the Müllerian (paramesonephric) ducts. These anomalies can range in severity from an arcuate uterus, which is heart-shaped or mildly indented at the fundus, to uterus didelphys, which is a complete lack of fusion of the duct systems, resulting in two separate uterine horns, cervices, and vaginas.

50. D. Uterine anomalies arise when errors occur during the fusion of the Müllerian (paramesonephric) ducts. These anomalies can range in severity from an arcuate uterus, which is heart-shaped or mildly indented at the fundus, to uterus didelphys, which is a complete lack of fusion of the duct systems, resulting in two separate uterine horns, cervices, and vaginas.

BLOCK 2

51. A 34-year-old at 11 weeks gestation is seen in the emergency room with nausea and vomiting, and you are called to evaluate her. You ask her about her pregnancy and she tells you she took clomiphene citrate in order to conceive. Which of the following describes the mechanism of action of clomiphene citrate?

    A. Restoration of the hypothalamic-pituitary-ovarian axis
    B. Acts as an anti-estrogen and stimulates pulsatile GnRH release
    C. Restores ovulation in cases of premature ovarian failure
    D. Improves cervical mucus
    E. Builds up the endometrial lining

52. A 17-year-old G_1P_1 is 2 hours status post a vaginal delivery. You are a medical student asked by the nurse to assess her continued vaginal bleeding. When you report to the chief resident, she asks you to quantitate the amount of vaginal bleeding. Postpartum hemorrhaging is defined as the loss of greater than what amount of blood in the first 24 hours after vaginal delivery?

    A. 100 mL
    B. 300 mL
    C. 500 mL
    D. 700 mL
    E. 1000 mL

53. A woman 2 weeks postpartum develops a fever to 39.0°C and a 4 × 3-cm area of tender erythema on the lateral aspect of her left breast. She is diagnosed with uncomplicated mastitis of the left breast and prescribed outpatient antibiotics. Additional management involves which of the following?

    A. Pumping her breast milk and discarding it
    B. Continuing to breastfeed the infant
    C. Neither breastfeeding nor pumping the milk from the left breast and allowing the milk to reabsorb from the left breast
    D. Pumping the left breast and sterilizing the milk before feeding it to the infant
    E. Continuing to breastfeed the infant, but treating the infant with antibiotic drops to prevent infection of the infant

54. A 22-year-old college student comes to your office for her routine Pap smear and exam. She tells you that her best friend recently had an abnormal Pap smear and is going to have biopsies of her cervix taken to make sure that she does not have cancer. Your patient is now fearful that her Pap smear might also be abnormal. She wants to know what causes abnormal Pap smears. You tell her that which of the following is associated with an increased risk for development of cervical carcinoma?

    A. Age of 25 at first intercourse
    B. A high fat diet
    C. A prior Pap smear with "metaplastic change"
    D. Frequent candidal infections
    E. Infection with human papilloma virus (HPV)

55. A 60-year-old woman complains that "something is wrong with the skin around my vagina." She states that her vulva constantly burns. She is not sexually active and has not attempted to visualize her vagina. Before performing an examination you create a mental differential diagnosis. Which of the following would you include in your differential diagnosis prior to examining your patient?

    A. Acne vulgaris
    B. Rosacea
    C. Eczema
    D. Pemphigus vulgaris
    E. Lichen planus

The next two questions (items 56 to 57) correspond to the following vignette.

A 21-year-old woman presents to the emergency department with vaginal spotting and right lower quadrant pain. She thinks she may be pregnant since she is two weeks late for her period. She reports her menses are regular and monthly, but is uncertain of the exact timing of her last menstrual period (LMP). She has a history of pelvic inflammatory disease (PID) and she smokes a half pack of cigarettes each day. She also complains of nausea and vomiting and is currently unable to void. She reports that her last pregnancy ended at 6 weeks with a miscarriage. Her blood pressure is 102/71 and her pulse is 93. She has right lower quadrant tenderness, no rebound or guarding, and her pelvic examination is notable for right adnexal tenderness.

56. Which of the following is the first test or study to order?

    A. Pelvic ultrasound
    B. Blood type and screen
    C. Serum quantitative β-hCG
    D. Complete blood count (CBC)
    E. Computed tomography (CT)

57. In addition to the above risk factors for ectopic pregnancy (PID, cigarette smoking), you elicit that she had an asymptomatic *Chlamydia* infection 3 months ago, which was treated, as well as an ectopic pregnancy treated with surgery 3 years ago. Which of the following increases her risk of ectopic pregnancy the most?

    A. History of PID
    B. History of asymptomatic *Chlamydia* infection
    C. History of ectopic pregnancy
    D. Cigarette smoking
    E. History of first trimester spontaneous abortion

End of Set

58. A 41-year-old G_3P_2 at 5 3/7 weeks presents to the emergency department (ED) with cramping and vaginal bleeding for 12 hours. She has a history of 2 normal spontaneous vaginal deliveries at term with the last occurring 8 years ago. She reports that the cramping is worsening, and she denies passage of tissue. Her physical examination is significant for bleeding from the cervical os and cervical dilation to 2.5 cm. There is no adnexal tenderness or palpable masses on exam. Ultrasound shows an intrauterine gestational sac. Which of the following is the correct diagnosis?

    A. Missed abortion
    B. Threatened abortion
    C. Completed abortion
    D. Incomplete abortion
    E. Inevitable abortion

59. A 19-year-old G_1P_0 has a follow-up clinic visit after an uncomplicated dilation and curettage for a missed abortion. She wonders if something she did caused her fetus to die. You tell her that the most common cause for first trimester abortions is which of the following?

A. Chromosomal abnormalities
B. Tetrachloroethylene
C. Uterine cavity abnormalities
D. Antiphospholipid antibody syndrome
E. Cervical incompetence

60. A 21-year-old G_1P_0 at 39 6/7 weeks presents to labor and delivery complaining of mild uterine contractions every 8 minutes that last about 30 seconds. She also reports a large "gush" of clear fluid. She denies vaginal bleeding and notes fetal movement. The fetal heart rate tracing (FHT) is notable for a baseline of 150 with moderate variability and two 15 by 15 accelerations in 20 minutes. The uterine contraction monitor shows contractions every 6 to 10 minutes She asserts that she would like to spend the early part of labor at home in her bath tub. Which of the following is the next most appropriate step in management?

    A. Admit to labor and delivery for oxytocin augmentation
    B. Admit to labor and delivery for observation and administration of intravenous antibiotics
    C. Discharge her to home with instructions to return with painful contractions
    D. Perform a sterile speculum examination
    E. Perform a cervical examination, check for the fetal presentation with ultrasound, and check the amniotic fluid index

61. A 37-year-old G_3P_2 at 42 0/7 weeks gestation presents for labor induction due to post-term gestation. She reports good fetal movement and denies vaginal bleeding, uterine contractions, and leakage of amniotic fluid. In addition to monitoring the fetus via FHT and uterine contractions with an external tocometer, you find her cervix to be 1.5-cm dilated, 50% effaced, fetal vertex at −3 station, soft consistency, and posterior position. Which of the following is the correct Bishop score (Table 2-61)?

    A. 4
    B. 5
    C. 7
    D. 8
    E. 9

The next two questions (items 62 to 63) correspond to the following vignette.

■ TABLE 2-61   The Bishop Score

Points	Dilation (cm)	Effacement (%)	Station	Cervical Consistency	Cervical Position
			Factor		
0	Closed	0 – 30	−3	Firm	Posterior
1	1 – 2	40 – 50	−2	Medium	Midposition
2	3 – 4	60 – 70	−1, −2	Soft	Anterior
3	>= 5	>= 80	+1, +2	–	–

Figure 2-62 is a FHT of a 31-year-old G_3P_2 in the active phase of labor with painful uterine contractions for 8 hours. Her membranes spontaneously ruptured approximately 6 hours ago, and her last cervical examination was 8-cm dilated, 100% effaced, and −1 station.

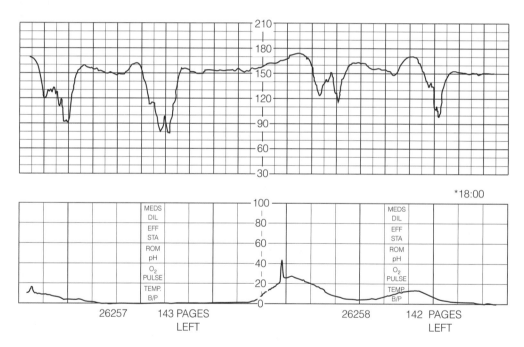

Figure 2-62 • Reproduced from Callahan TL, Caughey AB. Blueprints Obstetrics & Gynecology, 4th ed. Baltimore: Lippincott Williams & Wilkins, 2007. Fig. 4-7, p. 43.

62. What is the next best step in the management of this FHT?

A. Place an intrauterine pressure catheter (IUPC) for better contraction monitoring
B. Place a fetal scalp electrode for better fetal heart rate monitoring
C. Perform a forceps assisted vaginal delivery
D. Continue expectant management
E. Perform a cesarean section

63. Which of the following fetal heart rate deceleration categories is correctly matched with the etiology?

A. Variable deceleration—umbilical cord compression
B. Variable deceleration—uteroplacental insufficiency
C. Late deceleration—fetal head compression
D. Late deceleration—umbilical cord compression
E. Variable deceleration—maternal hypotension

End of Set

64. The two types of episiotomies are depicted in Figure 2-64. Which of the following statements regarding the use of episiotomies in modern obstetrics is most correct?

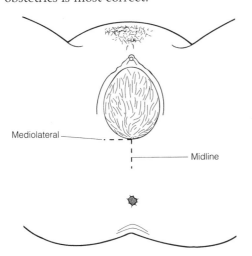

Figure 2-64 • Reproduced from Callahan TL, Caughey AB. Blueprints Obstetrics & Gynecology, 4th ed. Baltimore: Lippincott Williams & Wilkins, 2007. Fig. 4-14, p. 49.

A. Mediolateral episiotomy is associated with less pain when compared to midline episiotomy
B. Midline episiotomy has fewer third- and fourth-degree extensions when compared to mediolateral episiotomy
C. Patients should have an episiotomy to prevent pelvic relaxation
D. Mediolateral episiotomy results in less blood loss when compared to median episiotomy
E. Use of episiotomy is indicated when a clinician needs to hasten delivery or in the setting of a shoulder dystocia

65. A 23-year-old G_1P_0 presented in active labor and had normal progress in the first stage of labor. She has an epidural for pain management. Now in the second stage of labor, she has been pushing effectively for 2 hours. Which of the following is an indication for an operative vaginal delivery?

A. The fetus is at 0 station in the occiput anterior position
B. The fetus is at +3 station and the mother is exhausted
C. The fetus is having repetitive moderate variable decelerations
D. The mother has poor pain control
E. The fetus is at +3, and position is uncertain, either LOA or ROA

The next two questions (items 66 and 67) correspond to the following vignette.

A 47-year-old African American woman presents to you for her overdue annual gynecology examination. She reports that her mother and both of her sisters have fibroids, and she is concerned that she may also have fibroids given symptoms that have developed over the past several years.

66. Her most likely symptom is:

A. Dysmenorrhea
B. Abnormal uterine bleeding
C. Incontinence
D. Infertility
E. Constipation

67. Evaluation of this patient will include a Pap smear and pelvic exam. Figure 2-67 shows the various locations in which fibroids can occur. Which of the following diagnostic modalities is most commonly used to identify fibroids?

A. MRI
B. Saline infusion sonography
C. Hysterosalpingogram (HSG)
D. Ultrasound
E. Hysteroscopy

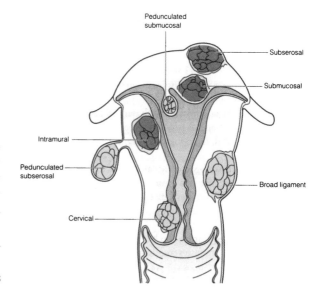

Figure 2-67 • Reproduced from Callahan TL, Caughey AB. Blueprints Obstetrics & Gynecology, 4th ed. Baltimore: Lippincott Williams & Wilkins, 2007. Fig. 14-2, p. 156.

End of Set

68. A 29-year-old woman complains of painful lesions near her vagina. She notes that they appeared to be fluid filled, were painful, and some of them "erupted." Her partner has no complaints. On examination there are multiple fluid filled vesicles on her perineum. Which of the following is the "gold standard" for the diagnosis of genital herpes?

    A. Viral culture of the affected area
    B. Tzanck smear of the fluid from several of the lesions
    C. IgG and IgM antibodies to HSV-2
    D. IgA and IgG antibodies to HSV-1
    E. Darkfield microscopy

The response options for items 69 to 72 are the same. You will be required to select one answer for each item in the set.

    A. HPV serotypes 6 and 11
    B. *Treponema pallidum*
    C. *Calymmatobacterium granulomatis*
    D. *Chlamydia trachomatis*, L serotypes
    E. *Haemophilus ducreyi*
    F. Herpes simplex virus (HSV)
    G. Molluscum contagiosum
    H. Behçet's syndrome

For each disease presentation, select the most likely etiologic agent.

69. A 17-year-old recent immigrant from Africa presents with painful inguinal adenopathy, fever, headache, malaise, and anorexia. She has not noticed any ulcerations and her physical examination is significant for painful, large inguinal adenopathy.

70. A 22-year-old sexually active woman presents complaining of a painful ulcer on the skin near her genitalia. On examination, she has a single painful, demarcated nonindurated ulcer on the skin immediately next to her left labium majus. You note left greater than right inguinal adenopathy.

71. A 25-year-old woman complains of "raised bumps" on her genitalia. On examination you note multiple lesions of the vulva and vagina resembling cauliflower shaped raised warts.

72. A 31-year-old woman presents with "bumps" on the skin near her genitalia. On examination, she has 20 solitary papules approximately 3 to 5 mm in diameter each with an umbilicated center.

End of Set

73. A 57-year-old nun presents without complaint for her routine annual exam and mammogram. On inspection of the vulva you notice a 1 × 1 cm area of ulceration on the left labia majora. The lesion is painless. In addition to drawing a rapid plasma reagin (RPR) to rule out the diagnosis of syphilis, you should:

    A. Do nothing until the RPR results return
    B. Perform a punch biopsy
    C. Perform cryotherapy on the lesion
    D. Prescribe a topical steroid
    E. Inject the lesion with subcutaneous steroids

74. You are in your GYN anatomy study section reviewing the structural changes of the cervix during puberty. The professor explains that during puberty, the prepubertal squamocolumnar junction (SCJ) everts, creating a new and mature SCJ. The area between the prepubertal and postpubertal SCJs is the area where most dysplasia arises and is termed the:

    A. Endocervical canal (EC)
    B. Transformation zone (TZ)
    C. Posterior fornix
    D. Squamo-squamo junction (SSJ)
    E. Puberty junction

75. A 19-year-old G_1P_0 at 37 3/7 weeks reports possible leakage of fluid for the past day. Which of the following tests can help differentiate between spontaneous rupture of membranes (ROM) and stress incontinence?

    A. Pooling of fluid in the vagina and ferning of a fluid sample
    B. Pooling of fluid in the vagina, ferning of a fluid sample, ultrasound examination revealing oligohydramnios
    C. Pooling of fluid in the vagina, ultrasound examination revealing oligohydramnios, positive nitrazine test
    D. Pooling of fluid in the vagina, ferning of a fluid sample, positive stream test, positive nitrazine test
    E. Pooling of fluid in the vagina, ferning of a fluid sample, positive nitrazine test, ultrasound examination revealing oligohydramnios, positive tampon test

The response options for items 80 to 83 are the same. You will be required to select one or more answers for each item in the set.

A. Effacement
B. Fetal presentation
C. Cervical consistency
D. Dilation
E. Fetal position
F. Cervical position
G. Anterior fontanelle
H. Station
I. Posterior fontanelle
J. Biparietal diameter

For each item regarding labor and delivery, select the appropriate answer(s). Answers may be used more than once.

76. The Bishop score is comprised of these components (SELECT 5)

77. A description of the presenting part of the fetus (SELECT 1)

78. A description of the relationship of the fetal head to the maternal pelvis (SELECT 1)

79. The widest part of the fetal head (SELECT 1)

End of Set

80. What is the correct order of the cardinal movements of labor?

A. Descent, engagement, internal rotation, extension, external rotation, flexion, delivery
B. Descent, flexion, internal rotation, engagement, extension, external rotation, delivery
C. Engagement, descent, flexion, internal rotation, extension, external rotation, delivery
D. Engagement, descent, flexion, external rotation, extension, internal rotation, delivery
E. Engagement, extension, internal rotation, descent, flexion, external rotation, delivery

The response options for items 81 to 83 are the same. You will be required to select one or more answers for each item in the set.

A. Occiput anterior
B. Right occiput anterior
C. Right occiput transverse
D. Right occiput posterior
E. Occiput posterior
F. Left occiput posterior
G. Left occiput transverse
H. Left occiput anterior

For each diagram, select the correct fetal position. Answers may be used more than once.

81. Figure 2-81.

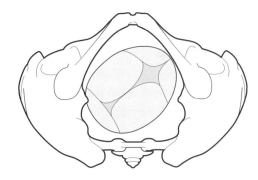

Figure 2-81 • Reproduced from Callahan TL, Caughey AB. Blueprints Obstetrics & Gynecology, 4th ed. Baltimore: Lippincott Williams & Wilkins, 2007. Fig. 4-5, p. 40.

82. Figure 2-82.

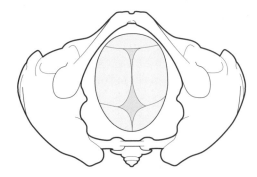

Figure 2-82 • Reproduced from Callahan TL, Caughey AB. Blueprints Obstetrics & Gynecology, 4th ed. Baltimore: Lippincott Williams & Wilkins, 2007. Fig. 4-5, p. 40.

83. Figure 2-83.

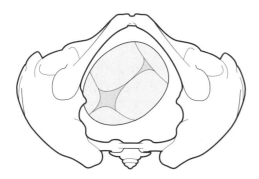

Figure 2-83 • Reproduced from Callahan TL, Caughey AB. Blueprints Obstetrics & Gynecology, 4th ed. Baltimore: Lippincott Williams & Wilkins, 2007. Fig. 4-5, p. 40.

End of Set

84. A 29-year-old G_2P_2 had vaginal birth complicated by a postpartum hemorrhage with an estimated blood loss of 1000 mL. The hemorrhage was attributed to a uterine inversion in the third stage of labor. Which of the following is a risk factor for uterine inversion?

    A. Twin gestation
    B. Excessive umbilical cord traction
    C. Succenturiate lobe of the placenta
    D. Pitocin administration
    E. Forceps-assisted delivery

85. You are a chief resident on labor and delivery called to assist an intern with a patient who has had a uterine inversion. In order to replace the uterine fundus, uterine relaxation must be facilitated. Which of the following can be used as a uterine relaxant?

    A. Metoprolol
    B. Nitroglycerine
    C. Lidocaine
    D. Hydralazine
    E. Pitocin

The response options for items 86 to 89 are the same. You will be required to select one or more answers for each item in the set.

    A. Circumvallate placenta
    B. Placenta previa
    C. Placenta accreta
    D. Placenta increta
    E. Placenta percreta
    F. Vasa previa
    G. Placental abruption
    H. Velamentous placenta
    I. Succenturiate placenta

For each item regarding placentas, select the appropriate answer(s). Answers may be used more than once.

86. These are major causes of antepartum hemorrhaging (**SELECT 2**)

87. An abnormality of placentation that can lead to antepartum hemorrhaging and is characterized by invasion of the placenta through the uterine serosa and possibly into adjacent organs such as the bladder or rectum (**SELECT 1**)

88. Insertion of blood vessels between the amnion and the chorion rather than directly into the placenta, leaving exposed vessels subject to compression or injury (**SELECT 1**)

89. Abnormal placental location over the cervix as depicted in Figure 2-89 (**SELECT 1**)

End of Set

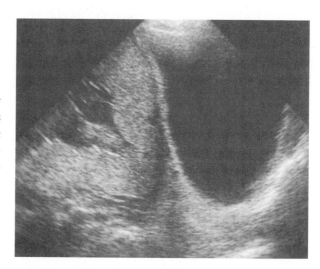

Figure 2-89 • Image Provided by Departments of Radiology and Obstetrics & Gynecology, University of California, San Francisco.

90. A 22-year-old G_3P_1 at 24 1/7 weeks presents with painful uterine contractions and cervical dilation of 2 cm. You examine her prenatal chart and realize that her LMP results in a gestational age of 24 1/7 weeks while a 6-week ultrasound would give her an estimated gestational age (EGA) of 22 6/7 weeks. Which of the following is correct?

A. The EGA of the fetus is 24 1/7 weeks because the ultrasound is consistent with the LMP
B. The EGA of the fetus is 22 6/7 weeks because in this case, the ultrasound is more accurate than an LMP
C. The EGA of the fetus is 23 4/7 weeks because you should average the two when they are within 10 days
D. The EGA of the fetus is 22 6/7 weeks because ultrasound is always more accurate than LMP dating
E. The EGA of the fetus is 24 1/7 weeks because a sure normal LMP is more accurate than a first trimester ultrasound

91. You are seeing a 34-year-old G_1P_0 at 28 weeks with systemic lupus erythematosus (SLE) who is asymptomatic. Over the course of her prenatal care you have relayed test results and educated her on the importance of prenatal care, labor, and delivery. Which of the following requires further work-up during her pregnancy?

A. Result of the 50-gm glucose load test (GLT) of 128 mg/dL
B. Blood type AB+, antibody negative
C. RPR positive, fluorescent treponemal antibody absorption (FT-ABS) nonreactive, lupus anticoagulant (LAC) negative, and anticardiolipin antibody (ACA) positive
D. PPD+, chest radiograph negative for active tuberculosis, status post 6 months of isoniazid for prophylaxis of tuberculosis
E. No history of chicken pox

92. A 17-year-old woman who has recently become sexually active comes to your office to discuss contraceptive options. She is in a monogamous relationship with her boyfriend of 7 months, and is only concerned about preventing pregnancy. She says many of her friends use "the pill" and seem to be satisfied, but she wants to know more about how they work. Which of the following best explains the primary mechanism of action of daily combined oral contraceptive pills?

A. They provide a mechanical barrier to fertilization of the egg by sperm
B. They prevent the development of a dominant ovarian follicle and subsequent ovulation
C. They inhibit uterine implantation of the embryo

D. They arrest the movement of sperm until the egg is no longer viable for fertilization
E. They stop the migration of the zygote from the Fallopian tube to the uterus

93. A 33-year-old G_3P_3 woman expresses a desire to begin long-term contraception. She is in the process of narrowing her options and is currently leaning toward an intrauterine device (IUD). However, she is worried about the side effects and adverse reactions of this method. Which of the following is accurate regarding the side effects of IUD use?

A. IUDs can cause unintended permanent sterility if used for long periods of time
B. She has a 15% increased chance of developing uterine cancer
C. She could experience vaginal bleeding between periods
D. IUDs are associated with vaginal dryness and decreased libido in some women
E. She may develop weight gain and breast tenderness

94. A couple approaches you to discuss options for permanent sterilization. They have 4 children and are sure they do not want more. After discussing techniques employed to sterilize women, including tubal ligation and hysterectomy, the discussion turns toward vasectomy. The husband has many questions regarding this procedure, and wants your opinion. What can you accurately tell him about vasectomy?

A. A vasectomy is easier to reverse than most female sterilization procedures
B. Vasectomy poses greater risk for adverse outcomes compared to tubal ligation
C. There is a 13% failure rate associated with vasectomy
D. The procedure typically requires an operating room and general anesthesia
E. Most men need 1 to 2 months of androgen supplementation following the procedure

95. A 34-year-old woman who underwent a Pomeroy tubal ligation one year ago now presents with a positive pregnancy test. She reports that a repeat test done the next day was also positive. What diagnosis must always be suspected when you find a positive pregnancy test in a patient who has previously undergone tubal ligation?

A. The fetus has Down's syndrome

B. The patient has an undetected tumor that is secreting β-hCG

C. The woman suffers from a psychiatric illness

D. The pregnancy is ectopic

E. The results are false positives

96. A single father accompanies his 10-year-old daughter to an annual well-child visit. He reports that his daughter has noted breast growth in the last few months. She would like to know what changes to expect over the next few years. In the course of your discussion, you explain that the pubertal milestone with the *latest onset* is usually:

A. Adrenarche

B. Gonadarche

C. Menarche

D. Pubarche

E. Thelarche

97. A 28-year-old G_0 woman with tubal factor infertility develops ovarian hyperstimulation syndrome after being treated with gonadotropins for ovulation induction. Her serum estradiol level is markedly elevated at 5000 pg/mL. Which of the following best describes the cellular origin and hormonal control of estradiol production in the nongravid patient (whether or not ovulation is exogenously induced)?

A. Produced by theca interna cells, in response to luteinizing hormone (LH) stimulation

B. Produced by theca interna cells, in response to follicle simulating hormone (FSH) stimulation

C. Produced by theca interna cells, in response to human chorionic gonadotropin (hCG) stimulation

D. Produced by granulosa cells, in response to LH stimulation

E. Produced by granulosa cells, in response to FSH stimulation

98. A 31-year-old G_0 woman presents to your office after a positive home pregnancy test. Her LMP was 6 weeks ago. In addition to many questions about her pregnancy, she is curious about the hormone detected by the home pregnancy test. Which of the following best describes the *direct* effect of hCG?

A. Causes a midcycle LH surge

B. Triggers ovulation

C. Maintains the corpus luteum

D. Maintains the endometrial lining

E. Stimulates growth of ovarian follicles

99. A 28-year-old G_0 woman presents to your clinic because she would like to conceive and would like to time intercourse to optimize her chances for conception. She has previously been using barrier contraception, and has had regular 34-day menstrual cycles for several years. Which of the following is the most likely day of ovulation for this patient?

A. Cycle day 12

B. Cycle day 14

C. Cycle day 16

D. Cycle day 18

E. Cycle day 20

100. A 24-year-old G_0 woman presents with a 3-year history of infertility. She reports that she has had three to four periods a year since menarche, with the last one occurring 4 months ago. On physical exam, the patient is obese, and facial hair is noted. She has normal female secondary sexual characteristics and a normal pelvic exam. Transvaginal ultrasound reveals multiple ovarian follicles bilaterally. The pathologic process causing this patient's oligomenorrhea and infertility is most likely to decrease production of which of the following?

A. Estrogens

B. Androgens

C. Sex hormone binding globulin (SHBG)

D. LH

E. Insulin

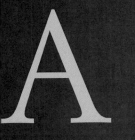

Answers and Explanations

51. B	68. A	85. B
52. C	69. D	86. B, G
53. B	70. E	87. E
54. E	71. A	88. G
55. E	72. G	89. B
56. C	73. B	90. B
57. C	74. B	91. E
58. E	75. E	92. B
59. A	76. A, C, D, F, H	93. C
60. D	77. B	94. A
61. A	78. E	95. D
62. D	79. J	96. C
63. A	80. C	97. E
64. E	81. D	98. C
65. B	82. A	99. E
66. B	83. H	100. C
67. D	84. B	

51. **B. Clomiphene citrate works at the level of the hypothalamus by preventing negative feedback and stimulating FSH and LH production in response to pulsatile GnRH, thereby stimulating ovarian follicular development.**

    A. In order to be an effective therapy, the axis already needs to be intact.
    C. Once ovarian failure has occurred, treatment with clomiphene will not induce ovulation.
    D. Mucus quality may change, but this is not the primary mechanism of action.
    E. The endometrium is affected by the increase in estrogen production, but this is not the primary mechanism of action.

52. **C. Postpartum hemorrhaging is defined as the loss of 500 mL or more of blood in the first 24 hours after a vaginal delivery or 1000 mL or greater after a cesarean delivery. This amount is commonly underestimated, and some reports indicate that a much higher percentage of vaginal deliveries have 500 mL of bleeding or more. Risk factors for postpartum hemorrhage fall into four major categories: (1) uterine atony, (2) retained placental tissue, (3) lacerations, and (4) uterine inversion. Uterine atony is associated with a distended uterus from a macrosomic fetus or multiple gestations, poor myometrial contraction from infection or prolonged labor, and higher number of parity.**

    A, B, D, E. See explanation for C.

53. **B. Mastitis (mammary cellulitis) is a common infection of the lactating breast. It occurs in approximately 2% to 3% of breastfeeding mothers. The most common organism is *Staphylococcus aureus*. The etiologic organism most commonly arises from the oropharynx of the nursing infant and enters the breast via cracks or fissures. Since the infant is already colonized, no precautions need to be taken to protect the infant from the mother's mastitis. Patients should be encouraged to continue breastfeeding the infant from the infected breast, as routine emptying of the infected breast will expedite treatment of the infection and prevent breast engorgement. Uncomplicated mastitis is treated on an outpatient basis with oral antibiotics, most commonly dicloxacillin or erythromycin if there is a penicillin allergy. Approximately 10% of** women with mastitis will develop a breast abscess, which often requires surgical incision and drainage.

    A. The infant should continue to breastfeed. The mother should be reassured that her mastitis will not cause any infection in her infant. She should be encouraged to first put the infant on the infected breast to assure that she fully empties the infected breast at each feeding.
    C. In mastitis it is important that the infected breast be emptied frequently to avoid engorgement and abscess formation. The preferred method of emptying is for the infant to breastfeed. However, occasionally the breast is so painful that the mother cannot stand the infant's suckling. In such cases, she should be encouraged to either pump or manually express the milk from her breast until she can tolerate return of infant suckling.
    D. The infant should continue to consume unaltered breast milk from both breasts. The milk does not need to be sterilized before the infant consumes it.
    E. Most etiologic organisms of mastitis arise from the mouth of the nursing infant. Thus, the infant will not become "infected" from continued consumption of breast milk. The infant does not need to be treated with antibiotics. However, some of the mother's antibiotics will be excreted into her breast milk. It is not uncommon for the breastfed infant to develop oral candidiasis ("thrush") when the mother takes antibiotics.

54. **E. Risk factors for development of cervical carcinoma include HPV infection, young age at first intercourse, multiple sex partners, cigarette smoking, immunosuppressed state, early child bearing, low socioeconomic status, and a high-risk male consort (male partners whose prior female partners have developed cervical neoplasia).**

    A. First act of intercourse at a young age is a risk factor for development of cervical carcinoma. Most authorities consider 17 years of age at the time of first intercourse to be young. In general, the younger the age at first intercourse, the higher the risk. Women who have never had sex have a very low rate of developing cervical cancer.

B. Although a high fat diet is generally not good for one's health, it has not specifically been associated with an increased risk for cervical cancer. There is some weak evidence suggesting that a diet high in folic acid and vitamin C may reduce a woman's risk for cervical cancer development. Women with cervical dysplasia are often counseled to consume 4 mg of folic acid. However, sound scientific evidence that this reverses dysplasia and/or prevents progression of disease is lacking.

C. Metaplasia is a benign process that occurs at the transformation zone when cells transform from mucus-secreting glandular cells to non-mucus-secreting squamous cells; metaplasia confers no increased risk for cervical cancer.

D. Frequent candidal infections have not been associated with an increased risk for cervical cancer. A woman who has frequent candidal infections should be screened for diabetes mellitus. She should also be counseled to avoid douching, use of perfumed soaps or vaginal deodorizers, and to wear cotton undergarments.

55. **E. Lichen planus usually occurs as a desquamative lesion of the vagina, but can involve the inner labia minora and vestibule as well. The lesions appear violaceous or red and patchy with a white lacy border. Patients typically complain of chronic vulvar burning and insertional dyspareunia. Treatment includes steroids and topical Tacrolimus (FK508). Other common vulvar dermatoses include psoriasis, lichen simplex chronicus, and lichen sclerosis. Psoriasis presents as slightly raised patches with silver scales on an erythematosus base. Lichen simplex chronicus arises from a local irritant that stimulates excoriation, which triggers hyperkeratosis, which in turn causes further itching and excoriation and perpetuates the vicious cycle. Lichen sclerosis is characterized by vulvar pruritus and diffusely involves the vulva. Lesions are thin and whitish, commonly termed "onion skin" lesions.**

A. Acne vulgaris usually arises on the face, commonly in the "T zone" where sebaceous secretions are greatest. The upper back and chest are also common sites of acne.

B. Rosacea is commonly called "adult acne" and consists of persistent redness in the center of the face that may progress to the cheeks, forehead, and chin. As the disease progresses, small blood vessels and pimples arise in the areas of erythema. However, unlike in acne vulgaris, there are no blackheads. Rosacea does not occur on the vulva.

C. Eczema may look different from person to person; however, it is most often characterized by dry, red, extremely itchy patches on the skin. Eczema is often called "the itch that rashes," since the itch, when scratched, results in the appearance of the rash. Eczema can occur on just about any part of the body. However, in infants, eczema typically occurs on the forehead, cheeks, forearms, legs, scalp, and neck. In children and adults, eczema typically occurs on the face, neck, and the insides of the elbows, knees, and ankles. Eczema does not commonly occur on the vulva.

D. Pemphigus vulgaris is a serious autoimmune system dermatologic disease that often affects the oral mucus membranes. It presents as large, fluid-filled bullae that are prone to rupture. Pemphigus vulgaris carries a high mortality rate and rarely presents on the vulva.

56. **C. This patient is unable to void and she is at high risk for an ectopic pregnancy. Due to the emergency room setting and the importance of triage, the first test to check is a serum β-hCG level and not wait for a urine pregnancy test.**

A. A pelvic ultrasound may be necessary if she has a positive β-hCG to search for the location of the pregnancy. If no intrauterine pregnancy exists and her level of β-hCG is greater than 1500 to 2000 mIU/mL (depending on the ultrasound sensitivity, this is when an intrauterine pregnancy can potentially be visualized with transvaginal ultrasound), then the possibility of ectopic pregnancy must be evaluated.

B, D. The type and screen and CBC are also appropriate for evaluation of this young woman. If she is pregnant and Rh negative, then she should be administered Rhogam since she is bleeding. Additionally, if she has an ectopic pregnancy, then the CBC is important to evaluate for intra-abdominal blood loss and is useful to know if she needs surgery.

E. A CT scan may be helpful in the diagnosis of other causes of right lower pain (e.g., appendicitis). However, her risk factors and presentation place ectopic pregnancy at the top of the differential diagnosis.

57. **C.** Prior history of ectopic pregnancy considerably increases her risk (up to 15% depending on the treatment) of a current ectopic pregnancy. Other risk factors considered "high risk" include history of any type of tubal surgery or congenital abnormalities (e.g., in utero exposure to diethylstilbestrol [DES]).

    A, B. PID, gonorrhea, and chlamydia certainly increase the risk of ectopic pregnancy. A history of infertility with clomiphene or gonadotropin use is associated with a similar ectopic risk.

    D. Smoking causes a small increase in the risk of ectopic pregnancy secondary to derangement of tubal cilia function.

    E. Previous spontaneous abortion is not known to contribute to ectopic pregnancy.

58. **E.** This patient is having what is commonly referred to as a miscarriage. The definition of inevitable abortion is vaginal bleeding before 20 weeks without expulsion of the products of conception but with cervical dilation. We can be certain that the products of conception are not expelled because the ultrasound shows a gestational sac in the uterus.

    A. Missed abortion occurs when there is death of the embryo before 20 weeks with complete retention of all products of conception. These are often diagnosed at ultrasound when the embryo or fetal size is several weeks less than dates without cardiac activity.

    B. Threatened abortion is diagnosed with any vaginal bleeding at <20 weeks gestational age. There is neither cervical dilation nor expulsion of products.

    C. Completed abortion is when all products are expelled and the cervix closes again. Often patients report that they had cramping and bleeding, then the cramping worsens and when they go to the bathroom a mass of tissue and blood clot is expelled. Patients report improvement in their bleeding and pain typically within a few hours.

    D. Incomplete abortion is diagnosed when some but not all of the products of conception are expelled.

59. **A.** The most common cause of a first trimester pregnancy loss is a chromosomal abnormality.

Estimates of up to 50% of all pregnancies may end in early loss, many of which are unrecognized. As the number of losses increases, the chance that the chromosomal abnormality is inherited increases. In fact, after three losses 3% to 8% of couples have a chromosomal abnormality.

    B. Environmental and occupational hazards such as anesthetic gases and agents used in dry cleaning (tetrachloroethylene) can cause pregnancy loss. However, chromosomal abnormalities still account for most first trimester losses.

    C. Anatomical causes such as a septate uterus, in utero DES exposure, or leiomyomata result in recurrent pregnancy loss less frequently than chromosomal abnormalities.

    D. Endocrine factors (e.g., thyroid hormone abnormalities) and hematologic disorders can lead to pregnancy loss but account for fewer cases than chromosomal abnormalities.

    E. Cervical incompetence is a cause for second trimester pregnancy loss.

60. **D.** Regardless of the gestational age when a patient presents with possible rupture of the amniotic membranes, a sterile speculum examination (SSE) must be performed to confirm this possibility. If the membranes are broken, the amniotic fluid may collect in the posterior vaginal fornix, termed pooling. Additionally, the pH of the vagina is typically acidic (pH = 4), but amniotic fluid is basic and will turn nitrazine paper blue. Once amniotic fluid dries on a slide and is observed under a microscope, it crystallizes and appears like the blades of a fern, termed ferning. Of note, blood and semen can cause a false positive nitrazine test and cervical mucus may fern in a similar pattern as amniotic fluid. Thus, the sample should be taken from the posterior fornix and not from the cervix.

    A. Admission in early labor is unwarranted for oxytocin augmentation with a reassuring FHT without a diagnosis of ROM. However, with ROM many clinicians would augment with oxytocin.

    B. This patient has a term fetus. If the patient had a viable but preterm fetus, admission for observation and intravenous antibiotics would be indicated.

C. Expectant management either at home or in the hospital has been shown to be associated with an increased rate of maternal infection and less patient satisfaction. However, some patients will prefer this management despite recommendations to the contrary. In this setting, rupture of membranes still needs to be confirmed with a SSE.

E. This is a reasonable course of action if the speculum examination is negative for evidence of ROM.

61. **A. This patient has a Bishop score of 4. The Bishop score encompasses the five components of the cervical exam (see Table 2-61). A "favorable" score is 8 or more, which indicates the likelihood for successful spontaneous or induced labor. This patient is dilated to 1.5 cm and 50% effaced, which are both good for 1 point. Also, she receives 2 points for the soft consistency. She gets zero points for the posterior position and high (–3) station. Of note, patients with a Bishop score of 5 or less typically undergo cervical ripening with prostaglandin agents as an initial approach to their induction.**

    B, C, D, E. See explanation for A.

62. **D. This FHT illustrates mild and moderate variable decelerations. Variable decelerations are characterized by a rapid onset to nadir, often in less than 30 seconds, with a rapid return to the baseline. Unless repetitive and severe, they are not concerning for fetal well-being. Therefore, the appropriate management is expectant.**

    A. An IUPC is appropriate when documentation of the timing and strength of contractions is important. For example, when contractions are persistent but no cervical change is made or there are late-shaped decelerations but uterine contractions are challenging to monitor externally, an IUPC is instrumental in determining if uterine forces are adequate or if the decelerations are late in reference to the contractions.

    B. The fetal scalp electrode is utilized if it is difficult obtain the FHT.

    C, E. There is no indication for delivery based on the information we are given. Furthermore, the patient is not completely dilated. Thus, a forceps assisted delivery is not an option.

63. **A. Variable decelerations are usually due to umbilical cord compression.**

    B. Variable decelerations are not secondary to placental insufficiency

    C, D. Late-shaped decelerations are due to uteroplacental insufficiency.

    E. Maternal hypotension can cause uteroplacental insufficiency, and thus may cause late decelerations. This is often observed after epidural placement for pain management when the sympathetic tracts are blocked causing maternal hypotension.

64. **E. Episiotomy is indicated when the delivery needs to be hastened (e.g., terminal bradycardia) or in the setting of a shoulder dystocia to facilitate delivery of the neonate.**

    A. When an episiotomy is indicated, there are two choices: a mediolateral and median. The mediolateral is an oblique incision from 5 or 7 o'clock laterally (see Figure 2-70). This type of incision is associated with fewer third- and fourth-degree lacerations but a higher incidence of postpartum infection and pain including dyspareunia.

    B. The midline episiotomy is cut vertically at 6 o'clock and results in less pain and infection when compared to a mediolateral episiotomy. However, midline episiotomies more commonly have extensions secondary to the birth process into the external sphincter or rectal mucosa, causing third- and fourth-degree lacerations.

    C. The episiotomy, like a surgical incision, is often easier to repair than the ragged edges of a perineal laceration. However, episiotomy is associated with an increased incidence of rectal and sphincter lacerations.

    D. Mediolateral episiotomy is associated with greater blood loss when compared to midline episiotomy.

65. **B. There are many indications for an operative vaginal delivery, including prolonged second stage, fetal heart rate abnormalities, and maternal exhaustion. In this scenario, the patent has an epidural and is nulliparous, which by convention would allow for her to continue pushing but she is exhausted. For an operative delivery to be performed safely several criteria**

must be met: experienced operator, complete cervical dilation, ruptured membranes, knowledge of fetal position, no evidence of cephalopelvic disproportion, adequate anesthesia, and an empty urinary bladder. In addition, most providers are not adequately experienced to perform midpelvic deliveries (from 0 to +2 station) so most clinicians restrict their practice to low (>/= +2 station) and outlet (scalp visualized at the vaginal introitus) operative deliveries.

A. The fetal station and position are requirements, not indications for operative delivery. In this case, if a delivery was attempted, it would be an elective operative delivery. Furthermore, it would be a midpelvic delivery, which is usually not attempted in the nonemergent setting.

C. Repetitive moderate variables are not an indication for delivery.

D. Adequate analgesia is required for an operative delivery.

E. For either vacuum or forceps delivery, correct ascertainment of fetal position is imperative. In this case, with confusion between LOA and ROA, either a more experienced examiner should determine position or operative delivery should not be performed.

66. **B. Abnormal uterine bleeding, often in the form of menorrhagia, is the most common symptom associated with uterine leiomyomata or fibroids. The other options can also be associated with fibroids, but bleeding is the MOST likely.**

A. Dysmenorrhea can result from fibroids but is less common.

C, E. Incontinence and constipation may be caused by the mass effect the tumors can have on the neighboring bladder and rectum.

D. Infertility can be secondary to fibroids if they impinge on the uterine cavity, block the fallopian tubes or cervical canal, or if the embryo attempts to implant on or over a fibroid.

67. **D. Ultrasound is the most commonly used diagnostic tool secondary to the widespread availability of ultrasound and reasonable resolution of fibroids. The other options are viable choices but not as commonly used due to expense, degree of invasiveness, and accessibility.**

A. MRI has high resolution but is a costly option for the evaluation of fibroids.

B, C, E. Hysterosalpingogram, saline infusion sonography, and hysteroscopy are all excellent options to evaluate the degree of impingement or distortion submucosal fibroids may have on the endometrial cavity, which may be of importance in an infertility evaluation.

68. **A. The gold standard for the diagnosis of genital herpes caused by HSV is a viral culture of a representative lesion; however, the overall sensitivity is about 50%.**

B. A Tzanck smear may reveal multinucleated giant cells but is not as sensitive as the culture.

C. Antibody titers can be used to identify the causative strain of HSV (HSV-1 vs. HSV-2) and also identify whether the infection is primary (+IgM, −IgG) or recurrent.

D. IgA does not indicate systemic infection of HSV.

E. Darkfield microscopy is used in the diagnosis of syphilis.

69. **D. This patient presents with systemic symptoms (fever, malaise, etc.) and painful inguinal adenopathy consistent with the secondary stage of lymphogranuloma venereum. Patients often do not notice the painless and transient ulceration of the primary stage of the disease. The tertiary stage consists of proctocolitis occasionally with fistula formation and elephantiasis. Advanced disease may be averted if treated with doxycycline for 3 weeks. The etiologic agents responsible are the L serotypes of *Chlamydia trachomatis*.**

70. **E. This patient suffers from Chancroid and the agent responsible is *Haemophilus ducreyi*. Patients present with painful ulcerations and adenopathy. Diagnosis is often made clinically (along with screening for other STDs), as culture is not reliable. Treatment is with antibiotics such as a cephalosporin (e.g., ceftriaxone), a macrolide (e.g., azithromycin), or a fluoroquinolone (e.g., ciprofloxacin).**

71. **A. Condyloma acuminata, or genital warts (Figure 2-71), is caused by HPV and results in warts in the anogenital area. This sexually transmitted infection can be treated with topical therapy such as trichloroacetic acid (TCA), imiquimod, 25% podophyllin, and 5% 5-fluorouracil cream. Alternatively, the lesions can be treated with cryotherapy or CO_2 laser.**

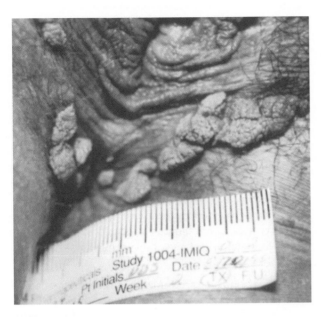

72. **G.** The patient has *Molluscum contagiosum* (Figure 2-72) caused by the pox virus by the same name. This virus does not grow on mucous membranes, and is thus found on the vulvar skin in the form of small (1 mm to 5

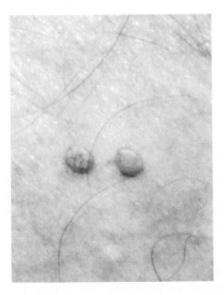

mm) umbilicated papules. The waxy material found inside a papule can be expressed onto a slide and with Wright's or Giemsa stain, intracytoplasmic molluscum bodies are observed.

B. *Treponema pallidum* is the causative agent in syphilis. In secondary syphilis, there are often lesions on the vulva called condyloma latum, which appear as large raised, gray-white lesions. Other characteristic features of secondary syphilis are mucous patches of the oropharynx and a generalized maculopapular rash, often located on the palms of the hands and the soles of the feet.

C. Donovanosis is a bacterial infection caused by the gram negative bacillus *Calymmatobacterium granulomatis*. It usually affects the groin region and can start as a small nodule and progress to a serpiginous ulceration. Donovanosis is more commonly diagnosed in developing countries with a focus in Papua, New Guinea. Proper identification requires a tissue smear. Various antibiotics have been used to treat it over the last few decades and currently azithromycin is the most cost effective.

F. HSV infections are characterized by clustered vesicles, which are preceded by a prodromal "tingling" phase. The lesion then progresses to a painful, pruritic cluster of vesicles. The vesicles will normally burst and lead to a wet ulcer. This is followed by a healing phase with a characteristic dry, crusted ulcer. Tender lymphadenopathy is typical and helps to distinguish HSV infections from the painless adenopathy associated with *Treponema pallidum*. HSV is typically treated with acyclovir.

G. Behçet's syndrome is a noninfectious, systemic inflammatory disease characterized by aphthous-like ulcers of the genitalia and mouth. It is usually distinguished from HSV infection when multiple HSV cultures return with negative results.

73. **B.** The lesion described could be a squamous cell cancer of the vulva. Any suspicious lesion on the vulva should be punch biopsied at the time of presentation. Most vulvar carcinomas arise in postmenopausal women in the posterior two-thirds of either labium majus. The most common symptom is vulvar pruritus.

A. It is inappropriate to potentially delay diagnosis while awaiting the results of the RPR. Further, it is unlikely that a 57-year-old nun has primary syphilis, although not impossible. The classic vulvar lesion of primary syphilis is a painless chancre.

C. Cryotherapy is a treatment modality and would not yield a tissue diagnosis. A vulvar lesion should only be treated with cryotherapy before a tissue diagnosis is obtained if its presentation is classic for genital warts or molluscum contagiosum.

D. Although topical steroids are a mainstay of dermatologic treatment, it would be inappropriate to prescribe a topical steroid for either a squamous cell carcinoma or syphilis lesion.

E. Very few dermatologic disorders are treated with intralesional steroid injections. Again, it would be inappropriate to prescribe steroid for either a squamous cell carcinoma or a syphilis chancre.

74. **B. The TZ is the area between the prepubertal SCJ and the postpubertal mature SCJ where metaplasia occurs. As the cervix and uterus grow during puberty, the SCJ rolls out, or everts, from its prepubertal location just inside the cervical os. As the SCJ everts, the endocervical cells behind the original SCJ are brought to the surface of the ectocervix where they undergo squamous metaplasia in response to the new surrounding secretions, irritants, and hormones. The TZ is where approximately 95% of squamous intraepithelial lesions arise.**

A. The EC consists of glandular and columnar cells that can undergo dysplastic changes. However, the incidence of dysplasia in the EC is far less than that of the cervix.

C. The posterior fornix is part of the vagina, not the cervix. Large cervical cancers can spread to encompass the posterior fornix of the vagina, but do not arise in the posterior fornix.

D, E. There is no anatomic region of the cervix referred to as either the squamo-squamo junction or the puberty junction.

75. **E. Pooling of fluid in the vagina, ferning of a fluid sample, positive nitrazine test, ultrasound examination revealing oligohydramnios, and positive tampon test can all be utilized to evaluate spontaneous ROM. The first three tests are carried** out with a sterile speculum exam via observation of a pool of fluid, and sampling of the fluid to see if upon drying, a characteristic ferning pattern is observed microscopically (ferning) and to test the pH of the fluid on nitrazine paper, which will turn blue in the presence of alkaline fluids. In a woman with a recently documented normal amount of amniotic fluid, an ultrasound revealing oligohydramnios (i.e., low amount of amniotic fluid) is suggestive of ROM. A tampon test is used in unclear situations where an accurate diagnosis of ROM is necessary. Indigo carmine dye is injected into the amniotic sac via amniocentesis, and a tampon is placed in the vagina to evaluate for leakage of dye-stained fluid from the cervix.

A. Pooling and ferning are components of amniotic fluid evaluation, but not the only ones.

B, C. In a woman with a recently documented normal amount of amniotic fluid, an ultrasound revealing oligohydramnios (i.e., low amount of amniotic fluid) is suggestive of ROM. However, other available tests exist and are discussed above.

D. There is no such thing as a stream test.

76. **A, C, D, F, H. The Bishop score is a systematic way of describing a cervical exam and was originally used to characterize the favorability of a cervix and thus predict the likelihood of a successful induction of labor. It is composed of cervical dilation, effacement, station, position, and consistency.**

77. **B. Fetal presentation is characterized by the part of the fetus that presents to the maternal pelvis (e.g., head, buttocks, foot). The terms used to describe presentation are breech, transverse, or cephalic. Breech presentations are further characterized depending on the type of breech (footling, complete, or frank). Additionally, cephalic presentation can be more specifically described as vertex presentation if the head is flexed and the vertex is truly presenting.**

78. **E. Fetal position is often confused with fetal presentation and describes only the *relationship* of the fetal presenting part to the maternal pelvis. Breech presentations are not as common as cephalic presentations and are described using the fetal sacrum as the reference point to the left**

or right, and anterior or posterior maternal pelvis. Cephalic presentations are determined using the fetal occiput as the reference point to the left or right, and anterior or posterior maternal pelvis. There are eight potential cephalic positions, ranging from occiput anterior to occiput posterior.

79. J. The biparietal diameter is the largest diameter of the fetal head and is typically 10 cm wide at term. Thus, 10-cm cervical dilation is generally required for delivery.

80. C. The cardinal movements of labor describe the fetal movements necessary for vaginal delivery. Engagement is entry of the fetal presenting part (generally the head) into the pelvis. Descent then follows as the fetal head flexes to allow the smallest diameter to present to the pelvis. Internal rotation involves the rotation of the fetal head from an occiput transverse position to either an occiput anterior or occiput posterior position. Extension occurs as the head passes beneath the pubic bone, and external rotation (also called restitution) follows delivery of the head and precedes delivery of the shoulders and the remainder of the infant.

    A, B, D, E. See explanation for C.

81. D. The anterior fontanelle is diamond-shaped and represents the intersection of the two frontal bones and the two parietal bones. The posterior fontanelle is generated by the intersection of the two parietal bones and the occipital bone. The suture connecting the two fontanelles is the sagittal suture. The relationship of these landmarks within the maternal pelvis allows the examiner to determine the fetal position as described by the relationship of the fetal occiput to the left or right, and anterior or posterior maternal pelvis.

82. A. See explanation for D.

83. H. See explanation for D.

84. B. Uterine inversion is a rare complication of the third stage of labor occurring in approximately 1 in 25,000 deliveries. Uterine inversion occurs more commonly in multiparous women and in the presence of a placenta accreta. However, the greatest risk factor for uterine

inversion is excessive umbilical cord traction before completion of uteroplacental separation. Uterine inversion is associated with postpartum hemorrhage and bradycardic shock secondary to a vagal response. It is first noted by the appearance of the placenta at the introitus attached to a mass (the uterus). Treatment is rapid reversal of the inversion by applying inward pressure around the leading portion. Uterine relaxants are often required for successful return of the uterus to its anatomic position.

A. Twin gestations are associated with many increased risks as compared to singleton gestations, including postpartum hemorrhaging. However, a twin gestation does not increase the risk of uterine inversion.

C. A succenturiate lobe is not associated with an increased risk of uterine inversion. Succenturiate lobes can be left behind in the uterus and result in increased postpartum blood loss. The placenta should always be carefully inspected after its delivery to ensure that it has been removed in its entirety.

D. Pitocin is a synthetic version of oxytocin and causes uterine contractions. Its administration is not associated with an increased risk of uterine inversion.

E. The use of forceps is not associated with an increased risk of uterine inversion. However, forceps are associated with an increased risk for postpartum hemorrhage secondary to genital tract lacerations.

85. B. Nitroglycerine (IV or sublingual) can be used for rapid uterine relaxation. Nitroglycerine also lowers blood pressure so the patient must have close cardiac monitoring when nitroglycerine is administrated. Another agent that is commonly used is terbutaline (subcutaneous or IV), a β-2 agonist, which promotes uterine relaxation.

A. Metoprolol is a β-blocker used for hypertension and is not a uterine relaxant.

C. Lidocaine is used as a local anesthetic or as an antiarrhythmic agent. It has no uterine relaxation qualities.

D. Hydralazine is a direct peripheral dilator and used for hypertension. It does not cause uterine relaxation.

E. Pitocin is used to stimulate uterine contractions rather than relax the uterus.

86. **B, G.** Placenta previa is the implantation and development of the placenta over the internal cervical os, preventing delivery of the fetus. The previa is further characterized as complete, partial, or marginal in location. Placenta previa accounts for approximately 20% of antepartum hemorrhaging while an additional 30% is attributable to placental abruption, which is the premature separation of a normally implanted placenta from the uterine wall.

87. **E.** Placenta percreta is the most severe form of placenta accreta and can lead to antepartum hemorrhage. Delivery should be via cesarean section, where treatment of the placenta percreta is careful dissection and hysterectomy.

88. **G.** Velamentous insertion of vessels can result in vessel injury and hemorrhage that can be detrimental to the fetus.

89. **B.** Placenta previa. See explanation for 86.

90. **B.** Dating in a pregnancy is important and implied in this scenario is the question of viability (i.e., the ability of the fetus to potentially survive if delivered; typically, a gestational age of 24 weeks). In general, the EGA can be determined using several factors. Very early in pregnancy (up to 7 or 8 weeks), ultrasound dating by crown-rump length is accurate to 3 to 5 days. Ultrasound is often employed for dating when the LMP is unsure or irregular. Ultrasound is quite accurate and generally is within 7 days in the first trimester, 10 to 14 days in the second trimester, and 21 days in the third trimester.

    A. In this scenario, the patient's menses and ultrasound dating are disparate by 9 days. Therefore, the most accurate EGA is 22 6/7 weeks by the first trimester ultrasound.
    C. Different estimated gestational ages should never be averaged to determine an EGA.
    D. Ultrasound is not always more accurate than a LMP as there is an error of approximately 8% at any gestational age. As such, the LMP can be consistent with ultrasound dating if it is within 3 to 5 days early in the first trimester, 10 to 14 days in the second trimester, and 21 days in the third trimester. If calculated EGAs are within these ranges, LMP dating should be used. However, deviations from these ranges should favor the ultrasound for dating.

    E. The LMP often gives the appropriate gestational age when the patient has regular monthly menses. However, in this case the early ultrasound, which is accurate to 3 to 5 days, is different by 9 days. Thus, the dating is most accurate by the ultrasound.

91. **E.** In patients with no known exposure to chicken pox or the varicella zoster virus (VZV), a titer should be obtained. If no antibodies exist, the patient should avoid exposure to known contacts.

    A. The 50-gm GLT is a screening test for gestational diabetes. Currently, the cutoff is 140 mg/dL for a positive screen, which would prompt the 100-gm 3-hour glucose tolerance test.
    B. The Rh and antibody status is important to avoid isoimmunization in future pregnancies. If the patient were Rh–, she would need Rhogam during her prenatal care.
    C. Approximately 2% of patients have a false-positive test for syphilis. Many patients with lupus have antibodies to anticardiolipin and have a false-positive RPR result. The RPR and Venereal Disease Research Laboratory (VDRL) tests are nontreponemal serologic tests for syphilis, which detect antibodies to a cardiolipin-cholesterol-lecithin antigen. The direct treponemal tests, fluorescent treponemal antibody absorption test (FT-ABS), and microhemagglutination test for antibodies to *Treponema pallidum* (MHA-TP) detect antibodies to the treponemal components. Since this is a false-positive test, these antibodies would not be present in the patient's serum.
    D. The patient has been exposed to tuberculosis and has appropriately received prophylaxis with isoniazid.

92. **B.** Combined oral contraceptive pills contain the hormones estradiol and progesterone. Depending on the brand, they come in several different formulations. Progesterone is the main contraceptive agent, suppressing LH secretion and thus ovulation. Estradiol works by decreasing FSH secretion, thereby preventing the development of a dominant follicle. These actions together are more than 99% effective in preventing pregnancy in patients who take the pill every day. The most common cause of failure is in patients who forget to take the pill daily.

A. Mechanical barriers to fertilization include such devices as condoms, diaphragms, cervical caps, foam, and spermicide. They work by physically preventing sperm from gaining access to the egg. Rates of efficacy vary considerably in this contraceptive class as they are highly dependent on the application technique and consistency of the user.

C. Inhibition of implantation is accomplished by the IUD, postcoital (emergency) oral contraceptives, and induced menstruation or abortion. Daily combined oral contraceptive use does not exert any effect on implantation, since its main mechanism of action involves prevention of zygote formation before implantation can even take place.

D. Oral contraceptive pills are known to induce thickening of cervical mucus, thus making sperm penetration into the uterus and fallopian tubes more difficult. However, combined oral contraceptive pills do not exert their effects directly on sperm, and thickened cervical mucus does not "arrest" sperm movement; it only slows it down.

E. Again, daily combined oral contraceptive pills do not exert their effects directly on formed gametes or products of conception. While some studies show that combined oral contraceptive pills can decrease fallopian tube peristalsis, this is not the main mechanism of action. In addition, peristalsis does not cease completely, and therefore, these pills do not stop the migration of a zygote to the uterine cavity.

93. **C. A common side effect of IUD use is vaginal bleeding or spotting between menstrual periods. Other common reactions include menstrual cramping and disruption of the menstrual cycle. Other more serious complications include spontaneous expulsion, uterine perforation, and increased incidence of ectopic pregnancy and pelvic infection.**

A. IUDs are believed to work mainly by creating an inflammatory response in the uterine cavity, thus making it hostile to zygote implantation. These changes are not permanent, and therefore do not cause permanent sterility.

B. There is no documented association between IUD use and uterine cancer.

D, E. There are no such effects associated with IUD use.

94. **A. While care should be taken to ensure that the couple is firm in their desire for permanent sterilization before undergoing any procedure, a vasectomy does offer the best chance of successful reversal compared to all female methods except the fallopian tube clip. This also translates to a higher failure rate, which can approach 1% (similar to the failure rate of clipping). Any other female sterilization procedure is more lasting because it involves permanent damage to all or part of the tubes, or complete removal of reproductive structures.**

B. Because vasectomy involves manipulation of structures outside the abdominal cavity, risks for adverse outcomes such as bowel perforation, uncontrolled hemorrhage, and death are markedly lower in men as compared to women.

C. See explanation for A.

D. Vasectomy involves removing a piece of the vas deferens and sealing the open ends with suture, cautery, or clip. It is generally done via a small incision into the scrotum. Because of the relatively noninvasive nature of the procedure, a vasectomy is usually done as an outpatient in the office under local anesthesia.

E. The aim of this procedure is solely to prevent sperm from being transported from the site of production (testes) to the site of release (urethra). There is no interruption in the production or transport of testosterone due to this procedure, and therefore no androgen supplementation is needed.

95. **D. Tubal ligations are more than 99% effective overall. Of the few pregnancies that do happen, about one-third of them are ectopic. However, due to the extremely dangerous situation an ectopic pregnancy can create for the mother, this worst case scenario must always be placed at the top of the differential until proven otherwise. Most cases are due to the scarring and structural damage fallopian tubes endure from the procedure as well as from microscopic fistulae that form between the disturbed segment and the peritoneal cavity.**

A. Tubal ligation has no effect on oogenesis, and thus does not increase the incidence of trisomy 21 pregnancies.

B. While this is certainly possible, few β-hCG-secreting tumors have been characterized. Also, the likelihood of occult malignancy is much lower than the likelihood of ectopic pregnancy in a healthy patient.

C. Psychiatric illness should always be a diagnosis of exclusion in patients without overt signs of psychosis or altered mental status. It should not be your first assumption.

E. Home pregnancy tests are considered almost 100% accurate, especially if two consecutive tests concur. False-positive results should not be assumed in this situation.

96. **C. Menarche is typically the pubertal milestone with the latest onset, typically occurring between ages 12 and 13. The hormonal changes of puberty begin well before the development of perceptible secondary sexual characteristics, with adrenarche and gonadarche. Subsequent phenotypic changes overlap, but onset is typically in the order of thelarche, pubarche, then menarche.**

A. Adrenarche is the regeneration of zona reticularis in the adrenal cortex and typically occurs between ages 6 and 8 years. Along with gonadarche, it is one of the hormonal changes of puberty that begins well before the development of perceptible secondary sexual characteristics.

B. Gonadarche is the GnRH-stimulated release of FSH and LH from the anterior pituitary. It typically occurs around age 8.

D. Pubarche is the development of pubic and axillary hair and typically occurs around age 12, after thelarche but before menarche.

E. Thelarche is breast development and typically occurs around age 10 to 11, followed by pubarche and menarche.

97. **E. Estrogen is produced in the ovary in a "two-cell" process: Theca interna cells produce androstenedione in response to LH stimulation, and granulosa cells aromatize androstenedione to estradiol in response to FSH stimulation.**

A, B, D. See explanation for E.

C. hCG is a hormone unique to pregnancy and does not play a role in estrogen production in the nongravid patient.

98. **C. hCG is a trophoblast-produced glycoprotein unique to pregnancy (although it bears considerable structural similarity to LH). The primary role of hCG is to maintain the corpus luteum, which in turn produces estrogen and progesterone until the placenta is able to assume synthetic responsibility for these hormones. Without fertilization and subsequent hCG production, the corpus luteum regresses and hormonal support for the endometrium is lost, leading to menstruation.**

A. Elevated estradiol triggers the midcycle LH surge.

B. The midcycle LH surge triggers ovulation.

D. Progesterone maintains the endometrial lining.

E. FSH, fittingly, stimulates the growth of ovarian follicles.

99. **E. Despite individual variation in the length of the follicular phase of the menstrual cycle, the luteal phase is generally consistent in all women: Menses occurs 14 days after ovulation. Ovulation occurs on day 14 of the common 28- day cycle, but on day 20 of a 34-day cycle.**

A, B, C, D. See explanation for E.

100. **C. This patient presents with classic features of polycystic ovarian syndrome (PCOS); production of SHBG is decreased in this process. PCOS is a self-perpetuating cycle in which chronic anovulation leads to increased levels of androgen production by the ovaries and adrenal cortex. These androgens are peripherally converted into estrone, increasing estrogen levels. Elevated androgens lead to a decrease in the production of SHBG, which leads to even higher levels of free estrogens and androgens. Elevated estrogens lead to increased LH levels, an increased LH-to-FSH ratio, abnormal follicular development, anovulation, and increased androgen production, thus perpetuating the cycle. The etiology initiating this cycle is not clear.**

A, B, D. See explanation for C.

E. Many patients with PCOS are insulin-resistant, and become hyperinsulinemic. The incidence of type II diabetes is increased in these patients.

BLOCK 3

The next three questions (items 101 to 103) correspond to the following vignette.

A 43-year-old G_2P_2 presents for her annual gynecologic visit. She has been unsuccessfully trying to conceive a third child for several years (but has declined any fertility diagnosis or treatment). She reports several months of irregular periods, and is concerned that she is having symptoms of menopause. The patient's physical exam is unremarkable, with no signs of vaginal atrophy.

101. The patient asks if menopause at her age would be abnormal. In the course of your explanation, you tell her that the average age of menopause in the United States is closest to:

    A. 35 years
    B. 40 years
    C. 45 years
    D. 50 years
    E. 55 years

102. Which of the following laboratory test profiles would be expected if this patient was indeed menopausal?

    A. High follicle stimulating hormone (FSH), low luteinizing hormone (LH)
    B. High FSH, high LH
    C. Low FSH, low LH
    D. Low FSH, high LH
    E. Low FSH, LH within normal limits

103. The patient reports that her older sister is taking hormone replacement therapy (HRT), and she is confused by conflicting information about its risks and benefits. According to the best available current evidence, HRT is most likely to *decrease* the risk of which of the following?

    A. Thromboembolic events
    B. Myocardial infarction
    C. Hip fracture
    D. Breast cancer
    E. Ovarian cancer

End of Set

104. A 59-year-old G_0 complains of occasional spotting over the past 2 months. She underwent menopause at age 54 and previous to that had infrequent, irregular menstrual cycles most of her adult life. Her medical history is significant for hypertension, hyperlipidemia, and obesity. On exam, she is moderately obese with a normal pelvic exam. An ultrasound shows an endometrial stripe that is thickened, shown in Figure 2-104. Suspicious of endometrial hyperplasia or cancer, you perform an endometrial biopsy, which returns grade 1 endometrial cancer. The patient subsequently undergoes surgical staging, total abdominal hysterectomy, and bilateral salpingo-oophorectomy. Which of the following is a risk factor for endometrial cancer?

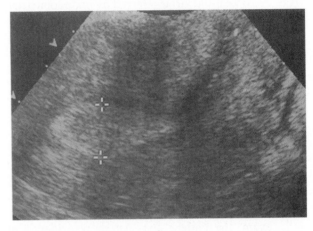

Figure 2-104 • Image Provided by Departments of Radiology and Obstetrics & Gynecology, University of California, San Francisco.

    A. Obesity
    B. Late onset of menarche
    C. Multiparity
    D. Cyclic progestin therapy
    E. Early age of menopause

105. A 43-year-old G_0 reports several episodes of painless postcoital bleeding over the past month. She also notes some vulvar pruritus and an increase in a white, clumpy vaginal discharge. Her gynecological history is significant for no history of abnormal Pap smears or sexually transmitted diseases, and she is in a mutually monogamous relationship with her husband. Which of the following can be excluded from the differential diagnosis based on history?

    A. Cervical polyp
    B. Yeast vaginitis
    C. Cervical cancer
    D. Vulvar intraepithelial neoplasia
    E. Submucosal fibroid

The response options for items 106 to 109 are the same. You will be required to select one answer for each item in the set.

    A. Hypothalamic-pituitary dysfunction
    B. Gonadal dysgenesis (primary ovarian failure)
    C. Müllerian agenesis
    D. Testicular feminization (androgen insensitivity)
    E. Imperforate hymen

For each vignette, select the most likely cause of primary amenorrhea that is consistent with the findings.

106. A 16-year-old girl is referred by her pediatrician because she has never had a menstrual period. She has no known medical or surgical history and is not taking any medications. On physical exam, she shows evidence of breast development. Pelvic exam demonstrates a patent vagina, but no uterus is palpated on physical exam or visualized by ultrasound. A karyotype is obtained and is found to be 46,XY.

107. A 16-year-old girl is referred by her pediatrician because she has never had a menstrual period. She has no known medical or surgical history and is not taking any medications. On physical exam, the patient does *not* show evidence of breast development. Pelvic exam demonstrates a normal uterus and vagina. Her karyotype is 46,XX and her FSH level is low.

108. A 16-year-old girl is referred by her pediatrician because she has never had a menstrual period. She has no known medical or surgical history and is not taking any medications. On physical exam, the patient does *not* show evidence of breast development. Pelvic exam demonstrates a normal uterus and vagina. Her karyotype is 46,XX and her FSH level is markedly elevated.

109. A 16-year-old girl is referred by her pediatrician because she has never had a menstrual period. She has no known medical or surgical history and is not taking any medications. She reports monthly cyclical pelvic pain. On physical exam, the patient has breasts and pubic hair. On perineal exam, you see a suburethral bluish bulge. Rectal exam notes a midline fullness. Ultrasound demonstrates a normal-appearing uterus.

End of Set

110. A 33-year-old G_2P_1 presents with 3 months of amenorrhea after previously normal menstrual cycles (every 28 days, with light flow lasting 4 days). She is otherwise without complaint, and her physical exam is unremarkable. A serum level of which of the following is the most appropriate initial step in her evaluation?

    A. Human chorionic gonadotropin (hCG)
    B. Thyroid stimulating hormone (TSH)
    C. Prolactin
    D. Insulin
    E. FSH

The next two questions (items 111 and 112) correspond to the following vignette.

A 30-year-old G_0 woman presents with 7 months of amenorrhea. She previously had fairly regular cycles (every 30 days, occasionally missing a period). She has no previous medical or surgical history and is not currently taking any medications. A urine pregnancy test is negative.

111. The patient is given oral medroxyprogesterone for 7 days and experiences vaginal bleeding 2 days after the end of this treatment. Based on this finding, which of the following is the most likely cause of this patient's secondary amenorrhea?

    A. Hypogonadotropic hypogonadism (hypothalamic-pituitary dysfunction)
    B. Hyperprolactinemia
    C. Hypoestrogenism secondary to ovarian failure
    D. Asherman's syndrome (intrauterine adhesions)
    E. Cervical stenosis

112. Which of the following, if found in laboratory testing, would prompt an MRI as the most appropriate next step in the management of this patient?

    A. Elevated serum TSH level
    B. Elevated serum prolactin level
    C. Elevated serum FSH level
    D. Elevated serum free estrogens
    E. Elevated serum free androgens

End of Set

113. A 33-year-old G_0 woman presents with a 2-year history of infertility. She has had irregular periods for the last several years, and reports that she has not had a period in the last 4 months. Which

one of the following conditions is most likely to result in a positive progesterone withdrawal test (i.e., vaginal bleeding in response to medroxyprogesterone administration)?

A. Pregnancy
B. Ovarian failure
C. Pituitary failure
D. Müllerian agenesis
E. Polycystic ovary syndrome (PCOS)

114. A 17-year-old G_0 woman presents to your clinic reporting a 2-year history of severe pain, cramping, and nausea occurring on the first and second days of her menstrual cycle. These symptoms frequently cause her to miss school. She achieves minimal relief from several nonsteroidal anti-inflammatory drugs (NSAIDs) that she has tried, even at high doses. She has no significant medical or surgical history and has recently had negative culture results for common pelvic infections. She is currently using barrier contraception. A pelvic exam is unremarkable, and ultrasound shows a normal-sized uterus with no masses. Which of the following is the most appropriate next therapeutic step?

A. OCPs
B. Cervical dilation
C. Neurectomy
D. Leuprolide injections
E. Reassurance and expectant management

115. A 26-year-old G_0 presents with several months of regular, heavy menstrual bleeding (1 pad per hour) lasting for several days. Her cycles remain regularly spaced at 29 days, and she does not experience spotting between periods. A urine pregnancy test is negative. Which of the following terms best describes this patient's abnormal uterine bleeding?

A. Hypomenorrhea
B. Menorrhagia
C. Metrorrhagia
D. Menometrorrhagia
E. Oligomenorrhea

The next two questions (items 116 and 117) correspond to the following vignette.

A 55-year-old G_3P_3 presents to your office complaining of vaginal bleeding. Her last menstrual period was 3 years ago. She is not currently on HRT.

116. Which of the following is the most likely cause of this patient's bleeding?

A. Vaginal and/or endometrial atrophy
B. Endometrial polyp
C. Endometrial malignancy
D. Cervical malignancy
E. Vaginal malignancy

117. Among the following, what is the most appropriate next step in the management of this patient?

A. Hysterectomy
B. Dilatation and curettage (D&C)
C. Endometrial biopsy
D. Endometrial ablation
E. Intermittent progestin therapy

End of Set

118. A 28-year-old woman with a dichorionic/diamniotic twin gestation at term is admitted for induction of labor. You perform a brief physical exam and note that her blood pressure (BP) is 150/80. You also note mild bilateral lower extremity edema and diaphoresis on exam. You are concerned that this patient may have gestational hypertension and check preeclampsia labs. Which of the following findings meets the clinical definition of gestational hypertension?

A. Systolic BP greater than 130 mm Hg
B. Diastolic BP greater than 90 mm Hg
C. Gestational diabetes
D. Obesity
E. Bilateral lower extremity edema

119. A 26-year-old G_4P_2 comes to you for contraceptive counseling. She states that she does not want to have another child for at least 4 years. Her history is notable for the following: (1) a history of trichomonas at age 18; (2) a DVT in her left leg at age 24 while on a 30-µg ethinyl estradiol-containing oral contraceptive (she is no longer on anticoagulation); and (3) two prior cesarean deliveries for arrest of descent during the second stage of labor. She has no history of hypertension, diabetes mellitus, cardiovascular disease, or cerebrovascular accident. She does not smoke. Of the following, which would you most recommend to this patient?

A. Low-dose combined OCPs
B. Ortho Evra transdermal patch (norelgestro-min/ethinyl estradiol)
C. Mirena IUD (levonorgestrel)
D. Nuva Ring (etonogestrel/ethinyl estradiol)
E. Laparoscopic tubal ligation

120. A 24-year-old nonpregnant woman presents with progressively worsening, severe labial pain for 3 days that is not relieved with ibuprofen. She has never had this pain before and reports that it is on her right labia, enlarging, and making it difficult to walk. She is sexually active with one partner and uses the birth control patch for contraception. On physical exam, she has a temperature of 100.0°F, tender lymphadenopathy in the right inguinal region, and her labia are shown in Figure 2-120. The likely diagnosis is:

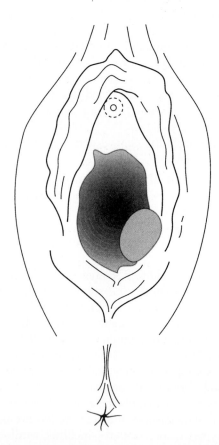

Figure 2-120 • Reproduced with Permission from Callahan T. Blueprints Obstetrics & Gynecology, 3rd ed. Blackwell Publishing, 2004. Fig. 13-4, p. 126.

A. Chancre
B. Bartholin's gland abscess
C. Vulvar candidiasis
D. Lichen sclerosus
E. Condyloma acuminata

The next two questions (items 121 and 122) correspond to the following vignette.

An 18-year-old G_1P_0 at 36 2/7 weeks by LMP presents to your office for a prenatal visit. At this time, you find that her BP is elevated at 166/98. You test her urine and find that it contains 3+ protein. She also exhibits moderately edematous upper and lower extremities bilaterally. Another BP 6 hours later reveals a pressure of 165/95. Based on this information, you suspect preeclampsia.

121. What additional historical information or objective finding would further suggest a diagnosis of preeclampsia in this patient?

A. Left lower quadrant pain
B. Increased urine output
C. Platelet count of 900,000
D. Complaints of blind spots in vision
E. Unexplained diarrhea

122. The patient is admitted for labor induction and magnesium sulfate seizure prophylaxis. However, she suffers an eclamptic seizure later that day. When you arrive to assess the patient, she is no longer seizing. Fetal heart rate monitoring exhibits decreased variability but no decelerations. What is the most appropriate next step in the management of this patient?

A. Provide supportive care (airway, breathing, circulation, etc.)
B. Administer diazepam or similar fast-acting anticonvulsant immediately
C. Deliver the baby immediately
D. Type and cross 2 units of packed red blood cells (RBC) for transfusion
E. Administer tocolytics

End of Set

123. A 29-year-old woman comes to your office with complaints of increased hair growth on her abdomen, lower back, and face, as well as "hoarseness" in her voice. Her menstrual periods

are regular, she has no history of chromosomal abnormality, and her past medical history is negative. On exam, she has increased terminal hair on her lower abdomen and lower back and increased facial hair. She also exhibits some mild temporal balding. Which of the following conditions could have caused these findings in this patient?

A. Grave's disease
B. Menopause
C. Use of spironolactone diuretic
D. Decreased levels of sex hormone-binding globulin (SHBG)
E. Deficiency in 5α-reductase activity

124. A 22-year-old woman presents to your office for her annual exam. During the examination, you notice that she has slightly increased hair growth on her abdomen, and her voice is deeper than you remember. She denies any major changes in her menstrual cycle or body. Nonetheless, you proceed with a workup for a virilizing syndrome and find that her testosterone levels are slightly above the normal range, with normal adrenal and ovarian functions. You decide that the increased testosterone is probably due to increased peripheral (extraglandular) production of androgen. Where does this peripheral production of testosterone from androstenedione primarily take place?

A. Hepatocytes
B. Type II alveolar cells
C. Vascular endothelium
D. Hair follicles
E. Adipocytes

The next two questions (items 125 and 126) correspond to the following vignette.

A 19-year-old G_1P_0 woman at 27 3/7 weeks GA by last menstrual period (LMP) comes to you for a routine prenatal visit. As you perform the physical exam, the patient mentions that her older sister had undergone gestational diabetes mellitus (GDM) screening during her pregnancy and the patient is now wondering whether she needs it as well.

125. Which of the following must be present in a patient to warrant a 1-hour glucola test for GDM screening?

A. Persistent glucose in the urine
B. Obesity
C. Strong family history of diabetes
D. History of giving birth to a large infant
E. GDM screening is done in all pregnancies regardless of risk factors or objective findings

126. You find that the patient meets your criteria for testing, and you perform the test. The result comes back positive with a blood glucose level of 154 mg/dL. Considering this result, what is the most appropriate next step in her management?

A. Initiation of an appropriate insulin regimen
B. Administration of a 3-hour glucose tolerance test (GTT)
C. Carbohydrate restriction diet
D. A second glucola test as two abnormal values are required for diagnosis
E. Ultrasound to assess the extent of the effects of this condition on the fetus

End of Set

127. A 22-year-old G_2P_1 woman at 34 weeks by LMP presents with dysuria and urinary frequency of 2 days' duration. She reports a slight fever, but no chills, nausea, or vomiting. She has not had sexual intercourse in 2 weeks. On exam she has no costovertebral angle tenderness. A urinalysis shows 12 white blood cells (WBC) per high power field, and urine culture grows 100,000 colonies of *Escherichia coli*. Other than pregnancy itself, which of the following factors has been shown to increase the incidence of urinary tract infections (UTI) during pregnancy?

A. GDM
B. Hyperemesis gravidarum
C. Ptyalism
D. GBS infection
E. Preeclampsia

128. A 25-year-old woman and her husband come to see you because they have not been able to conceive a child despite trying for over 13 months now. The husband has no problems with maintaining an erection or with ejaculation. The woman denies menstrual irregularity or any history of sexually transmitted disease. They are not on any chronic medications, do not smoke, and maintain a regular exercise regimen. She has recorded her basal body temperature over the

last month and reports a normal biphasic temperature shift in the middle of her cycle. Based on these findings, which of the following diagnostic tests should be initiated first?

A. Hysterosalpingogram
B. Huhner-Sims (postcoital) test
C. Testicular biopsy
D. Diagnostic laparoscopy of wife's genital tract
E. Semen analysis

129. You have recently diagnosed a 26-year-old woman with infertility due to anovulation. She agreed to a trial of clomiphene citrate to induce ovulation, but subsequently failed 5 cycles. She and her partner are aware of the many other options available to them and are eager to continue trying to conceive. What, based on the failure of clomiphene citrate, is the most appropriate next step in this patient's management?

A. In vitro fertilization (IVF)
B. Trial of human menopausal gonadotropin (exogenous FSH)
C. Intrauterine insemination (IUI)
D. Use of donor ova
E. Referral to an adoption agency

130. A couple in their early 30s presents with an inability to conceive for over 1 year. The wife was told that a frequent cause of female infertility is anovulation, and as a result she recorded her basal body temperature over the preceding 28 days to assess her cycle. The data reflected fluctuations in body temperature that occurred over the course of her menstrual cycle, as shown below. Based on the graph in Figure 2-130, at what point did ovulation most likely occur?

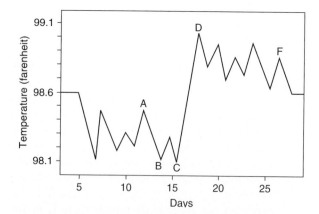

Figure 2-130 • Basal Body Temperature Graph.

A. A
B. B
C. C
D. D
E. E

131. A 19-year-old G_2P_1 at 26 weeks by LMP presents to your clinic for a routine prenatal visit. She denies any problems with the pregnancy aside from some lower back discomfort and frequent urination. She also notices that she has not grown in size nearly as much as she did with her first pregnancy. You assess her fundal height to be about 22 cm and send her for an ultrasound. The findings yield size less than dates by 5 weeks, suggesting intrauterine growth restriction (IUGR). What is the most common cause of IUGR in the United States?

A. Smoking
B. Hypertension
C. GDM
D. Fetal chromosomal abnormality
E. Maternal infection

132. A 22-year-old G_1P_0 at 8 weeks by LMP undergoes pregnancy termination via D&C. After the procedure, the patient has lingering questions about the possible adverse effects of this procedure. What do you tell her regarding the possible sequelae of an induced abortion?

A. An intrauterine device (IUD) will be a less effective means of contraception than before
B. She could develop Asherman's syndrome as a result of this procedure
C. Undergoing pregnancy termination via D&C will preclude use of any medical pregnancy termination techniques in the future
D. This procedure now increases her risk of midtrimester loss in a subsequent pregnancy
E. There is no evidence of any sequelae occurring after an abortion

133. A 24-year-old G_2P_1 woman at 27 weeks by LMP presents for a routine prenatal visit. She has no complaints other than some mild back discomfort. Her physical exam is normal, including an appropriate fundal height and amniotic fluid index (AFI). As part of routine prenatal care, the patient undergoes the 1-hour glucola screen for gestational diabetes. Which of the following is the highest plasma glucose level this patient could have with this test and still be considered normal?

A. 84 mg/100 mL
B. 109 mg/100 mL
C. 129 mg/100 mL
D. 154 mg/100 mL
E. 179 mg/100 mL

134. A 34-year-old obese woman was recently diagnosed with PCOS. She suffers from menstrual irregularity, anovulation, mild acne, and hirsutism. On exam, the most striking feature is significant terminal hair growth on the chin, lower back, and chest. She agrees to your plan to start her on combined OCPs to treat her PCOS, and asks you what she can expect in the long term regarding her hair growth. Which of the following statements is most accurate concerning hair growth in PCOS?

    A. She can expect complete resolution of all abnormal hair growth if she remains strictly compliant with her medication regimen
    B. Definitive treatment for her hirsutism can only be achieved via oophorectomy
    C. OCPs have not been shown to affect the hirsutism component of PCOS
    D. Treatment will prevent future hair growth, but will have little effect on existing hair
    E. Her hair growth will likely worsen, even with continued OCP use

135. A couple in their late 20s has been seeing you for an ongoing infertility workup. They have been trying to conceive for over 15 months now without success. So far, they have undergone semen analysis, a hysterosalpingogram, and endocrine testing of androgen, thyroid, and gonadotropin levels. All were normal. Given that they have no history of chronic medication use, do not smoke or use illicit substances, and have never had any sexually transmitted diseases, you decide to try the Huhner-Sims postcoital test. Which of the following is true of the Huhner-Sims test?

    A. The test should be done after ovulation has already occurred
    B. The couple should have had sexual intercourse approximately 24 hours before the scheduled exam
    C. 8 to 10 motile sperm per high power field in thin endocervical mucus is considered normal
    D. The test involves a Pap smear to detect cervical abnormalities
    E. Studies have shown this test to be 90% sensitive for identifying the cause of infertility

The next two questions (items 136 and 137) correspond to the following vignette.

A 19-year-old G_0 college woman comes to your office requesting a referral to a dermatologist for her acne and for laser hair removal. She complains of excessive dark hairs on her chin, around her nipples, and abdomen. On further questioning, she has irregular periods, menstruating every 2 to 3 months. She also expresses distress with her weight, stating that she has been "dieting my whole life" with essentially no weight loss. On physical exam she is 5'2" tall, weighs 160 lbs, BP is 118/73, and P = 64. She has moderate hirsutism consistent with her complaints, as well as facial and back pustular acne. Her voice is normal, and she has no evidence of balding, no clitoromegaly, no striae, no proptosis, and no galactorrhea. The rest of her exam is noncontributory and her pregnancy test is negative.

136. What is the most common cause of hirsutism in young women?

    A. Adrenal hyperplasia
    B. Iatrogenic testosterone excess
    C. PCOS
    D. Adrenal neoplasms
    E. Sertoli-Leydig cell tumors

137. At the hair follicle, testosterone is converted to the more potent androgen dihydrotestosterone (DHT) by which of the following enzymes?

    A. 21-hydroxylase
    B. 5α-reductase
    C. Dihydrotestosterase
    D. 11-β-hydroxylase
    E. 17-ketosteroid reductase

End of Set

138. A frantic 23-year-old G_1P_0 at 19 weeks by LMP presents to urgent care saying that her "water broke" 2 hours ago while standing in the kitchen. She was not engaged in any strenuous activity and did not sustain trauma to the abdomen. She is also experiencing intermittent cramping pain for the last hour that is growing in intensity. She denies fever, dizziness, oliguria, or active vaginal bleeding. On exam, her cervix is dilated to 4 cm, 50% effaced, and some blood is noted in the vaginal vault. A smear of the fluid obtained from the vault is shown below. Based on Figure 2-138 and the history, what is the likely diagnosis?

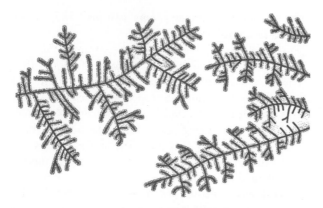

Figure 2-138 • Reproduced with Permission from Marbas, L. Blueprints Clinical Procedures. Blackwell Publishing, 2004. Fig. 60-1, p. 174.

A. Threatened abortion
B. Inevitable abortion
C. Incomplete abortion
D. Septic abortion
E. Missed abortion

139. A 33-year-old G_4P_3 woman at 11 weeks by LMP wishes to terminate her pregnancy. She has three living children and has never had to consider such a decision before. As a result, she knows very little about the abortion process and has many questions regarding how it works, what arrangements need to be made, and where she can obtain one. In order for an abortion to be performed appropriately, which of the following must be established by a health professional?

A. An approved contraceptive method was used and failed during intercourse
B. The fetus has a documented chromosomal abnormality
C. The patient is a resident of the state in which she will have the abortion
D. Medical abortion was not already attempted prior to a surgical approach being initiated
E. The patient has received education concerning options available to her other than abortion

The next two questions (items 140 and 141) correspond to the following vignette.

A 17-year-old female is brought to your office for evaluation because she has not yet had her first menses. She has normal vital signs, normal stature, normal facial and neck features, Tanner stage 3 breast development, and no evidence of virilization. She does not have terminal hair growth in her axilla and denies shaving. She did not want to come to the doctor's office in the first place and declines a pelvic examination. Her mother reports that her genitals "looked like a normal little girl" when she was young.

140. This type of amenorrhea is known as?
    A. Secondary amenorrhea
    B. Primary amenorrhea
    C. Juvenile amenorrhea
    D. Prepubertal amenorrhea
    E. Iatrogenic amenorrhea

141. If you were to do a pelvic examination on the above young woman, you would expect which of the following findings?

    A. A normal vagina, cervix, uterus, and adnexa/ovaries
    B. An imperforate hymen
    C. A blind-ending pouch, no cervix, no uterus, and small masses low in the abdomen
    D. A normal vagina, cervix, uterus, and absent or "streak" ovaries
    E. Clitoromegaly, and normal cervix, uterus, and adnexa

End of Set

The next two questions (items 142 and 143) correspond to the following vignette.

A 14-year-old girl is brought to your office by her mother for evaluation because she is worried that something is wrong with her daughter because she has not had her first menses yet. On examination the patient is 5'4" tall, weighs 105 lbs, and has normal vitals. She has moderate axillary hair and a Tanner stage 3 pubic hair pattern. Her breasts are Tanner stage 4. Her vulva, vagina, cervix, uterus, and adnexa are all within normal limits.

142. Which is the normal sequence of sexual maturation in a female?

    A. Adrenarche, menarche, thelarche
    B. Menarche, adrenarche, thelarche
    C. Thelarche, menarche, adrenarche
    D. Thelarche, pubarche, menarche
    E. Pubarche, thelarche, menarche

143. During puberty, which of the following hormones is released in a pulsatile manner from the hypothalamus and drives the hypothalamic-pituitary-gonadal (H-P-G) axis?

    A. FSH
    B. TSH
    C. Gonadotropin releasing hormone (GnRH)
    D. Vasopressin
    E. Prolactin

End of Set

144. A 26-year-old G_1P_1 is 2 days postpartum from an uncomplicated normal spontaneous vaginal delivery of a healthy daughter. She is successfully breastfeeding and plans on combining breast and bottle feeding when she returns to work in 6 weeks. She wishes to space her children about 3 years apart and inquires about an appropriate form of contraception before leaving the hospital to avoid an unintended pregnancy. Which of the following would you recommend to her?

    A. She does not need an additional method of contraception until she stops breastfeeding
    B. A combined 20 µg estrogen and progesterone OCP
    C. A combined 30 µg estrogen and progesterone OCP
    D. A progestin-only "mini" pill
    E. The Ortho Evra (norelgestromin/ethinyl estradiol) transdermal patch

145. A 29-year-old G_1P_1 woman presents to the emergency department (ED) complaining of weakness, lightheadedness, and persistent vaginal bleeding soaking 2 large pads per hour for the past 6 hours. The patient reports she had a home birth 1 hour ago of an $8^1/_2$-lb infant that was significant for a 2-day labor followed by $4^1/_2$ hours of pushing. Physical exam reveals an afebrile, tachycardic woman who exhibits orthostatic hypotension. Her perineum is intact with a repaired first degree laceration that is hemostatic. Sterile speculum exam reveals steady bleeding from the cervical os and bimanual exam reveals a boggy uterus with the fundus 2 cm above the umbilicus. A bedside ultrasound shows an unremarkable postpartum uterus with a thin endometrial stripe. Which of the following is the likely cause of this woman's postpartum hemorrhage?

    A. Uterine rupture
    B. Uterine inversion
    C. Retained products of conception (POC)
    D. Uterine atony
    E. Vaginal laceration

146. A 59-year-old $G_5 P_5$ woman presents to the ED reporting "something came out between my legs when I coughed." She is quite anxious as this has never occurred before. She denies pain, fever, discharge, dysuria, bleeding, or trauma. However, she does report involuntary loss of urine, which has been stable for years. Her past medical history is significant for bronchitis with chronic cough, and her past gynecological history is significant for 5 vaginal deliveries at term. She became menopausal at age 51 and has not been sexually active or seen her gynecologist for years. Physical exam is significant for uterine prolapse, with the cervix protruding 2 cm from the introitus. She also has a moderate cystocele as depicted in Figure 2-146. Despite her prolapse, she is able to void without difficulty. In this patient who wishes to avoid surgery, which of the following would be appropriate initial management?

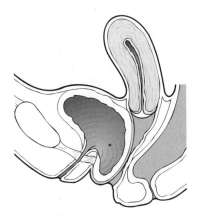

Figure 2-146 • Reproduced with Permission from Callahan TL, Caughey AB. Blueprints Obstetrics & Gynecology, 4th ed. Baltimore: Lippincott Williams & Wilkins, 2007. Fig. 18-2, p. 194.

    A. Oral estrogen
    B. Pessary
    C. Abdominal hysterectomy
    D. Vaginal hysterectomy
    E. Burch culposuspension

The response options for items 147 to 149 are the same. You will be required to select one answer for each item in the set.

    A. Overflow incontinence
    B. Stress incontinence
    C. Urge incontinence
    D. Total incontinence

For each scenario, select the appropriate type of incontinence.

147. A 49-year-old G_1P_1 presents for her routine annual exam. She reports occasional involuntary loss of urine and notes the odd history that it occurs most often when she arrives home but can't seem to get the door open in time before she experiences incontinence.

148. A 63-year-old G_4P_4 complains of severe involuntary loss of urine that is affecting her lifestyle. She has decreased her public outings because she loses urine every time she coughs or laughs. Despite wearing 4 pads a day, she still has the occasional severe accident in which she has to change her clothes.

149. A 54-year-old type II diabetic woman reports occasional involuntary loss of urine several times a day. Urine loss sometimes occurs with cough and straining, but she mostly notices it before she gets out of bed in the morning and at the end of the day. She works as a bus driver and rarely stops to use the bathroom.

End of Set

150. A 40-year-old G_2P_2 complains of gradually worsening menorrhagia and dysmenorrhea. She denies intermenstrual bleeding and reports a past gynecological history significant for 2 uncomplicated vaginal deliveries at term. On exam, a serum pregnancy test is negative and her uterus is mildly tender and feels diffusely enlarged, but without distinct masses. Her adnexa and the remainder of her exam are within normal limits. A pelvic ultrasound reveals an enlarged uterus with a normal endometrial stripe and without distinct masses on the uterus or adnexa. You start her on a trial of NSAIDs, which only minimally improves her symptoms. The patient ultimately elects for a hysterectomy. What would you expect to find on pathologic examination of the uterus?

    A. Fibroids
    B. Endometrial tissue in the myometrium
    C. Polycystic ovaries
    D. Hydrosalpinx
    E. Paratubal cysts

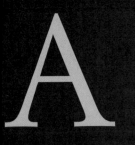

A Answers and Explanations

101. D	118. B	135. C
102. B	119. C	136. C
103. C	120. B	137. B
104. A	121. D	138. B
105. E	122. A	139. E
106. D	123. D	140. B
107. A	124. E	141. C
108. B	125. E	142. D
109. E	126. B	143. C
110. A	127. A	144. D
111. A	128. E	145. D
112. B	129. B	146. B
113. E	130. B	147. C
114. A	131. B	148. B
115. B	132. B	149. A
116. A	133. C	150. B
117. C	134. D	

101. **D. 50 to 51 years is the average age of menopause in the United States. Menopause before 40 years is formally considered premature menopause, often resulting from idiopathic premature ovarian failure.**

    A, B, C, E. See explanation for D.

102. **B. Menopause is a hypergonadotropic state. The gonadotropins— FSH and LH—are made in the anterior pituitary in response to pulsatile GnRH stimulation from the hypothalamus. They stimulate production of ovarian hormones which, in turn, control hypothalamic-pituitary secretion by negative feedback. With menopausal ovarian failure, estrogen production diminishes, FSH and LH are released from this negative feedback, and their levels are consequently high. Clinically, FSH alone is typically used to diagnose menopause (and is commonly used to quantify "ovarian reserve" in women seeking fertility treatment).**

    A, C, D, E. See explanation for B.

103. **C. Combination estrogen/progesterone HRT reduces the risk of osteoporosis, and thereby reduces the risk of hip fracture. According to current United States Preventive Services Task Force Guidelines (USPSTF), there is now fair or good evidence that the benefits of HRT include increased bone mineral density, reduced risk of fracture, and reduced risk of colorectal cancer. The USPSTF concluded that these benefits are outweighed by the risks associated with HRT (see below)** *in terms of prevention of chronic disease.* **Assessment of the impact of HRT on quality of life (e.g., menopausal symptoms and genitourinary atrophy) is not a part of this analysis; decisions about HRT should be patient-specific, accounting for personal preference and individual risk factors for chronic disease.**

    A. There is evidence that HRT increases the risk of venous thromboembolism and stroke.

    B. There is evidence that HRT increases the risk of coronary heart disease. An increased risk of cardiovascular mortality has not been demonstrated.

    D. There is evidence that HRT increases the risk of breast cancer. An increased risk of breast cancer-related mortality has not been demonstrated.

    E. The current evidence on HRT and ovarian cancer is conflicting, with some studies concluding that risk is increased, and others concluding that it is unchanged. Current evidence does not support a decreased risk of ovarian cancer.

104. **A. Endometrial cancer generally results from unopposed estrogen's effects on the endometrium, causing it to proliferate. Factors that increase estrogen exposure include: obesity, exogenous estrogen use, nulliparity, early age of menarche, late age of menopause, and chronic anovulation. Obesity increases a woman's estrogen via peripheral conversion and production of estrogens in adipocytes. Other risk factors include hypertension and diabetes.**

    B. Prolonged estrogen exposure is associated with breast cancer and endometrial cancer, but this would be seen in early onset of menarche.

    C. Nulliparity or low parity generally means that a woman undergoes more menstrual cycles as compared to multiparous women, which potentially increases her exposure to estrogen and endometrial proliferation. Thus, multiparity would decrease the risk of endometrial cancer.

    D. Unopposed estrogen leads to increased risk of endometrial cancer; progestins decrease the risk and can be used as conservative treatment for endometrial hyperplasia.

    E. Late onset of menopause would increase the risk of endometrial cancer.

105. **E. Submucosal fibroids usually cause menorrhagia with an increase in both length and volume of menstrual flow. They are not associated with postcoital bleeding.**

    A. Cervical polyps are generally benign growths on the cervix that can be broad-based or pedunculated. They are typically asymptomatic but can bleed or obstruct the cervical canal and should therefore be removed.

    B. While cervical lesions are more likely to cause postcoital bleeding, inflammation and irritation from yeast vaginitis can also lead to bleeding, even if the candidiasis is otherwise asymptomatic.

    C. Cervical cancer can present with postcoital bleeding. Despite the fact that this patient has had normal Pap smears, she should still be evaluated for cervical malignant and premalignant conditions.

D. Vulvar cancer and vulvar intraepithelial neoplasia (VIN) will present most commonly with vulvar pruritus or pain and a lesion. They can also present with postcoital bleeding, though the bleeding is from the lesion rather than the vagina. Certainly, this patient's history deserves inspection of the vulva for lesions.

106. **D. Testicular feminization (androgen insensitivity) results from dysfunction or absence of the testosterone receptor. Patients will have a male karyotype (46,XY) but a female phenotype because development of male secondary sexual characteristics is testosterone-dependent. Because secretion of Müllerian-inhibiting factor (MIF) is independent of testosterone, MIF will be produced and these patients will lack Müllerian-derived structures, including the uterus. Estrogen is usually produced (directly by the testes and by peripheral conversion), leading to breast development.**

A. Hypothalamic-pituitary dysfunction results from a defect in hypothalamic GnRH production (e.g., Kallman's syndrome), transport and pulsatile release of GnRH (e.g., anorexia, stress, hyperprolactinemia), or pituitary production and release of gonadotropins in response to GnRH stimulation (e.g., neoplasm, hemochromatosis, pituitary infarct). Both estrogen levels and gonadotropin levels (LH, FSH) are low: Amenorrhea is secondary to *hypo*gonadotropic hypogonadism.

B. Primary ovarian failure (gonadal dysgenesis) results in low levels of estradiol and elevated levels of gonadotropins—*hyper*gonadotropic hypogonadism—as is seen in the normal process of menopause. Multiple etiologies can cause primary ovarian failure and primary amenorrhea, including Turner syndrome (45,XO karyotype and rapid ovarian atresia), defects in enzymes for steroid synthesis, and Savage's syndrome (defect in ovarian receptors for FSH and LH).

C. Müllerian agenesis is an isolated failure of the Müllerian system to develop in a genotypic female despite otherwise normal endocrine function. This diagnosis would be likely in a patient presenting as above, but with the female karyotype (46,XX).

E. Imperforate hymen is an outflow tract obstruction that prevents egress of menses. It commonly presents with pelvic pain as menses accumulate above this level, and a bulging membrane can sometimes be seen on exam. This large suburethral bluish bulge, which can be palpated rectally as a midline mass, is a vagina full of menstrual blood (hematocolpos). The endocrine axis is functional and this patient has appropriate secondary sexual characteristics. The treatment is to incise the imperforate hymen and allow for normal menstrual flow. (A transverse vaginal septum, higher in the vagina, is another possible outflow tract obstruction.)

107. **A. Hypothalamic-pituitary dysfunction results from a defect in hypothalamic GnRH production (e.g., Kallman's syndrome), transport and pulsatile release of GnRH (e.g., anorexia, stress, hyperprolactinemia), or pituitary production and release of gonadotropins in response to GnRH stimulation (e.g., neoplasm, hemochromatosis, pituitary infarct). Both estrogen levels and gonadotropin levels (LH, FSH) are low: Amenorrhea is secondary to *hypo*gonadotropic hypogonadism.**

B. Primary ovarian failure (gonadal dysgenesis) results in low levels of estradiol and elevated levels of gonadotropins—*hyper*gonadotropic hypogonadism—as is seen in the normal process of menopause. Multiple etiologies can cause primary ovarian failure and primary amenorrhea, including Turner syndrome (45,XO karyotype and rapid ovarian atresia), defects in enzymes for steroid synthesis, and Savage's syndrome (defect in ovarian receptors for FSH and LH).

C. Müllerian agenesis is an isolated failure of the Müllerian system to develop in a genotypic female despite otherwise normal endocrine function.

D. Testicular feminization (androgen insensitivity) results from dysfunction or absence of the testosterone receptor. Patients will have a male karyotype (46,XY) but a female phenotype because development of male secondary sexual characteristics is testosterone-dependent. Because secretion of MIF is independent of testosterone, MIF will be produced and these patients will lack Müllerian-derived structures, including the uterus. Estrogen is usually produced (directly by the testes and by peripheral conversion), leading to breast development.

E. Imperforate hymen is an outflow tract obstruction that prevents egress of menses. It commonly presents with pelvic pain as menses accumulate above this level, and a bulging membrane can sometimes be seen on exam. This large suburethral bluish bulge, which can be palpated rectally as a midline mass, is a vagina full of menstrual blood (hematocolpos). The endocrine axis is functional and this patient has appropriate secondary sexual characteristics. The treatment is to incise the imperforate hymen and allow for normal menstrual flow. (A transverse vaginal septum, higher in the vagina, is another possible outflow tract obstruction.)

108. **B. Primary ovarian failure (gonadal dysgenesis) results in low levels of estradiol and elevated levels of gonadotropins—*hyper*gonadotropic hypogonadism—as is seen in the normal process of menopause. Multiple etiologies can cause primary ovarian failure and primary amenorrhea, including Turner syndrome (45,XO karyotype and rapid ovarian atresia), defects in enzymes for steroid synthesis, and Savage's syndrome (defect in ovarian receptors for FSH and LH).**

A. Hypothalamic-pituitary dysfunction results from a defect in hypothalamic GnRH production (e.g., Kallman's syndrome), transport and pulsatile release of GnRH (e.g., anorexia, stress, hyperprolactinemia), or pituitary production and release of gonadotropins in response to GnRH stimulation (e.g., neoplasm, hemochromatosis, pituitary infarct). Both estrogen levels and gonadotropin levels (LH, FSH) are low: Amenorrhea is secondary to *hypo*gonadotropic hypogonadism.

C. Müllerian agenesis is an isolated failure of the Müllerian system to develop in a genotypic female despite otherwise normal endocrine function.

D. Testicular feminization (androgen insensitivity) results from dysfunction or absence of the testosterone receptor. Patients will have a male karyotype (46,XY) but a female phenotype because development of male secondary sexual characteristics is testosterone-dependent. Because secretion of MIF is independent of testosterone, MIF will be produced and these patients will lack Müllerian-derived structures, including the uterus. Estrogen is usually produced (directly by the testes and by peripheral conversion), leading to breast development.

E. Imperforate hymen is an outflow tract obstruction that prevents egress of menses. It commonly presents with pelvic pain as menses accumulate above this level, and a bulging membrane can sometimes be seen on exam. This large suburethral bluish bulge, which can be palpated rectally as a midline mass, is a vagina full of menstrual blood (hematocolpos). The endocrine axis is functional and this patient has appropriate secondary sexual characteristics. The treatment is to incise the imperforate hymen and allow for normal menstrual flow. (A transverse vaginal septum, higher in the vagina, is another possible outflow tract obstruction.)

109. **E. Imperforate hymen is an outflow tract obstruction that prevents egress of menses. It commonly presents with pelvic pain as menses accumulate above this level, and a bulging membrane can sometimes be seen on exam. This large suburethral bluish bulge, which can be palpated rectally as a midline mass, is a vagina full of menstrual blood (hematocolpos). The endocrine axis is functional and this patient has appropriate secondary sexual characteristics. The treatment is to incise the imperforate hymen and allow for normal menstrual flow. (A transverse vaginal septum, higher in the vagina, is another possible outflow tract obstruction.)**

A. Hypothalamic-pituitary dysfunction results from a defect in hypothalamic GnRH production (e.g., Kallman's syndrome), transport and pulsatile release of GnRH (e.g., anorexia, stress, hyperprolactinemia), or pituitary production and release of gonadotropins in response to GnRH stimulation (e.g., neoplasm, hemochromatosis, pituitary infarct). Both estrogen levels and gonadotropin levels (LH, FSH) are low: Amenorrhea is secondary to *hypo*gonadotropic hypogonadism.

B. Primary ovarian failure (gonadal dysgenesis) results in low levels of estradiol and elevated levels of gonadotropins—*hyper*gonadotropic hypogonadism—as is seen in the normal process of menopause. Multiple etiologies can cause primary ovarian failure and primary amenorrhea, including Turner syndrome (45,XO karyotype and rapid ovarian atresia), defects in enzymes for steroid synthesis, and Savage's syndrome (defect in ovarian receptors for FSH and LH).

C. Müllerian agenesis is an isolated failure of the Müllerian system to develop in a genotypic female despite otherwise normal endocrine function.

D. Testicular feminization (androgen insensitivity) results from dysfunction or absence of the testosterone receptor. Patients will have a male karyotype (46,XY) but a female phenotype because development of male secondary sexual characteristics is testosterone-dependent. Because secretion of MIF is independent of testosterone, MIF will be produced and these patients will lack Müllerian-derived structures, including the uterus. Estrogen is usually produced (directly by the testes and by peripheral conversion), leading to breast development.

110. **A. Pregnancy is the most common cause of secondary amenorrhea in a sexually active woman of childbearing age. Although this patient does not meet the definition of secondary amenorrhea (>6 months of amenorrhea in a woman who has had prior menses), ruling out pregnancy is the first step before any further workup.**

B. Hypothyroidism can cause secondary amenorrhea, but is far less likely than pregnancy, especially in a patient with normal cycles until 3 months ago and no other signs of hypothyroidism.

C. Hyperprolactinemia can cause secondary amenorrhea, but is far less likely than pregnancy, especially in an asymptomatic patient (e.g., no galactorrhea).

D. PCOS can cause secondary amenorrhea, but is less likely than pregnancy. In addition, although PCOS can lead to insulin resistance and hyperinsulinemia, a random insulin level is not diagnostically useful.

E. Premature menopause will lead to amenorrhea, but is far less likely than pregnancy in a young patient with no menopausal symptoms (e.g., vasomotor flushing).

111. **A. Hypogonadotropic hypogonadism (hypothalamic-pituitary dysfunction) is the cause of secondary amenorrhea in the setting of a positive progesterone withdrawal test. A positive test (experiencing a withdrawal bleed after treatment with medroxyprogesterone) indicates that endogenous estrogen production is** adequate and that the outflow tract is unobstructed. **After pregnancy, anovulation due to hypogonadotropic hypogonadism is the most common cause of secondary amenorrhea in a woman of reproductive age.**

B. Hyperprolactinemia has multiple etiologies, including pituitary tumor, medications, and hypothyroidism. Since prolactin secretion is inhibited by dopamine, and dopamine abnormalities can result in abnormal gonadotropin (FSH and LH) secretion, amenorrhea or other menstrual irregularities are common sequelae of hyperprolactinemia. This patient, however, has no signs or symptoms of hyperprolactinemia.

C. A positive progesterone withdrawal test demonstrates adequate endogenous estrogen and gonadotropin production. Thus, this patient's amenorrhea is not caused by hypergonadotropic hypogonadism (ovarian failure). Hypoestrogenism is suspected when, after a negative progesterone withdrawal test, a combined estrogen/progesterone challenge results in bleeding.

D, E. A positive progesterone withdrawal test rules out an outflow tract obstruction as the cause of amenorrhea. An outflow tract obstruction is suspected when, after a negative progesterone withdrawal test, combined estrogen/progesterone still does not result in bleeding. Common obstructive processes include Asherman's syndrome (endometrial synechiae or adhesions, usually secondary to surgery or infection) and cervical stenosis.

112. **B. Hyperprolactinemia has a variety of possible etiologies (e.g., hypothyroidism, medications, tumor, breastfeeding), but any patient with elevated prolactin levels should have an imaging study to rule out prolactinoma. Macroadenomas often require surgical resection, and microadenomas can often be treated with a dopamine agonist (e.g., bromocriptine), which can lead to tumor regression and ovulation.**

A. Imaging is generally not useful in the diagnosis of hyperthyroidism.

C. Imaging is generally not useful in the diagnosis of hypergonadotropic hypogonadism.

D, E. Imaging is generally not useful in the diagnosis of PCOS.

113. E. PCOS is characterized by anovulation and an abundance of circulating estrogen. The endometrial lining is stimulated to proliferate by the endogenous estrogen, but endogenous progesterone is not produced in the setting of anovulation. Thus, exogenous administration of progesterone will result in withdrawal bleeding.

    A. Withdrawal bleeding will not occur in pregnancy, since endogenous progesterone is already abundant (produced by the corpus luteum in the first trimester, and the placenta thereafter).
    B. In ovarian failure, estrogen is not present to stimulate endometrial proliferation, and exogenous progesterone will not cause withdrawal bleeding.
    C. Without gonadotropin stimulation, estrogen will not be produced in amounts sufficient to stimulate endometrial proliferation, and exogenous progesterone will not cause withdrawal bleeding.
    D. In Müllerian agenesis, the uterus is not formed.

114. A. NSAIDs are usually first-line treatment for primary dysmenorrhea. OCPs are the next step for patients refractory to this therapy (and who do not desire pregnancy). Dysmenorrhea is defined as severe painful cramping in the lower abdomen during or just before menses, often accompanied by other symptoms, including sweating, tachycardia, headaches, nausea, vomiting, and diarrhea. Primary dysmenorrhea is the diagnosis given when no pathologic condition (e.g., endometriosis, fibroids, cervical stenosis, pelvic adhesions) can be identified. There is evidence that primary dysmenorrhea may be caused by prostaglandin-mediated uterine contractions. Prostaglandin production is inhibited both by NSAIDs and by the progesterone in combination with OCPs.

    B, C. Surgical therapies such as cervical dilation and neurectomy have been used in the past, but do not generally play a role in the current management of primary dysmenorrhea.
    D. Leuprolide (Lupron; a GnRH analog) is a treatment option for endometriosis. However, a trial of oral contraceptives should be attempted first.
    E. This patient is experiencing debilitating pain, and although primary dysmenorrhea often decreases as a patient gets older, it would be inappropriate not to attempt alternate treatment.

115. B. Menorrhagia refers to heavy or prolonged menstrual bleeding. It is formally defined as total blood loss per cycle greater than 80 mL (average: 35 mL) or bleeding for greater than 7 days. A history of soaking through more than 1 pad per hour is also commonly used. Menorrhagia can be caused by fibroids, adenomyosis, endometrial hyperplasia, endometrial polyps, complications of pregnancy, or endometrial or cervical malignancy.

    A. Hypomenorrhea refers to periods with abnormally light flow, usually secondary to an atrophic endometrium. It is commonly caused by hypogonadotropic hypogonadism (e.g., athletes, anorexics), outflow tract obstruction (e.g., Asherman's syndrome, cervical stenosis), or oral contraceptive use.
    C, D. Metrorrhagia refers to irregular bleeding (i.e., between periods, or such that cyclicity cannot be identified), if bleeding is not excessive or prolonged. Menometrorrhagia refers to irregular bleeding that is excessive or prolonged. Metrorrhagia and menometrorrhagia can be caused by endometrial polyps, complications of pregnancy, or endometrial or cervical malignancy. This patient's bleeding is heavy, but it is regular.
    E. Oligomenorrhea refers to periods that are greater than 35 days apart. The causes are similar to those for secondary amenorrhea (e.g., disruption of the hypothalamic-pituitary-ovarian axis). The most common cause of oligomenorrhea is pregnancy. Polymenorrhea refers to periods occurring less than 24 days apart.

116. A. Atrophy is the most common cause of postmenopausal vaginal bleeding (occurring in more than half of women with this presentation). Hypoestrogenism, secondary to the ovarian failure of menopause, results in a thin lining of the uterus and lower reproductive tract that is prone to bleeding. Having said this, it is vital to rule out malignancy in all cases of postmenopausal bleeding.

    B. Endometrial polyps, benign growths of unknown etiology, account for another 10% of postmenopausal bleeding.
    C. Although endometrial malignancy accounts for only about 10% of postmenopausal bleeding (depending on age and other risk factors), further testing is always necessary in this population.

D. Cervical cancer is a less common (1%) cause of postmenopausal bleeding.

E. Although vaginal malignancy does present with vaginal bleeding, it is much less common than the other choices.

117. **C. Vaginal bleeding in a postmenopausal woman is considered malignancy until proven otherwise; sampling of the endometrium via endometrial biopsy is usually used to make this diagnosis. Transvaginal ultrasound to evaluate the thickness of the endometrial stripe is another useful modality (though not offered as an answer choice), but it does not provide a tissue diagnosis. A Pap smear should also be performed for this patient to evaluate the possibility of cervical malignancy.**

A. Hysterectomy would be indicated for adenocarcinoma of the endometrium (or atypical endometrial hyperplasia), but diagnosis is needed before treatment. Hysterectomy is also occasionally used to treat nonmalignant causes of dysfunctional uterine bleeding (in women of reproductive age) refractory to other therapies.

B. Although D&C would lead to a diagnosis, an endometrial biopsy can be done more easily in the office and with less discomfort to the patient.

D. Endometrial ablation is used for severe, symptomatic uterine bleeding in the absence of endometrial pathology. It is appropriate for women of reproductive age who are refractory to other therapies, but would not be appropriate in a postmenopausal woman where a tissue diagnosis is necessary.

E. Hormonal therapy may be appropriate for this patient, but a pathologic diagnosis of the endometrium must be made before treatment is initiated.

118. **B. Hypertension in pregnancy is defined as either systolic BP above 140 mm Hg or diastolic BP above 90 mm Hg that is recorded on two separate occasions at least 6 hours apart. Only one of these criteria needs to be satisfied for the diagnosis of gestational hypertension.**

A. See explanation for B. Only systolic BPs above 140 mm Hg meet the criteria for gestational hypertension.

C. While gestational diabetes increases the risk for hypertension, it is not a requirement for the diagnosis of gestational hypertension.

D. While obesity increases the risk for hypertension, it is not a requirement for the diagnosis of gestational hypertension.

E. Edema is common in pregnancy and is not a formal diagnostic criterion for hypertension. However, nondependent edema (e.g., hands and face) is considered abnormal and concerning for preeclampsia.

119. **C. This patient has a history of a deep vein thrombosis (DVT) while on OCPs. Elevated levels of estrogen, exogenous or secondary to pregnancy, place a woman in a hypercoagulable state and increase her risk of deep vein thromboses. A history of a DVT is generally a contraindication to OCPs or any form of contraception that contains an estrogen component. The Mirena IUD releases 20 µg of levonorgestrel per day and does not contain estrogen. The Mirena can be easily placed in the office and lasts for 5 years, although it can be removed at any point. The levonorgestrel IUD prevents pregnancy by producing a decidualized endometrium and gland atrophy, thickened cervical mucus, impaired sperm entry, and partial inhibition of ovulation. Approximately 15% of patients with Mirena IUDs will not ovulate. The Mirena IUD has also been shown to significantly reduce menstrual cramps and blood loss (up to 90% by 1 year).**

A, B, D. All of these methods contain estrogen. Estrogen has many effects on coagulation. Estrogen increases protein C, fibrinogen, factors II, VII, VIII, IX, X, XI, and vWF, and decreases protein S and anti-thrombin III. This patient has a history of a DVT while on an estrogen-containing contraceptive method and is thus not a good candidate for an estrogen-containing agent. The relative risk of developing a DVT while on oral contraceptives in premenopausal women is 4.

E. A laparoscopic tubal ligation would be a poor choice in this woman because she does not desire permanent sterilization. Should she decide her family is complete, a laparoscopic tubal would be a very reasonable option. In addition to the contraceptive counseling, she should be counseled regarding the risk of anesthesia and DVT before the surgery.

120. **B.** This is the classic presentation for a Bartholin's gland abscess. They arise from the Bartholin's glands, which are located bilaterally on the labia majora at the 4 and 8 o'clock positions. These glands normally secrete mucus, but can become obstructed, leading to Bartholin's cysts, which can be asymptomatic if small in size. However, cysts can evolve into abscesses, which should be treated with drainage and either placement of a Word catheter or marsupialization in order to allow the cyst to epithelialize and prevent recurrence.

   A. Chancres are painless lesions caused by *Treponema pallidum*, the organism that causes syphilis.
   C. Candidiasis, or yeast infections, can cause marked pruritus and erythema in the vagina and on the vulva, which is not the case for this patient.
   D. Lichen sclerosus is a benign lesion of the skin that is frequently found on the vulva. It can occur at any age and begins as small, white spots that can develop into larger patches of thin, delicate skin that are susceptible to tearing and discoloration. Affected skin can also atrophy and lead to narrowing of the vagina. Treatment involves topical steroids.
   E. Condyloma acuminata are also known as genital warts and are caused by human papilloma virus (HPV). They are typically painless, raised papillomatous, spiked, or cauliform growths on the cervix, vagina, vulva, perineum, or anus. Treatment includes excision, cryotherapy, and topical treatments such as trichloroacetic acid, podophyllin, imiquimod, and 5-fluorouracil.

121. **D.** Preeclampsia is a disorder of pregnancy typically characterized by hypertension (BP > 140/90) and proteinuria ≥300 mg in 24-hour urine collection) with or without nondependent edema. It usually manifests after the twentieth week of gestation and is more common in multiple gestations. It is also more common in first-time mothers at either end of the reproductive age spectrum. Other signs and symptoms of preeclampsia include visual changes usually in the form of scotomata, headache, oliguria, pulmonary edema, right upper quadrant or epigastric pain, and thrombocytopenia. Severe preeclampsia also manifests as the above, but is defined as a BP of ≥160/110 and/or 24-hour urine protein >5000 mg.

   A. Abdominal pain is usually limited to the upper quadrants, primarily the right, and is believed to be due to subcapsular hepatic hemorrhage or stretching of Glisson's capsule due to edema. The lower quadrants are generally not affected.
   B. Decreased urine output, not increased, is seen in preeclampsia, presumably due to decreased effective circulating volume secondary to edema.
   C. Hematologic abnormalities associated with preeclampsia include thrombocytopenia, not thrombocythemia. This is likely the result of hepatic dysfunction, probably due to the factors described in A. Elevated liver transaminases are also sometimes observed.
   E. Diarrhea is not typical in preeclamptic patients. However, nausea and vomiting can occur.

122. **A.** Eclampsia is the occurrence of nonepileptic seizures in the setting of preeclampsia. Although the seizures are almost always self-limited, they pose significant risks to the mother including musculoskeletal injury (e.g., biting of the tongue), aspiration, intracerebral hemorrhage, and hypoxia. The risks to the fetus are equally serious, including fetal heart rate decelerations and decreased variability. While these fetal heart rate abnormalities are usually self-limited, any persistent nonreassuring fetal status may necessitate immediate delivery. Initial management of seizures should include the ABCs (i.e., airway, breathing, circulation, etc.). Intravenous access is equally important to manage fluid status. Other measures that must be taken include assessment of metabolic changes such as acidosis and possible continuous EKG if heart conditions arise.

   B. As exhibited by this patient, seizures are generally self-limited. Therefore, the goal is to prevent further seizure activity with magnesium sulfate. Anticonvulsive agents such as diazepam are used sparingly to stop active seizures. Of note, diazepam can cause respiratory depression, hypotonia, temperature homeostasis difficulties, and kernicterus in the fetus.
   C. While delivery has been shown to be the most definitive cure for preeclampsia, delivery during an eclamptic episode poses significant risk to the mother and baby, and should only be undertaken once maternal condition is stabilized and if fetal status is deemed nonreassuring.

D. Blood transfusion is not needed during an eclamptic episode. While thrombocytopenia is a complication of preeclampsia, it is usually not severe enough to warrant blood products, and even if it were, packed RBCs would not be the appropriate choice.

E. Transient uterine hyperactivity is sometimes seen in eclampsia and can lead to fetal heart rate abnormalities. However, this uterine hyperactivity is generally transient and rarely requires the use of tocolytics.

123. **D. This is a classic case of female endocrine-mediated virilization. There are myriad causes of virilization and hirsutism in women, but they all have in common a generalized increase in circulating levels of free testosterone. These androgens are produced in the adrenal gland, ovaries, and adipose tissue and released into the bloodstream, with the vast majority (97% to 99%) bound to SHBG. This bound form keeps testosterone in an inactive state, but the remaining 1% to 3% is free (unbound) and able to exert its effects on the body. Thus, whenever there is a decrease in the amount of circulating SHBG due to hepatic compromise or decreased estrogen levels, the proportion of free testosterone in the blood rises accordingly and causes the symptoms described above.**

A. Grave's disease, also known as autoimmune thyroiditis, is a disorder of hyperthyroid activity due to autoantibody stimulation of TSH receptors. Common symptoms include thinning of the hair, infiltrative ophthalmopathy (exophthalmos), and pretibial myxedema, as well as the less common sequelae of diabetes mellitus, myasthenia gravis, and pernicious anemia. However, no virilizing changes have been observed in this disorder.

B. While menopause can sometimes cause changes in hair growth and in skin, these changes are not nearly as pronounced as those manifest in this patient. Also, at age 29 and with normal menses, it is very unlikely that this patient is menopausal.

C. Spironolactone is a diuretic that works by binding aldosterone receptors in renal tubules to prevent them from exerting their antidiuretic effect. Spironolactone also competitively binds androgen receptors in hair follicles and decreases production of testosterone. Therefore, use of this drug would be expected to cause feminizing signs and symptoms, not virilization.

E. 5α-reductase works in the periphery to convert testosterone to DHT, an even more potent androgen. Therefore, a decreased amount of this enzyme in the body would not be expected to cause hirsutism or virilization.

124. **E. The major sites of androgen production are the adrenal glands and the ovaries. Peripheral conversion of androstenedione to testosterone also occurs in adipocytes. Due to this latter phenomenon, obesity can sometimes lead to virilizing changes in women.**

A. Hepatocytes synthesize a staggering array of hormones and enzymes. In this case, the relevant peptide is SHBG, which binds testosterone and keeps it in an inactive state. Hepatocytes do not participate in testosterone production, however.

B. Type II alveolar cells produce surfactant, which decreases the surface tension of water and prevents alveolar collapse. These cells do not produce testosterone.

C. Vascular endothelial cells do not participate in testosterone production.

D. Hair follicles possess testosterone receptors and contain the 5α-reductase enzyme that converts testosterone to its more potent form DHT, but they do not participate in the conversion of androstenedione to testosterone.

125. **E. Almost half of all women with GDM do not show any overt signs or symptoms of diabetes and usually do not have a family history of the disease. However, even subclinical diabetes can be harmful to both the mother and the developing fetus, and must be diagnosed and controlled as early as possible. Therefore, all pregnant women, regardless of risk factors, are tested for GDM as standard practice. This is done between 24 and 28 weeks GA, as insulin resistance becomes more prevalent in the third trimester and detection at this time allows early intervention.**

A. Persistent glucosuria is a finding concerning for GDM. However, glucosuria is also present in many nondiabetic pregnant women due to increased renal blood flow and subsequent increases in tubular glucose concentrations. Thus, it is not a sensitive enough measure for use in diagnostic and treatment decisions.

B. Most cases of GDM resemble type II diabetes, where the disorder is more a function of insulin resistance, not decreased production. Therefore, obesity does play a role in the development of GDM in pregnancy. However, even slender women can develop GDM, and thus all women must be screened.

C. A strong family history of diabetes is considered a risk factor for GDM. However, as mentioned in E, lack of a family history does not prevent GDM from occurring and therefore is not used to guide screening decisions.

D. A history of macrosomia or elevated weight of the newborn is also considered a risk factor for GDM. Again, because of the high incidence of GDM in women without this history, all women should be screened for GDM.

126. **B. The 1-hour glucola test consists of an oral 50-gm glucose solution challenge followed by a blood glucose determination 1 hour later. It is performed on all pregnant women between 24 and 28 weeks GA, even if they have no risk factors or symptoms, and any value above 140 mg/dL is considered abnormal. However, this test is meant as an initial screening only, and does not by itself diagnose GDM. An abnormal value must therefore be confirmed with the more definitive 3-hour GTT. This second test is done after the patient has followed a 3-day carbohydrate loading diet (e.g., all the pasta and starch she can eat in a meal plus one candy bar per day). A fasting level is drawn, followed by ingestion of a 100-gm glucose challenge. Blood glucose values are obtained hourly for the next 3 hours. One abnormal value suggests GDM, but two or more make the diagnosis. Only after this step has yielded a positive result would a patient have to initiate a treatment regimen, usually beginning with diet control and measurement of glucose values.**

A. Insulin is employed in cases of GDM that cannot be adequately controlled by diet. However, this patient does not yet have a diagnosis of GDM and requires further evaluation via a GTT. As mentioned, other treatment modalities for GDM include carbohydrate and fat restriction, and exercise to reduce weight (and thus insulin resistance). These focused and sustained lifestyle changes can dramatically reduce the severity of the disease and its complications. Oral hypoglycemic agents may be appropriate alternatives to insulin in select patients.

C. If the diagnosis of GDM was made, changes in diet would be indicated.

D. As above, the glucola test is a screening test only, and not meant to be diagnostic. Generally, only one administration of this test is required to determine what further action needs to be taken. However, the glucola can be administered in the first trimester in patients with risk factors and repeated again at the start of the third trimester if previously normal.

E. Unlike pregestational diabetics, congenital anomalies are not typically seen with GDM. Thus, an ultrasound exam beyond what is typical in routine prenatal care is not indicated.

127. **A. Approximately 2% to 7% of pregnant women will show an asymptomatic bacteriuria (i.e., asymptomatic presence of bacteria in the urinary tract), regardless of diabetic status. This is three times the nonpregnant rate. Also, more cases of asymptomatic bacteriuria progress to UTI and pyelonephritis in pregnant women than nonpregnant women. One factor that causes this bacteriuria is pregnancy-associated urinary stasis (due to mechanical compression of the ureters and decreased ureteral tone secondary to increased progesterone levels). Glucosuria also predisposes to bacteriuria. While normal pregnant women exhibit glucose in the urine due to increased renal flow and inability of glucose transporters in the tubules to accommodate the increased glucose load, women with GDM have an even greater amount of glucose in the urine, leading to an increased incidence of UTI in this group.**

B. Hyperemesis gravidarum is a condition of excessive nausea and vomiting beyond traditional "morning sickness." The etiology is unknown, although sequelae can be severe including weight loss, dehydration, metabolic disturbance, and ketosis. This condition has not been shown to increase the incidence of UTI, however.

C. Ptyalism is a condition of excessive salivation, as high as 1 L/day seen in some pregnancies. The etiology is unknown, but tincture of belladonna or atropine may alleviate symptoms. This condition does not lead to UTI.

D. GBS is usually an asymptomatic colonizer of the genital tract and poses little risk of UTI to the mother. Infection of the newborn, however, may cause devastating problems such as neonatal sepsis, pneumonia, or meningitis. Thus, GBS carriers are given intrapartum antibiotics to reduce the incidence of such complications.

E. Preeclampsia is a disorder of hypertension and proteinuria with or without edema. It is of concern because it may lead to eclampsia, which includes all of the above plus nonepileptic seizures. The latter may lead to grave complications for the fetus including hypoxia, metabolic acidosis, and even death. Preeclamptic states are not known, however, to increase the incidence of UTIs in pregnant women.

128. E. The main objectives in fertility testing are to be as thorough and noninvasive as possible. Initial evaluation should include a comprehensive history and physical to identify risk factors for infertility, followed by baseline labs. The female partner is likely ovulating given her basal body temperature recordings and regular menses. However, lab studies should still be undertaken and include checking a prolactin level, TSH, and basic prenatal labs. Obtaining menstrual cycle day 2 or 3 levels for estrogen and FSH can indicate ovarian reserve, while checking a midluteal (days 21 to 23) progesterone can assess ovulation. However, neither of these is an answer choice. Lab evaluation of the male partner should include semen analysis to assess semen volume, sperm count, motility, viscosity, morphology, WBC count, and presence of antisperm antibodies.

A. A hysterosalpingogram (HSG) is a contrast X-ray study to examine the architecture and integrity of the female genital tract. It can detect tubal non patency, anatomic abnormalities of the uterine cavity or tubes, or the presence of any foreign objects or masses. This is a very useful, minimally invasive test for fertility. However, the initial lab studies discussed in the explanation for E generally precede HSG.

B. The Huhner-Sims test (postcoital test) examines the characteristics of endocervical mucus aspirated shortly after intercourse. This test provides information on coitus, ejaculation, sperm pickup, motility, and storage in the endocervical canal. Given the invasiveness and relative inconvenience of this test as well as lack of proven utility, it should not be used as a first-line test.

C. Testicular biopsy is not a normal part of an infertility workup unless a mass or tumor is detected. Semen analysis should be performed first.

D. Due to its considerable invasiveness, diagnostic laparoscopy of the female genital tract is only undertaken if there is evidence of a uterine or tubal abnormality based on hysterosalpingogram or a thorough infertility evaluation is otherwise negative. This procedure provides information on the external surfaces of reproductive organs (e.g., presence of endometriosis) and complements the information obtained about internal surfaces from the hysterosalpingogram.

129. B. Whenever possible, the goal of treatment in an anovulatory patient is to restore natural ovulation using existing induction agents. Generally, when clomiphene citrate fails, the next step is to introduce exogenous FSH, since a deficiency in this hormone is a likely cause of the problem. Exogenous gonadotropins can be purified from the urine of postmenopausal women (menotropins or human menopausal gonadotropins [HMG]) and successfully given to anovulatory women. With expert administration, this treatment is 85% to 90% effective in inducing ovulation.

A. IVF is always an option for infertile couples. However, it is prohibitively expensive for many and should therefore be tried after other appropriate options have been attempted.

C. Artificial insemination involves the placement of sperm in either the uterine cavity or at the external os of the cervix and is indicated in cervical factor infertility or cases where ejaculation is problematic but semen analysis is normal. This method can only work if the patient is ovulating normally, however, and is therefore inappropriate for this patient.

D. Donor gametes are never the first-line therapy, and are only used if all reasonable attempts at autologous conception have failed.

E. Adoption is an option for any infertile couple, but that route is premature in this case.

130. **B. Almost 90% of women, when meticulously recording their temperature at the same time each morning, will show the similar biphasic temperature pattern depicted in the graph. The shift in temperature is due to the increased production of progesterone by the corpus luteum after ovulation. However, this change in temperature does not manifest itself until 2 days after the follicle has ruptured, reflecting the time it takes for the progesterone level to build to sufficient quantity to exert its thermal effect. In this case, that shift occurs at point C, corresponding to day 16. Therefore, ovulation must have occurred on day 14, marked as point B in the graph. The flat lines reflect a stable body temperature during the period of menses, depicted here as spanning 6 days. All other points are of no particular significance, and simply outline the normal daily variation that occurs in an individual during the month.**

A, C, D, E. See explanation for B.

131. **B. While there are over a dozen known causes of IUGR, underlying chronic maternal hypertension has been implicated in 25% to 30% of cases. It is believed that vasospasm leads to diminished uterine flow leading to decreased fetal nutrition. It is thus important to manage any hypertensive conditions as aggressively as possible to ensure a healthy outcome for the fetus.**

A. Smoking in pregnancy is a severe problem for a plethora of reasons, including causing a decrease in fetal weight by as much as 50%. However, it is not the most common cause of IUGR.

C. GDM causes the opposite problem of macrosomia due to increased glucose utilization by the fetus during development. This condition can be as problematic as IUGR for the fetus and mother and must likewise be managed carefully.

D. Fetal chromosomal abnormalities account for a large number of first-trimester miscarriages. They are also responsible for IUGR, although the incidence is less than 10%.

E. Maternal infection can also cause fetal growth restriction, although it is a rare cause of IUGR (less than 5% of pregnancies).

132. **B. Asherman's syndrome, or intrauterine synechiae, is a disorder where the endometrium is scarred, usually due to overaggressive curettage or dilation and evacuation (D&E) that strips away too much of the endometrial layer from the uterus. Typical symptoms are recurrent miscarriage, infertility, pain, and irregular menses, or amenorrhea. Surgical lysis of the synechiae plus estrogen to rebuild the endometrium is sometimes a successful treatment. Of note, it is unlikely that a patient would develop Asherman's after one procedure.**

A. There is no evidence that any form of contraception becomes less efficacious after an induced abortion.

C. There is no data to suggest that once a woman has undergone surgical pregnancy termination that subsequent pregnancy terminations cannot be performed using medical regimens such as mifepristone or misoprostol.

D. Some studies have shown that two or three induced abortions can increase the likelihood of subsequent spontaneous midtrimester abortions or premature deliveries. However, a single uncomplicated D&C poses no additional risk of adverse outcomes in future pregnancies.

E. See explanations for B, C, and D. Adverse events are certainly possible both during and after a D&C, including those listed above, as well as uterine or bowel perforation, infection, hemorrhage, and all complications that can result from a general operative procedure.

133. **C. GDM is a serious disorder that affects nearly 2% of all pregnancies. Because it can develop at any time during the pregnancy and not manifest any overt symptoms, universal testing for**

this disorder is vital to ensure a healthy pregnancy. If patients do not demonstrate any risk factors or symptoms, they are usually tested between 24 and 28 weeks GA, as this is the time when most cases are detectable. The test involves consumption of 50 gm of glucose solution (Glucola) and assessment of the plasma glucose concentration 1 hour later. In most labs, any value of 140 mg/dL and above is considered positive and requires further testing via the 3-hour GTT. Some clinicians consider values greater than 135 mg/dL to be positive. Of note, the patient does not need to be fasting for the Glucola test to be accurate.

A, B, D, E. See explanation for C.

134. D. The unfortunate consequence of hirsutism is that once hair has converted from vellus to terminal hair, the follicles are now permanently stimulated to grow. Treatment of this patient's PCOS will help keep androgen production under control, which will both slow the rate of terminal hair growth and prevent new vellus hair from growing. However, OCPs cannot reverse follicular stimulation once it has occurred, and the only permanent solution for excess terminal hair growth is electrolysis or depilation procedures.

A. See explanation for D. Terminal hair growth cannot be reversed with OCP therapy alone.
B. Oophorectomy cannot reverse terminal hair growth.
C, E. OCPs can help prevent new hair growth and can keep current hair growth in check as long as they are working to treat the underlying PCOS problem.

135. C. The Huhner-Sims test, or postcoital test, is another way to detect abnormalities in sperm motility and density, as well as the interaction of sperm with the endocervical canal. The test is ideally performed 8 hours after intercourse and involves a speculum examination of the female partner and aspiration of the endocervical mucus to be examined under light microscopy. Eight to ten motile sperm per high-power field (HPF) seen in thin, acellular mucus is normal. Anything different implies problems with sperm density or motility, endocervical mucus that is not conducive to sperm survival or transport, or poor testing technique.

A. The ideal time to perform this test is immediately prior to ovulation, as this is the ideal time for conception to occur. It is also the time when the endocervical mucus is abundant and best at facilitating sperm movement and survival.
B. See explanation for C. The test is normally performed 8 hours after intercourse.
D. While a speculum exam is performed to visualize the cervix and aspirate mucus, a Pap smear is not a part of this test.
E. There is scant scientific data on the accuracy, sensitivity, or utility of this test in determining the cause of infertility. For this reason, the test is not performed as frequently as it used to be.

136. C. Hirsutism is defined as excessive terminal body hair and should be distinguished from virilization. Virilization is the masculinization of a woman as manifested by clitoromegaly, a deepened voice, temporal balding, breast involution, and a remodeling of the limb-shoulder girdle. The most common cause of hirsutism is PCOS. PCOS is a syndrome characterized by oligomenorrhea/amenorrhea (anovulation), hirsutism, obesity, acne, and infertility. These women typically have a complex metabolic disorder that results in a hyperandrogenic state. Biochemical variations in women with PCOS include: (1) increased LH:FSH ratio; (2) higher levels of estrone than estradiol; (3) androstenedione at the upper limits of normal; (4) testosterone at, or slightly above, the upper end of normal; (5) impaired glucose tolerance (a significant proportion of women with PCOS eventually develop type II diabetes mellitus); (6) low serum progesterone levels (anovulation); and (7) hyperlipidemia.

A. Adrenal hyperplasia affects approximately 2% of the population and is the result of an alteration in the 21-hydroxylase enzyme gene, which ultimately leads to increased levels of dihydroepiandrostenedione sulfate (DHEA-S). In severe forms, a female infant may be virilized. In mild forms, patients may have acne, hirsutism, oligomenorrhea, and infertility. 21-hydroxylase deficiency is diagnosed by measuring increased levels of DHEA-S and androstenedione. Adrenal hyperplasia is less often secondary to 11β-hydroxylase deficiency. An elevated level of deoxycorticosterone is diagnostic of this deficiency.

B. Iatrogenic testosterone excess is most commonly intentionally achieved in genetic females who are undergoing gender reassignment for the purpose of virilization. Iatrogenic androgen excess can also be secondary to administration of Danazol (an attenuated androgen) for the treatment of endometriosis or to oral contraceptives (the progestins in OCPs are impeded androgens).

D. Adrenal neoplasms are very rare causes of hirsutism. The workup of a suspected adrenal neoplasm should include a CT scan of the adrenals. DHEA-S is often elevated in patients with adrenal neoplasms.

E. Sertoli-Leydig cell ovarian tumors (also known as an androblastomas) are also an uncommon cause of hirsutism. They typically arise in women 20 to 40 years of age and are unilateral. In addition to hirsutism, these women usually demonstrate defeminization followed by masculinization. These changes may occur in less than 6 months time. Laboratory findings included markedly elevated testosterone, decreased FSH, LH, and androstenedione. The treatment is surgical resection.

137. B. 5α-reductase locally converts testosterone to DHT in the hair follicle. It is thought that women with constitutional hirsutism have elevated levels or activity of 5α -reductase at the hair follicles. This enzyme is also responsible for virilization of the genetically male fetus and its deficiency leads to a female phenotype in a genetically male fetus. At the time of puberty, male virilization begins via additional steroid pathways.

A. 21-hydroxylase converts progesterone and17-α-hydroxyprogesterone to deoxycorticosterone and compound S. Its deficiency causes adrenal hyperplasia.

C. There is no dihydrotestosterase enzyme in the steroidogenesis pathway.

D. 11-β-hydroxylase catalyzes the conversion of deoxycorticosterone to cortisol. Its deficiency leads to mild congenital adrenal hyperplasia with excess androgens. It is often manifested by hypertension and mild hirsutism.

E. 17-ketosteroid reductase converts testosterone to androstenedione, not to DHT.

138. B. This is an inevitable abortion because the gestational age is less than 20 weeks. In order for an abortion to be considered inevitable, two or more of the following must apply: moderate cervical effacement, cervical dilation >3 cm, rupture of membranes, bleeding >7 days, cramping even with narcotics, or other signs of pregnancy termination. In this patient, the slide of the collected fluid demonstrates the characteristic "ferning" pattern of amniotic fluid, which makes it likely that the patient did experience a rupture of membranes. The cervical effacement and open external os to 4 cm are also positive signs, as is the presence of cramping. The absence of passage of POC (indicated by the lack of active vaginal bleeding) distinguishes this patient's condition from an incomplete abortion, while the open cervical os suggests this is not a complete, missed abortion, or threatened abortion. Treatment includes type and cross for possible blood transfusion, oxytocin to aid in fetal expulsion and to minimize blood loss, and D&C for possible retention of products of conception.

A. In a threatened abortion, the pregnancy is in danger of termination. It is marked primarily by first-trimester menstrual bleeding. Cramping may be present, but the membranes have not yet ruptured and the external os remains closed in contrast to inevitable abortion. Lack of passage of intrauterine contents rules out complete or incomplete abortion. Treatment consists primarily of expectant management. Patients are typically counseled to restrict their activity, which seems logical, but it should be noted that there are little data to support the efficacy of such management. Progesterone administration is a controversial treatment and not universally implemented.

C. Incomplete abortion is a loss of pregnancy with partial retention of POC, including parts of the fetus, amnion, or placenta. Continued bleeding, pain, an open cervix, and an enlarged uterus after passage of material characterizes this condition. Treatment is essentially the same as for inevitable abortion and focuses on control of hemorrhage and evacuation of fetal and placental remains.

D. Septic abortion is a serious condition marked by pregnancy loss or termination accompanied with intrauterine infection manifested by fever, malodorous vaginal discharge, pain, suprapubic tenderness, cervical tenderness, jaundice, shock, renal failure, and/or peritonitis. Treatment almost always involves hospitalization with invasive monitoring for sepsis, IV antibiotics, D&C, examination to rule out serious uterine trauma, and supportive care.

E. In a missed abortion, fetal death has occurred but the pregnancy is retained for a prolonged period, generally more than two menstrual cycles. Hypotheses as to why this occurs include viable placental function and prolonged progesterone effects. Typical signs of a missed abortion are decreased uterine size, loss of pregnancy symptoms, and possibly brownish vaginal discharge. The cervix is closed and no intrauterine contents are passed, distinguishing this from complete, incomplete, and inevitable abortions. Treatment includes expectant management, or evacuation of uterine contents either via D&C or medical means.

139. **E. In order to assure that the patient is fully informed regarding this process, she must be made aware of all possible options available to her. This includes adoption, first- or second-trimester abortion, and continuation of the pregnancy. Any procedure that is performed without discussion of all possible options violates the patient's autonomy and right to be fully informed regarding her care and is inappropriate.**

A. There is no legal provision that the pregnancy must be the result of failure of contraception. The law grants a woman the right to an abortion without conditions.

B. While chromosomal abnormalities are a common reason women choose to terminate pregnancies, especially those pregnancies that will result in significant disability or early death, having a fetus with an abnormal condition is not a requirement for a legal abortion.

C. Different states have unique laws regarding where, how, when, and to whom an abortive procedure can be given. However, these state laws only apply to the borders of the state, and not to the people in that state. Therefore, state law (including the right to an abortion) applies to all individuals physically present in that state regardless of their state of residence.

D. To the contrary, surgical abortion is frequently used as a failsafe when medical abortion is not successful. Medical abortion refers to the practice of using hormones or drugs to induce uterine contractions, create a hostile uterine environment, cause problems with placental attachment, or render other effects that will ultimately lead to fetal demise and expulsion. There are instances, however, when these methods fail to cause fetal death, or fail to lead to complete passage of the POC after fetal death has occurred. When this is the case, surgical techniques must be employed in order to ensure complete evacuation of POC.

140. **B. Primary amenorrhea is the absence of menarche by the age of 16. The mean age for menarche in North America is 12.8 years of age. This patient is 17 years of age and has not yet had menarche, thus, she has primary amenorrhea. Primary amenorrhea affects <0.1% of the population. Primary amenorrhea can be secondary to anorexia nervosa, gonadal dysgenesis, chromosomal abnormalities (Turner's or Swyer's), imperforate hymen, hypogonadotropic hypogonadism, testicular feminization, cystic fibrosis, craniopharyngioma, hypothyroidism, congenital adrenal hyperplasia, or pregnancy.**

A. Secondary amenorrhea is defined as cessation of menses for 6 months or more in a woman with previously normal menses. The most common cause of secondary amenorrhea is pregnancy. Always check a pregnancy test in a patient presenting with secondary amenorrhea. Additional causes of secondary amenorrhea include lactation, GnRH deficiency (can be secondary to severe psychiatric or physical illness), PCOS, hypothyroidism, hyperprolactinemia, and premature ovarian failure.

C. Juvenile amenorrhea is not a recognized medical term or diagnosis.

D. Prepubertal amenorrhea is not a recognized medical term or diagnosis. However, prior to puberty, girls should not experience vaginal bleeding. Any prepubertal girl who presents with vaginal bleeding should be thoroughly evaluated for underlying medical conditions as well as evaluated for sexual abuse or trauma.

E. Iatrogenic amenorrhea is amenorrhea secondary to medical intervention, such as administration of oral contraceptives, Depo-Provera contraceptive injections, use of a Mirena (levonorgestrel) IUD, Asherman's syndrome following a D&C, or endometrial ablation. Iatrogenic amenorrhea is a form of secondary amenorrhea.

141. C. The clinical description is that of a patient with androgen insensitivity syndrome, formerly known as testicular feminization. Patients with androgen insensitivity have an XY karyotype and produce normal androgens; however, they are resistant to the actions of the androgens. The resistance can be complete, as in the above patient, or it can be partial and result in ambiguous genitalia. Complete androgen insensitivity occurs in 1 in 20,000 live births. These patients have no Müllerian structures (they produce MIF), and thus have no cervix, uterus, or adnexa. The vagina is a short, blind-ending pouch. The intraabdominal masses described are intraabdominal testes; undescended testes need to be removed secondary to an increased risk for malignancy. The testes may be in the labia in these patients.

A. The clinical description of the above patient is consistent with androgen insensitivity syndrome and these patients do not demonstrate normal female genital and gonadal findings.

B. Primary amenorrhea may be secondary to an imperforate hymen and blockage of menstrual flow. These patients often give a history of cyclic cramps and PMS symptoms. Some patients may notice a cyclic vulvar bulge or sense of pressure as the menstrual flow pools behind the hymen. Treatment involves incision of the hymen, or a hymenectomy, to allow for efflux of the menstrual flow.

D. Again, the clinical description is of a patient with androgen insensitivity syndrome. The findings in this answer choice are not consistent with androgen insensitivity syndrome. Also, "streak ovaries" are not detectable on a simple bimanual exam. A normal vagina, cervix, uterus, and absent or "streak" ovaries might be found in a patient who is a Turner's mosaic. However, such a patient would undoubtedly also demonstrate other findings that would suggest the diagnosis of Turner's syndrome.

E. Clitoromegaly in the setting of other completely normal genitalia and Müllerian structures is a sign of virilization, and these patients should be evaluated for the etiology of the androgen excess. These patients will likely display additional signs of virilization, such as voice-deepening, facial and chest hair, a restructured shoulder girdle, and breast involution. Clitoromegaly is not seen in patients with complete androgen insensitivity syndrome. Some clitoromegaly may be seen in incomplete androgen insensitivity.

142. D. In the normal sequence of sexual maturation, thelarche (breast development; Figure 2-142) precedes pubarche (pubic hair growth), which precedes menarche (the first menstruation). On average, thelarche begins between 10 and 11 years of age, pubarche begins between 10.5 and 11.5 years of age and menarche occurs between 11.5 and 13 years of age. Many factors influence the age at which puberty begins in normal individuals, including ethnicity, family history, nutrition, weight and percent body fat, population crowding, optic exposure to sunlight, and the ability to obtain adequate sleep.

A, B, C, E. None of these are the correct sequence for normal sexual maturation.

143. C. GnRH is released from the hypothalamus in a pulsatile manner during puberty, as well as subsequent ovulatory cycles. The hypothalamus is considered the central command center of the reproductive axis, often referred to as the H-P-G axis. The H-P-G axis begins functioning by day 50 to 55 of gestation and remains active during the first year of life in both females and males. After the first year of life the H-P-G axis is turned off until puberty when it is reactivated. The exact stimuli that reactivate the axis are not completely understood. The pulsatile release of GnRH is essential to the function of the H-P-G axis; if GnRH is continuously administered, the pituitary gonadotrophs become desensitized and the H-P-G axis shuts down and anovulation ensues.

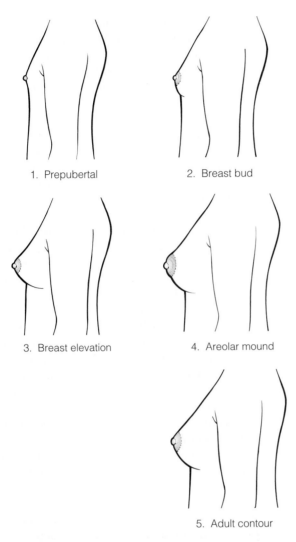

1. Prepubertal

2. Breast bud

3. Breast elevation

4. Areolar mound

5. Adult contour

Figure 2-142 • Reproduced with Permission from Callahan TL, Caughey AB. Blueprints Obstetrics & Gynecology, 4th ed. Baltimore: Lippincott Williams & Wilkins, 2007. Fig. 20-2, p. 214.

A. FSH is released from the anterior pituitary, not the hypothalamus. The release of FSH is cyclic, corresponding to the menstrual cycle, and is somewhat pulsatile in response to the pulses of GnRH.

B. TSH is released from the anterior pituitary by the thyrotrophs, not the hypothalamus.

D. Vasopressin is released by the posterior pituitary gland, not the hypothalamus. Vasopressin is not thought to play a critical role in the initiation or progression of puberty.

E. Prolactin is released by the anterior pituitary, not the hypothalamus. Recall that prolactin secretion is spontaneous from the anterior pituitary and that its release is inhibited by the release of dopamine from the hypothalamus.

144. **D. In women who are lactating and desire a more reliable method of contraception, a progesterone-only "mini pill" method is preferred. Estrogen-containing oral contraceptives can diminish the quantity and quality of breast milk. Other options for breastfeeding women include depot medroxyprogesterone acetate (Depo-Provera), an IUD, or barrier methods.**

A. Lactational amenorrhea is an effective method of contraception in 98% of women who exclusively breastfeed at regular intervals (including at nighttime) for the first 6 months. This is equivalent to oral contraceptive efficacy. At 1 year of exclusive breastfeeding the contraceptive efficacy is 92%. However, if a woman is going to combine breast and bottle feeding, she can no longer rely on lactational amenorrhea as a contraceptive method. It is imperative that the infant suckle at frequent intervals around the clock to inhibit the H-P-G axis from initiating an ovulatory cycle.

B, C. Although detailed studies comparing the effect on breastfeeding of a 20 μg to 30 μg combined oral contraceptive have not been reported, it is generally felt that either dose could negatively influence a woman's ability to successfully breastfeed her infant. See explanation for D.

E. The Ortho Evra transdermal patch contains both an estrogen and progesterone component. Specific studies on the effect on lactation have not been reported. One might hypothesize that since it is delivered via a transdermal route and bypasses first-pass hepatic metabolism, could have a different impact on breastfeeding than orally administered contraceptive pills. However, until further studies prove otherwise, it is generally assumed to have a similar impact on breast milk as the combined oral contraceptives.

145. **D. Postpartum hemorrhage is defined as blood loss greater than 500 mL following a vaginal delivery and 1000 mL following a cesarean**

delivery. If the hemorrhage occurs beyond 24 hours after delivery, it is called a delayed postpartum hemorrhage. Uterine atony is the primary cause of postpartum hemorrhage and risk factors include increased uterine distention (e.g., multiple gestation, macrosomia), uterine infection, exposure to magnesium sulfate, uterine abnormalities preventing adequate uterine contractions, and grand multiparity (i.e., history of more than five deliveries). Treatment includes uterine massage and administration of agents to increase uterine tone (e.g., oxytocin, Methergine [methylergonovine], or Hemabate [prostaglandin $F_{2\alpha}$]). If bleeding is refractory to medical management, a D&C should be performed to evaluate for possible retained POC. Uterine artery embolization is a potential treatment if medical management and D&C fail. Finally, laparotomy is reserved for bleeding refractory to the above measures and can involve ligation of major vessels, compression stitches (e.g., B-Lynch suture), or hysterectomy.

A. Uterine rupture is a rare cause of postpartum hemorrhage, occurring in 0.5% to 1% of women with a prior uterine scar (e.g., prior cesarean section, myomectomy), and in 1 of 20,000 women with no prior uterine scar. While hemorrhage typically occurs in the immediate postpartum period, the diagnosis should be considered in any woman with bleeding and any of the following risk factors: breech extraction, history of uterine surgery, and high parity. Treatment involves operative repair of the rupture site, possibly necessitating hysterectomy.

B. Uterine inversion is a rare obstetric emergency, occurring in 1 of 2500 deliveries, and can result in catastrophic hemorrhage due to the inability of the uterus to contract when inverted. It is more likely to be associated with immediate postpartum hemorrhage rather than delayed postpartum hemorrhage. Treatment involves manual replacement of the uterus to its anatomic position with the aid of uterine relaxants. If this is unsuccessful, replacement via laparotomy may be necessary.

C. Retained POCs refers to fragments of placenta or membranes that were not completely evacuated from the uterus following delivery of the fetus. Treatment involves removal of retained POCs via manual exploration after delivery or D&C. Retained POCs is an unlikely etiology in this patient with a thin endometrial stripe on ultrasound. However, this diagnosis should be considered if medical treatment fails.

E. Bleeding from vaginal lacerations can lead to postpartum hemorrhage. Thus, evaluation must include inspection of the perineum and vagina for lacerations, which are then treated via repair and suture ligation of bleeding vessels.

146. **B. This patient has uterine prolapse due to pelvic relaxation. Her risk factors include menopause and chronically increased intraabdominal pressures due to chronic cough. Additionally, five vaginal deliveries likely contributed to her pelvic laxity. Most women with pelvic relaxation will develop one or more of the following symptoms: urinary incontinence or other urinary symptoms, pelvic pressure, low back pain, or dyspareunia. In addition to uterine prolapse, cystoceles (i.e., herniation of the anterior vaginal wall due to the bladder) and rectoceles (i.e., herniation of the posterior vaginal wall due to the rectum) can also occur and exacerbate symptoms. Due to embarrassment, some women may not seek medical care until symptoms become unbearable. Pelvic relaxation is a structural support issue and therefore can be treated surgically via hysterectomy, culdoplasty, and colporrhaphy (i.e., removal of excess vaginal mucosa and plication of the underlying fascia) as appropriate. Patients wishing to avoid surgery can try more conservative therapies such as pessaries to provide support. Pessaries are intravaginal devices that provide mechanical support and attempt to restore pelvic structures to their anatomic position.**

A. While systemic estrogens may provide some improvement in pelvic relaxation by promoting healthier tissue, they are unlikely to significantly improve this patient's prolapse. Further, long-standing oral estrogens are not currently recommended because of concerns of increasing the risk of thromboembolic disease and breast cancer. Estrogen cream would be a possibility to gain local estrogenic effects

C, D. While hysterectomy followed by anterior colporrhaphy would be a definitive treatment for this patient, an immediate hysterectomy is not warranted in a patient wishing to avoid surgery.

E. Burch culposuspension is used in the setting of bladder neck relaxation and genuine stress urinary incontinence. At this time, this patient does not suffer from incontinence.

147. C. Urge incontinence is urine leakage due to involuntary and uninhibited bladder contractions. It is also known as detrusor instability.

148. B. Stress incontinence is urine leakage with exertion or straining. It is typically associated with pelvic relaxation and displacement of the urethrovesical junction.

149. A. Overflow incontinence occurs due to poor or absent bladder contractions that lead to urinary retention with overdistention of the bladder. As the bladder becomes overdistended, urine "overflows" the bladder and incontinence occurs.

D. Total incontinence is urine leakage that is continuous and usually the result of a urinary fistula.

150. B. The patient has adenomyosis, which is the presence of endometrial tissue in the myometrium. Adenomyosis affects approximately 15% of women and is usually found in parous women in their 30s or 40s. Potential symptoms include menorrhagia, dysmenorrhea, dyspareunia, dyschezia, and metrorrhagia. While mild symptoms can be treated with NSAIDs, oral contraceptives, or progestins, definitive treatment (and diagnosis) can only be made with hysterectomy.

A. While it is possible for a patient to have both fibroids and adenomyosis simultaneously, this patient's uterus and ultrasound examinations are not consistent with that of fibroids.

C. This patient's history of menorrhagia and dysmenorrhea as well as the exam are not consistent with that of polycystic ovaries.

D. A hydrosalpinx is a fluid-filled fallopian tube and is typically associated with infection or tubal trauma. They can result in tubal factor infertility, but are not associated with menorrhagia.

E. Paratubal cysts are generally benign cysts found along fallopian tubes. If they get large, they can cause pelvic pain due to torsion, but are most often incidental findings. They would not explain this patient's symptoms.

BLOCK 4

151. A 19-year-old woman presents to your office with complaints of vulvar and vaginal pruritus. She reports being treated for a urinary tract infection with amoxicillin 10 days earlier. She denies abdominal pain or fever. On physical exam you note some erythematous punctate macular lesions bilaterally near the perineum, but no papular or vesicular lesions. On speculum exam, there is a white discharge that has a negative whiff test and a potassium hydroxide (KOH) prepared slide reveals the image in Figure 2-151. What is the treatment of choice?

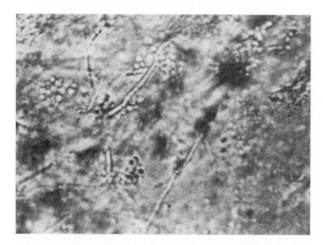

Figure 2-151 • Reproduced with Permission from Crissey, JT. Manual of Medical Mycology. Blackwell Science, 1995: 90.

A. Oral acyclovir
B. Topical acyclovir applied to the lesions
C. Oral metronidazole (Flagyl)
D. A longer course of amoxicillin
E. Antifungal vaginal cream

152. A 22-year-old G_0 Caucasian woman presents with complaints of increased body and facial hair. She has noticed increased hair growth on her upper lip, chin, upper back, and lower abdomen for about 6 weeks. Upon review of systems, she also notes deepening of her voice and enlargement of her clitoris. None of the other women in her family have any of these symptoms, and she feels quite self-conscious as a result. She underwent menarche at age 13, has irregular menses every 25 to 45 days, and has never been sexually active. On physical exam, she is 5'6" tall and weighs 114 lbs. She has some generalized acne on her face and back in addition to acanthosis nigricans. There are a few terminal hairs on her back as well as some stubble on her cheeks and upper lip. Her escutcheon is diamond-shaped. A pelvic ultrasound shows a large adnexal mass that has both cystic and solid components as well as septations. Her most likely diagnosis is:

A. Sertoli-Leydig cell tumor
B. Congenital adrenal hyperplasia (CAH)
C. Testicular feminization
D. Polymenorrhea
E. Polycystic ovarian syndrome (PCOS)

153. A 33-year-old G_4P_2 patient at 38 5/7 weeks GA has been in the second stage of labor for 3 hours when you are called for the delivery. She presented with contractions about 12 hours ago and was 3 cm dilated. She made reasonable progress, becoming fully dilated over the ensuing 10 hours with oxytocin augmentation. Her antenatal course was complicated only by diet-controlled gestational diabetes. Her last two births were 7 and 5 years ago, both vaginal, with fetal weights of 8.5 and 9 lbs, respectively. As the fetus is beginning to crown, you are prepared to:

A. Perform a forceps delivery
B. Perform a vacuum delivery
C. Perform a cesarean delivery
D. Manage a shoulder dystocia
E. Manage a uterine inversion

154. A 54-year-old woman presents for an exploratory laparotomy and total abdominal hysterectomy-bilateral salpingo-oophorectomy (TAH-BSO) for a large left pelvic mass that is shown in Figure 2-154. Upon entering the abdomen, peritoneal washings are taken. The mass is isolated to the left ovary with no evidence that it is broken beyond the capsule. Upon examination of the uterus, tubes, and contralateral ovary, there is no gross evidence of disease. Upon palpation of the pelvic and aortic lymph nodes, they seem entirely normal. There is no evidence of any lesions on the bowel, omentum, or diaphragm either. Final pathology returns consistent with the above gross findings, but with positive malignant cells in the washings. Given the above tumor and the positive peritoneal washings, what is the stage of this ovarian cancer?

A. Ia
B. Ib
C. Ic
D. IIb
E. IIIc

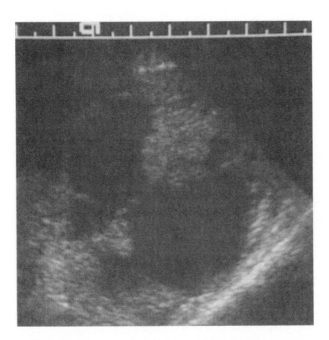

Figure 2-154•Image Provided by Departments of Radiology and Obstetrics & Gynecology, University of California, San Francisco.

155. A 46-year-old G_0 obese woman with chronic hypertension and diabetes presents with infiltrating ductal carcinoma of the breast. She undergoes a wide local excision and axillary lymph node dissection. Surgery is performed without complications and there is no evidence of metastatic disease on frozen section. You go to the postoperative area to discuss these findings with her. She is quite bitter about her diagnosis, but glad that she got the disease at age 46 rather than at age 36 like her sister, who had bilateral disease requiring mastectomies. She asks you why she got breast cancer. Which of the following was her strongest risk factor?

A. Obesity
B. Nulliparity
C. Hypertension
D. Family history
E. Diabetes

156. A 33-year-old G_1P_0 is seen in clinic at 36 weeks gestational age (GA). Her fundal height measures 32 cm. You send her for ultrasound, which shows an estimated fetal weight of 2800 gm, an amniotic fluid index (AFI) of 3.0, and normal uterine artery Doppler's. Which of the following can lead to oligohydramnios of a fetal etiology?

A. Tracheoesophageal fistula
B. Rupture of membranes (ROM)
C. Gestational diabetes
D. Renal agenesis
E. Fetal hydrops

157. A 27-year-old presents 2 months past her last menstrual period (LMP). She is in a stable, monogamous relationship with her boyfriend. They were regularly using condoms, but recently began to use the withdrawal method. Your office urine pregnancy test is positive. She wishes to terminate her pregnancy. Which of the following is true regarding pregnancy termination?

A. In 1972 maternal mortality from illegal abortions was 52%; in 1974 it was 6%
B. General anesthesia is now the major cause of mortality from pregnancy termination
C. A single, induced abortion does not cause pregnancy complications or sterility
D. Cervical dilation in the second trimester cannot safely be achieved by using laminaria
E. Surgical termination is associated with a greater blood loss than medical termination

158. A 28-year-old G_1P_0 comes to you at 10 weeks gestation for her first pregnancy visit. She feels that she is much larger than her friends have been at this stage of pregnancy. Her periods are regular, and she feels certain of her date of conception. On exam, her fundus measures approximately 16 week's size. On ultrasound, you diagnose diamniotic-monochorionic twins. The approximate age at which the embryo split is:

A. 0 to 3 days
B. 3 to 8 days
C. 8 to 13 days
D. 13 to 15 days
E. Beyond 15 days

The response options for items 159 to 162 are the same. You will be required to select one or more answers for each item in the set.

A. Lactate dehydrogenase (LDH)
B. Testosterone
C. Estrogen
D. Human chorionic gonadotropin (hCG)
E. Alpha fetoprotein (AFP)
F. CA-125

For each type of ovarian tumor, select the most commonly associated tumor marker(s) or hormone. Answer choices may be used more than once.

159. Choriocarcinoma **(SELECT 1)**

160. Endodermal sinus tumor **(SELECT 1)**

161. Dysgerminoma **(SELECT 2)**

162. Granulosa cell tumor **(SELECT 1)**

End of Set

163. You have been following a 62-year-old G_1P_1 woman in your office for a small left labial lesion that was first noticed 1 month ago because of pruritus and discomfort. The lesion is white with an irregular border. You prescribed a trial of low-dose topical steroid, but the symptoms have not improved. What is the appropriate next step?

    A. Increase the dose of steroid
    B. Biopsy
    C. Wide local excision of the lesion
    D. Laser ablation
    E. Cryotherapy

164. A 28-year-old G_0 reports worsening cyclic pelvic pain as well as dyspareunia that are minimally improved with NSAIDs. You initiate an infertility evaluation because she has been trying unsuccessfully to conceive for the past $1\frac{1}{2}$ years despite regular menses and timed intercourse. Her labs and a hysterosalpingogram are all normal. You presume endometriosis and recommend either continuous oral contraceptives (OCPs) for symptom control or laparoscopic surgery. Which of the following is true about endometriosis?

    A. Severity of symptoms can vary in the estimated 60% of affected women
    B. It is the presence of ovarian tissue in the uterus
    C. Definitive diagnosis can only be made via direct visualization
    D. It is not a cause of infertility
    E. Only surgical therapy is effective

165. A 66-year-old G_3P_3 complains of three episodes of light vaginal bleeding in the past month. She is not sexually active and denies vaginal discharge, trauma, history of exogenous estrogen usage, or other complaints. Her past medical history is noncontributory. On exam, she is a thin woman with a slightly atrophic vagina but

no obvious lesions are visible on speculum exam. She had a normal Pap smear 6 months ago and her cervix appears normal. A pelvic ultrasound shows an appropriately small uterus with a 1-cm lesion in the cavity and no adnexal masses. What is the most likely diagnosis?

    A. Endometrial polyp
    B. Endometrial cancer
    C. Atrophy
    D. Cervical cancer
    E. Hemorrhoids

The response options for items 166 to 169 are the same. You will be required to select one or more answers for each item in the set.

    A. Clue cells
    B. Pseudohyphae
    C. Motile flagellated organisms
    D. Thin, dry vaginal mucosa
    E. Frothy, malodorous green-gray discharge
    F. Cottage cheese-like discharge
    G. Slightly increased gray malodorous discharge

A 26-year-old G_0 presents to clinic complaining of vaginal itching and burning. You obtain a wet prep. For each of the finding(s) in vaginitis, select the most likely diagnosis. Answers may be used more than once.

166. Atrophic vaginitis **(SELECT 1)**

167. *Candida* vaginitis **(SELECT 2)**

168. *Trichomonas vaginalis* **(SELECT 2)**

169. Bacterial vaginosis **(SELECT 2)**

End of Set

170. A 17-year-old G_0 patient presents to the emergency department (ED) with complaints of fever and lower abdominal pain. On physical exam she has a temperature of 101.2°F and bilateral lower abdominal tenderness. On bimanual exam she has cervical motion tenderness with bilateral adnexal tenderness. There is a slight fullness on her right that is difficult to assess because of her discomfort. She is admitted to the hospital with the diagnosis of pelvic inflammatory disease (PID) and started on cefoxitin and doxycycline. After 48 hours of this therapy, she still has fevers to 101.6°F. Which of the following is the next best step in management?

A. Laparoscopy
B. Laparotomy
C. Await final cultures
D. Pelvic ultrasound
E. Change antibiotics to ampicillin and gentamicin

171. A 26-year-old G_2P_0 woman presents for her first prenatal appointment. She is generally healthy with seasonal allergies and no history of prior surgeries. She reports that her menstrual periods occur every month, and the last one was about 5 months ago. When you ask her to be more specific about the day, she can only answer that it was between the first and the ninth days of that month. You order an ultrasound to help with the dating of the pregnancy. Which of the following is the best method to date a pregnancy when used alone?

A. LMP
B. First-trimester ultrasound
C. Second-trimester ultrasound
D. Third-trimester ultrasound
E. Quantitative β-hCG correlated with dates

172. A 26-year-old G_1P_0 woman presents at 18 weeks gestation complaining of increased vaginal discharge. She began noticing an increase in a clear, nonodorous discharge two days ago. She notes no fevers, chills, changes in bowel or urinary function, and no abdominal pain. She has had an uncomplicated pregnancy up to this point. On speculum exam, you note that the external os of the cervix looks slightly open. You take cultures and slide preparations of the vaginal discharge. There is no evidence for ruptured membranes, trichomoniasis, or bacterial vaginosis. You return to the bedside and perform a sterile vaginal exam. Her cervix is 1 cm dilated and 2 cm long. At this point, her management could include which of the following?

A. Oral metronidazole (Flagyl)
B. Cerclage placement
C. Amniocentesis for chromosomal abnormalities
D. Tocolysis with magnesium sulfate
E. Betamethasone for fetal lung maturity

The response options for items 173 to 176 are the same. You will be required to select one or more answers for each item in the set.

A. Metronidazole
B. Estrogen cream
C. Antifungal agents
D. Clindamycin

For each diagnosis, select the most appropriate possible treatment(s). Answers may be used more than once:

173. Atrophic vaginitis (**SELECT 1**)

174. *Candida* (**SELECT 1**)

175. *Trichomonas vaginalis* (**SELECT 1**)

176. Bacterial vaginosis (**SELECT 2**)

End of Set

177. A 24-year-old woman comes to see you in clinic to discuss her difficulty getting pregnant. She has been trying for almost 2 years, and she is getting frustrated and concerned that she will never be able to have children. You ask her about her menstrual cycle and the timing of intercourse to determine if there is an obvious reason that she has had difficulty getting pregnant. The patient believes there is "something wrong" with her. You remind her that male factors contribute to what percent of infertility?

A. 5%
B. 15%
C. 25%
D. 40%
E. 55%

178. A couple presents to your office for evaluation of infertility after 13 months of attempting to conceive. You take a medical history from both partners. The wife's history is noncontributory. In your discussion of potential ovulatory etiologies, you explain that disruption of the hypothalamic-pituitary-ovarian axis is the cause of female infertility in 15% to 20% of cases and is directly related to impairment in folliculogenesis, ovulation, and which of the following?

A. Endometrial development
B. Tubal dilation
C. Cervical dilation
D. Basal temperature
E. Uterine growth

The response options for items 179 to 182 are the same. You will be required to select one answer for each item in the set.

A. Klinefelter syndrome
B. Trisomy 13
C. Turner syndrome
D. Cri du chat syndrome

E. Cystic fibrosis
F. Tay-Sachs disease
G. β-thalassemia
H. Sickle cell disease
I. Trisomy 18
J. Down syndrome

For each statement or population, select the syndrome or disease with the greatest carrier frequency. Answer choices may be used more than once.

179. African-American populations **(SELECT 1)**

180. Ashkenazi Jews **(SELECT 1)**

181. Most common newborn autosomal disorder **(SELECT 1)**

182. Mediterranean populations **(SELECT 1)**

End of Set

183. A 30-year-old G_2P_0 at 8 weeks GA comes in for her initial prenatal visit. She reveals to you that she started consuming more alcohol ever since she lost her job about 6 months ago. She was drinking up to a bottle of wine most evenings. She has been struggling to cut back over the past few weeks since she found out she was pregnant. She has felt very anxious and feels like she needs a drink to "take the edge off." She says she wants to do what is best for the baby but is having such a hard time dealing with her own life. In addition to admission to a rehabilitation program, which of the following is the most appropriate treatment for this patient?

A. Treatment with a benzodiazepine to manage her symptoms of withdrawal
B. Treatment with a barbiturate to manage her symptoms of withdrawal
C. Reassure her that her baby will likely be fine because the risk of teratogenic effects increases later in pregnancy
D. Insist that she stop drinking immediately and avoid any symptomatic relief for her symptoms of withdrawal to avoid further fetal effects
E. Inform her that any damage to the fetus is likely done and therefore she should not put such pressure on herself to quit now

184. A 26-year-old woman is in for her routine gynecological visit. She is currently taking OCPs for birth control but says she and her husband have

been talking about having children. Before she is 30, she wants to go back to school but wants to have a child first. She has a friend who had a hard time having a baby and wants to know her chances of getting pregnant in the next year. What percentage of couples will get pregnant after trying to conceive for 1 year?

A. 55%
B. 65%
C. 75%
D. 85%
E. 95%

The response options for items 185 to 188 are the same. You will be required to select one or more answers for each item in the set.

A. Metronidazole
B. Clindamycin
C. Erythromycin
D. Trimethoprim/sulfamethoxazole
E. Azithromycin
F. Acyclovir
G. Zidovudine
H. Ampicillin
I. Miconazole
J. Cephazolin

For each infection, select the most appropriate treatment(s) during pregnancy. Answers may be used more than once.

185. Group B *Streptococcus* (GBS) **(SELECT 4)**

186. Bacterial vaginosis **(SELECT 2)**

187. HIV **(SELECT 1)**

188. *Varicella* **(SELECT 1)**

End of Set

189. A 29-year-old G_2P_1 at 39 2/7 weeks GA presents in active labor. She has been contracting for 4 hours and on admission is contracting painfully every 2 to 3 minutes. Her cervix is 4 cm dilated and the fetal head is at −1 station. The fetal heart rate (FHR) tracing is reassuring. By Leopolds, the estimated fetal weight is 3500 gm and the position is left occiput posterior (LOP). The patient's prior labor lasted 13 hours and culminated in a spontaneous vaginal delivery of a 7 lb, 8 oz boy (3400 gm) after a 60-minute second stage. The

patient progresses slowly in labor, dilating approximately 1 cm every 1 to 2 hours during the next 6 hours. When she is 8 cm dilated, she requests an epidural, which is placed without complication. Over the next 4 hours, the patient slowly changes to full dilation. On exam, she is fully dilated, +1 station, and right occiput transverse (ROT) position. She begins the second stage. After pushing for 2 hours, she is +3 station, and right occiput anterior (ROA) position, as depicted in the Figure 2-189. She requests assistance with a forceps or vacuum delivery because of exhaustion. Which of the following is unnecessary for a low forceps delivery of this fetus?

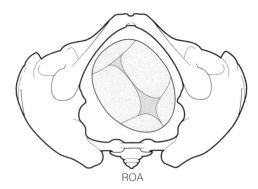

ROA

Figure 2-189 • Reproduced with Permission from Callahan TL, Caughey AB. Blueprints Obstetrics & Gynecology, 4th ed. Baltimore: Lippincott Williams & Wilkins, 2007. Fig. 4-5, p. 40.

A. Anesthesia
B. Knowledge of station at or beyond +2
C. An estimate of fetal weight that is not macrosomic
D. Direct occiput anterior position (OAP)
E. Skilled operator

190. A 31-year-old G_2P_1 presents in active labor at 39 5/7 weeks GA. She is 5 cm dilated, 90% effaced, and at +1 station. The FHR tracing is reassuring with no decelerations, and the tocometer reveals contractions every 2 to 3 minutes. She has had an uncomplicated prenatal course. Her obstetrical history is remarkable for a cesarean delivery 4 years ago for failure to progress past 7 cm dilation. On labor and delivery, she requests an epidural, which is placed without complication. On her next examination 2 hours later, she is 7 cm dilated and +2 station, but her contractions have decreased to every 5 to 7 minutes. She is begun on oxytocin for augmentation. An hour and half later, the nurse calls you for a prolonged FHR deceleration. She has already stopped the pitocin, given oxygen by face mask, and changed the patient's position. The FHR tracing is shown in Figure 2-190. On examination, the cervix is 8 to 9 cm dilated, but the fetal head cannot be easily palpated, indicating that it is at least above –3 station. The next step in management of this patient is:

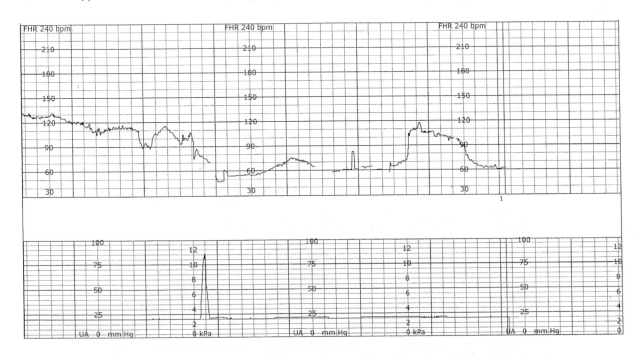

Figure 2-190 • Image Provided by the Department of Obstetrics & Gynecology, University of California, San Francisco.

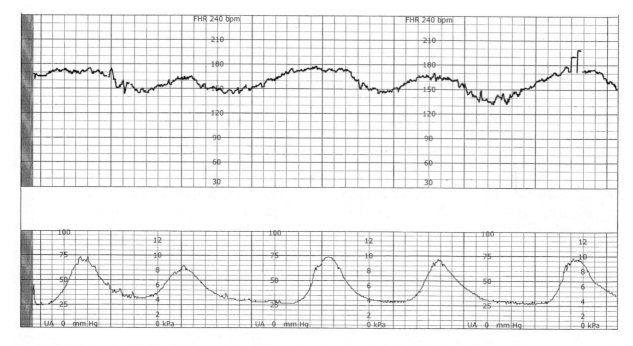

Figure 2-191 • Image Provided by the Department of Obstetrics & Gynecology, University of California, San Francisco.

A. Fetal scalp pH
B. Cesarean delivery
C. Forceps delivery
D. Expectant management
E. Restart pitocin to help bring the head back down

The next two questions (items 191 and 192) correspond to the following vignette.

191. A 27-year-old G_2P_1 presented at 37 weeks with PROM 2 hours ago. Her cervix was 2 cm dilated and 50% effaced, and the fetal head was at –3 station. The FHR tracing was reactive and an induction of labor with pitocin was begun. During the last 20 minutes, the FHR tracing has begun to show the pattern shown in Figure 2-191. This pattern represents:

A. Early decelerations
B. Cord compression
C. Variable decelerations
D. Fetal bradycardia
E. Late decelerations

192. The patient in the previous question declines intervention. One hour later she is afebrile, her pulse is 80 beats/minute, and she is 5 cm dilated. The FHR tracing is shown in Figure 2-192. The tracing demonstrates:

A. Fetal bradycardia
B. Maternal pulse
C. Loss of information
D. Second stage head compression
E. Variable deceleration

End of Set

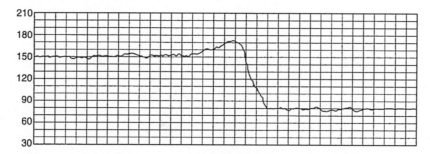

Figure 2-192 • Reproduced with Permission from Caughey, A. Blueprints Q&A Step 3 Obstetrics & Gynecology, 1st ed. Blackwell Science, 2002. Fig. 89, p. 55.

193. A 23-year-old G_1P_0 presents at 11 weeks gestation with spotting. She undergoes ultrasound to rule out an ectopic pregnancy or missed abortion. A large cystic hygroma is identified, as shown in Figure 2-193. The patient undergoes chorionic villus sampling (CVS), which reveals Turner syndrome (45,XO). The patient's risk for recurrence of this syndrome in a subsequent pregnancy is:

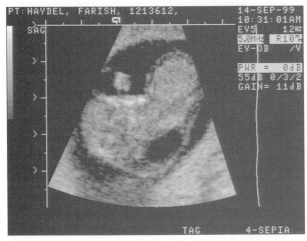

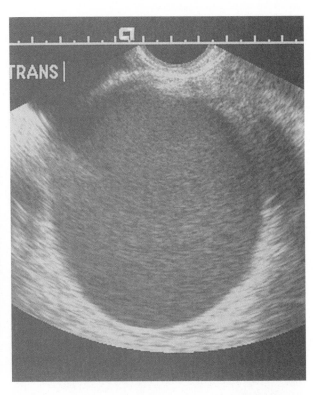

Figure 2-193 • Image Courtesy of Dr. Richard Barth, Lucille Packard Children's Hospital, Palo Alto, California.

A. 10%
B. 25%
C. 50%
D. 70%
E. Not increased

194. A 37-year-old G_0 presents to clinic for evaluation because she and her husband are attempting to conceive. She is concerned because she is 37 years old and not yet pregnant after 2 cycles. Which of the following is true regarding fertility?

A. Approximately 10% of couples have unexplained infertility
B. Smoking does not affect fertility
C. Caffeine does not affect fertility
D. The normal fecundability rate is 20%
E. Male factor infertility accounts for 15% of infertility

195. A 27-year-old G_0 complains of constant, mild pelvic pain that worsens with her menses. She has experienced dyspareunia for the last 2 years. An ultrasound (Figure 2-195) reveals evidence of endometriosis in her ovary in the form of an endometrioma, a common finding in endometriosis. What is the test of choice to diagnose endometriosis?

Figure 2-195 • Image Provided by Departments of Radiology and Obstetrics & Gynecology, University of California, San Francisco.

A. Trial of OCPs
B. GnRH-agonists
C. Laparoscopy
D. Laparotomy
E. Danazol

196. A 21-year-old with an unknown LMP undergoes an ultrasound for dates. Duodenal atresia is identified, as shown in Figure 2-196. The most

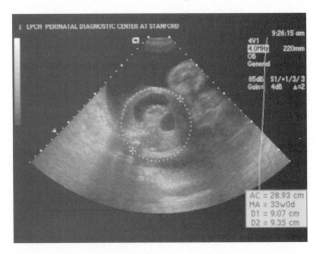

Figure 2-196 • Image Courtesy of Dr. Richard Barth, Lucille Packard Children's Hospital, Palo Alto, California.

frequent chromosomal abnormality associated with duodenal atresia is:

A. Turner syndrome (XO)
B. Trisomy 13
C. Trisomy 18
D. Trisomy 21
E. Trisomy 16

197. A 32-year-old G_1P_0 presents for a dating ultrasound. She has no medical problems and her pregnancy has been unremarkable. During her ultrasound an omphalocele is identified as shown in Figure 2-197. You counsel her that:

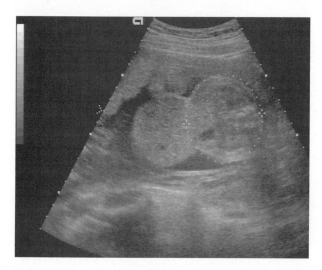

Figure 2-197 • Image Courtesy of Dr. Richard Barth, Lucille Packard Children's Hospital, Palo Alto, California.

A. In contrast to gastroschisis, omphaloceles are associated with chromosomal abnormalities
B. Omphaloceles are caused by a herniation of abdominal contents lateral to the umbilicus
C. In contrast to gastroschisis, omphaloceles are not associated with syndromes
D. Repair of omphaloceles typically involves bowel resection
E. Patients with fetuses with omphaloceles should deliver by cesarean section

198. A 16-year-old G_0 presents to clinic with primary amenorrhea. She is 5'2" inches tall, well-nourished, has normal breast development and pubic hair, and no evidence of hyperandrogenism. On exam, her ovaries are palpable but her vagina ends blindly and the uterus is absent. Her serum testosterone level is normal. What additional test should be sent?

A. Karyotype
B. Intravenous pyelogram
C. Thyroid stimulating hormone (TSH)
D. Follicle stimulating hormone (FSH)
E. Luteinizing hormone (LH)

199. A 34-year-old G_2P_2 presents for her annual Pap smear. She hesitates before leaving, and then asks to discuss sexual problems that she's been having with her husband. Which of the following is the most common cause of sexual dysfunction among women?

A. Arousal disorder
B. Decreased lubrication
C. Vaginismus
D. Medical illness
E. Hypoactive sexual desire

200. A 28-year-old G_0 presents to clinic complaining of intermittent left-sided pelvic pain that began 24 hours ago. The pain has worsened during the last 3 hours, and she has developed nausea. Her LMP was 3 weeks ago. She is monogamous with her boyfriend and uses timed withdrawal for contraception. She is afebrile and appears moderately uncomfortable. Her abdomen is soft, without rebound tenderness, but she guards when you examine the left side. Her cervical exam is unremarkable. You perform an office ultrasound, which reveals a 6 cm $\times$ 5 cm $\times$ 5 cm simple left-sided ovarian cyst and no free fluid in the cul de sac. The most likely etiology of her pain is:

A. Ruptured ovarian cyst
B. Chlamydial cervicitis
C. PID
D. Ovarian torsion
E. Cyst pain

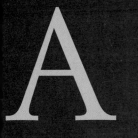

A Answers and Explanations

151. E	168. C, E	185. B, C, H, J
152. A	169. A, G	186. A, B
153. D	170. D	187. G
154. C	171. B	188. F
155. D	172. B	189. D
156. D	173. B	190. B
157. C	174. C	191. E
158. B	175. A	192. A
159. D	176. A, D	193. E
160. E	177. B	194. D
161. A, F	178. A	195. C
162. C	179. H	196. D
163. B	180. F	197. A
164. C	181. J	198. B
165. A	182. G	199. E
166. D	183. B	200. D
167. B, F	184. D	

151. E. The patient has vulvovaginal candidiasis secondary to treatment with the amoxicillin for her UTI. Vulvovaginal candidiasis may present with pruritus, a white discharge, and may be triggered by changes in sexual habits, undergarments, or a course of antibiotics. Treatments for this condition include over-the-counter antifungal preparations (Monistat), prescription topical agents (Terazole cream), and oral fluconazole (Diflucan). The oral treatment consists of a one-time dose, is >85% effective, and is much more convenient than the topical agents.

   A. Oral acyclovir would be used to treat or prophylax against herpes simplex virus (HSV) lesions.

   B. Topical acyclovir is more often used for herpes labialis or herpetic lesions on the upper lip rather than herpes vaginalis or vulvar lesions.

   C. Metronidazole can be used to treat bacterial vaginosis. Common dosing regimens include 500 mg PO BID and 250 mg PO TID.

   D. The patient has been treated for her UTI, so she does not need anymore amoxicillin.

152. A. This patient presents with acute hirsutism as well as virilism (e.g., deepening of the voice, male pattern baldness, clitoromegaly). Ovarian tumors that can lead to hirsutism and virilism include the sex-cord mesenchymal tumors, granulosa-theca cell tumors, germ cell tumors, and the Sertoli-Leydig cell tumors. These tumors can all secrete testosterone and lead to virilization.

   B. CAH results from a constellation of enzyme deficiencies, the most common being an absence in 21-hydroxylase, which results in excess 17-α-hydroxyprogesterone and can lead to the complete inability to synthesize cortisol or mineralocorticoids. Adult-onset CAH can be quite mild with anovulation and androgenization but should still have elevated dehydroepiandrosterone sulfate (DHEA-S) and/or testosterone. CAH usually presents in early childhood, but can present in adults. It rarely presents as acutely as seen in this patient, and would not have an associated ovarian tumor.

   C. Testicular feminization is most commonly related to the absence or dysfunction of the testosterone receptor. These patients are genetically 46,XY but are phenotypically female. Because of the testosterone receptor dysfunction, they cannot become hirsute or virilized.

   D. Polymenorrhea is menstruation more frequently than every 21 days. This patient has irregular, less frequent menses.

   E. PCOS is also known as polycystic ovarian disorder (PCOD) or simply PCO. This condition first described by Stein and Leventhal in the setting of hirsutism, virilism, anovulation, amenorrhea, and obesity presents as a chronic condition. It is also associated with insulin resistance and hence, type II diabetes. This patient's symptoms are too acute to be PCOS.

153. D. In this patient with gestational diabetes and a history of a macrosomic birth, you should be prepared for the possibility of a shoulder dystocia. This includes alerting the nursing staff of your suspicion, having extra help in the room, flexing the patient's thighs for delivery, and having someone ready to apply suprapubic pressure after delivery of the head, if necessary.

   A, B. A forceps delivery is unnecessary in this case. Further, given your suspicion for macrosomia, the use of forceps or vacuum to perform an operative vaginal delivery is inadvisable.

   C. A cesarean delivery is unnecessary at this point with vaginal delivery being imminent. Rarely, if a severe shoulder dystocia cannot be resolved after 5 to 6 minutes of maneuvers, the fetal head is pushed back into the maternal pelvis and a cesarean delivery is performed. This is called a Zavanelli maneuver and is the procedure of last resort in a shoulder dystocia.

   E. Uterine inversion is more common in multiparous women and with macrosomic fetuses. It is uncommon, and it is unlikely to occur in this patient.

154. C. Ovarian cancer stage I is as follows: Ia is confined to one ovary; Ib involves both ovaries; Ic is either a or b with rupture of the ovary, disease outside the capsule, or positive peritoneal washings.

   A, B, D, E. See Table 2-154.

■ TABLE 2-154 Staging of Ovarian Carcinoma

Stage I – Growth Limited to Ovaries	
a	Limited to one ovary. No ascites. Capsule intact
b	Limited to both ovaries. No ascites. Capsule intact
c	a or b plus positive washings or disease beyond the capsule
Stage II – Disease Extends to the Pelvis	
a	Malignant cells in the uterus or fallopian tubes
b	Malignant cells elsewhere in the pelvis
c	a or b plus positive washings or disease beyond the capsule
Stage III – Disease Extends to the Abdomen	
a	Only microscopic disease
b	Metastases < 2 cm in size
c	Metastases > 2 cm in size or any positive pelvic or para-aortic nodes
Stage IV – Distant Metastases Include Positive Pleural Effusion, and Disease in the Liver Parenchyma	

155. **D.** A first-degree relative with bilateral, premenopausal disease confers an eight-fold increase in breast cancer risk. This family history is the strongest risk factor in any patient, and management usually entails annual mammograms starting 10 years prior to when the relative was first diagnosed with disease.

   A. Obesity carries a relative risk of 2.
   B. Nulliparity is associated with a three-fold risk of disease when compared to parous patients.
   C. Hypertension appears associated with breast cancer, with an odds ratio of 1.2 to 1.5.
   E. Diabetes, similar to hypertension, is weakly associated with breast cancer.

156. **D.** Amniotic fluid is produced primarily by the fetal kidneys and less by the fetal lungs. Thus, renal agenesis leads to oligo- or anhydramnios. Amniotic fluid provides an acoustic window for ultrasound, which is quite limited within the setting of anhydramnios or severe oligohydramnios. Ultrasound with Doppler can be used to identify the renal arteries, which suggests the presence of kidneys. The absence of the renal arteries suggests the absence of kidneys.

   A. During the second trimester onward, fetal swallowing and urination result in continuous circulation of amniotic fluid. Disorders of the gastrointestinal tract, such as tracheoesophageal fistulas, generally result in polyhydramnios, not oligohydramnios.
   B. ROM must always be ruled out in any patient with oligohydramnios, regardless of GA. However, it is not a fetal cause of oligohydramnios.
   C. Gestational diabetes that is not controlled can be associated with fetal macrosomia and polyhydramnios similar to pregestational diabetes.
   D. Fetal hydrops is more commonly associated with polyhydramnios.

157. **C.** One or more prior abortions are unlikely to be associated with an increased risk of adverse outcomes in subsequent pregnancies. A history of three or more induced abortions appears to be associated with pregnancy complications such as placental abruption, PROM, low birth weight, preterm delivery, and bleeding in the first and third trimesters when compared with women with a history of two or fewer induced abortions.

   A. Illegal abortions resulted in significant maternal mortality (39% prior to legalization of abortion) but the rate was not as high as 52%. A mere 2 years after the passage of *Roe V. Wade* in 1972, maternal mortality fell dramatically to 6%, largely due to increased access to procedures performed sterilely in adequate medical facilities by trained, accountable practitioners.
   B. General anesthesia is rarely needed, except in cases of extreme anxiety, mental retardation, or psychotic disorders, and poses the greatest risk to a woman undergoing pregnancy termination. Most terminations of pregnancy are performed with the use of a paracervical block, often in combination with a sedative.
   D. Laminaria, often composed of hygroscopic seaweed, are placed into the cervix to facilitate cervical dilation prior to the procedure. The laminaria take on liquid, which results in their expansion and gentle dilation of the cervix. Gradual dilation reduces the risk of cervical trauma and is safe for use in both first- and second-trimester terminations.
   E. Medical termination is associated with more bleeding than surgical termination. However, overall blood loss from both procedures is low.

158. **B. The presence of a single chorion means that the twins are monozygotic. Monozygotic twins may divide over a period of a couple of weeks, and the timing of division determines the degree of the split. A split during the first 3 days results in 2 amnions and 2 chorions, or diamniotic-dichorionic twins. If the split occurs between day 3 and 8, the split is less "complete" and a single chorion (placenta) results.**

  A. See explanation for B.
  C. A split between 8 and 13 days results in a monoamniotic pregnancy, with twins in a single, shared amniotic sac. Monoamniotic twins are at high-risk of acute cord accident and death.
  D, E. Beyond 13 days, twins cannot split entirely, resulting in conjoined twins. Seventy-five percent of conjoined twins are thoracopagus, facing each other and often sharing a sternum, diaphragm, upper abdominal wall, gastrointestinal tract, pericardium, and liver. Three-quarters of thoracopagus twins have a shared heart, which makes the prognosis for separation very poor.

159. **D. Choriocarcinoma is most commonly associated with elevated hCG. Occasionally, choriocarcinoma has been associated with elevated LDH.**

160. **E. Endodermal sinus tumor is most commonly associated with AFP. Occasionally it may be associated with increased LDH.**

161. **A, F. Dysgerminoma is associated with elevated LDH and CA-125. It is the most common malignant germ cell neoplasm. Teratomas are by far the most common germ cell neoplasm.**

162. **C. Granulosa cell tumors are sex-cord stromal tumors. While they are capable of synthesizing estrogen, testosterone, and other androgens, granulosa cell tumors most commonly synthesize estrogen.**

163. **B. Any vulvar lesion, particularly in a postmenopausal woman, that is not responsive to a short trial of topical steroids should be biopsied to evaluate for neoplastic lesions of the vulva.**

  A. It is inappropriate to increase the steroid dose without a diagnosis as you could be delaying the diagnosis of a malignant lesion.
  C. Wide local excision is the treatment for premalignant or malignant vulvar lesions. However, this diagnosis should first be made via biopsy.
  D, E. It is inappropriate to use laser or cryotherapy to ablate a vulvar lesion if malignancy has not been ruled out.

164. **C. The diagnosis of endometriosis is often made clinically as not every patient undergoes surgical treatment, during which time endometriosis implants, scarring, or endometriomas can be visualized.**

  A. While severity of symptoms does vary and the extent of disease does not necessarily correlate with a patient's symptoms, the incidence of endometriosis is estimated to be 10% to 15% of reproductive age women. This incidence is higher in with infertility.
  B. Endometriosis is the presence of endometrial tissue (i.e., implants) outside of the endometrial cavity. The can be found anywhere in the pelvis including the ovaries, pelvic peritoneum, uterus, and rectum.
  D. Endometriosis has been associated with infertility, but the mechanism is unclear. Potential mechanisms include tubal scarring and obstruction and distortion of pelvic architecture.
  E. Surgical therapy involves ablation of endometriosis implants. However, these can return. Definitive therapy involves total abdominal hysterectomy, bilateral salpingo-oophorectomy, ablation of implants, and lysis of adhesions. However, this is not an option for those desiring fertility. Medical options do exist but are generally only temporary solutions due to desire for fertility or long-term side effects. These include NSAIDs, OCPs, Danazol (an androgen derivative), and GnRH agonists such as leuprolide acetate (Lupron), which create a state of pseudomenopause.

165. **A. Endometrial polyps are generally benign lesions that can cause abnormal bleeding. In this thin woman without risk factors for endometrial cancer and with an identifiable lesion on ultrasound, the most likely diagnosis would be an endometrial polyp. Endometrial biopsy or hysteroscopy could be used for diagnostic purposes. Despite the likelihood of this being a polyp, postmenopausal bleeding must always be evaluated for possible endometrial cancer.**

B. See explanation for A.
C. Atrophy of the vagina and genital tissues can certainly lead to vaginal bleeding due to irritation and erosion, but these lesions are often visible on speculum exam.
D. Cervical cancer is not likely in this woman with a recently normal Pap smear as well as a normal appearing cervix.
E. Bleeding from hemorrhoids can sometimes be confused with vaginal bleeding. Thus, physical exam should include evaluation of the anus to rule out rectal bleeding, which is not noted in this patient.

166. D. Estrogen deficiency can lead to atrophic vaginitis, characterized by a thin, dry vaginal mucosa. Vaginal rugae are decreased and may be absent. Common symptoms include dyspareunia, vaginal itching, and dryness. Atrophic vaginitis is typically seen in post-menopausal women.

167. B, F. Yeast infections are caused by *Candida,* which appear as pseudohyphae on wet mount. Symptoms classically include vaginal and vulvar itching and cottage cheese-like discharge. All complaints of abnormal discharge should be investigated with a wet mount swab of the discharge in normal saline and KOH solutions.

168. C, E. *Trichomonas vaginalis* is characterized by copious, frothy, malodorous green-gray discharge and, on wet mount, motile, flagellated organisms, or trichomonads. *Trichomonas* is transmitted through sexual contact so any patient with the diagnosis should be screened for other sexually transmitted infections.

169. A, G. Clue cells, which are vaginal epithelial cells filled with coccobacilli that distort the epithelial cell's borders, strongly suggest infection with bacterial vaginosis. The causative organism is *Gardnerella vaginalis.* Typically the vaginal pH is greater than the normal pH of <4.5.

170. D. With presumed PID and no resolution of symptoms or signs after 48 hours of appropriate treatment, the patient is at risk for a tubo-ovarian abscess (TOA). This is best diagnosed by pelvic ultrasound. Furthermore, given the possible mass on her pelvic exam in the ED, pelvic ultrasound should probably have been performed on admission to rule out TOA. Figure 2-170 shows findings associated with chronic PID.

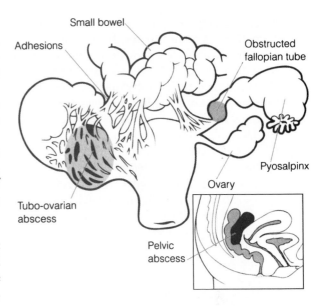

Figure 2-170 • Reproduced with Permission from Callahan TL, Caughey AB. Blueprints Obstetrics & Gynecology, 4th ed. Baltimore: Lippincott Williams & Wilkins, 2007. Fig. 17-2, p. 188.

A. Laparoscopy is used in some facilities to diagnose PID, and can also differentiate it from TOA. However, it is more invasive than beginning with an ultrasound, which is useful for characterization of TOAs.
B. If the patient has a TOA that does not respond to more aggressive antibiotics, she may require surgical treatment. Because she is a young woman, and surgical management often involves salpingo-oophorectomy, conservative management with antibiotics is usually first-line therapy.
C. Cultures from the cervix can be useful to fine tune antibiotic treatment. In this patient who is not responding to medical therapy, broadening treatment is likely to be more effective than waiting for culture results.
E. While broadening coverage may be necessary, ampicillin and gentamicin would need to be given with clindamycin for coverage of chlamydia and anaerobic organisms.

171. B. First trimester ultrasound utilizing mean sac diameter or crown-rump length is the most consistent way to date a pregnancy. In general, first trimester ultrasound is considered to be within 4 to 7 days of accurate dating. Thus, if the dating by LMP is off by a week or more in the first trimester, dating should be recalculated based upon the ultrasound.

A. LMP can be quite accurate, particularly in a patient with a certain LMP and regular menstrual cycles. However, this form of dating needs to be substantiated by ultrasound because irregular menses, poor documentation of the LMP, and ovulation other than on day 14 of the cycle can lead to poor dating.

C. Second-trimester ultrasound uses biometry of the biparietal diameter, head circumference, abdominal circumference, and femur length to help determine dating. Generally, this form of dating is felt to be within 7 to 14 days.

D. The third-trimester ultrasound is a notoriously inaccurate form of dating. Estimates of the due date or estimated date of confinement (EDC) can be off by as much as three weeks.

E. While β-hCG values have been used to determine whether a pregnancy is normal, they are not well associated with exact dating of GA.

172. B. This patient presents most likely with incompetent cervix, which is silent, painless dilation of the cervix without contractions, usually occurring in the mid- to late second trimester. Unfortunately, most diagnoses of incompetent cervix are made when it is too late to intervene to benefit the current pregnancy. Future management is to place a prophylactic cerclage between 12 and 14 weeks of gestation. In this pregnancy, because her cervix is still of reasonable length and only 1 cm dilated, a rescue cerclage can be placed. Because there are no randomized controlled trials for rescue cerclages, which have been associated with infection and rupture of the membranes, expectant management and bedrest is also a reasonable alternative.

A. While bacterial vaginosis (BV) is associated with preterm delivery, this patient does not have BV.

C. There is no particular association between chromosomal abnormalities and incompetent cervix. Furthermore, clinically, this patient is likely at higher risk of complications from amniocentesis than an uncomplicated patient. Thus it would be a poor idea to perform amniocentesis at this time.

D. This patient has had no contractions, making tocolysis unnecessary at this time.

E. Betamethasone and dexamethasone (corticosteroids) have been shown to decrease rates of respiratory distress syndrome in neonates when given between 24 and 34 weeks of gestation. At this GA, the fetus is previable. Thus, it is of little use to give antenatal corticosteroids at this point.

173. B. Atrophic vaginitis may be treated with estrogen cream or oral estrogen replacement therapy. If hormonal therapy is contraindicated, patients may use alternatives such as vaginal lubricants to alleviate symptoms.

174. C. *Candida* is treated with antifungal agents such as miconazole, butoconazole, and terconazole. These agents are topical and applied in a cream or a suppository. Oral agents, such as fluconazole, are available and provide the option of one-time dosing.

175. A. *Trichomonas vaginalis* is treated most effectively with metronidazole. Both the patient and her partner should be treated, and should be advised to avoid alcohol during treatment because of a disulfuram-like reaction.

176. A, D. Bacterial vaginosis may be treated with either metronidazole or clindamycin. Oral preparations and vaginal creams are available.

177. B. Forty percent of infertility is related to male factors, another 40% due to female factors, and in the remaining 20% the cause is unknown. Male factor infertility is related to the quantity and quality of the spermatozoa in the semen. Problems include decreased production, abnormal morphologic types, and decreased motility. Female factor infertility can include poor or absent ovulation, scarring or blockage of the fallopian tubes, or problems with the intrauterine environment and implantation.

A, B, C, D. See explanation for E.

178. A. Endometrial development is dependent on appropriate estrogen production in response to FSH during the follicular phase of the menstrual cycle. Thus, while many patients with a disruption in the hormonal axis will have anovulation, even those who do ovulate can have infertility secondary to lack of implantation.

B. Tubal dilation does not change in response to hormone levels throughout the menstrual cycle and occlusion is related to prior scarring of the tubes.

C. Cervical dilation also does not change and stenosis is usually related to prior cervical procedures (e.g., LEEP).

D. Basal body temperature is a marker of ovulation, not a cause of dysfunction.

E. Uterine growth is not related to the hypothalamic-pituitary-ovarian axis.

179. **H.** The carrier frequency for sickle cell disease among black populations is approximately 1 in 10, making it the most common hemoglobinopathy of clinical significance in the United States. Sickle cell disease is autosomal recessive and is caused by a mutation in the beta-globin gene. Affected individual's experience "sickling" of hemoglobin in situations of decreased oxygenation, leading to hemolysis and anemia with painful vasoocclusive crises.

180. **F.** The carrier frequency for Tay-Sachs disease among the Ashkenazi Jewish population is approximately 1 in 30. Tay-Sachs is a devastating, progressive, autosomal recessive neurodegenerative lysosomal storage disease that leads to death in the first decade.

181. **J.** Trisomy 21, or Down syndrome, is the most common autosomal disorder seen at birth, with an incidence of 1 in 800 liveborns. Other autosomal disorders may be more common *in utero* but do not survive as often as those with Down syndrome. All affected individuals have mental retardation, although the degree ranges widely and is impossible to predict prenatally.

182. **G.** β-thalassemia is seen much more commonly among Mediterranean populations, where the carrier frequency is 1 in 25.

183. **B.** Barbiturates are safe during pregnancy and will increase the patient's chances of being able to tolerate the period of acute alcohol withdrawal. She will need other support systems to maintain her sobriety.

A. Benzodiazepines are potentially teratogenic and should be avoided during pregnancy.

C. The developing fetus is at high risk of toxic injury early in pregnancy during embryogenesis. The cumulative effect is very important, and the sooner the patient quits drinking, the better her chances of having a good outcome.

D. The primary goal is to help your patient stop drinking. Treatment of her acute withdrawal symptoms may be necessary in order to achieve that goal.

E. Fetal effects from alcohol exposure are cumulative, and thus the patient should be encouraged to quit drinking for her health and that of the fetus.

184. **D.** Of all women trying to get pregnant, 80% to 85% will conceive in 1 year and 90% will conceive within 18 months. Once a woman has tried to conceive for 1 year and has failed, she is considered to have infertility and deserves a thorough work-up.

A, B, C, E. See explanation for D.

185. **B, C, H, J.** The goal of GBS prophylaxis is to reduce neonatal GBS sepsis. In August 2002, the Centers for Disease Control and Prevention revised its screening and treatment guidelines, and recommended culture-based screening of all pregnant women between 35 and 37 weeks of pregnancy, and those at risk for preterm delivery. Patients should be treated in labor if they screen positive. Also treated are those with preterm PROM, threatened preterm delivery, and those with a history of an infected neonate. Penicillin is the recommended treatment for GBS prophylaxis, with ampicillin recommended as an alternative. Because of the high incidence of strains resistant to clindamycin and erythromycin, and GBS sensitivity to penicillin and ampicillin, patients with a history of penicillin allergy should be questioned regarding the nature of their allergy. Those not at high risk for anaphylaxis should be treated with cephazolin. GBS sensitivity testing to clindamycin and erythromycin should be obtained among patients at high risk for anaphylaxis; if GBS is sensitive, these drugs may be used. If it is resistant, vancomycin should be used.

186. **A, B.** Metronidazole or clindamycin are used to treat bacterial vaginosis (BV) during pregnancy. Each one is about 85% to 90% effective at treating BV. Concerns, which are not supported by data, have been raised about the use of metronidazole during pregnancy.

187. G. Zidovudine is recommended during pregnancy to reduce neonatal transmission of HIV. Studies have shown that when patients and neonates were treated with zidovudine, transmission of HIV was 8% compared to 25% among those given a placebo. Today, highly active antiretroviral therapy (HAART) can further decrease transmission to 0% to 2% among compliant patients with responsive viral strains. Patients with AIDS should receive prophylaxis against *Pneumocystis carinii* with trimethoprim/sulfamethoxazole regardless of pregnancy if CD4 counts are <200/ml, and mycoplasma prophylaxis with azithromycin for CD4 counts <50/ml.

188. F. *Varicella* infection is concerning during pregnancy, and in any adult, because of the risk of *varicella* pneumonia, which confers a significant risk of death. Acyclovir is the treatment of choice for *varicella*.

189. D. A low forceps delivery is defined as at least +2 station, meaning that the fetal skull is at least 2 cm below the ischial spines. Outlet forceps is when the fetal scalp is visible without separating the labia. A mid-forceps is when the head is between 0 and +2 station and engaged. Anything above a mid-forceps is a high forceps, which are no longer practiced in the United States because of association with fetal injury. Position of the fetal head does not need to be direct OAP in order to perform a forceps-assisted delivery. However, knowing the position of the fetus is essential to proper placement of the forceps in order to minimize fetal and maternal injury.

A. Adequate anesthesia is essential for operative vaginal delivery and is usually in the form of an epidural, but it can also be a pudendal or rarely a spinal.
B. See explanation for D.
C. Because operative vaginal delivery is a risk factor for shoulder dystocia, operative vaginal delivery should not be undertaken, or should only be done with extreme caution, on a fetus that is estimated to be macrosomic.
E. An obstetrician who is familiar with the indications and limitations of the use of obstetric forceps is essential for a safe operative vaginal delivery. Since the advent of the vacuum extractor, increasingly fewer obstetricians are trained in the use of forceps.

190. B. While variable decelerations and even prolonged decelerations are a relatively common phenomenon during labor, the sudden change of the fetal station from +2 to impalpable and high is abnormal and highly concerning. In this setting of a patient undergoing a trial of labor having had a prior cesarean delivery, the most likely diagnosis is a uterine rupture. Other common signs and symptoms associated with uterine rupture include a maternal "popping" sensation in the abdomen, extreme abdominal pain, palpation of fetal parts outside of the uterus, gush of vaginal bleeding, and maternal hypotension secondary to intra-abdominal bleeding. Even with the FHR improving, a rapid cesarean delivery is indicated.

A. This would be a reasonable next step if the fetal head was palpable.
C. Forceps cannot be used with a fetal head this high or a cervix that is not fully dilated.
D. Expectant management would be reasonable if uterine rupture was not suspected. If the head were still at +2 station and there were no recurrences of the prolonged decelerations, the patient would hopefully be completely dilated soon and could be delivered vaginally.
E. As with expectant management, if you did not suspect uterine rupture, you would restart the pitocin about 20 to 30 minutes after the prolonged deceleration.

191. E. The FHR tracing demonstrates repetitive late decelerations, suggestive of uteroplacental insufficiency and possibly fetal hypoxia. Late decelerations are seen in association with contractions with the nadir following the peak of the contraction. They are characterized by a gradual decrease of the FHR prior to return to baseline, with an onset-to-nadir interval lasting ≥30 seconds.

A. Similar to late decelerations, early decelerations are characterized by a gradual decrease and return to baseline of the FHR as well as an onset-to-nadir interval of ≥30 seconds. The two types of decelerations are distinguished by the timing, with the nadir of the early deceleration occurring *with* the peak of the contractions as opposed to *following* the contractions, as seen with late decelerations. Early decelerations represent compression of the fetal head and are not concerning.

B, C. Variable decelerations represent umbilical cord compression and are characterized by an abrupt decrease in the FHR. Unlike late and early decelerations, the onset to nadir of variable decelerations occurs in <30 seconds. The FHR slows more than 15 beats/minute below the baseline, and the deceleration lasts between 15 seconds to <2 minutes from onset to return to baseline. Variable decelerations may be seen with transient umbilical cord compression, which occurs more frequently with oligohydramnios.

D. Fetal bradycardia describes a FHR baseline of <110 beats/minutes lasting 2 minutes or more, which is not seen in the FHR tracing shown. Fetal tachycardia refers to a baseline FHR of >160 beats/minute.

192. **A. The pattern shown is consistent with a fetal bradycardia. The FHR had been in the 150s, and is well-recorded as it falls to 80. A fetal bradycardia is defined by a FHR of <110 beats per minute lasting for more than 2 minutes. This pattern is worrisome and should prompt an emergent delivery by cesarean section to prevent fetal asphyxia if it doesn't resolve within several minutes more.**

B. The maternal pulse is also 80 and is sometimes confused with the FHR. However, in this case, the descent of the FHR is well-recorded. When the fetus moves, the electrode recording the FHR reverts to the nearest signal, which may be the maternal pulse. One generally one sees an abrupt change in the recorded heart rate as the electrode records the fetal and then the maternal heart rate, as opposed to the gradual, continuously recorded tracing shown.

C. Fetal movement may disrupt the signal from the electrode, resulting in loss of information, which does not appear to be the case here.

D. Head compression patterns, whether seen during the second stage of labor or any other time, involve decelerations which last more than 30 seconds from onset to nadir, return to baseline, and coincide with contractions. The pattern shown demonstrates a terminal bradycardia.

E. Variable decelerations are characterized by an abrupt drop in the FHR. The time of onset to nadir occurs within 30 seconds, with return to baseline within 2 minutes. While the drop in the FHR shown is abrupt, it lasts for more than 2 minutes and represents a fetal bradycardia

rather than a variable deceleration. The persistence of this pattern suggests fetal asphyxia rather than transient cord compression.

193. **E. Sex chromosome abnormalities like Turner syndrome are generally sporadic. The risk of recurrence is not increased from that of the general population.**

A, D. Turner syndrome occurs in approximately 1 in 4000 female live births. Because the syndrome occurs sporadically, this is the patient's risk of recurrence.

B. Autosomal recessive conditions carry a 25% risk of producing an affected individual when both partners carry the recessive trait. Cystic fibrosis is an example of such a condition.

C. Autosomal dominant conditions confer a 50% risk of producing an affected offspring when one partner has the disease. If both partners are affected, they risk producing a fetus with a double-dominant mutation, which is often lethal. Therefore, the risk that a survivor is affected with the disease is approximately two-thirds, or 66%.

194. **D. The natural fecundability rate, or chance of pregnancy per cycle attempted, is 20%. It is important to educate patients about this rate, as well as give them information about the optimal time of conception, preconceptional use of folic acid, and screen for rubella immunity. Nonimmune women should be vaccinated. Because of decreased fertility after the age of 35, such women should be instructed to return for evaluation after 6 months of unsuccessful timed intercourse, as opposed to 1 year for women under the age of 35.**

A. Approximately 10% of couples have infertility that is attributed to multiple etiologies. In approximately 10% of patients with infertility, the cause is not identifiable or unexplained. Among all couples, infertility is unexplained in approximately 1%. About half of couples in this group may achieve pregnancy naturally.

B, C. Both smoking and caffeine may slightly decrease fertility, which should be explained to the patient.

E. Male factors account for approximately 40% of the causes of infertility. Male factor infertility may be caused by abnormal anatomy, infection, or chromosomal problems leading to decreased number or function of sperm.

195. C. Endometriosis is diagnosed by laparoscopy through direct visualization and biopsy of the affected areas.

A, B, E. OCPs, GnRH-agonists, and rarely danazol are used to suppress estrogen levels, causing necrosis and eventual resorption of endometriosis implants. While they may be relatively effective long- or short-term treatments, they are not used to make the diagnosis of endometriosis.

D. With the widespread availability of minimally invasive surgery such as laparoscopy, laparotomy is not the procedure of choice to diagnose endometriosis.

196. D. The finding depicted in the image is the "double-bubble" sign seen with duodenal atresia which, when associated with chromosomal anomalies, is seen most frequently with trisomy 21, or Down syndrome. Approximately 12% of fetuses with Down syndrome also have gastrointestinal anomalies. A fluid-filled stomach is normally visualized as hypoechoic. The atretic duodenum causes fluid to fill the duodenum proximally, resulting in the second "bubble." Other anomalies are frequently found in individuals with Down syndrome, the most common of which are cardiac, seen in approximately 40% of cases.

A. Gastrointestinal anomalies are not commonly seen with Turner syndrome. Rather, short stature and defective ovarian development are commonly found. Eighty percent have congenital lymphedema, which may be seen in utero or at any age.

B. Individuals with trisomy 13 are affected by multiple anomalies, and 82% die within the first year of life. The most common anomalies seen are cardiac defects (80%) and cleft lip (60% to 80%).

C. Individuals with trisomy 18 are affected by severe mental retardation, and only 5% to 10% survive the first year. Affected individuals generally have multiple anomalies. Characteristics seen in more than half of affected individuals include cardiac defects, polyhydramnios, single umbilical artery, growth restriction, clenched hands, and cryptorchidism (among males).

E. Trisomy 16 is a lethal chromosomal malformation and affected fetuses do not survive to birth.

197. A. Omphalocele is characterized by a central defect in the anterior abdominal wall. Skin, muscles, and fascia are missing, and the peritoneum and amnion create a membranous covering of the herniated organs, which are primarily bowel. The umbilical cord inserts into the membrane. Omphalocele is associated with chromosomal abnormalities and syndromes, of which Beckwith-Wiedemann syndrome is more frequently seen. Because of the increased possibility of a chromosomal abnormality, amniocentesis is offered when an omphalocele is identified by ultrasound.

B. Gastroschisis, rather than omphalocele, is a ventral wall defect involving herniation of the abdominal contents lateral to the umbilical ring, as opposed to the central defect found with omphalocele. With gastroschisis, the umbilical cord inserts normally into the abdominal wall and the herniation nearly always occurs on the right side.

C. Gastroschisis is often an isolated anomaly, with an increased incidence found among younger women and smokers. The incidence of chromosomal anomalies and syndromes is not increased with gastroschisis.

D. Repair of omphaloceles is accomplished through surgical closure. Primary closure is preferred; for larger omphaloceles, a staged reduction using a silo is preferred.

E. The mode of delivery for omphalocele and gastroschisis has been a source of controversy for many years. With the possible exception of very large (>5 cm) omphaloceles, cesarean delivery does not appear to provide additional benefit when compared to vaginal delivery, and the mode of delivery should be determined by the usual obstetric indications.

198. B. The patient described has primary amenorrhea due to a Müllerian anomaly, which accounts for 20% of cases of primary amenorrhea. Gonadal failure is the most common cause of primary amenorrhea, constituting about 33% of cases. Renal anomalies are seen in approximately 40% of females with Müllerian agenesis, and therefore an IVP is indicated. Mayer-Rokitansky-Kuster-Hauser syndrome is an example of uterovaginal agenesis.

A. A karyotype would be indicated if the patient's serum testosterone levels were in the male range, suggesting a diagnosis of testicular feminization or androgen insensitivity syndrome. Such patients may also have a blind-ending vagina, and often absence of pubic and axillary hair. Affected individuals are phenotypically female, with an XY karyotype.

C, D, E. TSH, FH, and LH are not indicated and would not change management.

199. **E. Hypoactive sexual desire is the most common complaint related to sexual dysfunction seen today. Lack of desire often results from anger, resentment, or dissatisfaction with the partner, although it can also result from other problems with any of the stages of sexual response such as lack of arousal or lack of orgasm. Patients are often hesitant to discuss sexual dysfunction and do not generally raise such problems, highlighting the need to include this topic, when appropriate, while taking a medical history.**

A. Three phases of sexual response are sometimes used to assess dysfunction and include desire, arousal, and orgasm. Disorders in any of the phases can create sexual dysfunction, and a careful, sensitive history should be taken.

B. Decreased lubrication is not an uncommon complaint, often related to diminished foreplay, or hormonal changes such as the hypoestrogenic state caused by lactation or menopause. This complaint can be addressed by recommending increased foreplay or a lubricant.

C. Vaginismus involves the involuntary contraction of the lower third of the vagina, resulting in painful, difficult, or impossible intercourse. The sexual response, including desire and orgasm, is intact.

D. Medical illness may result in sexual dysfunction and should be ruled out.

200. **D. The patient's intermittent, worsening pain in the setting of a large ovarian cyst is highly concerning for ovarian torsion. A large ovarian cyst can predispose to torsion and eventual ovarian ischemia. Suspected ovarian torsion merits a diagnostic laparoscopy.**

A. A ruptured ovarian cyst may cause significant pain at the time of rupture. Often, free fluid is visible in the posterior cul de sac on ultrasound, representing cyst fluid or blood due to the rupture. In this case, the patient has pain in the setting of a large ovarian cyst, and rupture is unlikely to be the source of her pain.

B, C. Chlamydial cervicitis and PID may cause vaginal and pelvic pain, and are certainly possibilities in anyone who is sexually active. However, the patient's cervix is nontender and she is afebrile, suggesting a noninfectious cause of her pain.

E. A large ovarian cyst can certainly cause pain through distension of the capsule. However, such pain tends to be nonacute, which is inconsistent with the patient's symptoms.

Section

3 Pediatrics

BLOCK 1

1. An 8-year-old girl is brought in to the hospital while actively seizing. She has been hospitalized many times before for status epilepticus. She is receiving valproic acid at home to control the seizures. The first step in the management of this patient is to:

   A. Administer 20 mL/kg 0.9% normal saline
   B. Establish secure intravenous access and administer an anticonvulsant
   C. Administer activated charcoal via NG tube
   D. Stabilize airway and provide 100% oxygen
   E. Perform gastric lavage

2. An 8-year-old, 40-kg child presents with a history of vomiting for 3 days. There is no fever or diarrhea. Her mother reports bedwetting and increased fluid consumption for the same period. Her vital signs are as follows: HR 140, RR 35, and BP 94/60. Available laboratory data include Na 114 mEq/L, K^+ 4.0 mEq/L, Cl 95 mEq/L, HCO_3^- less than 5 mEq/L, serum glucose 1200 mg/dL, BUN 45, and creatinine 1.6 mg/dL. The most likely cause for these electrolyte abnormalities is:

   A. Syndrome of inappropriate antidiuretic hormone (SIADH)
   B. Renal salt wasting
   C. Acute tubular necrosis
   D. Diabetic ketoacidosis (DKA)
   E. Hemolytic-uremic syndrome (HUS)

3. A 1-year-old child presents with severe, watery diarrhea for the last 4 days. You suspect rotaviral diarrhea. His eyes are sunken, the pulse is 190 beats/minute, and his extremities are cool. His weight on admission is 10 kg. His serum sodium is 175 mEq/L. Assuming body water is 60% of the total body weight and his normal serum sodium is 140 mEq/L, which of the following is closest to this child's calculated free water deficit?

   A. 500 mL
   B. 750 mL
   C. 1000 mL
   D. 1500 mL
   E. 2000 mL

4. A mother is concerned that her baby might be sharing a room in the hospital with an infant who has RSV. She is asking for a private room. To reassure her, you counsel her that the most important measure that can be taken to prevent the spread of RSV disease in a hospitalized patient is:

   A. Wearing a mask in the room of an infected patient
   B. Wearing a paper gown when entering the room of an infected patient
   C. Keeping the patient in respiratory isolation for the first 24 hours on appropriate antibiotics
   D. Testing all children with respiratory illnesses for RSV during the winter respiratory viral season
   E. Hand washing

5. You are seeing a 4-month-old (Figure 3-5) for a well-child checkup. The child has been gaining weight well and has some mild motor developmental delays. His head circumference plots out at the 95th percentile, his weight plots at the 10th percentile, but his height is well below the 5th percentile. He is accompanied by his mother,

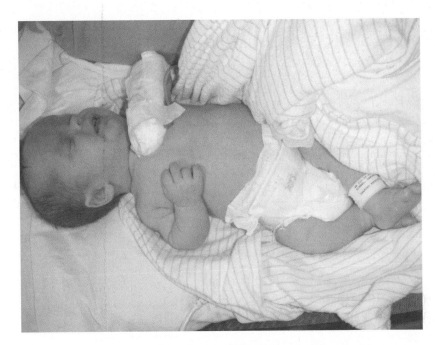

Figure 3-5 • Image Courtesy of the Phoenix Children's Hospital, Phoenix, Arizona.

who is affected with the same condition, and his father who appears unaffected. She is known to have vertebral problems and has had a shunt placed for hydrocephalus. Which of the following best accounts for this condition's inheritance pattern?

A. Autosomal recessive mutation
B. Autosomal dominant mutation
C. X-linked recessive mutation
D. Random mutation
E. X-linked dominant mutation

6. A 3-year-old child is being seen in your clinic for follow-up of hepatitis A. The mother is concerned about the 1-year-old brother becoming ill. The diagnosis was made in the 3-year-old 5 days ago. The correct management for postexposure prophylaxis in the child's brother is:

A. Hepatitis A vaccine only
B. Immunoglobulin only
C. Both hepatitis A vaccine and immunoglobulin
D. Observation only
E. Serologic testing for hepatitis A

7. A 1-year-old child is being seen with a history of nausea, vomiting, and severe abdominal pain. There is no history of fever or rash. The mother reports no history of trauma. The physical exami-

nation is pertinent for significant, diffuse abdominal pain to palpation with no rebound tenderness. The laboratory evaluation is significant for an amylase of 1400 U/L and a lipase of 3000 U/L. What is the most likely etiology of this patient's disease?

A. Gallstones
B. Trauma
C. Annular pancreas
D. Coxsackie B virus
E. Cystic fibrosis

8. A 6-month-old, previously normal infant is brought in because he seems to be having trouble feeding. He has not had a bowel movement in 4 days, and his eyes have started drooping in the last 24 hours. He is afebrile with a normal heart rate and respiratory rate. Although his lungs are clear, his oxygen saturations are in the 80s. However, there are no retractions or other signs of increased work of breathing. His precordium is not hyperdynamic and he has no murmur; pulses are normal in all four extremities. The liver and spleen are not enlarged. Neurologic examination is significant for severe hypotonia and ptosis. When supplemental oxygen is given in the office, his saturations increase into the high 90s. Additional testing reveals absent DTRs. Which of the following is the most likely diagnosis?

A. Ventricular septal defect (VSD)
B. Infant botulism
C. Tetralogy of Fallot
D. RSV bronchiolitis
E. Lyme disease

9. A 6-month-old infant was delivered at 33 weeks gestation. The neonatal course was complicated by grade II intraventricular hemorrhage on the left and initial slow feeding. The baby required ventilation for 3 days and was weaned off of oxygen after 10 days. The baby has been growing well but is noted to have weakness on the right side and increased DTRs in the right lower extremity. You suspect cerebral palsy. The correct diagnosis in this case is:

A. Diplegia
B. Hemiplegia
C. Extrapyramidal cerebral palsy
D. Quadriplegia
E. Dystonic cerebral palsy

10. A 2-week-old infant is admitted with a history of troubled breathing. The parents report that this child has had a stuffy nose since birth. Since their discharge home after delivery, they report that their child is congested. He struggles to breathe and can eat only 1 oz of his bottle at a time. The parents have been taking turns getting up to feed him every hour. You attempt to suction the nares and find that the catheter cannot be advanced. The most likely diagnosis is:

A. Nasal polyps
B. Fractured nasal cartilage
C. Choanal stenosis
D. Snuffles
E. Nasal encephalocoele

11. A 10-year-old boy is struck by a car while riding through an intersection on his bicycle. The boy was not wearing a helmet at the time of the accident. Initial evaluation finds him unconscious and unresponsive, although he is breathing and has a palpable pulse. After his arrival at the hospital, the diagnosis of closed head injury is made. Which of the following is a true statement about this situation?

A. Females are just as likely as males to sustain serious head injury
B. This child has more than a 90% chance of having a seizure
C. Brain hemorrhage is more likely to be intraparenchymal when it occurs after head trauma

D. This child is likely to have amnesia for the accident
E. Prolonged coma in these patients is predictive of motor, but not cognitive, deficits

The next two questions (items 12 and 13) correspond to the following vignette.

You are seeing a 1-month-old infant in your office. The birth history reveals that the mother is HIV positive. The child has been doing well and tolerating AZT. The physical examination is unremarkable except for some mild thrush.

12. Which laboratory test would help rule out infection in this infant?

A. HIV DNA qualitative PCR
B. HIV RNA quantitative PCR
C. HIV ELISA/Western blot
D. HIV viral load
E. HIV culture

13. The most common side effect of AZT treatment to be expected in this patient is

A. Myopathy
B. Pancreatitis
C. Anemia
D. Diarrhea
E. Rash

End of Set

14. A 3-week-old infant is hospitalized with fever, poor feeding, and fussiness for the last 2 days. The fever increased to 102°F on the day of admission. Maternal history is unremarkable and the delivery was uneventful. The mother is breastfeeding. Her diet is unremarkable, although she does use an unprocessed cheese that she procures at a local market. On examination, the infant is fussy with a full fontanelle. The lungs are clear and there is no skin rash. CSF examination shows 350 WBCs, 2 RBCs, and the Gram stain is positive for white cells and a few Gram-positive rods. The most likely organism causing meningitis in this infant is:

A. *Escherichia coli (E. coli)*
B. *Haemophilus influenzae*
C. *Staphylococcus aureus*
D. *Listeria monocytogenes*
E. *Clostridium perfringens*

15. A 19-year-old female you have followed for 6 years in your practice has recently married. She and her 22-year-old husband are planning to start a pregnancy. You advise her to start taking a multivitamin with folic acid. This advice is important to help prevent:

    A. Prematurity
    B. Skull defects
    C. Chromosomal defects
    D. Neural tube defects
    E. Osteopenia

16. A 3-year-old boy is brought to your office with the complaint of persistent rhinorrhea for the past 6 weeks. Otherwise, the patient has been asymptomatic. On physical examination, you note that the patient is mouth breathing and has dark circles under the eyes. Examination of the nose reveals a watery discharge and edematous, boggy, bluish mucous membranes with no erythema. The most likely diagnosis is:

    A. Chronic upper respiratory infection
    B. Sinusitis
    C. Nasal foreign body
    D. Allergic rhinitis
    E. CSF leak

17. The mother of a 6-year-old boy with a history of multiple hospitalizations for reactive airway disease comes to your office. She is pregnant and wants to know what can be done to decrease the chances that her next child will have such severe asthma. The best advice for her is:

    A. There is no evidence that smoking during pregnancy can cause asthma in the baby
    B. If a baby gets many upper respiratory infections (URIs), he or she may actually have a lower risk of developing asthma
    C. Her baby should get palivizumab to prevent RSV bronchiolitis, a condition that can lead to reactive airway disease
    D. She should start feeding her baby meats and eggs at an early age to strengthen the immune system
    E. There really is nothing that she can do to prevent or lessen the severity of asthma

18. A 10-day-old baby presents to your office with a 1-day history of unilateral conjunctivitis. The upper and lower eyelids are mildly swollen, the sclera is inflamed and red, and there is a mucopurulent discharge. The baby is acting well and has no fever. The mother denies any sexually transmitted diseases (STDs) during pregnancy. In the delivery room, the baby received prophylactic erythromycin eye drops. The most likely cause of this child's problem is:

    A. Chemical conjunctivitis
    B. Gonococcal conjunctivitis
    C. Chlamydial conjunctivitis
    D. Allergic conjunctivitis
    E. Dacryostenosis

19. You are asked to consult on a 12-year-old male who has been admitted for the last 72 hours with profuse, watery diarrhea. Fluid management has become difficult because the patient is noted to be hypertensive despite massive amounts of diarrhea and marginal urine output. On physical examination, this child appears healthy but has multiple (14) light brown, pigmented lesions on the extremities, back, and trunk. The diagnosis that best explains these findings is:

    A. Severe anxiety and neurodermatitis related to hospitalization
    B. Adrenal carcinoma with associated catecholamine release
    C. Tachycardia and hypertension due to hyperthyroidism
    D. Renovascular hypertension secondary to neurofibromatosis
    E. Tuberous sclerosis with intrarenal and intracardiac tubercles

20. A 5-year-old girl is seen in the ED because of fever, sore throat, and respiratory distress that developed rapidly over the past 3 hours. She is drooling and holding her neck in a hyperextended position. She has mild inspiratory stridor but does not have a barky cough. Because of the family's religious beliefs, she has received no immunizations. This patient most likely has:

    A. Viral croup
    B. Spasmodic croup
    C. Epiglottitis
    D. Bacterial tracheitis
    E. Reactive airway disease (asthma)

21. A 3-month-old baby comes to your office for a routine visit. He is growing well and his weight is 5.5 kg (25th percentile for age). His diet consists exclusively of cow's milk formula with iron. His

mother wants to know if he is getting an adequate amount of formula. A baby this size should be taking approximately how many ounces of formula per day?

A. 11 oz
B. 15 oz
C. 20 oz
D. 28 oz
E. 40 oz

22. A 9-year-old boy comes to your office because of progressive, generalized, bilateral lower extremity weakness and ataxia. He has also been complaining of some diminished sensation in his fingers and toes. On physical examination, you cannot elicit DTRs in his legs, and there appears to be mild facial weakness. Aside from a URI about 10 days ago, he has been healthy. CSF shows elevated protein with minimal pleocytosis. What is the most likely diagnosis?

A. Viral meningitis
B. Tick paralysis
C. Enteroviral encephalitis
D. Guillain-Barré syndrome
E. Acute lymphoblastic leukemia

23. A 9-month-old infant who was previously healthy and gaining weight was recently discharged from the hospital. The hospitalization was the result of a bout of severe rotavirus diarrhea that required rehydration with IV fluids. Four days later, he is brought to your office because he continues to have loose stools after each feeding. He is now drinking his regular cow's milk–based formula well. On physical examination he appears to be happy and well hydrated. A repeat rotavirus test is negative. What is the most likely reason for the baby's continued loose stools?

A. Cow's milk protein allergy
B. Starvation diarrhea
C. Secondary lactose intolerance
D. Viral gastroenteritis
E. Cystic fibrosis

24. A 24-month-old child is brought to your office for evaluation of a nasal discharge that has been present for 4 days. The mother has been using a drugstore decongestant but there has been no improvement. Immediately on entering the examining room, you notice a foul odor. On physical examination, you discover a purulent unilateral nasal discharge. The most likely diagnosis is:

A. Viral URI
B. Allergic rhinitis
C. Sinusitis
D. Nasal foreign body
E. Nasal polyp

25. An obese, 12-year-old, African-American boy comes to your office because of a painful limp that has been present for 1 week. There is no history of trauma. The patient has had no fever or other signs of illness. Radiographs of the boy's hips are obtained (Figure 3-25). The most likely diagnosis is:

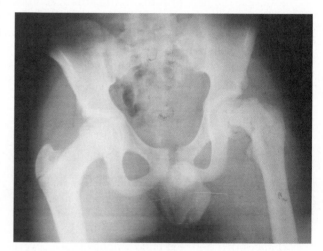

Figure 3-25 • Image Courtesy of the Department of Radiology, Phoenix Children's Hospital, Phoenix, Arizona.

A. Osteomyelitis
B. Legg-Calvé-Perthes disease
C. Septic hip
D. Slipped capital femoral epiphysis
E. Limp secondary to growing pains

26. A 15-month-old boy comes to your office because of bloody diarrhea that started today. The previous night he was seen in the local emergency room for management of a febrile seizure. The child had no previous history of convulsions. You collect a stool sample for microscopic examination and note that the stool contains many polymorphonuclear cells. Which organism is most likely responsible for this child's illness?

A. Group A *Streptococcus*
B. *Staphylococcus aureus*
C. *E. coli*
D. Shigella
E. Rotavirus

27. A 10-year-old boy is brought to your office because of intermittent, unexplained fevers over the past 18 months. His mother is especially concerned because she thinks her son has stopped growing. In fact, when you look at the boy's growth chart, you note no height increase since age 8 and his height percentile has fallen from the 25th percentile to well below the 5th percentile for his age. A CBC demonstrates very mild anemia, but the patient's erythrocyte sedimentation rate (ESR) is elevated. The urine pH is 5 and the serum bicarbonate is normal. The mother's height and father's height both fall at the 25th percentile of the adult range. What is the most likely diagnosis?

    A. Constitutional growth delay
    B. Familial short stature
    C. Inflammatory bowel disease (IBD)
    D. Renal tubular acidosis
    E. Pituitary tumor and growth hormone deficiency

28. An 18-month-old child is admitted to the hospital because of a 2-day history of fever and extreme irritability. The CSF analysis shows 2000 WBCs of which 90% are polymorphonuclear cells. The spinal fluid glucose is markedly depressed. The patient is started on cefotaxime and vancomycin. Eight hours after admission, the child has a generalized convulsion. What would be your next course of action?

    A. No additional diagnostic tests or treatment are needed
    B. Start aggressive antipyretic treatment to decrease the chance of febrile seizures
    C. Change antibiotics to provide a broader spectrum of coverage
    D. Order a set of electrolytes
    E. Order a computerized scan of the head to rule out a brain abscess

29. A mother brings her 2-month-old baby girl for a regular checkup. She says that a friend told her she should always put the baby to sleep on her belly to prevent choking, in case the baby spits up. With regard to infant sleeping position, how should you counsel the mother?

    A. Place baby on the belly (prone)
    B. Place baby on the side

C. Place baby on the back (supine)
D. Elevate head of infant's crib
E. Elevate foot of infant's crib

30. A 4-month-old boy comes to your office for a well-baby checkup. His mother expresses concern about his slow growth and poor motor development that she has noticed over the last month. There is no history of constipation. On physical examination, the baby appears to be hypotonic and weak. You are unable to elicit DTRs. There is visible atrophy and fasciculations of the tongue, but no ptosis or facial weakness. The most likely diagnosis is:

    A. Guillain-Barré syndrome
    B. Infant botulism
    C. Hypothyroidism
    D. Spinal muscular atrophy
    E. Myasthenia gravis

31. An 11-year-old male is brought in by his mother because he has recently developed acne. The mother is concerned because her brother developed numerous scars due to acne in his teenage years. She reports discovering that her son has recently been eating chocolate bars at lunch and drinking soda at night. Which of the following is true regarding the causes of acne breakouts?

    A. A diet high in greasy foods and chocolate will contribute to acne breakouts
    B. Scrubbing the skin and using an exfoliating skin cleanser will help prevent blackheads and acne breakouts
    C. A genetic factor is involved in how much trouble a teen will have with acne
    D. Sexual activity contributes to acne lesions
    E. The use of cosmetics and lubricating lotions and creams will aggravate acne

32. On one of your rare days off, you go to watch your niece's soccer team in the championship playoffs. While you are cheering her on, a 9-year-old suddenly collapses on the field during the soccer game. The child is not breathing and is pulseless. The best first response is:

    A. Open the airway and give two rescue breaths
    B. Call 911
    C. Do not use an automated external defibrillator (AED) because the child is only 9 years old
    D. Start chest compressions immediately
    E. Administer abdominal thrusts, as she may have aspirated her gum

33. A 5-month-old baby presents to the Urgent Care Center with a fever and history of a chronic, draining ear. You note a severe diaper rash, cradle cap, and a scaling, purpuric, papular rash appearing over the trunk on your thorough physical examination. Your diagnosis is:

    A. Otitis externa from the bath water
    B. Contact dermatitis from the laundry detergent
    C. Langerhans cell histiocytosis
    D. Atopic dermatitis
    E. Scabies

34. The parents of a 6-month-old Caucasian boy report that the child has been "turning blue" since birth. In the first few weeks of his life, they noted that his fingers and toes seemed bluish, although that condition has resolved. Now they notice that the skin around his mouth is blue, especially when he is outside in cool air. The child has been otherwise well, growing, gaining weight, and developing appropriately. Vital signs and physical examination are normal, with normal pulses in all extremities and no audible murmurs or abnormal cardiac sounds. What is the next step in evaluating this child?

    A. Echocardiogram
    B. Electrocardiogram
    C. Cardiology consult
    D. Reassurance only
    E. Chest radiograph

35. A 14-month-old boy is seen in your office because his mother is concerned about his bowlegs. He began walking at 10 months, and since then she has noticed that his gait is becoming worse. On examination, you find he does have significant leg bowing bilaterally, and x-rays reveal evidence of rickets. Regarding his diagnosis, which one of the following is true?

    A. Rickets of any kind is always associated with low serum calcium
    B. Alkaline phosphatase is high in all forms of rickets
    C. Parathyroid hormone is high in all forms of rickets
    D. This boy cannot have vitamin D–resistant rickets if his mother is normal
    E. Patients with vitamin D–deficiency rickets frequently have normal serum phosphorus

36. A child is found lying unconscious at the base of a tree. A ladder is observed to be propped up against the trunk of the tree. The child appears to be cyanotic and not breathing. The best first step to take is:

    A. Call 911 immediately
    B. Perform a head tilt and chin lift to open the airway and give two rescue breaths
    C. Start chest compressions
    D. Perform a tongue-jaw lift and blind finger sweep of the throat to remove an aspirated foreign body obstruction
    E. Perform a jaw thrust to open the airway and give two rescue breaths

37. You are evaluating a newborn infant on the postpartum floor. The mother had several prenatal visits 3 to 4 months ago, but was then lost to follow-up. At that time the mother was noted to have a positive RPR. The mother tells you she believes that she was treated with one injection of penicillin. There is no documentation of this treatment available in the chart. An RPR done at the time of delivery is 1:8. What is the first step in the further evaluation of this baby?

    A. Long bone films
    B. Spinal tap and CSF VDRL
    C. RPR on the baby
    D. CBC, platelet count, and liver function tests
    E. Initiating IM injections of penicillin

38. A 3-year-old boy was brought into the ED via EMS after his older sister found him floating in the pool. Early resuscitation was begun by the family and continued by the EMS team, en route to the children's hospital. After being placed on a mechanical ventilator and admitted to the ICU, the patient shows neurological improvement over the first 24 hours and is weaned off the ventilator. However, over the ensuing 48 hours the patient displays a slow but steady decline in his pulmonary function, becomes comatose, and dies despite renewed resuscitative efforts in the ICU. Which of the following is the best description for this patient's outcome?

    A. Drowning
    B. Near drowning
    C. Secondary drowning
    D. Immersion injury
    E. Water intoxication

39. A 6-year-old boy comes to your office for a well-child checkup. His mother tells you that she is concerned about his nightly bedwetting. The boy has never had a prolonged period of nighttime dryness, and he never has "accidents" while awake. He has no dysuria and his urinary stream is normal. What is the most common cause of primary nocturnal enuresis?

    A. UTI
    B. Vesicoureteral reflux
    C. Psychological problem
    D. Normal developmental variant
    E. Unstable bladder

40. You are seeing a 10-year-old boy for his well-child checkup and notice that he is hypertensive. He has otherwise been doing well. When looking back through his old chart, you realize that his previous blood pressures were normal. What would be your next course of action?

    A. Urinalysis
    B. Renal ultrasound
    C. 24-hour blood pressure monitoring
    D. Rechecking his blood pressure in 1 week
    E. Basic metabolic panel

41. While reviewing laboratory results in your office, you receive a message regarding an abnormal newborn screening test on one of your patients. The 6-day-old infant is reported to have an abnormal screening test for congenital hypothyroidism. The most likely etiology of this result is:

    A. Maternal Graves's disease treated with propylthiouracil
    B. Maternal antithyrotropin antibodies
    C. Iodine deficiency
    D. Ectopic or hypoplastic thyroid gland
    E. Newborn screen performed at 12 hours of age

42. A 7-month-old male is being seen in your office after being hospitalized with *Streptococcus pneumoniae* bacteremia and pneumonia. When looking through his chart, you notice that he has had multiple otitis media, and both his height and weight are at the 5th percentile. Which of the following is the most likely diagnosis?

    A. X-linked agammaglobulinemia
    B. Wiskott-Aldrich syndrome
    C. Chronic granulomatous disease
    D. Chediak-Higashi syndrome
    E. Leukocyte adhesion defect

43. A mother calls in to the office at 8 AM, concerned that her 2-month-old baby has been screaming for the last 2 hours. This is unusual for her baby and she feels this is a cry of pain. Nothing she has tried will comfort the baby. You request that she bring the baby in for an examination. After undressing the baby, you notice that her second toe is swollen. The most likely diagnosis is

    A. Hair entrapment
    B. Colic
    C. Osteomyelitis
    D. Fractured toe
    E. Scorpion sting

44. You are seeing a 2-week-old infant who appears jaundiced. He is growing well without any problems and is exclusively breastfed. His physical examination is notable only for some scleral icterus and jaundice to the upper chest. Your next course of action would be

    A. Abdominal ultrasound
    B. Fractionated bilirubin
    C. Observation with a follow-up appointment at 1 month
    D. Liver function tests
    E. Urine culture

45. A 5-year-old boy presents with a history of grossly bloody urine, puffy eyes, and headache for 1 day. He has been a well child, but he did have a fever and sore throat about 10 days ago, which resolved without treatment. The most likely diagnosis is:

    A. Acute cystitis
    B. IgA nephropathy
    C. Acute pyelonephritis
    D. Postinfectious glomerulonephritis
    E. Benign hematuria

46. A 2-month-old infant is admitted with constipation and an abdominal mass. Birth history was unremarkable. The infant was noted to have a patent rectum and passed meconium at 32 hours of life. The mother reports difficulties with constipation since birth and has tried multiple remedies without great success. The infant has had a fever for the last 2 days and has been very fussy and feeding poorly. He has vomited intermittently for the last 2 days. Abdominal films are consistent with marked dilatation of the proximal and distal colon with a partial bowel obstruction. A barium enema shows the findings in Figure 3-46. The most important next step in the care of this infant is:

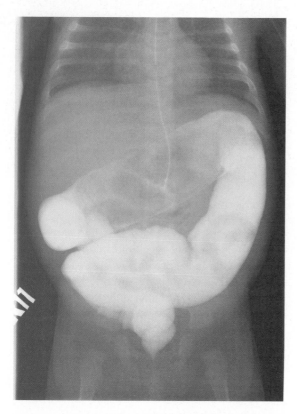

Figure 3-46 • Image Courtesy of the Department of Radiology, Phoenix Children's Hospital, Phoenix, Arizona.

A. Surgical consult for rectal biopsy
B. Fleet enema and Golytely drip
C. IV fluid rehydration and IV antibiotics
D. Colostomy
E. Manual decompression

47. A 3-month-old infant has developed increasing numbers of episodes that consist of his head turning to the right, staring, and stiffening of the extremities. There has been no history of fever or trauma and the child had been growing well. Because of the increasing numbers of these episodes, the child is now feeding poorly and has been hospitalized for further evaluation and consideration for nighttime drip feeds. An EEG demonstrates diffuse, high-voltage slow waves and multiple spike-and-wave discharges; consistent with hypsarrhythmia. This EEG is typically associated with the diagnosis of which of the following:

A. Petit mal seizures
B. Myoclonic seizures
C. Akinetic seizures
D. Pseudoseizures
E. Infantile spasms

The response options for items 48 to 50 are the same. You will be required to select one answer for each item in the set.

A. 2 months
B. 4 months
C. 6 months
D. 9 months
E. 12 months
F. 18 months
G. 24 months

For each patient described, select the most accurate developmental age.

48. A new Asian family to your clinic brings in an infant boy. On examination, you find he is able to lift his head off of the examination table while prone. He will fix on the otoscope light and track it from side to side as you hold it in front of him. When held by his dad, he will turn toward the voice and smile when the dad says his name.

49. While working in the ED, you examine a toddler for an earache. She can go up and down the two steps of the play slide in the waiting area by herself. She engages in parallel play with the other children in the waiting area. In the exam room, you hand her a book, and she can turn the pages one at a time. She is able to understand two-step commands during the examination.

50. During continuity clinic, you examine a child for a well-child checkup. She has mastered pulling to a stand and is just beginning to take her first steps alone. She enjoys picking things up with a mature pincer grasp and dropping them. She has just begun to use a couple words other than "mama" and "dada."

End of Set

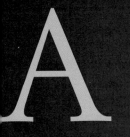

A Answers and Explanations

1. D	18. C	35. B
2. D	19. D	36. E
3. D	20. C	37. C
4. E	21. D	38. C
5. B	22. D	39. D
6. B	23. C	40. D
7. B	24. D	41. D
8. B	25. D	42. A
9. B	26. D	43. A
10. C	27. C	44. B
11. D	28. D	45. D
12. A	29. C	46. C
13. C	30. D	47. E
14. D	31. C	48. A
15. D	32. B	49. G
16. D	33. C	50. E
17. B	34. D	

1. D. The first step in the stabilization of ANY patient in acute distress is to evaluate and ensure a stable airway and provide 100% oxygen. The ABCs of stabilization stand for airway, breathing, and circulation, and must be attended to before any other aspect of patient management is addressed. Therefore, this child's airway must first be determined to be stable and secure, the adequacy of her breathing assessed, and her circulation evaluated by checking her heart rate, blood pressure, central and peripheral pulses, extremity color and temperature, and capillary refill. If these are all adequate, further management, such as securing IV access and administering an anticonvulsant, is then indicated.

A. Obtaining IV access and providing fluids is important in the emergency room or in the ICU, but would not supersede airway management. A fluid bolus would be helpful in a dehydrated patient.
B. IV access is important to establish once airway and pulses are assessed.
C. Activated charcoal is used for patients who have ingested toxic substances. The charcoal binds these substances and assists them to pass outside the body before being absorbed.
E. Gastric lavage is used for patients with an ingestion or gastrointestinal bleed.

2. D. The patient's serum glucose of 1200 mg/dL, significant metabolic acidosis with a bicarbonate of less than 5 mEq/L, and clinical history of polyuria (bedwetting) and polydipsia (fluid consumption) indicate DKA. The low serum sodium results from a factitious laboratory reporting of low sodium due to the high serum glucose (pseudohyponatremia), and as the serum glucose resolves, the reported serum sodium will normalize.

A. Hyponatremia is present in SIADH, but inappropriate ADH secretion would not explain the hyperglycemia and elevated BUN and creatinine. A history of oliguria is expected in patients with SIADH.
B. Renal salt wasting is a cause of hyponatremia and may, indeed, present with polyuria, but would not explain the hyperglycemia and elevated BUN and creatinine.
C. Acute tubular necrosis might result in an elevated BUN and creatinine, but would not be associated with significant hyperglycemia and the clinical history of polyuria and polydipsia.

E. HUS is the most common cause of acute renal failure in children and would present with elevated BUN and creatinine as well as oliguria. It commonly follows an episode of gastroenteritis with *E. coli* 0157:H7 as the offending pathogen. The diagnosis is confirmed by thrombocytopenia, acute renal failure, and a microangiopathic hemolytic anemia.

3. D. Rotavirus results in a significant loss of free water from stools. The total body sodium content will remain unchanged. The predehydration total body water can be determined from the equation: dehydrated sodium × dehydrated body water = normal serum sodium × normal body water. From this equation:

$$175 \text{ mEq/L} \times (60\% \times 10 \text{ kg}) = 140 \text{ mEq/L} \times \text{normal body water}$$
$$\text{Normal body water} = 175 \times 6 \text{ L}/140$$
$$\text{Normal body water} = 7.5 \text{ L}$$

His deficit is then Normal body water − dehydrated body water or

$$7.5 \text{ L} − 6 \text{ L} = 1.5 \text{ L or } 1500 \text{ mL.}$$

A, B, C, E. These are incorrect calculations. See explanation for D.

4. E. RSV is spread via contact with the droplets and secretions of an infected patient. Handwashing is the most effective preventive measure to decrease contact with viruses that spread via droplet contamination.

A. RSV is not aerosolized, so wearing a mask just to enter a room is not necessary unless close patient contact is anticipated.
B. Wearing a gown when entering the room of an RSV-infected patient is necessary only if close contact will occur.
C. RSV is a virus. Placing the patient on antibiotics would not be indicated.
D. Testing all children with respiratory illnesses for RSV may help to cohort patients in hospital rooms, but RSV may still spread throughout the hospital unless proper infection control techniques, such as good handwashing, are vigorously practiced.

5. B. The patient in this scenario has achondroplasia or classic dwarfism. It is inherited in an autosomal dominant fashion, in this case from the

mother. Patients with achondroplasia have short trunks and limbs, macrocephaly with frontal bossing, and often vertebral anomalies. They are sometimes prone to hydrocephalus secondary to an obstructed and small foramen magnum. During infancy they are often hypotonic and have mild motor delays that are regained by 2 to 3 years of age.

A, C, D, E. None of the other inheritance patterns listed is correct for achondroplasia.

6. **B. The use of immunoglobulin (Ig) within 2 weeks of hepatitis A exposure is more than 85% effective at preventing any symptomatic infection. It is recommended in all previously unimmunized people with close contact with the index case, defined as household and/or sexual contacts. Since this child is less than 2 years of age, only the Ig is indicated.**

A. In patients with a recent exposure (less than 2 weeks), rapid protection can occur with Ig injection. Hepatitis A vaccine alone will take longer to provide protection. In addition, hepatitis A vaccine is not indicated for children less than 2 years of age and would not be appropriate in this 1-year-old patient.

C. If the child were older than 2 years of age, the Ig as well as the hepatitis A vaccine would be recommended now, with a second dose of hepatitis A in 6 months.

D. Since preventive measures are available, observation alone would not be the best course.

E. Serologic testing of contact cases is not recommended and may delay the appropriate management as detailed in the explanation for B.

7. **B. Blunt abdominal trauma is a common cause of pancreatitis in younger children and infants. The absence of any report of trauma does not rule out child abuse as the underlying etiology. A strong suspicion for abuse must be considered in unexplained cases of pancreatitis in very young children.**

A. Although gallstones account for a large proportion of pancreatitis in adults, they are uncommon in the healthy infant or child unless there is an underlying history of hemolytic disease, liver disease, or TPN dependence with biliary sludge.

C. Annular pancreas is an uncommon etiology of pancreatitis. It occurs due to incomplete rotation of the ventral side of the pancreas, resulting in bowel obstruction. It can be associated with intestinal atresias and Down syndrome.

D. Although viral illnesses such as Coxsackie virus, Epstein-Barr virus, and cytomegalovirus are common causes of pancreatitis, there is no history of prodromal illness or fever in this case.

E. Cystic fibrosis is certainly a cause of pancreatitis, especially in children with gastrointestinal involvement. Those children tend to have a long history of failure to thrive and large, smelly stools and may have respiratory symptoms.

8. **B. Botulism in infants presents with progressive motor weakness, which is generally preceded by several days of constipation. It is caused by the ingestion of *Clostridium botulinum* spores. Exposure may result from ingestion of contaminated honey or airborne spores in dusty, windy areas. The difficulty feeding and ptosis in this patient are evidence of cranial nerve involvement. The absent DTRs are evidence of peripheral nerve involvement, which often presents as hypotonia. The hypoxia with clear lungs and lack of increased effort points to respiratory muscle weakness, a complication of botulism that may require intubation.**

A. A VSD may cause congestive heart failure and present with poor feeding. However, there is usually a murmur unless the defect is so large that LV and RV pressures are the same. In that situation, the patient's heart should be hyperdynamic.

C. Tetralogy of Fallot is a cyanotic heart disease that virtually always has a murmur from the pulmonic stenosis (PS). It typically includes VSD, PS, RV hypertrophy, and overriding aorta. Neither of these two heart defects, however, could explain this patient's neurologic findings.

D. RSV bronchiolitis that is severe enough to produce hypoxia presents with increased work of breathing and an abnormal auscultatory examination of the lungs.

E. Lyme disease can cause Bell's palsy, but does not cause generalized hypotonia.

F. Muscular dystrophy presents with skeletal muscle weakness, but it is more of a slowly progressive disorder.

9. **B. This child has spastic cerebral palsy. The involvement of one side with the upper extremity more involved than the lower is called hemiplegia. Treatment includes physical and occupational therapy.**

   A. Diplegia refers to bilateral lower extremity spasticity.

   C. Extrapyramidal cerebral palsy is characterized by movement abnormalities, such as ataxia, chorea, or dystonia.

   D. Quadriplegia refers to involvement of all the extremities, more prominent in the lower extremities.

   E. Dystonic cerebral palsy results in uncontrollable jerking, writhing, or posturing movements.

10. **C. Choanal stenosis is the most common cause of nasal obstruction in infants. Most often there is a bony and membranous septum between the nose and the pharynx. It may be associated with other congenital anomalies. The classic presentation of an infant with choanal stenosis is difficulty breathing at birth or shortly thereafter. Crying may relieve cyanosis or distress by allowing air passage through the mouth. Infants may breathe well through the mouth, but then have significant distress when feeding. Attempts to pass a catheter through the nostrils will be unsuccessful.**

    A. Nasal polyps are very rare in infants. They are much more common in older children or adolescents and may be associated with cystic fibrosis, allergic rhinitis, or chronic sinusitis.

    B. Fractured nasal cartilage is unusual in infants. It could occur as a result of a difficult delivery with a face presentation. More typical findings of a fractured nasal cartilage include swelling of the nose with misalignment of the nasal bridge.

    D. Snuffles is severe rhinorrhea and nasal stuffiness associated with congenital syphilis. Introduction of a nasal suction tube should not encounter resistance.

    E. A nasal encephalocele is brain tissue that extends into the nasal cavity. There might be a visible mass within the nose or extruding from the nose.

11. **D. Retrograde and/or anterograde amnesia is common in patients with concussion or closed head injury.**

    A. Males are much more likely to suffer from head trauma.

    B. The chance of developing a seizure is about 10% in children hospitalized after head trauma.

    C. Subdural and epidural hemorrhages are much more common than intraparenchymal hemorrhages.

    E. The risk of cognitive and motor deficits is increased in patients with prolonged coma.

12. **A. HIV DNA PCR is the correct answer. This is a qualitative test that detects the presence of viral DNA material within blood cells. It becomes more sensitive as the child's age increases from about 30% at 2 weeks to 90% at 1 month and 99% by 4 months. HIV infection can be excluded in an infant with two negative HIV DNA PCR assays, providing one result is at 1 month or older AND the second result is obtained at 4 months or older.**

    B. HIV RNA PCR is a quantitative test. In the presence of HIV infection, the result will yield the number of copies of virus/mL of blood. It is not a diagnostic test, and may report an undetectable level in the presence of well-controlled disease.

    C. HIV Elisa/Western blot is the standard HIV testing method. It relies on the detection of antibodies to HIV. Exposed infants will typically have a positive antibody test due to transplacental transfer of maternal antibody.

    D. The HIV viral load is the same as HIV RNA PCR.

    E. Isolation of HIV by culture is expensive, not readily available, and may require as many as 28 days for positive results. It has no current role in the management of perinatally HIV-exposed infants. HIV DNA PCR has virtually replaced this older form of testing.

13. **C. Anemia is the most common side effect of AZT, due to bone marrow suppression.**

    A. Myopathy is a less common side effect of AZT.

    B, D, E. Pancreatitis, diarrhea, and rash are much less common side affects in newborns receiving AZT, but are more common side effects of other HIV antiretrovirals.

14. **D.** *Listeria monocytogenes* is a Gram-positive rod that can cause neonatal meningitis. The most common bacteria involved in meningitis in neonates are group B *Streptococcus, E. coli, L. monocytogenes,* and *Klebsiella. Listeria* can be associated with contaminated dairy products, including some forms of contaminated unprocessed cheeses, such as Jalisco cheese.

   A. *E. coli* is a Gram-negative rod and is the most common cause of neonatal bacterial meningitis. The organism is usually acquired during passage through the maternal birth canal.
   B. *Hemophilus influenzae* is a Gram-negative rod that is an uncommon cause of meningitis in neonates. Most cases of *H. influenzae* occur in children over 5 months of age. *Hemophilus meningitis* is much less common now because of the HIB vaccine.
   C. *Staphylococcus aureus* is a Gram-positive coccus and is a less common cause of neonatal meningitis.
   E. *Clostridium perfringens* is a Gram-positive rod, but would be an unusual cause of neonatal meningitis.

15. **D.** Closure of the neural tube occurs very early in gestation, usually within the first 2 to 3 weeks of development. Defects in the formation and closure of the neural tube have been associated with folic acid deficiency. Abnormalities such as anencephaly, myelomeningocele, and spina bifida can result. These lesions are associated with persistent leaking of alpha-fetoprotein (AFP) into the amniotic fluid, so that measurement of maternal AFP levels is an effective screening test for neural tube defects. Initiation of good nutrition and folic acid supplementation before the onset of pregnancy has been shown to significantly decrease the incidence of these types of lesions.

   A. Although good nutrition is extremely important in maintaining a healthy pregnancy, folic acid supplementation does not decrease the number of premature births.
   B. Skull defects unrelated to neural tube closure are not prevented with folic acid use.
   C. Chromosomal defects can be associated with neural tube defects, but folic acid has not been shown to prevent other lesions.
   E. Osteopenia may be related to vitamin or mineral deficiencies, but is not related to folic acid.

16. **D.** This patient's examination is typical of allergic rhinitis. The allergic gape (continuous open-mouth breathing) and allergic shiners (dark circles under eyes) are classic findings. The watery discharge and nonerythematous mucous membranes are also typical. Many patients with allergic rhinitis will have conjunctival erythema and itching. Children with allergic rhinitis may have related sinusitis, otitis media, eczema, or asthma.

   A. The membranes in a patient with URI are usually inflamed and erythematous.
   B. In sinusitis, the nasal discharge is usually thick and purulent. The patient may also have fever, headache, and/or halitosis, which are not common in allergic rhinitis.
   C. A nasal foreign body usually causes a purulent, malodorous, or bloody nasal discharge from one nostril only. These children may also have a generalized body odor known as bromhidrosis.
   E. CSF otorrhea or rhinorrhea may occur with severe head injury and skull fracture. Although CSF leaks are an indication for hospitalization, they are rarely a neurosurgical emergency; the leak will usually resolve by 3 to 7 days.

17. **B.** Recurrent episodes of rhinitis (that are not associated with lower respiratory tract disease) have actually been shown to decrease the risk of developing asthma. Children who are exposed to many viruses because they are from large families or that attend day care at an early age have a much lower than average chance of becoming asthmatic. Exposure to livestock or a farm environment may also decrease the risk of developing asthma.

   A. Maternal smoking during pregnancy doubles or triples the chance of the baby developing reactive airway disease.
   C. Children who develop bronchiolitis from RSV have an increased chance of having future wheezing from airway hyperresponsiveness. Palivizumab, however, is usually used for premature infants with chronic lung disease. A positive family history of asthma is not an indication to use this very expensive medication.
   D. Feeding a baby meats and eggs before the age of 6 to 9 months can cause food allergy. Food allergy and eczema are highly correlated with the development of asthma and wheezing.
   E. Avoiding cigarette smoke (in utero and in the home) and delaying introduction of highly allergenic foods may decrease the risk of developing asthma.

18. **C. The most common cause of ophthalmia neonatorum is *Chlamydia trachomatis*. The onset is usually 5 to 12 days postpartum. The diagnosis is made with a *Chlamydia* antigen test or a culture. Although instillation of antibiotic eye drops will cure the conjunctivitis, many of these children will continue to carry the organism in their nasopharynx, which puts them at risk for developing pneumonia. For this reason, the eye infection (and nasopharygeal carriage) should be treated with oral erythromycin.**

A. Chemical conjunctivitis is most commonly caused by prophylactic silver nitrate instilled at the time of delivery. It usually resolves by 36 hours of age.

B. Gonococcal conjunctivitis typically presents 2 to 4 days after delivery. This child did not develop symptoms until 9 days of age.

D. Allergic conjunctivitis generally is not a problem in the newborn. The discharge tends to be watery more than purulent. Itching is common.

E. Dacryostenosis, a blocked tear duct, causes a watery discharge that often dries and forms a crust on the lower lid. The sclera is generally not inflamed. Tear duct massage may help, but the problem usually resolves spontaneously. Some children might need tear duct probing by an ophthalmologist if the problem does not resolve by 1 year of age.

19. **D. This child has multiple caféau lait macules consistent with the diagnosis of neurofibromatosis. The patient is hypertensive despite profuse diarrhea and dehydration related to an acute infectious process. This paradoxical finding can be explained by underlying renovascular hypertension, which is associated with neurofibromatosis. Patients with neurofibromatosis type I can have renal artery stenosis, resulting in hypertension.**

A. Patients who are hospitalized may be tachycardic or hypertensive due to anxiety or pain. In this case, the pigmented lesions are café au lait macules, seen in neurofibromatosis.

B. Adrenal carcinoma is extremely rare in children and would not explain the skin findings.

C. Hyperthyroidism could cause tachycardia and hypertension, but would not result in hyperpigmented lesions.

E. Tuberous sclerosis is associated with hypopigmented macules, not hyperpigmented macules.

20. **C. Epiglottitis is a potentially lethal condition in which a child may develop air hunger, restlessness, cyanosis, and coma in just hours. Typically, the patient will present with fever, sore throat, and drooling. The child often keeps the neck in a hyperextended position to keep the airway open. Patients with epiglottitis do not have the typical barky cough seen in viral croup. Stridor is a late finding and may not be present until the airway is nearly completely obstructed. Anxiety-provoking interventions should always be avoided in patients with epiglottitis. Phlebotomy, IV line placement, supine placement of the child, or direct visualization of the oral cavity should be delayed until the airway is secure. The classic finding on lateral neck radiographs is the "thumb sign." Patients suspected of having epiglottitis should never be taken to the radiology department until after endotracheal intubation is performed to prevent complete airway obstruction. The flu vaccine has nearly eradicated this illness.**

A. Viral croup is preceded by a URI and progresses at a much slower pace than epiglottitis. The typical presentation includes the characteristic "barky" cough, hoarseness, inspiratory stridor, and low-grade fever. Patients are usually under 3 years of age.

B. Spasmodic croup tends to occur in the evening or nighttime and is preceded by coryza and hoarseness. The child awakens with a barky cough, stridor, and may appear anxious. The patient is usually afebrile. This condition may be an allergic reaction to viral antigens, but the exact cause is unknown.

D. Bacterial tracheitis is a life-threatening condition, often caused by *Staphylococcus*, in which there are purulent secretions in the trachea. Patients present with a brassy cough, stridor, fever, and toxicity, but they generally do not drool or have dysphagia.

E. Reactive airway disease is a problem that primarily involves the lower airways. The prominent physical finding is expiratory wheezing and prolongation of the expiratory phase of respiration. Upper airway obstruction, such as viral croup and epiglottitis, usually causes inspiratory noises known as stridor.

21. **D. To do this calculation, the pediatrician must know that (1) standard cow's milk formula contains 20 kcal per ounce and (2) the daily**

energy requirement for an infant is approximately 100 kcal per kilogram of body weight. Therefore, this baby requires 550 kcal per day, which will be supplied by about 27 to 28 oz of formula.

A, B, C, E. These calculations are incorrect. See explanation for D.

22. **D. Guillain-Barré syndrome generally causes an ascending paralysis with absent DTRs. This syndrome is thought to result from immune-mediated neuronal injury provoked by a respiratory or gastrointestinal infection (i.e., Epstein-Barr, *Varicella, Campylobacter jejuni*) or immunization. The most serious complications are respiratory failure and autonomic dysfunction (arrhythmia, hypertension, hypotension, GI motility disorders). Since respiratory failure can occur in 10% to 15% of cases, careful monitoring of respiratory effort is critical. For patients with severe symptoms, IV gamma globulin or plasmapheresis can be given. Approximately 85% of patients with Guillain-Barré syndrome will have a good recovery.**

A. The CSF in cases of viral meningitis would show pleocytosis, but one would not expect to find neurologic deficits, including areflexia.

B. Certain wood ticks and dog ticks produce a neurotoxin that can cause a picture of ascending paralysis and areflexia that mimics Guillain-Barré syndrome. When the tick is removed, the patient can recover very quickly.

C. Enteroviral encephalitis would be associated with a greater degree of mental status change than is seen in this patient. A patient with encephalitis would not generally demonstrate areflexia.

E. Leukemia may present with severe bone or joint pains, particularly in the legs. The paralytic pattern and absence of reflexes in this patient is not typical of leukemia.

23. **C. After a severe bout of viral gastroenteritis, many babies will develop villous atrophy with depletion of intestinal lactase. When these babies are given a formula containing lactose (including breast milk and cow's milk formulas), they may have watery stools resulting from sugar malabsorption. This problem usually resolves if the baby is fed a non-lactose–containing formula for a few weeks.**

A. Cow's milk protein allergy is relatively uncommon in babies. This condition would be expected to present prior to 9 months of age.

B. Starvation diarrhea can be the result of the prolonged use of oral electrolyte solutions. The intestine requires adequate nutrition to allow villi to regenerate and replenish lactase.

D. Several organisms may cause gastroenteritis. Although some organisms (rotavirus, coronavirus) can cause prolonged chronic diarrhea, most cases of viral gastroenteritis resolve spontaneously in just a few days.

E. Cystic fibrosis can cause chronic malabsorption, failure to thrive, and recurrent pneumonia. This patient's history is not typical of cystic fibrosis. Patients with cystic fibrosis frequently require treatment with pancreatic enzymes and close nutritional monitoring.

24. **D. A foul-smelling, purulent, unilateral discharge is the classic presentation of a nasal foreign body. Referral to an otolaryngologist may be needed if suctioning the secretions from the nose does not allow visualization and removal of the object.**

A. The discharge in URI is generally bilateral and not foul smelling. The turbinates are generally inflamed and erythematous.

B. The discharge in allergic rhinitis tends to be watery. The turbinates usually appear quite swollen and pale.

C. Sinusitis can cause persistent rhinorrhea, purulent discharge, and foul-smelling breath. The discharge itself is generally not foul smelling. The onset of sinusitis is generally more prolonged than in this case. Cough and fever may also be present.

E. Nasal polyps are often associated with long-standing conditions such as cystic fibrosis or chronic allergies. This child's course was much more acute. Furthermore, no polyp was seen on physical examination.

25. **D. Slipped capital femoral epiphysis (SCFE) is the most common hip disorder that presents during adolescence. The limp is painful and there may also be limb shortening. Lateral-view radiographs show displacement of the epiphysis inferiorly and posteriorly. The condition is twice as common in males as in females. It has been associated**

with obesity, renal disease, and hypothyroidism. Patients should be advised to be non–weight bearing and referred to an orthopedist immediately.

A. Plain radiography frequently does not detect osteomyelitis until the infection in the bone has been present for a week or longer. Patients often have fever and an elevated ESR.

B. Legg-Calvé-Perthes disease, or avascular necrosis of the femoral head, most often presents in children 5 to 10 years of age. It may first be noted as a painless limp, vague knee and hip pain, knee pain alone, or decreased range of motion around the hip. Treatment involves reduction of activities, NSAIDs, and the use of crutches. For severe cases or in older children, braces or surgical procedures may be needed.

C. Septic hip is usually associated with fever and an ill-appearing child. Blood cultures may be positive in about 40% of the cases. Joint space widening is seen on the plain radiograph.

E. Growing pains are recurrent nighttime leg aches in children 4 to 8 years old. Treatment includes massage, muscle stretching, and local heat application. This is a benign condition that resolves without complication.

26. **D. *Shigella* often causes seizures and bloody diarrhea in children. *Shigella* is a Gram-negative rod that can cause fever, headache, profuse watery diarrhea (with or without blood), cramps, and tenesmus. As with other bacterial gastroenteritis, the stools often contain blood and leukocytes. *Shigella* is commonly associated with neurologic manifestations (in 10% to 45%), such as a brief seizure, lethargy, confusion, hallucinations, and severe headache. CSF analysis is usually normal. Antibiotics do shorten the duration of *Shigella* diarrhea.**

A, B. *Streptococcus* and *Staphylococcus* do not commonly cause diarrhea in children.

C. *E. coli* can certainly cause bloody diarrhea, but this organism is generally not associated with an increased risk of seizures. *E. coli* is associated with an increased chance of developing HUS, particularly after exposure to antibiotics.

E. Rotavirus diarrhea is generally not bloody in nature. Rotavirus vaccine was recently released, but later recalled when it was found to be associated with intussusception.

27. **C. Inflammatory bowel disease (IBD), including ulcerative colitis and Crohn disease, may first present as short stature before any GI symptoms develop. The growth arrest, unexplained fevers, mild anemia, and elevated ESR are most consistent with this diagnosis. The stool should be checked for blood. Additional tests for IBD might include pANCA and ASCA (anti-*Saccharomyces cerevisiae* antibody). Imaging studies and referral to a gastroenterologist for possible endoscopy are warranted.**

A. In constitutional growth delay, the decrease in growth rate always occurs in the first 2 years of life. It would not be associated with abnormal lab test results or fever.

B. The complete growth arrest seen in this child is not consistent with a diagnosis of familial short stature. Based on the parents' heights, the child would not be expected to have a height below the 5th percentile.

D. Renal tubular acidosis can present with failure to thrive and short stature. The renal problem is often secondary to malnutrition. Serum bicarbonate level tends to be low and the urinary pH may be elevated.

E. The growth arrest pattern could be due to a brain tumor, but the laboratory abnormalities and fever in this case are more consistent with IBD.

28. **D. Children with bacterial meningitis may develop the syndrome of inappropriate antidiuretic hormone secretion, also known as SIADH. In this condition, excessive water is retained by the kidneys and the electrolytes become diluted. Because of the overhydration, the kidneys tend to excrete increased amounts of sodium. The result is hyponatremia, which is a common cause of seizure activity and can be evaluated with serum electrolytes. Treatment involves fluid restriction. Hypertonic saline solutions should be reserved for emergency situations with repeated seizures. Diuretics should not be used because they can worsen the hyponatremia.**

A. It is important to monitor the electrolytes and weight of a child with meningitis. SIADH may develop within 24–48 hours after the initial diagnosis of meningitis is made.

B. Antipyretic therapy may increase comfort in patients with high fevers.

C. Bacterial meningitis in children this age is most often caused by *Streptococcus pneumoniae, Neisseria meningitidis,* and *H. influenzae.* The antibiotic coverage is adequate.

E. Children with meningitis, especially neonates, may develop a brain abscess or subdural effusions. However, this complication typically occurs around 7 to 10 days from the initial presentation, and would be unlikely this early.

29. **C. Research has demonstrated that babies put to sleep in a prone position are at a 2 to 12 time's higher risk for sudden infant death syndrome (SIDS). Since the Academy of Pediatrics has been recommending supine sleep position, SIDS rates have fallen by about 40% to 50%. SIDS remains the most common cause of infant death beyond the neonatal period. Other risk factors for SIDS include maternal smoking during pregnancy, soft sleep surfaces, loose bedding, bed sharing, overheating, preterm birth, and low birth weight. The peak incidence of SIDS is 2 to 4 months of age. The cause remains incompletely understood and there actually may be several mechanisms. One hypothesis involves the delayed development of arousal or cardiorespiratory control in the central nervous system (arcuate nucleus).**

    A. Prone sleeping position has the highest risk for SIDS. Babies can and should be placed on their belly while awake. This will help with positional occipital plagiocephaly (flattening of the skull) that may result from lying on the back for long periods of time.

    B. While sleeping on the side appears to be less risky than prone sleeping, it still has a higher risk than the supine sleeping position.

    D, E. Elevation of the head or foot of the crib has not been associated with any increase or decrease in the rate of SIDS.

30. **D. Spinal muscular atrophy (SMA) is a disorder that causes progressive weakness. The early infantile form (type I, Werdnig-Hoffman) is usually diagnosed before 6 months of age. Most cases are inherited as an autosomal-recessive trait. The clinical findings include severe hypotonia, generalized weakness, small muscle mass, absent DTRs, and tongue atrophy and fasciculations. Infants with acute infantile SMA may have respiratory distress as well as sucking and**

feeding problems. Ptosis, ophthalmoplegia, and facial weakness are not common. DNA testing for the responsible mutation should be obtained initially. If normal, further work-up should include muscle biopsy and electromyography (EMG). There is currently no treatment and most babies with this condition die by age 3 years.

    A. While Guillain-Barré syndrome usually occurs in older children, it can cause hypotonia and areflexia in infants. Tongue fasciculations are not typical.

    B. Babies with botulism are often constipated. Unlike type I SMA, they may present with a masklike, expressionless face and ptosis of the eyelids. Again, tongue atrophy and fasciculations are not typical.

    C. Congenital hypothyroidism can cause hypotonia and delayed DTRs. These infants may also have hypothermia, large fontanelles, coarse facial features, and a hoarse cry. Unlike children with infantile SMA, the tongue tends to be large (macroglossia).

    E. Babies born to mothers with myasthenia gravis may have transient weakness and hypotonia due to the presence of maternal acquired antibodies against the acetylcholine receptor. There is also a rare congenital form. Ptosis and ophthalmoplegia may be early findings in either of these two forms of myasthenia gravis.

31. **C. Genetics is involved in the propensity and severity expected in a teen's acne development.**

    A. Research has proven that diet has little or nothing to do with acne breakouts.

    B. Cleansing the skin too harshly, by either scrubbing or the use of strong cleansers, irritates the skin and will only contribute to acne formation.

    D. Although a good scare tactic to use on your teen, it has no basis in truth.

    E. Controlled studies have also shown that the use of cosmetics and greasy vehicles on the face do not aggravate acne.

32. **B. In a witnessed collapse in which the patient is pulseless, the probability of a cardiac arrhythmia is much higher, even in a child. The faster you can get a defibrillator to the patient, the better chance you have of a successful resuscitation.**

A. Phone first, not fast, in a witnessed pulseless collapse, as it is a priority to get a defibrillator to the patient as quickly as possible.
C. AEDs can be used in children 8 years of age and older when indicated.
D. Activate the EMS system and establish the airway and breathing before starting chest compressions.
E. There is a higher probability of cardiac arrhythmia in this case of witnessed pulseless collapse, than of aspiration and airway obstruction.

33. **C. Langerhans cell histiocytosis often presents with chronic, draining otitis media; a seborrheic type of dermatitis of the scalp and diaper area; and a characteristic skin rash on the trunk. Histiocytosis is associated with skeletal involvement in 80% of patients. These skeletal lesions may be single or multifocal, most commonly involving the skull.**

A. Otitis externa is uncommon in infants and would not explain the rash or fever.
B. The fever and draining ear are unlikely associations with a contact dermatitis.
D. The morphology and distribution of the rash and the fever are not consistent with atopic dermatitis.
E. The fever and draining ear, scalp dermatitis, and diaper dermatitis are not typical of scabies.

34. **D. Reassurance only is the correct answer. Acrocyanosis in the newborn period is normal. Isolated circumoral cyanosis in an otherwise healthy child whose physical examination is normal is generally not a cause for concern. It is likely to be due to sluggish capillary blood flow, particularly when related to cold exposure. Circumoral cyanosis is more evident in fair skinned children.**

A. Echocardiography would be useful if there was a question of central cyanosis. Evidence of central cyanosis would raise suspicion for an intracardiac right-to-left shunt. Pulmonary hypertension with a resulting right-to-left shunt could be evaluated by echocardiography. However, this child has only limited peripheral cyanosis and no signs or symptoms of cardiac disease.
B. ECG would be useful in identifying ventricular or atrial hypertrophy and ventricular conduction disturbances as part of the diagnosis of congenital or acquired heart disease. As this child is healthy, with no signs or symptoms of cardiac disease, he does not need further cardiac evaluation.

C. Routine referral to a cardiologist is not necessary and may raise the family's anxiety and lead to a prolonged and expensive cardiac evaluation.
E. Chest radiograph would be indicated if there were any signs of respiratory distress, a murmur, or other signs of cardiac or respiratory disease.

35. **B. All forms of rickets are associated with high alkaline phosphatase activity. In rickets, osteoblasts are stimulated in an attempt to help with bone formation; these osteoblasts secrete large amounts of alkaline phosphatase.**

A. Vitamin D–resistant rickets and other forms of rickets secondary to phosphorus deficiency usually have normal serum calcium levels.
C. Parathyroid levels are high in only those forms of rickets with low serum calcium levels.
D. Vitamin D–resistant rickets is usually transmitted as sex-linked dominant, but there is a significant level of spontaneous new mutations. Therefore, his mother may not be affected, or she may have a partial expression with only low serum phosphorus.
E. Vitamin D–deficiency rickets may have normal phosphorus levels very early in the course, but usually phosphorus levels are low, and they are virtually always low when symptoms are manifest.

36. **E. In cases of suspected trauma, such as a fall from the tree or the ladder, the jaw thrust with simultaneous stabilization of the cervical spine is the correct method of opening the airway.**

A. Establishing an airway and 1 minute of CPR before activating the EMS system is indicated in infants and children—phone fast, not phone first.
B. In cases of suspected trauma, the head tilt and chin lift method of establishing the airway may cause further damage to an injured cervical spine.
C. The child is cyanotic and not breathing. Attention to the airway and reestablishing respiration is indicated before attention to circulation.
D. The tongue-jaw lift may further injure the cervical spine in cases of trauma. A blind finger sweep is never indicated.

37. **C. It is unclear if this mother has been thoroughly treated for syphilis. Therefore, it is possible she may have transmitted syphilis to the baby. Adequate treatment for mothers should include penicillin treatment at least 4 weeks prior to**

delivery, and the mothers should show a serologic response to treatment, including a fourfold or better improvement in their titers. Evaluation of the infant should also include a thorough physical examination looking for snuffles (nasal discharge), hepatosplenomegaly, or a papulosquamous rash. It is important to draw an RPR on the baby. If the baby's titer is higher than that of the mother, it is very suggestive of active infection. The RPR can also be used to monitor response to treatment, if indicated.

A. Long bone films may show metaphyseal lesions secondary to osteochondritis.

B. CSF should be evaluated in infants when there is a concern for congenital syphilis. A negative CSF VDRL does not exclude neurosyphilis, but a positive CSF VDRL is diagnostic.

D. Congenital syphilis can cause anemia, leukopenia, and/or thrombocytopenia. It is helpful to check these values to assess for symptomatic infection. Liver function tests are also commonly elevated in infected infants.

E. Treatment of congenital syphilis requires high-dose IV therapy for 10 days.

38. C. "Secondary drowning" occurs after an initial immersion injury that results in successful immediate resuscitation, but progresses to death after a period of 24 hours (or more) from the initial event, typically due to progressive pulmonary dysfunction. Even though some near drowners will regain a degree of neurologic function after initial stabilization, this is often misleading to both providers and family members, and has been referred to as a "honeymoon phase" in the literature. Following this phase, a portion of patients will ultimately progress to a vegetative state or to death. Physiologically, many large aspirations (such as drownings) result in a final common pathway of alveolar inflammation, exudate, atelectasis, hypoxia, pulmonary hypertension, and pulmonary edema. The net result is a picture very similar to ARDS.

A. A "drowning" is defined as an immersion injury resulting in immediate asphyxia and death.

B. A "near drowning" is defined as an immersion injury that results in at least temporary survival. In fact, many near drowners live for many years after the event, with varying degrees of morbidity.

D. An "immersion injury" is a generic term for any injury sustained after being submerged in a liquid substance (most often water). It implies nothing about the severity or outcome.

E. Water intoxication can be seen following fresh water drowning. The result is a hyponatremic state secondary to excessive free water which may cause cellular swelling and a clinical picture of cerebral edema and increased intracranial pressure.

39. D. The definition of nocturnal enuresis is the involuntary discharge of urine at night. The term "primary" is used when the child has never had a sustained period of nighttime dryness greater than 3 to 6 months. Approximately 85% to 90% of bedwetters simply have a developmental delay of bladder control and most will "outgrow" their problem without treatment. Although about 15% to 20% of 5-year-olds are enuretic, only 5% of 10-year-olds and 1% to 2% of children over 15 still wet their beds at night.

A. UTI is a rare cause of enuresis. Many experts do not feel a urinalysis or urine culture is required in the evaluation of a child with primary nocturnal enuresis, unless there are associated symptoms such as dysuria or a weak urine stream.

B. An anatomic abnormality of the urinary tract is an extremely rare cause of enuresis in a 6-year-old. Radiologic imaging of the urinary tract is not necessary in most cases of primary nocturnal enuresis.

C. Although some children with enuresis have some minor emotional problems secondary to their bedwetting, most enuretics have no significant behavioral problem.

E. Unstable bladder, also known as uninhibited bladder contractions, is a common cause of daytime (diurnal) enuresis. Only about 5% of all enuretics also wet in the daytime. Children with an unstable bladder usually have nocturnal enuresis in addition to their daytime "accidents."

40. D. Recheck his blood pressure in 1 week. True hypertension is defined as three blood pressure readings on different occasions that are greater than the 95th percentile for age, gender, and height.

A. Although a urinalysis would give you useful information about his kidneys, such as proteinuria or hematuria, it would not be necessary at this point. This is only one reading at a point in time and will need to be followed.

B. Renal ultrasound with Doppler would be extremely useful in the evaluation of a patient who has been shown to have true hypertension, but it is not indicated at this time.

C. Twenty-four-hour ambulatory blood pressure monitoring is useful in evaluating the patient who has already been shown to be hypertensive on several separate occasions in the office. It records multiple readings throughout the day and eliminates artificially elevated blood pressures resulting from anxiety at the doctor's office.

E. A basic metabolic panel to evaluate kidney function, in particular BUN and creatinine, would be warranted once true hypertension has been documented, as in the explanation for D.

41. **D. The most common cause of congenital hypothyroidism is the result of abnormal development of the thyroid gland. Patients may have aplasia/hypoplasia or ectopic thyroid gland tissue. This occurs in 1 in 4000 live births and accounts for 85% of cases.**

A. Maternal Graves's disease can be treated with antithyroid medications such as propylthiouracil (PTU) or methimazole. These drugs can cross the placenta and cause transient inhibition of thyroid hormone synthesis in the neonate. These infants may even develop a goiter.

B. Maternal antithyrotropin antibodies inhibit the binding of TSH to its receptor and may cross the placenta, producing transient hypothyroidism and an abnormal screening test result in newborns.

C. Maternal iodine deficiency is a rare cause of hypothyroidism in developed countries. In countries with widespread malnutrition, iodine deficiency is common.

E. The newborn screen tests for low T_4 levels and elevated TSH levels. A surge in TSH occurs shortly after birth in full-term infants. The levels normally decline rapidly within the first 24 hours, then gradually reach normal levels. A newborn screen performed before 24 hours of age may reflect this surge.

42. **A. X-linked agammaglobulinemia is a disorder found in males that presents early in infancy following the decline of maternal antibodies. As a consequence of no antibody production and minimal B-cell production, patients are susceptible to encapsulated organisms, such as *S. pneumoniae, H. influenzae,* and *N. meningitidis.* As with most immunodeficiencies, growth is often affected as well.**

B. Wiskott-Aldrich is also X-linked, but is a disorder of both T- and B-cell immunity that presents with atopic dermatitis and thrombocytopenia.

C. Chronic granulomatous disease is an X-linked disorder that is characterized by a deficiency in phagocytosis. Patients often present with cutaneous infections, deep skin abscesses, and recurrent lymphadenitis.

D. Chediak-Higashi syndrome is an autosomal-recessive disease. It is also a disorder of phagocytosis that presents with partial albinism, photophobia, and nystagmus.

E. Leukocyte adhesion defect is another disorder of phagocytosis. Newborns may present with delayed umbilical cord separation. There is a tendency toward skin and subcutaneous infections with poor wound healing.

43. **A. Unexplained crying in an infant can occur for a variety of reasons, and should lead to a thorough evaluation. If there is no obvious cause or evidence of illness, the evaluation should consider glaucoma, corneal abrasion, intussusception, and hair entrapment. This mother had very long, light-colored, silky hair. Several strands were found in the sleeper the baby had been wearing and one strand had encircled the toe tightly.**

B. Colic is a common condition characterized by repetitive episodes of crying in infants less than 3 months of age. The episodes typically occur daily, usually in the afternoon and evening and may last several hours. They may be exacerbated by increased stimulation or an alteration in the daily schedule. It rarely persists after 3 months of age.

C. Osteomyelitis could present with irritability and swelling of the affected toe. This is an uncommon location. Osteomyelitis is usually associated with other signs of illness such as fever, poor feeding, emesis, or other findings.

D. Fractures are uncommon in infants due to their lack of mobility. A fracture of the toe would be even more unusual. Child abuse should be considered in any infant with a fracture of unexplained cause.

E. Scorpion stings are fairly common in certain parts of the southwestern United States. Children and infants will certainly cry at the time of a sting. It is often very difficult to locate the sting site on physical examination. Other symptoms suggestive of a scorpion sting include stridor, respiratory distress, and uncontrolled, writhing movements of the extremities and tongue, as well as opsoclonus.

44. **B. Any infant who presents with jaundice at 2 weeks or more should have a fractionated bilirubin drawn to demonstrate that there is not a direct/conjugated component. A direct component greater than 2 mg/dL or greater than 20% of the total would be very suspicious for other pathologies, including biliary atresia or intrinsic liver disease. A significant direct component would lead away from the diagnosis of simple breast-milk jaundice, which results in an elevated indirect/unconjugated bilirubin level.**

A. An abdominal ultrasound would be useful if a significant direct hyperbilirubinemia had been present. This test could evaluate for structural anomalies, such as a choledochal cyst.

C. Observation with follow-up in 1 month would potentially delay the diagnosis of biliary atresia.

D. Liver function tests are not indicated at this time. There is no evidence of hepatomegaly or direct hyperbilirubinemia that would warrant further investigation.

E. Infants with UTIs can present with jaundice, but the absence of fever, irritability, or foul-smelling urine rule against this.

45. **D. This is the most common presentation of postinfectious glomerulonephritis. This condition is most often an immunologic reaction to a recent Group A β-hemolytic streptococcal throat or skin infection; thus, the term "poststreptococcal glomerulonephritis." The latency period is usually 7 to 14 days, and it occurs more often in boys between 4 and 14 years of age. The presentation is characterized by gross hematuria, edema, and hypertension.**

A. Acute cystitis can present with gross hematuria, but it is most often associated with a viral illness with bladder symptoms (frequency, urgency, dysuria, suprapubic pain).

B. IgA nephropathy may mimic poststreptococcal glomerulonephritis but is much less common, and generally does not present with hypertension and edema.

C. Acute pyelonephritis is usually a febrile illness, and gross hematuria is uncommon.

E. Benign hematuria is usually microscopic and unassociated with other symptoms.

46. **C. This child has Hirschsprung disease and is showing symptoms that are consistent with enterocolitis and toxic megacolon, a potentially life-threatening complication of Hirschsprung disease in infants. Mortality is very high in this condition. Treatment with IV fluids and IV antibiotics is critical to reestablishing intravascular volume and appropriate circulation as well as preventing overwhelming sepsis. Hirschsprung disease refers to the syndrome of congenital aganglionic megacolon. An abnormal migration of neural crest cells to the distal colon occurs, resulting in an aganglionic segment of the bowel. This results in an inability of the colon to mount a coordinated relaxation, leaving a hypertonic area with proximal dilatation.**

A. Immediately after instituting IV fluids and antibiotic therapy, it will be important to obtain a surgical consult to assist with further diagnosis and treatment. The diagnosis of Hirschsprung disease is confirmed by rectal biopsy showing the absence of ganglion cells in the distal colon.

B. Fleet's enema and Golytely drip would not be the treatment of choice in a child this young, with disease this severe. Surgical decompression would most likely be required.

D. Colostomy will commonly be performed in patients with Hirschsprung disease after the diagnosis is confirmed. Definitive surgery with eventual reanastomosis is usually planned after 8 to 12 months.

E. Manual decompression would be extremely difficult and likely unsuccessful in a child this age and would not be recommended.

47. **E. Hypsarrhythmia is the classic EEG finding in infantile spasms. Patients usually present with recurrent flexion-extension seizure episodes between 2 and 7 months of age. These seizures can occur multiple times per day and can be difficult to treat. They may be associated with underlying CNS abnormalities. The use of ACTH may be helpful in some patients.**

A. Petit mal seizures are associated with a spike-and-wave pattern at a frequency of 3 cycles/second. This pattern results in brief staring episodes in older children.

B. Myoclonic seizures consist of short, sharp jerking movements and are usually seen in patients with certain degenerative disorders or cerebral palsy.

C. Akinetic seizures are extremely brief episodes of the loss of motor movements or postural tone.

D. Pseudoseizures are not true seizures. They are typically seen in school-age or adolescent patients with severe behavioral issues. EEG findings in these patients are normal.

48. **A. A 2-month-old infant would be expected to lift his head off the table, follow objects past the midline, recognize his parents, and smile when engaged.**

49. **G. A 24-month-old child should walk up and down steps alone, turn book pages one at a time, understand two-step commands, and be able to engage in parallel play.**

50. **E. A 12-month-old child would be expected to begin to walk independently, demonstrate a mature pincer grasp, use a couple more words than "mama" or "dada," and imitate some actions of others.**

B. A 4-month-old child should be able to roll over, sit well with support, move arms in unison while grasping at an object, and regard his environment with excitement.

C. A 6-month-old infant should sit well without support, transfer objects between hands, use a raking grasp, babble, and recognize strangers.

D. A 9-month-old infant would be expected to crawl and creep and begin to pull to a stand while exploring his environment. A pincer grasp should have developed, as should an understanding of "no."

F. An 18-month-old toddler should be able to run, turn 2 to 3 book pages at a time, begin to feed himself with a spoon, say 10 to 20 words, and imitate the actions of his parents.

BLOCK 2

51. A 4-year-old, white male presents with 6 days of fever to 104°F, irritability, erythematous tongue and lips, nonexudative, bulbar conjunctivitis bilaterally, an erythematous, maculopapular rash predominantly on the trunk, and cervical lymphadenopathy. You make the diagnosis of Kawasaki disease (mucocutaneous lymph node syndrome). Which of the following is the most appropriate therapy?

    A. Prednisone (2 mg/kg/day)
    B. Nafcillin IV
    C. Intravenous immunoglobulin (IVIG) 2 g/kg
    D. Observation
    E. Aspirin (80–100 mg/kg/day)
    F. Prednisone (2 mg/kg/day) and aspirin (80–100 mg/kg/day)
    G. Nafcillin IV and IVIG 2 g/kg
    H. IVIG 2 g/kg and aspirin (80–100 mg/kg/day)

52. Because of the use of proper restraint systems, childhood deaths from automobile crashes have decreased significantly in recent years. A mother of two children, ages 11 months (22 lbs) and 5 years (47 lbs), asks you for advice about the best way to transport her children while she is driving the family car. Which one of the following statements is true?

    A. The 5-year-old should sit in a booster seat designed to position the car's lap and shoulder belts across the child's hips and chest
    B. The 5-year-old should sit in a rear seat with the shoulder belt placed behind the child to keep it off the neck
    C. The 11-month-old should sit in the front seat next to the mother so she can reach the child easily
    D. Whenever possible, children should be placed in front of the passenger side air bag for maximum protection
    E. The 11-month-old should sit in a front-facing, upright infant seat placed in the back seat of the car

53. A 14-year-old boy was hospitalized after sustaining a severe crush injury in an auto accident. His condition was stabilized during the first 6 hours in the hospital. However, his urine becomes brown in color, and he is found to be oliguric. Rhabdomyolysis is suspected. Which one of the following is frequently associated with rhabdomyolysis?

    A. Hypercalcemia
    B. Hypophosphatemia
    C. Hyponatremia
    D. Hypocalcemia
    E. Hypokalemia

54. You are seeing a 2-month-old infant for a well-child visit. The baby has been doing well with appropriate weight gain and development. His mother wants to know when she can start feeding her baby cereals and strained fruits and vegetables. The American Academy of Pediatrics recommends starting solid foods at age:

    A. 1 to 2 months
    B. 2 to 3 months
    C. 4 to 6 months
    D. 9 to 12 months
    E. 18 months

55. You are working in the pediatric ICU and receive an outside call about a 1-year-old child who is currently being intubated with chest compressions ongoing. The most likely cause of cardiorespiratory arrest during childhood is

    A. Cardiac arrhythmias
    B. Respiratory failure or arrest
    C. Drug reactions and interactions
    D. Drug ingestions
    E. Cardiovascular disease

56. An 8-year-old returns from a family vacation in Mexico, where they picked and enjoyed many of the local foods and fruits. Her mother brings her to your office with streaky, nonscaly, brown areas appearing on her chest, fingers, and chin. Some of these are forming blisters. On further examination, you note that there are none on her trunk, abdomen, or buttocks. Your diagnosis is which of the following?

    A. Physical child abuse
    B. Neurofibromatosis
    C. Phytophotodermatosis
    D. Fungal dermatosis
    E. Drug reaction to her sunscreen

57. A 4-year-old boy presents with insidious, generalized, dependent edema over the 2 weeks preceding this visit. He had previously been well, but his mother has noticed that he has not been urinating very much for several days. His examination reveals a prominent abdomen with some ascites, and 3+ pitting edema of the pretibial

areas bilaterally. His blood pressure is mildly elevated. His urine contains 4+ protein, trace blood, and specific gravity of 1.035. The most likely diagnosis is

A. Chronic renal failure
B. Minimal change nephrotic syndrome
C. Focal segmental glomerulosclerosis (FSG)
D. Acute glomerulonephritis
E. Membranous glomerulonephropathy

58. A worried mother calls in to report that her 2-day-old newborn is "bleeding from her bottom." Her prenatal and birth history were unremarkable. On physical examination in your office, you notice a bloody serosanguineous fluid oozing from the vagina and staining the diaper. There is no bruising or petechiae. The most likely diagnosis is

A. Hemophilia A
B. Child abuse
C. Birth trauma
D. Hemangioma of the vulva
E. Withdrawal bleeding

59. A 17-year-old female is brought into the ER by paramedics who were called to a dance club following an episode of syncope. She admits to taking multiple illicit drugs. In approaching her exam you recall various side effects of these drugs. Which of the following is consistent with an ecstasy ingestion?

A. Hypoadrenergic state
B. Decreased respirations and mental status
C. Rotary nystagmus
D. Tachycardia and hyperthermia
E. Miotic pupils

60. A 2-month-old boy is admitted to the hospital for nonbilious vomiting after feedings. He had been breastfeeding well until 2 weeks ago, when the vomiting became worse and the mother noted that the baby was having fewer bowel movements. On physical examination, the baby is found to have obvious jaundice. You can see gastric peristaltic waves, but you are unable to palpate any masses in the abdomen. The electrolytes show hypokalemic, hypochloremic alkalosis. The most likely diagnosis is:

A. Acute gastroenteritis
B. Duodenal atresia
C. UTI

D. Pyloric stenosis
E. Milk allergy

61. A 6-year-old Hispanic girl is brought to your office at the end of the summer with multiple, dark lesions on her legs and arms for the past month. The lesions are about 1 cm in size, much darker than the rest of her skin, nonpalpable, nontender, and not pruritic. The girl reports also having had a lot of mosquito bites over the summer. The lesions are most likely:

A. Impetigo
B. Postinflammatory hyperpigmentation
C. Henoch-Schönlein Purpura (HSP)
D. Eczema
E. Tinea corporis

62. A 10-year-old white female presents with pain and swelling in her left elbow and right knee for 3 days. Today her left elbow is no longer swollen. There is no redness or warmth to the joints. The arthritis was preceded by a 3-day history of fever of 102°F, approximately 2 weeks ago with a sore throat. Laboratory results reveal an elevated sedimentation rate, a negative ANA and rheumatoid factor, and an elevated antistreptolysin titer. The most likely diagnosis is:

A. Systemic lupus erythematosus (SLE)
B. Juvenile rheumatoid arthritis (JRA)
C. Rheumatic fever
D. Gonococcal arthritis
E. Lyme disease

63. A laboratory test used to detect Disease X has a sensitivity of 80% and a specificity of 80%. The prevalence of Disease X in the population of patients you test is known to be 20%. A patient has a positive test. How do you interpret this result?

A. All patients with a positive test have the disease
B. 75% of those with a positive test actually have the disease
C. 50% of those with a positive test actually have the disease
D. 25% of those with a positive test actually have the disease
E. There is not enough information to answer the question

64. A 2-year-old boy is admitted to the hospital with dehydration. He has had diarrhea for 2 to 3 days. The child is irritable with sunken eyes and a sunken fontanelle, there are few tears and the mucous membranes are dry. The pulse rate is increased and there has been little urine output today. Capillary refill is slow. A urinalysis reveals a negative test for protein, negative for blood, SG 1.025, 3+ ketones. Which one of the following laboratory tests would you likely find in this patient?

    A. Na^+ 140 mEq/L, K^+ 3.5 mEq/L, Cl^- 120 mEq/L, CO_2 8 mEq/L, BUN 25 mg/dL, creatinine 0.5 mg/dL
    B. Na^+ 138 mEq/L, K^+ 4.5 mEq/L, Cl^- 104 mEq/L, CO_2 20 mEq/L, BUN 25 mg/dL, creatinine 0.6 mg/dL
    C. Na^+ 140 mEq/L, K^+ 5.0 mEq/L, Cl^- 95 mEq/L, CO_2 24 mEq/L, BUN 25 mg/dL, creatinine 0.7 mg/dL
    D. Na^+ 142 mEq/L, K^+ 4.0 mEq/L, Cl^- 105 mEq/L, CO_2 8 mEq/L, BUN 80 mg/dL, creatinine 2.0 mg/dL

65. A 7-day-old infant is found to have a significantly elevated total bilirubin, but is otherwise well. The fractionated bilirubin reports a direct bilirubin of 3.0 mg/dL, and the indirect bilirubin is 6.0 mg/dL. Which one of the following should be considered in your differential diagnosis?

    A. Breast-milk jaundice
    B. Gilbert syndrome
    C. Congenital infection
    D. Congenital spherocytosis
    E. Crigler-Najjar syndrome

66. A 7-year-old girl is seen at your office because of significant joint pain and swelling for the past 2 weeks. She has had low-grade fever, is mildly anemic, and has had some malaise. There is no family history of arthritis. An ASO titer is negative, and her sedimentation rate is 80. One of your diagnostic considerations is JRA. Which one of the following statements regarding this diagnosis is correct?

    A. A rheumatoid factor is the best test to confirm the diagnosis of JRA
    B. Polyarticular JRA occurs with equal frequency in both sexes
    C. An ANA test would not be helpful in this case
    D. The prognosis in polyarticular JRA is generally good
    E. It is important to have an ophthalmologic consultation in polyarticular JRA

67. A 2-month-old female infant is seen in your office for a well checkup. While examining the hips, you find some resistance in abduction of the right hip. You apply the Ortolani and Barlow maneuvers to ascertain whether or not further investigation is necessary. Which one of the following statements is correct?

    A. In performing the Barlow maneuver, an attempt is made to dislocate the hip
    B. In performing the Ortolani maneuver, an attempt is made to dislocate the hip
    C. There seems to be no relationship between in-utero position and hip dysplasia
    D. In developmental hip dysplasia there is a 9:1 male predominance
    E. An audible "click" when performing the Ortolani test identifies a hip dysplasia

68. A 12-month-old male infant is seen for a well visit and is found to have some pallor. He has been fed Similac with iron since birth. His examination is otherwise normal except for a palpable spleen. His mother is of Greek ancestry. A blood count reveals the following: HB 9.9 g/dL, MCV 67, MCHC 32, RDW 13.5, reticulocyte count 1.5%, platelet count 240,000. Which one of the following is a true statement?

    A. A hemoglobin level of 9.9 g/dL is the lower limit of normal for this 12-month-old
    B. The dietary history is probably not true since this patient is iron deficient
    C. The reticulocyte count is high, suggesting a hemolytic process
    D. This infant must be losing blood, and the stools should be checked for occult blood
    E. A hemoglobin electrophoresis should make the diagnosis

69. A 2-year-old girl is seen with fever and right flank pain. Her examination is normal with the exception of right flank tenderness. A urinalysis has a positive test for nitrite, positive leukocyte esterase, many Gram-negative rods, and 20 to 30 leukocytes per high power field (HPF) on an uncentrifuged specimen. Your findings are consistent with acute pyelonephritis. Although multiple findings are consistent with UTI, which is the best single test that confirms the diagnosis of UTI in this child?

A. Pyuria greater than 10 WBCs/HPF in uncentrifuged urine

B. A catheterized urine culture with greater than 10^3 organisms per mL

C. Clinical findings of flank pain and tenderness

D. A midstream urine culture with greater than 10^5 organisms per mL

E. A positive nitrite and a positive leukocyte esterase test

The next two questions (items 70 and 71) correspond to the following vignette.

70. A 7-year-old Caucasian girl is seen in your office for her annual physical. Her physical examination is remarkable for a palpable goiter. The mother has a positive family history of hypothyroidism, requiring thyroid hormone replacement. The patient's growth chart is shown in Figure 3-70. What is the most likely diagnosis?

A. Hashimoto thyroiditis
B. Iodine deficiency
C. Thyroid adenoma
D. Brain tumor causing TSH deficiency
E. TRH deficiency

71. Which of the following laboratory studies is the most sensitive indicator of primary thyroid gland dysfunction and the most useful initial test to order in this case?

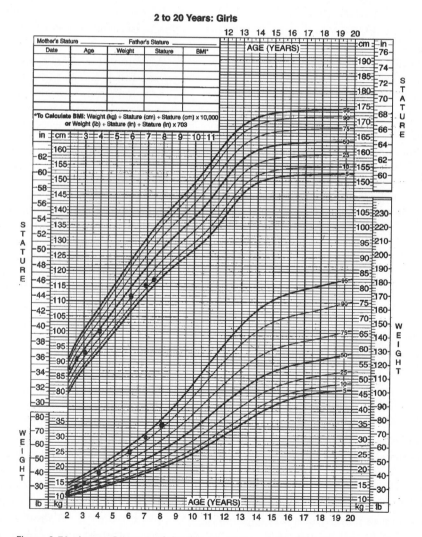

Figure 3-70 • Image Courtesy of the Phoenix Children's Hospital, Phoenix, Arizona. Source: Developed by the National Center for Health Statistics in Collaboration with the National Center for Chronic Disease Prevention and Health Promotion (2000). http://www.cdc.gov/growthcharts.

A. T_4
B. T_3
C. TRH
D. TSH
E. ACTH

End of Set

72. You are asked to see a 17-year-old male with a 1-month history of fatigue, lymphadenopathy, pharyngitis, and intermittent fevers. His examination is significant for palpable hepatosplenomegaly. You suspect that he may have Epstein-Barr virus (EBV). Which of the following malignancies is/are associated with EBV?

    A. Burkitt lymphoma
    B. Nasopharyngeal carcinoma
    C. Acute lymphocytic leukemia
    D. Hodgkin disease
    E. Burkitt lymphoma and acute lymphocytic leukemia
    F. Burkitt lymphoma, nasopharyngeal carcinoma, and acute lymphocytic leukemia
    G. Burkitt lymphoma, acute lymphocytic leukemia, and Hodgkin disease
    H. Burkitt lymphoma, nasopharyngeal carcinoma, and Hodgkin disease
    I. Burkitt lymphoma and Hodgkin disease

73. A 17-year-old female calls the office complaining of vaginal bleeding. She was just started on oral contraceptives (Cops) 2 weeks ago for dysfunctional uterine bleeding and is currently halfway through her pill pack. She is concerned about her vaginal spotting. She denies missing any of her pills and has not been sexually active for 6 months. A urine pregnancy test was negative 2 weeks ago. Which of the following is the most appropriate management?

    A. Stop taking the Cops
    B. Continue with her current pill pack and take one pill a day. Call the office if the bleeding increases significantly
    C. Throw away the current pill pack and start a new one
    D. Take 3 pills a day of a new pill pack for 3 days, then 2 pills a day for 2 days, then 1 pill a day until she has completed the entire pill pack and follow-up in the office
    E. Change to a different OCP with higher estrogen

74. A 13-year-old male presents to the office with complaints of pain just below his left knee for about 6 weeks. He denies any acute injury. He runs on the track team at school and has been very active for years. He also plays basketball during the weekends. He stopped running for about 10 days and the pain resolved. On examination, you find he has swelling and tenderness over the tibial tubercle and normal range of motion at the knee. Which of the following is the most likely diagnosis?

    A. Patellofemoral syndrome
    B. Slipped capital femoral epiphysis (SCFE)
    C. Subluxation of the patella
    D. Osteochondritis dissecans
    E. Osgood-Schlatter disease

75. You are seeing a 12-year-old female with a history of fever, arthritis, oral ulcers, malar rash, and photosensitivity. You suspect she may have an immunologic disease. Which of the following tests would be most specific for SLE?

    A. ANA
    B. Anti-double-stranded DNA
    C. C3
    D. Anti Ro
    E. Antihistone Ab

76. A mother is concerned that her 14-year-old daughter has not started menstruating. On physical examination, you detect that the girl has evidence of breast buds, slight widening of the areola, and breast tissue projecting as a small mound. Which of the following sexual maturity ratings (SRS) is appropriate for this patient?

    A. SMR 1
    B. SMR 2
    C. SMR 3
    D. SMR 4
    E. SMR 5

77. A 15-year-old female presents to the ED complaining of fever and abdominal pain. On further questioning you determine that she has been sexually active with two partners in the last 6 months and has used a condom only "some of the time." She has yellow, thick vaginal discharge and complains of dyspareunia. She denies any visible genital lesions. She is most likely infected with which of the following organisms?

A. *Trichomonas vaginalis*
B. *Candida albicans*
C. *Chlamydia trachomatis*
D. *Treponema pallidum*
E. *Gardnerella vaginalis*
F. Herpes simplex
G. Human papilloma virus

78. During a routine sports physical, you notice a cluster of large, hyperpigmented, macular lesions in the axilla of the patient, which extend down toward the axillary line and the upper chest in a dermatomal distribution. The lesions are not itchy or tender. There are no other lesions anywhere else on her body, and no one else in the family has any dark spots on their skin. The correct diagnosis is:

A. Contact dermatitis from her deodorant
B. Hyperpigmentation from a heat rash
C. Neurofibromatosis, segmental type
D. Hydradenitis suppurativa, a disorder of the sweat glands
E. Phytophotodermatosis

79. A 4-month-old infant is being seen in the emergency room. The child is in significant distress with profuse crackles bilaterally on lung exam and a barely audible heart beat. Where is the correct place to palpate for the presence of a pulse in this infant?

A. Femoral or brachial artery
B. Carotid artery
C. Radial artery
D. Dorsalis pedis artery
E. Posterior tibial artery

80. A 10-year-old boy is seen for a routine presort physical examination. He is asymptomatic and his blood pressure and examination are normal. His urine is found to have a 1+ reaction for hemoglobin and negative reaction for protein, and a microscopic sediment contains 10 to 20 RBCs/HPF. Which of the following would be your next step?

A. Measurement of his glomerular filtration rate
B. Renal ultrasound
C. Hearing test
D. Urinalysis on the parents
E. Serum BUN and creatinine

81. A mother brings in her 8-year-old child for treatment of severe sunburn. She is surprised this has happened since the day was cloudy, and she applied sun block before the children went swimming in their backyard pool. Which of the following is true regarding avoiding sun injury to the skin?

A. Sunscreen needs to be applied only before exposure
B. Sunscreens are the most important form of preventing sun injury to the skin
C. A sunburn can occur almost as easily on cloudy days as on sunny days
D. The time of day of sun exposure is not as important as wearing sunscreen
E. Sun exposure in childhood does not matter, as melanomas occur only in adults

82. A 16-year-old male presents to the clinic for routine health care. His social history is significant for two female sexual partners in the last 6 months with occasional condom usage. He smokes a half pack of cigarettes a day, drinks some alcohol on the weekends, and denies any IV drug use. Three months ago he had a friend help him with two tattoos on his legs. For the last 2 weeks he has noticed a decrease in his energy level but denies fever, history of jaundice, rash, pruritus, or abdominal pain. His appetite is normal. Screening labs reveal that his total bilirubin is normal, but his AST is 65 and his ALT is 70. GGT and lipase are normal. RPR is nonreactive and HIV is negative. Urine for gonorrhea and *Chlamydia trachomatis* is negative. Which of the following is the most likely diagnosis?

A. Hepatitis A
B. Hepatitis B
C. Hepatitis C
D. Hepatocellular carcinoma
E. Cholelithiasis

83. The mother of a 6-month-old boy has been feeding her baby infant formula with iron. He has been tolerating it well, but the mother wants to switch to whole cow's milk because she feels that "formula is much more expensive than milk." You suggest that she continue the formula with iron and wait to start whole milk until the baby is:

A. 6 months old
B. 9 months old
C. 12 months old
D. 15 months old
E. 18 months old

84. Your next patient in clinic is a 12-year-old boy with a chief complaint of chest pain. He is accompanied to the visit by both of his parents, who appear very anxious that he might have a "heart" problem. You counsel them that what proportion of chest pain in children is of cardio-vascular etiology?

A. 5%
B. 15%
C. 25%
D. 45%
E. 60%

85. A woman without prenatal care is admitted at 38 weeks by dates for the delivery of her third child. The 8 lb 13 oz infant is born vaginally and APGAR scores are 6 and 9. The pediatrician is called several hours later by the nursery staff to evaluate the left arm. The initial examination reveals an R-sided cephalohematoma. There is asymmetry of the upper limb movements with minimal movement of the left arm. The grasp is preserved. The most likely cause for this paralysis is:

A. Grade II intraventricular hemorrhage (IVH)
B. Hypoxic event during pregnancy secondary to drug abuse
C. Peripheral neuropathy associated with undi-agnosed gestational diabetes
D. Shoulder dystocia
E. CNS manifestations of syphilis

86. A 13-year-old female is seen for a well-child visit. The mother tells you that she was diagnosed with a ventricular septal defect and had had a delayed discharge after birth. The social history is signifi-cant for some academic difficulties in school. A thorough physical examination demonstrates scoliosis of the spine and the findings shown in Figure 3-86. Concerned with the overall picture, the resident refers the patient to genetics. Velocardiofacial syndrome or Shprintzen syn-drome is diagnosed. The geneticist describes the defect to the residents who learn that the loca-tion of the chromosomal defect is in the same region as the lesion in DiGeorge syndrome and may be a different manifestation of the same sequence. Old records are obtained. Of the fol-lowing, which was the most likely cause of the delayed discharge after birth?

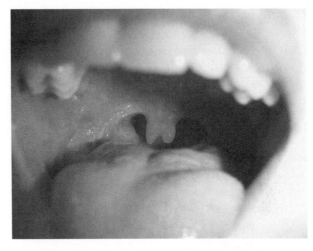

Figure 3-86 • Image Courtesy of the Phoenix Children's Hospital, Phoenix, Arizona.

A. Transient neonatal hypocalcemia
B. Transient hyperthyroidism
C. Acute renal failure secondary to postnatal fluid shifts
D. Superior vena cava (SVC) syndrome secondary to an enlarged thymus
E. Swallowing difficulty requiring special feed-ing nipples

87. An infant is delivered vaginally in the ED at a local county hospital. Prenatal care for the mother has been limited. The infant is macro-somic, but a thorough physical examination demonstrates no other abnormalities. The admitting nursery labs reveal a glucose of 40 at 2 hours of life. The blood sugar continues to decrease and ultimately an IV line with dex-trose is started. Of the following, what is the most likely laboratory abnormality that you might expect to encounter in this infant over the next few days?

A. Hypermagnesemia
B. Hypocalcemia
C. Elevated transaminases
D. Anemia
E. Elevated creatinine

88. A husband and wife are happy to learn that they are having fraternal twins. They would like to paint the nursery and ask about the possibility of the sexes. What advice do you give them?

    A. There is a 25% chance that there will be one boy and one girl
    B. There is a 50% chance that there will be two boys
    C. There is a 50% chance that there will be two girls
    D. There is a 50% chance that there will be one boy and one girl
    E. There is a 75% chance that there will be one boy and one girl

89. A 9-year-old girl is noted to have dozens of open and closed comedones on her face, but no inflammatory acne lesions or scars. Which of the following statements is true?

    A. This is not early acne, but rather a nevoid condition
    B. This is early acne and is normal in a 9-year-old girl
    C. This girl will go on to severe, scarring acne
    D. This is indicative of androgen excess, requiring further evaluation
    E. This would be more likely to happen in a boy than a girl

90. A 3000-g female is born at 38 weeks GA to a 19y G_1P_0 mother. The prenatal labs are all normal, except that the mother is positive for group B *Streptococcus* (GBS). It was a precipitous delivery, so the mother did not receive her GBS prophylaxis until just before the delivery. The baby's physical examination is normal. The most appropriate next step in management would be:

    A. Lumbar puncture
    B. Chest x-ray
    C. Observation for 48 hours
    D. CBC and blood culture
    E. Empiric IV antibiotics for 72 hours

91. An infant is crawling around on the floor of his home. Suddenly, he starts coughing and then becomes cyanotic. The next best step in responding to this witnessed event is:

    A. Call 911
    B. Abdominal thrusts
    C. Perform a blind finger sweep of his throat to search for and remove an aspirated foreign body

    D. Mouth-to-mouth resuscitation
    E. Back blows followed by chest thrusts

92. A 7-year-old boy is referred to you because he was found to have protein in his urine during an evaluation for vague abdominal pain. The pain resolved after treatment for his constipation, but the proteinuria has persisted. A urinalysis on a morning specimen at the referring office had a proteinuria of 2+, no hematuria, specific gravity 1.024. You check another urine in your office and find a 1+ reaction on dipstick, and again the urine is otherwise normal. His blood pressure was normal. Your next step in helping to identify significant proteinuria would be:

    A. IV urogram
    B. 24-hour urine containing greater than 2 g of protein
    C. A random urine with a protein/creatinine ratio greater than 0.2
    D. Ultrasound examination of the kidneys
    E. Serum BUN, creatinine, and albumin

93. Your patient is a 3-week-old African-American boy with a normal prenatal history. He was born at term with a birth weight at the 50th percentile. His newborn examination was normal. He now presents with a 4-day history of difficulty feeding with evidence of dyspnea and decreased urine output. He is afebrile but lethargic with skin pallor most notable in the lower extremities. Auscultation of his heart reveals a gallop rhythm; peripheral pulses are absent in the feet. The most likely cause of his current symptoms is:

    A. Bacterial sepsis
    B. Congenital viral infection
    C. Cardiogenic shock
    D. Sickle cell anemia
    E. Pneumonia

94. A 12-month-old boy is brought to your clinic because he is refusing to walk. His mother states that he began walking at 10 months of age, and has been doing well until this point. His vital signs are remarkable for a temperature of 39.2°C and a physical examination that reveals a moderately ill infant, with an externally rotated, left hip with limitation to passive and active motion. The most likely causative organism for this illness is:

A. *Neisseria gonorrhoeae*
B. Adenovirus
C. *Staphylococcus aureus*
D. Group A *Streptococcus*
E. Group B *Streptococcus*

95. During the course of your physical examination, it is noted that this 9-month-old infant strenuously objects to occlusion of the right eye, but allows occlusion of the left eye. The child tracks small toys with the right eye, but does not even follow a large toy with the left eye. The child was born after 38 weeks gestation. The pupils are equal and reactive, and the red reflex is symmetrical. The reflection of a penlight is centered on both pupils. The conjunctiva is quiet. The most likely diagnosis is:

A. Iritis
B. Strabismus
C. Phlyctenulosis
D. Amblyopia
E. Retinopathy of prematurity

96. A 7-month-old Caucasian female presents to your clinic for evaluation of failure to thrive. She was term at birth and weighed 7 lbs 3 oz. She initially gained weight well and was breastfed exclusively, but around 3 months began to lose percentiles on the weight and growth curves. She has been developing normally. Her parents also report a history of constipation since she was 2 months old. She stools every 3 to 4 days and they are firm, round balls. Parents intermittently use glycerin suppositories. She passed meconium in the first 24 hours of birth. They deny any polyuria. She is normotensive on exam. You obtain routine screening blood work that reveals a metabolic alkalosis. Her renal function, electrolytes, magnesium, and hepatic panel are otherwise normal with a decreased serum albumin of 2.8. The most likely diagnosis is:

A. Bartter syndrome
B. Cystic fibrosis

C. Gitelman syndrome
D. Renal tubular acidosis
E. Celiac disease

97. A 9-month-old female presents to your office for a routine well-child exam. During the physical examination, you notice a shortened fourth metacarpal, webbing of the neck and a II/VI systolic ejection murmur best heard at the left interscapular area. You suspect possible Turner syndrome. An echocardiogram is performed revealing which of the following cardiac defects?

A. Ventricular septal defect (VSD)
B. Atrial septal defect (ASD)
C. Coarctation of the aorta
D. Pulmonic valve stenosis
E. Mitral valve prolapse

The response options for items 98 to 100 are the same. You will be required to select one answer for each item in the set.

A. Randomized controlled trial
B. Cross-sectional survey
C. Longitudinal cohort study
D. Case control study
E. Meta-analysis

For each purpose description, select the most appropriate type of study.

98. Which primary study design is generally most useful in identifying the prognosis of a disease, such as breast cancer, picked up at an early stage?

99. Which primary study design would be most useful for testing the efficacy of a new drug treatment?

100. Which primary study design would be most useful in demonstrating whether a new diagnostic test is valid?

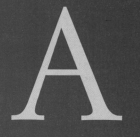

A Answers and Explanations

51. H	68. E	85. D
52. A	69. B	86. A
53. D	70. A	87. B
54. C	71. D	88. D
55. B	72. H	89. B
56. C	73. B	90. D
57. B	74. E	91. E
58. E	75. B	92. C
59. D	76. B	93. C
60. D	77. C	94. C
61. B	78. C	95. D
62. C	79. A	96. B
63. C	80. D	97. C
64. A	81. C	98. C
65. C	82. C	99. A
66. D	83. C	100. B
67. A	84. A	

51. H. IVIG 2 g/kg and aspirin (80–100 mg/kg/day). Patients with acute Kawasaki disease should be treated with IVIG and high-dose aspirin (80–100 mg/kg/day) as soon as the diagnosis is made, to help prevent the development of coronary artery aneurysms. The mechanism of action for IVIG is unknown. Treatment with IVIG and aspirin within the first 10 days of the illness reduces the prevalence of coronary disease to 2% to 4%.

A. The use of prednisone is controversial in the treatment of Kawasaki disease. Most patients are not treated with prednisone.
B. IV nafcillin can be used to treat toxic shock syndrome (TSS) caused by *Staphylococcus*
C, E. See explanation for H.
D. This patient is quite ill with Kawasaki disease. As rapid intervention as possible is important to prevent the development of coronary aneurysms. Observation is inappropriate.
F. While aspirin is part of the appropriate therapy, the use of prednisone, as in the explanation for A, is controversial.
G. Although aspirin is part of the appropriate therapy, nafcillin, as in the explanation for B, is used to treat TSS.

52. A. Booster seats are designed for older children weighing between 40 to 80 lbs. Unfortunately, recent studies show that the vast majority of children of the appropriate age do not use them. Without a booster seat, the car's lap and shoulder belts can cause abdominal and neck injuries in a crash. Compared to regular adult seat belts, booster seats decrease injuries in auto crashes by about 50%.

B. Adult lap and shoulder belts are not appropriate for children. When parents place the shoulder belt behind the child to keep the belt off the neck, children can slip out of the seat and be ejected from the car in a crash.
C. Because the safest place in the car is the back seat, children should be placed in the front seat only if no space is available in the back.
D. Children should NEVER be placed in front of an airbag. Even in a minor crash, the explosive force of the airbag can kill a child.
E. Until a child is over 12 months AND over 20 lbs, he or she should be transported in a reclined, rear-facing, infant seat that is placed in the back seat. The reclined position is necessary to provide adequate support for an infant's head and neck. When a child is over 12 months and 20 lbs, he or she graduates to a forward-facing child seat that is placed in the upright position in the back seat of the car.

53. D. Hypocalcemia commonly accompanies rhabdomyolysis, usually caused by the associated hyperphosphatemia that decreases the release of calcium from bone.

A. Hypocalcemia, not hypercalcemia, commonly accompanies rhabdomyolysis, usually caused by the associated hyperphosphatemia.
B. Hyperphosphatemia, not hypophosphatemia, frequently accompanies rhabdomyolysis secondary to the release of intracellular phosphorus into the extracellular fluid.
C. Hyponatremia is not a part of rhabdomyolysis, although it may result from the associated water retention in acute oliguric renal failure.
E. Hyperkalemia, not hypokalemia, may result from the release of intracellular potassium into the extracellular fluid.

54. C. Early introduction of solid foods may result in the development of food allergies. The early feeding of solids may also interfere with adequate intake of formula. For these reasons, the American Academy of Pediatrics suggests solid baby food not be started until 4 to 6 months of age. Many pediatricians delay the initiation of highly allergenic foods, such as eggs, until the baby is 9 months old or even longer in babies with a strong family history of allergy.

A, B, D, E. These ages are incorrect per the current AAP guidelines.

55. B. Respiratory failure or respiratory arrest is the most common cause of cardiorespiratory arrest in childhood. Recognizing and correcting the respiratory problem will very likely prevent progression to cardiac arrest.

A. Cardiac arrhythmias are unusual in the pediatric age group.
C. Children usually take many fewer drugs than adults. Cardiorespiratory arrest is a very uncommon side effect of most pediatric drugs.

D. Drug ingestions, although common in the pediatric population, uncommonly lead to cardiorespiratory arrest.

E. Children normally have healthy cardiovascular systems. The incidence of congenital heart disease approximates 1% in the pediatric population. Other cardiac conditions, such as myocarditis, may be responsible for arrest in children, but are much less common than respiratory illnesses.

56. **C. The hyperpigmented areas are a phytopho-todermatosis caused by the interaction of the sunlight with the psoralens in the local limes the children were picking and eating. Clues to the diagnosis are that the lesions are located only on sun-exposed areas, and the streaky pattern is consistent with the dripping of the juice.**

A. These lesions are only on sun-exposed areas. The color and pattern of the discolorations are not consistent with the lesions of physical abuse.

B. These lesions are new in onset and the distribution is unusual for neurofibromatosis.

D. Fungal dermatoses are typically annular and scaling.

E. Other areas where sunscreen was applied, such as the arms, face, and legs, would also be affected if the child was having a drug reaction to the sunscreen.

57. **B. Minimal change nephrotic syndrome (also known as idiopathic nephrosis of childhood) is the best answer. About 60% of patients develop nephrotic syndrome between 2 and 6 years of age. It is more common in boys than in girls. The condition is characterized by insidious edema, heavy proteinuria, minimal hematuria, hyperlipidemia, and occasional hypertension. It is not usually associated with renal failure.**

A. Chronic renal failure does not generally **present** with nephrotic syndrome, although nephrosis can occur in the course of chronic renal failure.

C. FSG can present this way, but is far less frequent. FSG accounts for less than 10% of childhood nephrosis and is more often present in the older nephrotic patient. FSG is also often resistant to the standard treatment for idiopathic nephrosis of childhood.

D. Acute glomerulonephritis usually presents with gross hematuria, edema that is not as dependent, and hypertension. On occasion, this may lead to nephrotic syndrome, but this is not an early manifestation of acute glomerulonephritis.

E. Membranous glomerulonephropathy is a cause of nephrotic syndrome in adults and is rare in children before adolescence.

58. **E. Vaginal bleeding is sometimes seen in new-born female infants. It results from withdrawal of estrogen exposure from the mother's bloodstream after delivery.**

A. Hemophilia A is characterized by Factor 8 deficiency, which results in clotting dysfunction and easy bleeding.

B. Child abuse with local trauma could result in vaginal bleeding but would not be a common diagnosis. The most common form of child abuse in infants is shaken baby syndrome.

C. Birth trauma to the vaginal area is unusual and would most likely result in visible bleeding at the time of delivery or shortly after. In addition, a laceration or hematoma might be associated.

D. Hemangioma of the vulva could be susceptible to injury and bleeding. This is uncommon and the hemangioma would be visible on inspection.

59. **D. Ecstasy is a synthetic compound with effects similar to amphetamines and has mild hallucinogenic properties. It would be expected to cause a hyperadrenergic state resulting in tachycardia and hyperthermia.**

A. Narcotics and opiates would be expected to cause a hypoadrenergic state.

B. Most opioids affect the Mμ receptors and result in altered mental status, pinpoint pupils, and respiratory depression.

C. Rotary nystagmus is a classic ocular finding in the setting of PCP intoxication.

E. Miotic or pinpoint pupils would be expected following a narcotic or opiate ingestion. Given its amphetamine-like properties, mydriatic, or dilated pupils, would not be expected following ecstasy ingestion.

60. **D.** Pyloric stenosis is a condition in which hypertrophy of the pylorus causes projectile (nonbilious) vomiting, decreased stool frequency, dehydration, and metabolic alkalosis. Occasionally it can be accompanied by jaundice. Pyloric stenosis usually occurs between 3 and 8 weeks of age and is four times more common in boys than in girls. A palpable "olive" may be felt in the midabdomen. Gastric peristaltic waves can be seen through the abdominal wall, shortly after eating. Hypochloremic alkalosis is typical. The diagnosis can be made by abdominal ultrasound.

   A. Acute gastroenteritis is usually associated with diarrhea.
   B. Duodenal atresia can cause vomiting, jaundice, and visible peristaltic waves. The vomitus is classically bilious, and the emesis is noted in the first day or two of life. Abdominal x-ray typically demonstrates the "double bubble" sign.
   C. UTIs can cause vomiting, dehydration, and jaundice in a small baby. Gastric peristaltic waves would not be seen.
   E. Milk allergy is often associated with diarrhea or bloody stools. Though not impossible, milk allergy is quite unusual in a breastfed baby. This condition is not associated with jaundice.

61. **B.** Postinflammatory hyperpigmentation is the most likely cause of these hyperpigmented lesions. These are most likely a result of scratching her mosquito bites.

   A. The lesions in impetigo are typically erythematous macules, with vesicles or bullae that release cloudy, yellow fluid and form a golden, thick crust.
   C. The lesions are not purpuric. Other symptoms of HSP, such as abdominal pain or arthritis, are not present.
   D. The lesions are not scaly or pruritic as seen in eczema.
   E. Tinea corporis lesions would be scaly and annular with a central clearing.

62. **C.** Migratory arthritis occurs in about 75% of patients with rheumatic fever. It typically involves the large joints and responds dramatically to salicylates. This patient meets the Jones Criteria with one major criteria—migratory polyarthritis—and three minor criteria—elevated ASO titer, ESR, and fever.

   A. Arthritis in patients with SLE commonly involves the small joints of the hands, wrists, elbows, shoulders, knees, and ankles and can be migratory. Joint pain is often severe, with minimal objective findings. Patients with SLE almost always have a positive ANA. SLE is a multisystem disease that can result in nephritis, hypertension, oral ulcerations, pleuritis, and pericarditis.
   B. Patients with JRA have swollen and warm joints that are painful with active motion. There are three particular types of JRA: pauciarticular, polyarticular, and systemic. Systemic disease often presents with constitutional symptoms of fatigue and weight loss. An elevated ASO titer is not associated with JRA.
   D. Gonococcal arthritis is usually monoarticular. The joint is red, warm, and swollen. The knee is the most commonly involved joint. Gonococcal arthritis is more typically found in the adolescent or sexually active population.
   E. Arthritis in Lyme disease is a late finding. It typically affects larger joints. There is no history of preceding erythema migrans or tick bite in this case.

63. **C.** Sensitivity is the percentage of diseased patients who have a positive test. Specificity is the percentage of patients without disease who have a negative test. In this example, 16% of the tested patients will have a true positive test. These are the patients with Disease X who have a positive test (80% sensitivity × 20% prevalence = 16%). In this example, 64% of the patients tested will have a true negative test. These are the healthy patients with a negative test (80% specificity × 80% healthy patients). The result is that 16% of the patients tested will have a false positive test. These are the healthy patients with a positive test (80% − 64% = 16%). The number of true positives (16%) is the same as the number of false positives (16%); therefore, only half of the patients with a positive test have Disease X. In this example, a positive test has a predictive value of 50%. In other words, only half of the patients with a positive test actually have Disease X. See Table 3-63.

   A, B, D, E. These answers are incorrect. See explanation for C.

■ **TABLE 3-63** Disease X Test Results		
	Disease	**Healthy**
Positive test	16% (true positive)	16% (false positive)	50% (+) predictive value
Negative test	4% (false negative)	64% (true negative)	94% (–) predictive value
	20% prevalence	80% healthy	

64. **A. There is a significant acidosis as would be expected in dehydration. The loss of bicarbonate in the stools stimulates renal tubular reabsorption of chloride, resulting in hyperchloremia. The unmeasured anions (anion gap) $Na^+ - (CL^- + CO_2)$ is elevated at 19, likely because of the serum ketones, which are anions. The elevated BUN is prerenal and expected in moderate to severe dehydration.**

   B. This would be the most likely finding if there were no ketosis and a normal anion gap. Diarrheal dehydration is always a nonanion gap acidosis (hyperchloremic) because of the bicarbonate wasting and increased renal tubular chloride reabsorption. A normal anion gap $Na^+ + (CL^- + CO_2)$ is less than 15.

   C. There is no acidosis here, which would be expected with severe diarrheal dehydration.

   D. Hypochloremia without acidosis would not be consistent with diarrheal dehydration.

   E. This picture of severe acidosis and a very large anion gap, with evidence of renal failure, is more typical of uremic acidosis, which is secondary to the retention of mineral and organic acids.

65. **C. Congenital infection is the best choice since all of the others cause indirect hyperbilirubinemia. This infant has a direct hyperbilirubinemia, which is defined as a direct fraction above 15% to 20% of the total bilirubin (when total bilirubin is above 2.0 mg/dL). This infant has either significant biliary obstruction or hepatobiliary disease. Congenital infections such as toxoplasmosis, CMV, syphilis, herpes, and rubella are all considerations. Other possibilities include biliary atresia, tyrosinemia, galactosemia, cystic fibrosis, and alpha$_1$-antitrypsin deficiency.**

   A. Breast-milk jaundice causes *indirect* hyperbilirubinemia secondary to a suspected inhibition of glucuronyl transferase. It is generally benign with total bilirubin reaching as high as 10 to 30 mg/dL during the second or third week of life.

   B. Gilbert syndrome causes indirect hyperbilirubinemia secondary to genetically low levels of bilirubin glucuronyl transferase, and is generally benign.

   D. Congenital spherocytosis causes indirect hyperbilirubinemia because of hemolysis. A combination of MCHC over 35.0 and an RDW over 14.5 is almost pathognomonic of congenital spherocytosis. Patients may have severe jaundice in infancy and may develop gallstones later in life. Cholecystectomy or splenectomy may be required in some cases.

   E. Crigler-Najjar syndrome is a genetic deficiency of bilirubin glucuronyl transferase activity. This syndrome produces very high levels of indirect hyperbilirubinemia and is associated with serious neurologic consequences including self-mutilation behaviors.

66. **D. The prognosis in polyarticular JRA is generally good. Only about 10% to 15% of children with polyarticular JRA will ultimately develop severe disabling disease.**

   A. Rheumatoid factor is rarely positive in early-onset JRA. Rheumatoid factor–positive patients are generally much older (late childhood and adolescence) and their clinical course resembles the adult disease.

   B. Polyarticular JRA has a 9:1 female predominance.

   C. ANA is positive in about 25% of cases of polyarticular JRA. In addition, lupus must still be a diagnostic consideration in patients with these symptoms.

   E. Chronic iridocyclitis occurs in 50% of pauciarticular JRA, and acute iridocyclitis occurs in 5% to 10% of cases of pauciarticular JRA with spondylitis. This problem is not generally seen with polyarticular JRA.

67. **A. The Barlow maneuver is performed by flexing and abducting the hip and applying a posterior force in an effort to dislocate an unstable hip.**

B. In performing the Ortolani maneuver, an attempt is made to reduce a dislocated hip by flexing and abducting the hip and applying anterior force behind the acetabulum.

C. In infants with developmental hip dysplasia, 30% to 40% are breech deliveries.

D. In developmental hip dysplasia there is a 9:1 **female** predominance.

E. In the Ortolani test, there is a "clunk" when a dislocated hip is reduced. This is not to be confused with a "click." Clicks are common and not usually pathologic, and are secondary to soft tissue or tendinous motion.

68. **E. An infant with microcytic anemia and a normal RDW is highly suspicious of β thalassemia trait, especially if the mother is of Greek ancestry. The hemoglobin electrophoresis will demonstrate a high hemoglobin α_2 globin, and many will also have elevated HB F.**

A. A 1-year-old infant should have a hemoglobin above 12 g/dL.

B. Although the feeding history could be false, there would seem to be no reason for the mother to be untruthful. It is unlikely that the child could become iron deficient due to the diet unless he had been consuming large amounts of cow's milk. A high RDW is more suggestive of iron deficiency.

C. A reticulocyte count at 1 year should be less than 1%. If the reticulocyte count is corrected for the anemia, the corrected value would be very close to 1%. To correct for the anemia, multiply the actual value times the actual hemoglobin divided by a normal hemoglobin, that is, 1.5% × (9.9/13) = 1.1%.

D. Blood loss as a cause of iron deficiency anemia should result in a high RDW. This can occur without overt or gross bleeding, especially in cow's milk enteropathy. The dietary history and the normal RDW rule against this.

69. **B. A catheterized urine culture, which grows a significant number of a single pathogenic organism, is the best test. A catheterized urine should normally contain no organisms, but, allowing for some contamination, a few organisms (perhaps fewer than 1000) might grow out of a catheterized urine.**

A. Pyuria is a consistent feature of UTIs, especially those that are symptomatic. However, some pyuria, up to 20 to 30 WBCs/HPF in an uncentrifuged urine, may be seen in febrile and dehydrated infants and children without UTIs.

C. Flank pain and tenderness in this febrile patient are certainly suggestive of UTI, but urinary calculus might also produce the same symptoms.

D. A midstream urine sample would be difficult to obtain without contamination in a sick 2-year-old, especially if you want to institute treatment before receiving the culture result. In older, toilet-trained children, a midstream specimen containing greater than 10^5 of a single organism is usually confirmatory, but not as good as a catheterized urine.

E. The positive predictive value (PPV) of having a UTI is good if both the nitrite and leukocyte esterase tests are positive (greater than 90%). This PPV is still not as good as a catheterized urine culture, which is close to 100%.

70. **A. Hashimoto thyroiditis is the most common form of thyroiditis and hypothyroidism. This is an autoimmune disorder. The antibodies in Hashimoto thyroiditis include thyroid peroxides (previously referred to as antimicrosomal), and antithyroglobulin antibodies. The most common manifestations include growth retardation (predominantly in stature) and goiter. It is found more frequently in girls than boys.**

B. Although multiple family members may be iodine deficient, this is more likely in Third World countries. Iodine supplementation would be the recommended treatment, rather than thyroid hormone.

C. Thyroid adenomas are uncommon in children. They can present with a rapidly growing thyroid mass. The majority of patients with adenomas are found to have normal thyroid function tests.

D. This patient did not have focal neurologic symptoms, headaches, or visual disturbances, which would be suggestive of a CNS etiology.

E. TRH and TSH deficiencies are tertiary and secondary causes of thyroid failure, and are less common than primary hypothyroidism.

71. **D. TSH is the most sensitive indicator of thyroid function in patients with primary hypothyroidism. It is the first indicator of thyroid**

hormone changes. The thyroid gland is maintained by a negative feedback loop that consists of TRH released from the hypothalamus in response to low serum thyroid hormone levels. TRH stimulates the anterior pituitary to produce and release TSH. TSH then stimulates thyroid hormone release mostly in the form of T_4. T_4 is converted peripherally to its more active form, T_3. Increased thyroid hormone levels feed back to the hypothalamus and pituitary, decreasing the serum TSH level. TSH is the first hormone to appear in the serum, indicating a change in thyroid hormone status and thus T_4, T_3, and TRH levels are less sensitive indicators.

A, B, C. See explanation for D.
E. ACTH or adrenocorticotropin is secreted from the anterior pituitary gland and acts on the adrenal gland to help regulate the synthesis of and secretion of cortico steroids and mineralocorticoids from the adrenal cortex.

72. H. Burkitt lymphoma, nasopharyngeal carcinoma, and Hodgkin disease. EBV was the first human virus to be associated with malignancy. Burkitt lymphoma is associated with EBV infection in children from equatorial East Africa and New Guinea. EBV increases the risk of Hodgkin disease by a factor of 2 to 4. It is associated with more than 50% of cases of mixed-cellularity Hodgkin disease. In southern China, nasopharyngeal carcinoma is the most common malignant tumor among adult men. Patients with this tumor have been found to have high titers of EBV.

A, B. Burkitt lymphoma and nasopharyngeal carcinoma are associated with EBV, but so is Hodgkin disease, making H the correct answer.
C. Acute lymphocytic leukemia has not been shown to be associated with EBV.
D. This is only partially correct. See explanation for H.
E. Burkitt lymphoma has been shown to be associated with EBV, but acute lymphocytic leukemia has not.
F. Burkitt lymphoma and nasopharyngeal carcinoma have been shown to be associated with EBV, but acute lymphocytic leukemia has not.
G. Burkitt lymphoma and Hodgkin disease have been shown to be associated with EBV, but acute lymphocytic leukemia has not.
I. This is only partially correct. See explanation for H.

73. B. Midcycle breakthrough bleeding is very common when initiating OCPs, particularly during the first 3 months. Pregnancy must always be considered, but the patient had a negative urine pregnancy test and is not sexually active.

A. If she stops her OCPs, her bleeding will increase.
C. Throwing away her current pills and restarting a new pack is not useful.
D. Since her vaginal bleeding is light, it is unnecessary to take multiple pills daily for several days to decrease bleeding; this method would be helpful to control heavy vaginal bleeding.
E. A different OCP could be considered if breakthrough bleeding continues for more than 2 to 3 months. However, at this point it will be helpful to allow her body to adjust to the new pill.

74. E. Osgood-Schlatter disease is painful enlargement of the tibial tubercle at the insertion of the patellar tendon. It is common in active, adolescent males during periods of rapid linear growth. Unilateral involvement is more common than bilateral involvement. The knee should have a normal range of motion.

A. Patellofemoral syndrome, or patellar malalignment syndrome, is a very common cause of knee pain in adolescents. The pain is characterized by a peri- or retropatellar location and is related to activity. Pain is worse with ascending or descending stairs. It is the result of abnormal biomechanical forces across the patella. A weakened quadriceps femoris muscle or a high-riding patella can result in these abnormal forces.
B. SCFE is seen in adolescents who are overweight, causing a chronic gradual slip of the epiphyseal plate. Pain is usually localized to the hip or groin and a limp can occur. Knee pain may be present secondary to obturator nerve referral.
C. Subluxation of the patella occurs when there is instability of the patellofemoral joint. Episodes occur while the quadriceps is contracting with the knee in flexion and the foot is fixed to the ground. There is pain at the patella with the feeling of the knee giving way.

D. Osteochondritis dissecans is a focal avascular necrosis in which bone and overlying articular cartilage separate from the medial femoral condyle or, less commonly, the lateral femoral condyle. The patient may walk with the tibia in external rotation on the affected side. Localized tenderness over the femoral condyles with the knee in 90-degree flexion is common.

75. **B. Anti-double-stranded DNA is specific for lupus and reflects the degree of disease activity.**

A. ANA is positive in the majority of patients with SLE, but patients can have a positive ANA in the absence of disease.
C. Complement levels of both C3 and C4 are typically low during an acute SLE flare, but they are not specific for SLE.
D. Anti Ro can be seen in patients with neonatal lupus and Sjögren syndrome.
E. Antihistone Ab is commonly seen in patients with drug-induced lupus, including with drugs such as procainamide and hydralazine.

76. **B. SMR 2 for breast development includes the findings described in this patient.**

A. SMR 1 is prepubertal.
C. In SMR 3, the entire breast is enlarged with no protrusion of the papilla or nipple.
D. SMR 4 has enlargement of the breast and projection of areola and papilla as a secondary mound.
E. SMR 5 has enlargement of the breast with protrusion of the nipple. The areola no longer projects separately from the remainder of the breast.

77. **C. This patient has PID caused by *Chlamydia trachomatis*. PID presents with fever, abdominal pain, and vaginal discharge in patients with high-risk sexual behavior. Gonorrhea can also cause this clinical picture. None of the other organisms listed lead to systemic illness with fever and significant abdominal pain.**

A. *Trichomonas vaginalis* is a flagellated protozoan that is sexually transmitted and causes pruritus, frothy green vaginal discharge, and dyspareunia.
B. *Candida albicans* causes about 85% of cases of vulvovaginal candidiasis. Patients present with intense burning and pruritus and a milky white vaginal discharge that has no odor.

D. *Treponema pallidum* causes syphilis, which can present with nonpainful ulcers in the genital area.
E. *Gardnerella vaginalis* causes bacterial vaginosis, which is diagnosed microscopically with clue cells and with a positive whiff test (amine is produced when vaginal discharge is tested with KOH). Patients typically have a grayish white, thin vaginal discharge sometimes with a fish odor.
F. Herpes simplex presents with vesicular genital lesions on an erythematous base that are painful, and tender inguinal lymphadenopathy. Primary infections can cause low-grade fever and myalgias.
G. HPV is a sexually transmitted virus responsible for causing genital warts. These can be small, flat-topped warts 1 to 4 mm in diameter to sessile growths with a pebble-like surface. HPV infection can lead to malignant changes in the cervix, vulva, and penis.

78. **C. Hyperpigmented macules in the axilla are pathognomonic for segmental neurofibromatosis. This is a rare form of neurofibromatosis in which genetic transmission has not been documented and is characterized by café au lait spots and/or neurofibromas limited to one dermatome.**

A. The lesions are larger and not rough or raised, like those of a contact dermatitis.
B. A heat rash is papulovesicular and usually pruritic.
D. Hydradenitis is papulopustular and tender.
E. This is not a sun-exposed area, as is necessary for a photodermatitis.

79. **A. In an infant, the femoral or brachial arteries are the easiest places to accurately palpate for a pulse.**

B, C, D, E. The other arteries listed (carotid, radial, dorsalis pedis, and posterior tibial) are too small or too difficult to palpate in a compromised child. Attempting to determine whether or not a pulse is present may result in an incorrect decision, if these smaller arteries are used.

80. **D. Minimal microscopic hematuria without proteinuria is generally benign. The condition of familial benign essential hematuria is frequently**

an autosomal-dominant condition, more often passed on by the mother and occasionally by the father. The parents' urine should be checked, and if microscopic hematuria is found, no further investigation is necessary. However, if the parents' urines are negative, further investigation may be warranted.

A. Measurement of the glomerular filtration rate would not be helpful. Any significant nephritis would be accompanied by significant proteinuria.

B. Renal ultrasound would be the second preferred test. This would rule out any occult tumor or significant urologic abnormality.

C. A hearing test might be justified if there is any family history of deafness or kidney disease. Alport syndrome (familial nephritis with deafness) may present with microscopic hematuria. However, virtually all cases of Alport syndrome in males will have significant proteinuria. In female carriers, the presentation may mimic benign hematuria.

E. Serum BUN and creatinine elevation are late manifestations of chronic renal disease, not a likely problem without significant proteinuria.

81. **C. Ultraviolet light still penetrates through the cloud layer and causes sunburns.**

A. Sunblock needs to be reapplied every few hours and after swimming to be effective.

B. Sun avoidance is the most important method of sun injury prevention.

D. From 11 AM until 3 PM are the hours of most intense sunlight, and exposure during these hours should be avoided.

E. Sun exposure before age 19 years is the most important risk factor for skin cancer occurring in the adult years.

82. **C. Hepatitis C may present with vague symptoms of fatigue, minimal or no elevation of AST/ALT, or absence of symptoms early in the disease. Risk factors for contracting hepatitis C include sharing IV needles, tattoos and body piercing, blood transfusions, solid organ transplantation, and any blood contact. This patient has two tattoos as a risk factor.**

A. Hepatitis A presents acutely with jaundice, hepatomegaly, nausea/emesis, and fatigue and is fecally/orally transmitted.

B. Hepatitis B can present acutely with hepatomegaly, jaundice, and AST/ALT elevation in the thousands or may also be more subacute. It can be transmitted via sexual contact, IV needles, blood transfusions, and vertically during birth.

D. Hepatocellular carcinoma is a complication of long-term hepatitis B and C infections and presents with fatigue, weight loss, and elevated AFP. Presentation during adolescence is uncommon.

E. With a normal GGT and total bilirubin, cholelithiasis is unlikely and there is no history of right upper quadrant pain following meals with high fat content.

83. **C. The AAP suggests that babies be fed formula containing iron until 12 months of age. Whole cow's milk contains inadequate amounts of iron. It also causes a small amount of chronic blood loss from the GI tract. Babies fed large amounts of whole cow's milk at a young age are prone to the development of iron deficiency anemia, as are older children if milk consumption exceeds 24 to 32 oz/day.**

A, B, D, E. These ages are incorrect per the current AAP guidelines. See explanation for C.

84. **A. Chest pain is a common complaint in children and adolescents, although cardiovascular etiologies comprise only 5%. The three most common causes of chest pain in children are costochondritis, musculoskeletal trauma, and cough (related to asthma or pneumonia). Psychogenic factors and GI disturbances are also relatively common causes of chest pain. Cardiovascular causes are rare and may include ischemic ventricular dysfunction, pericardial or myocardial inflammation, and arrhythmias.**

B, C, D, E. These percentages are incorrect. See explanation for A.

85. **D. This child has a brachial plexus injury. Brachial plexus injuries are seen following trauma to these nerves (fifth cervical to first thoracic) during delivery. They are often seen in macrosomic infants and infants presenting with shoulder dystocia.**

A. IVH is more commonly seen in premature infants and would not be associated with this type of Erb's palsy.

B. Hypoxic events should not result in this type of focal deficit with a preserved grasp.

C. Gestational diabetes could cause the macrosomia in this infant, but would not result in peripheral neuropathies directly.

E. Congenital syphilis would not be associated with this type of neurologic deficit.

86. **A. As stated in the case vignette, the chromosomal defect in Shprintzen syndrome and DiGeorge syndrome are in the same region. The presentations of the two syndromes may overlap. Neonatal hypocalcemia is common in the DiGeorge syndrome, due to thymic and parathyroid hypoplasia. Likewise, hypocalcemia may also occur in the neonatal period in those patients with Shprintzen syndrome. Learning disabilities are common later in life.**

B. Hyperthyroidism is not associated with these syndromes.

C. Fluid shifts are not associated with these syndromes.

D. Hypoplasia, not hyperplasia, of the thymus is seen.

E. Difficulty swallowing is a problem with some types of clefts, but bifid uvula is not associated with feeding difficulties. Although a bifid uvula is associated with many syndromes, it may also be an isolated finding without associated genetic syndromes.

87. **B. One of the most common causes of hypoglycemia in a macrosomic neonate is a diabetic mother. This mother most likely has gestational diabetes that was undetected and untreated due to her lack of prenatal care. Hypocalcemia and hypomagnesemia are common in the infants of diabetic mothers and must be considered in a lethargic, jittery, or sick infant. Routinely monitoring these labs is not recommended in an asymptomatic infant.**

A. Hypomagnesemia, rather than hypermagnesemia, would be expected.

C, D, E. Elevated transaminases, anemia, or elevated creatinine would not be expected in this infant.

88. **D. Unlike monozygotic or "identical twins," fraternal or dizygotic twins are the result of fertilization and implantation of two separate ova.**

Therefore, there is an equal chance for each ova to be a boy or a girl. Therefore, the various possible combinations available result in a 50% chance that there will be one boy and one girl. There is a 25% chance that there will be two boys and a 25% chance that there will be two girls.

A, B, C, E. These percentages are incorrect. See explanation for D.

89. **B. Comedonal acne is common in girls by 7 to 9 years of age.**

A. Open and closed comedones are seen in acne. Nevoid lesions include moles and other melanocytic or nevoid cell lesions.

C. Comedonal acne at this age can correlate with subsequent inflammatory acne, but not necessarily with scarring acne.

D. The acne seen in this child is a normal condition for this age. Further evaluation is not indicated at this time.

E. Acne occurs an average of 2 years later in boys than in girls.

90. **D. Because the duration of intrapartum prophylaxis was less than 4 hours, the AAP recommends a limited evaluation that includes a CBC and blood culture, in addition to 48 hours of observation in the hospital. No other studies are indicated at this time.**

A. A lumbar puncture would be indicated only for signs of neonatal sepsis or proven bacteremia.

B. Without any evidence of respiratory distress or hypoxia, a chest x-ray would not be useful.

C. Although the infant will most likely be observed for 48 hours in this scenario, a CBC and blood culture are recommended as well.

E. Empiric antibiotics should not be started before obtaining relevant cultures.

91. **E. This infant has most likely ingested and aspirated a foreign body. In an infant, the correct method of response to foreign-body aspiration is a series of back blows or chest thrusts.**

A. In children and infants, airway and respiratory support is needed before activating the EMS system—phone fast, not phone first. Quick respiratory support can often maintain or restore circulatory function.

B. Abdominal thrusts are not recommended for use in infants under 1 year of age.

C. Blind finger sweeps are never used in children, as they may push the aspirated object farther into the airway and cause further obstruction.

D. Mouth-to-mouth resuscitation would be used only in the unresponsive infant.

92. **C. A protein-to-creatinine ratio above 0.2 (above 0.5 in infants) would warrant a 24-hour urine collection to more accurately measure the amount of proteinuria. A ratio over 1.0 indicates nephrotic-range proteinuria.**

A. IV urogram would identify gross anatomic abnormalities of the kidneys and collecting system, but would not be helpful in quantifying significant isolated proteinuria.

B. A 24-hour urine protein would be the second test to order if the protein-to-creatinine ratio was elevated. Normal excretion in children is usually less than 150 mg, and levels above 1000 mg/24 hours would be reason for further investigation. Nephrotic syndrome rarely occurs when proteinuria is less than 2000 mg/ 24 hours.

D. Renal ultrasound would identify anatomic renal abnormalities, but would not be helpful in quantifying significant isolated proteinuria.

E. Serum BUN, creatinine, and albumin would be indicated only if the proteinuria was significant or if there was hypertension.

93. **C. This infant has signs and symptoms most consistent with severe coarctation of the aorta with acute cardiogenic shock. Coarctation occurs in 8% to 10% of all congenital heart defects. It is more common in males than in females. Infants may not be symptomatic until the ductus arteriosus closes completely. Differential cyanosis, with the lower half of the body predominantly affected, along with absent or diminished lower extremity pulses and evidence of congestive heart failure are best explained by a critical coarctation.**

A, E. Bacterial sepsis and pneumonia are less likely in the absence of fever, and do not explain the abnormal pulses, differential pallor, and cardiac murmur.

B. Children with a congenital viral infection are less likely to be normal at birth and less likely to have an acute decompensation.

D. Sickle cell anemia can be associated with an acute vascular crisis in the lungs causing respiratory compromise, but it does not usually present in the neonatal period, nor with such significant cardiac symptoms.

94. **C. *Staphylococcus aureus* is the correct answer. *S. aureus* is the most common cause of septic arthritis or septic hip as in this patient's case.**

A. *Neisseria gonorrhea* is a cause of septic arthritis to be considered in the adolescent patient.

B. Adenovirus can cause a toxic synovitis. However, the ill appearance and high temperature of this child are more suggestive of a bacterial infection than the more common, viral-induced toxic synovitis.

D. Group A streptococcal bacteremia can result in septic arthritis in this age group, but is less commonly seen than *Staphylococcus*.

E. Group B streptococcal infection is an important cause of septic arthritis in the neonatal period.

95. **D. Amblyopia is defined as abnormal visual acuity in one or both eyes. In a preliterate/preverbal child, amblyopia presents as poor tracking with the affected eye, and avoidance of occlusion of the better seeing eye. Amblyopia is usually asymptomatic, which stresses the need for continual visual screening, even in young infants.**

A. Iritis presents as a painful, red eye with photophobia.

B. Strabismus is a misalignment of the eyes. When checking the corneal light reflex, the light from a penlight reflects off of asymmetric parts of the eye's surface.

C. An inflamed, red eye with nodules on or near the cornea is typical of phlyctenulosis.

E. Retinopathy of prematurity can be a blinding condition, but does not occur in term infants.

96. **B. Cystic fibrosis can present with metabolic alkalosis, failure to thrive, and constipation without pulmonary symptoms. Cystic fibrosis causes a metabolic alkalosis due to urinary losses of potassium. The hypoalbuminemia is also a marker for malabsorption that is common in cystic fibrosis secondary to pancreatic insufficiency. A sweat chloride test and genetic studies for cystic fibrosis should be obtained to confirm the diagnosis.**

A, C. Both Bartter syndrome and Gitelman syndrome are autosomal recessive disorders that can present with metabolic alkalosis, hypokalemia, and elevated urinary chloride. Patients with Gitelman syndrome also have hypocalciuria and hypomagnesemia.

D. Renal tubular acidosis causes acidosis, not alkalosis.

E. Celiac disease, or gluten-sensitive enteropathy, can present with failure to thrive, hypoalbuminemia, constipation, or diarrhea, but a metabolic alkalosis is not a typically associated feature.

97. **C. Coarctation of the aorta is the most common cardiac defect associated with Turner syndrome. The murmur typically presents as a systolic murmur that is often heard best in the left interscapular area. On physical examination, the femoral pulses may be weak or absent. Elevated blood pressures in the arms compared to the legs may be seen. In 85% of patients with coarctation of the aorta, a bicuspid aortic valve is also present.**

A. A VSD on exam reveals a regurgitant, systolic, often holosystolic, grade II to V/VI blowing murmur heard best at the lower left sternal border.

B. An ASD on exam reveals a widely split and fixed S2 with a systolic ejection murmur, grade II/VI, often heard best at the upper left sternal border.

D. Pulmonic stenosis reveals a systolic ejection murmur grade II to V/VI with an ejection click at the second left intercostal space.

E. Significant mitral valve prolapse has a midsystolic click with a late systolic murmur.

98. **C. The value of a longitudinal cohort study is its ability to watch a disease process over time. For a question of prognosis, the group of interest is an inception cohort, a group of patients identified as being in the early phase of a disease. The goal is to follow the disease process, looking at morbidity, mortality, disease complications, and other factors.**

A. Randomization is not necessary; treatment effects are not the point of comparison.

B. Cross-sectional studies look at data at a single point in time, and cannot follow disease process to draw conclusions about prognosis.

D. Case-control designs generally compare those with a disease to a group without disease, and are used to look retrospectively for implications about disease etiology.

E. Meta-analysis is not a primary study design, but rather a secondary use of data.

99. **A. In a randomized, controlled trial, participants are randomly allocated to either one intervention or another, for example, placebo versus treatment. Both groups are followed and analyzed in terms of specified outcomes. Because the initial allocation is random, the groups are assumed to be identical apart from the intervention and any differences in outcome are assumed to be due to the intervention.**

B. Cross-sectional studies collect data at a single point in time, and are not used to follow patients to a specified outcome.

C. Longitudinal cohort studies can compare treatment options, but are generally not randomized. Cohorts may not be similar enough to compare outcomes between groups.

D. Case-control studies are used to ask retrospective questions about etiology, and are subject to significant bias in terms of case definition, control definition, and bias in recalling medical history.

E. Meta-analysis can be used to draw conclusions about the efficacy of a new treatment, but it is not a primary study design.

100. **B. The question of validity refers to whether or not we can trust a new diagnostic test, specifically in comparison to the established "gold standard" test. A cross-sectional survey in which both the new test and the gold standard test are applied to the same patient would be most efficient in evaluating the validity of the new test.**

A. Randomization is not necessary; because each subject undergoes exactly the same tests, there are no differences in interventions.

C. Longitudinal data are not necessary in this case, as the data point of interest is only the immediate results of the two tests being compared.

D. There is no need for a control group, as the only important comparison is within each subject.

E. Meta-analysis is not a primary study design, but rather a secondary use of data.

BLOCK 3

101. An 11-year-old boy is seen at your office for growth delay. He has gradually fallen off the growth curve from the 50th percentile to below the 3rd percentile for height over the past 2 to 3 years. His appetite has decreased and he is sleeping more than usual. He has also developed nocturia. His examination, in addition to his growth delay, reveals pallor and a BP of 180/110. He also has enlargement of his wrists and enlargement of the costochondral junctions. Which of the following is most likely to reveal the diagnosis?

    A. Measurement of the 1,20-dihydrocholecalciferol
    B. X-ray of the wrists
    C. Blood count
    D. Serum BUN and creatinine
    E. Serum calcium and phosphorus

102. During his annual physical, a 12-year-old boy with Marfan syndrome informs you that he wants to join one of the school sports teams. His parents are concerned for his health, and want you to make a recommendation. Which of the following choices would be most appropriate for this patient?

    A. Football
    B. Basketball
    C. Weight training
    D. Golf
    E. **Soccer**

103. You are seeing a 6-month-old infant for a well-child visit. Her growth chart is available for review (Figure 3-103). Her head circumference and length are both stable at the 50th percentile line. The mother tells you that she is both breastfeeding the baby and giving her 4 oz of formula in a bottle every 3 hours. On physical examination, you find the baby is happy, but spits up a little after you palpate her abdomen. The rest of the physical examination is normal. The best next step in management is:

    A. Morning cortisol determination
    B. CT of the abdomen, with special attention to the adrenal glands
    C. MRI of the brain, with special attention to the pituitary gland
    D. Advising the mother to stop the extra formula feedings
    E. Hemoglobin A1C determination

104. A 1-month-old girl is brought to the hospital with a history of decreased appetite. When the child is noted to be lethargic and barely responsive to stimulation, a CT scan of the head is performed, which shows multiple areas of intraparenchymal bleeding. A thorough retinal examination confirming shaken baby syndrome would typically show which of the following?

    A. Cherry red spot in the center of a bland, white retina
    B. Thick, white, cotton wool spots scattered about the posterior pole
    C. Midperipheral retina covered with dark, bone-speckled pattern
    D. Dozens of yellow-centered, oval hemorrhages
    E. Large patches of bloody white exudates thickening the choroids and retina

105. You are seeing a 13-month-old child for follow-up in clinic. Her last labs showed a hemoglobin of 9.2 g/dL, with basophilic stippling reported on her smear. You are concerned she may have lead poisoning. Which of the following is the most accurate information to give to her parents?

    A. Skeletal radiographs will be unremarkable
    B. Symptoms may include diarrhea and increased appetite
    C. Sources may include paint chips, soil, water, air, and food
    D. The CDC recommends screening for lead poisoning at age 6 months to 1 year
    E. Immediate chelation therapy will be needed to treat this patient

106. You receive a phone call from a 9-month-old child's mother. She has found a scorpion in his crib and is very concerned that he may have been stung. Which of the following is consistent with a scorpion envenomation?

    A. A necrotic area on the shin
    B. An ecchymotic area on the tip of the right index finger
    C. A rigid abdomen, hypertension, and emesis
    D. Tongue fasciculations, disconjugate eye movements, arching of the back, and hypersalivation
    E. Pinpoint pupils and hypoventilation

107. A 10-year-old child is being seen in your clinic for the evaluation of obesity. His development has been appropriate until this point and no major illnesses have been reported. His body

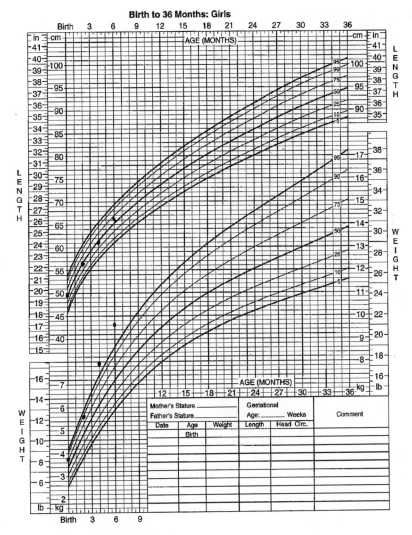

Birth to 36 Months: Girls

Figure 3-103 • Image Courtesy of the Phoenix Children's Hospital, Phoenix, Arizona. Source: Developed by the National Center for Health Statistics in collaboration with the National Center for Chronic Disease Prevention and Health Promotion (2000). http://www.cdc.gov/growthcharts

mass index is 32 kg/m². Which of the following statements is most accurate about obesity and its management?

A. The incidence of obesity is decreasing
B. Associated abnormal physical findings are common
C. Laboratory tests are usually not helpful in confirming the diagnosis
D. Weight reduction programs are unsafe for prepubertal patients
E. Family history is not important

108. A 5-year-old boy was injured after jumping from the monkey bars at school. He has significant pain and swelling over his right lower leg with a normal neurovascular exam. A radiograph is obtained (Figure 3-108). Which of the following best describes this fracture?

A. Salter-Harris type I fracture
B. Salter-Harris type II fracture
C. Salter-Harris type III fracture
D. Salter-Harris type IV fracture
E. Salter-Harris type V fracture

109. A 7-year-old girl presents with complaints of fever, decreased exercise tolerance, and arthralgias. Recent medical history is significant for a culture-proven diagnosis of streptococcal pharyngitis 3 months ago. The girl and her mother are not certain whether she finished the course of

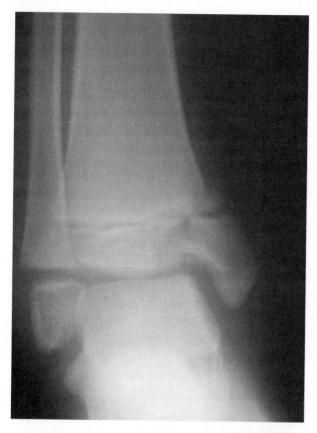

Figure 3-108 • Image Courtesy of the Department of Radiology, Phoenix Children's Hospital, Phoenix, Arizona.

amoxicillin you prescribed; they do remember that she felt better quickly. Physical examination is significant only for a new murmur: a moderately loud, pansystolic, high-pitched murmur that does not change with positioning. Given these findings and her recent history of streptococcal pharyngitis, you entertain a diagnosis of rheumatic heart disease. Which of the following groups of findings would meet criteria for a diagnosis of rheumatic heart disease?

A. Subcutaneous nodules, elevated ANA titers, thrombocytopenia
B. Erythema marginatum and chorea
C. Arthralgias and elevated C-reactive protein
D. Polyarthritis, ESR, anemia
E. Prolonged PR interval on ECG, leukocytosis, and fever

110. A mother is concerned about her 4-month-old infant. She has recently switched from breast milk to formula. Last week, the child developed several dry, scaling lesions on the arms and face.

The lesions are asymmetric with no central clearing, consistent with atopic dermatitis. There is a strong family history of atopic dermatitis. Which statement is true relative to childhood atopic dermatitis?

A. The prevalence of atopic dermatitis is decreasing
B. It is usually caused by dietary protein allergy
C. The condition usually improves by age 5 years
D. Atopic dermatitis is associated with dry skin and flexural lichenification
E. Atopic dermatitis is usually asymptomatic

111. You are caring for a 14-year-old Caucasian girl, who was admitted to the PICU with hypotension, tachycardia, and respiratory failure. Her history consists of 8 months of frequent episodes of nausea, abdominal pain, progressive fatigue, and diffusely increased pigmentation of her skin without tanning. She is thought to have adrenal crisis. What is the most likely cause of the disease in this patient?

A. Histoplasmosis
B. Adrenal hemorrhage
C. Meningococcemia
D. Adrenal tumor
E. Autoimmune adrenalitis

112. A 14-year-old male is being seen for a routine preparticipation sports physical. During his examination, you notice evidence of scoliosis without any other abnormalities. Which of the following is an accurate statement regarding idiopathic scoliosis?

A. Patients with a curve of less than 25 degrees require bracing
B. The incidence is higher in males
C. There is usually no associated significant pain
D. The family history is insignificant
E. MRI is routinely needed for further evaluation

113. A 3-week-old baby is brought to your office because of jaundice. The parents first noticed the color on day 3 of life. The mother is breast-feeding. She is concerned because the baby's stools are very light in color and the urine is darker than normal. The baby is feeding normally and is not acting ill. The total bilirubin level is 8.6 mg/dL with a direct component of 3.2 mg/dL. An abdominal ultrasound shows no gallbladder. The most likely diagnosis is:

A. Prolonged physiologic jaundice
B. Breast-milk jaundice
C. Neonatal hepatitis
D. Biliary atresia
E. Gilbert syndrome

114. A mother brings her 3-day-old baby for a new-born nursery follow-up visit. She is breastfeeding and also giving some supplemental cow's milk formula. Her older child had problems with severe dental decay and she wants to avoid the problem with this baby. The mother also has a history of multiple caries. What advice would you give the mother?

    A. Start fluoride drops
    B. Stop all bottle feeds
    C. Switch to a soy-based formula
    D. Advise the mother to avoid sugary foods, brush often, use fluoride, and see a dentist herself
    E. Suggest that the mother share utensils with baby to promote normal bacterial colonization

115. An infant girl is born with a rather severe talipes equinovarus (clubfoot) deformity of the right foot. Which one of the following is a true statement?

    A. Congenital clubfoot is almost always associated with other congenital abnormalities
    B. Clubfoot typically exhibits mild calf atrophy, with tibial and fibular hypoplasia
    C. Isolated congenital clubfoot is almost never bilateral
    D. There is no familial incidence of clubfoot, and there is no sex preponderance
    E. The deformity of clubfoot (equinovarus) typically shows equinus of the hindfoot, with abduction of the forefoot

116. The most frequent genetic abnormality in Down syndrome is trisomy 21. Which one of the following best describes the embryologic abnormality that causes trisomy syndromes?

    A. A fragment of one chromosome is lost in meiosis
    B. There is a mitotic nondisjunction in one chromosome
    C. A fragment of one chromosome attaches to another chromosome in meiosis
    D. Meiotic nondisjunction occurs in one chromosome
    E. A third chromosome forms in reduction division

117. A 17-year-old female presents to your office with a complaint of a missed period. Menarche occurred at age 13, and her periods have been regular for the last 18 months. She normally bleeds for 4 to 5 days with a moderate flow. Her last menses was 2 months ago. After performing a thorough history and physical examination, what would be the next step in her evaluation?

    A. CBC
    B. Urine β-hCG
    C. Serum quantitative-hCG
    D. LH level
    E. Serum testosterone level

118. You are seeing a 3-year-old child with a history of fatigue, pallor, and weight loss. A previous CBC revealed a hemoglobin of 5.2 g/dL. Repeat labs confirm the anemia with a reticulocyte count of 9% and positive direct Coombs test. The direct antiglobulin (Coombs) test detects:

    A. Antibody circulating in serum directed against RBC membrane proteins
    B. Antibody directed against RBC membrane proteins attached to the RBC
    C. The percentage of circulating fetal hemoglobin
    D. The percentage of RBCs in the circulation that are less than 1 day old
    E. The presence of coexisting SLE

119. A severely dehydrated child with a prolonged history of diarrhea is brought in for evaluation. The child is cyanotic, in distress, bradycardic, and hypotensive. Which one of the following must be present to make the diagnosis of shock?

    A. Only when hypotension is noted on blood pressure measurement
    B. Only when cardiac output is decreased
    C. Only when the child becomes unconscious or has diminished mental alertness
    D. Only when decreased tissue perfusion results in insufficient delivery of oxygen and substrate to meet the metabolic needs of the tissues and end organs
    E. Only when the patient is also bradycardic and cyanotic

120. During the first newborn examination of a full-term infant, you notice a microphallus and poor scrotal fusion. You suspect congenital adrenal hyperplasia (CAH). What study would most likely confirm your diagnosis?

    A. 21-hydroxylase enzyme level
    B. 17α-hydroxyprogesterone
    C. Karyotype
    D. Random cortisol level
    E. Rectal exam

121. A 10-year-old boy presents to clinic for a routine preparticipation sports physical. His height is at the 95th percentile for age; his weight is at the 50th percentile for age. He reports no recent illnesses or unusual symptoms. On physical examination, you hear a distinct systolic ejection murmur. It is loudest at the left lower sternal border and is low-pitched and somewhat musical in nature. Which of the following is the most likely diagnosis?

    A. Aortic valve stenosis
    B. VSD
    C. Vibratory innocent murmur
    D. Pulmonary valve stenosis
    E. ASD

122. It is a typically busy morning in your practice, and several patients have been brought to your office complaining of throat pain. Which of the following patients is most likely to have a streptococcal pharyngitis?

    A. A 6-year-old boy with sore throat, fever, severe cough, and coryza, but no cervical lymphadenopathy or tonsillar exudate
    B. A 4-month-old with poor feeding, fever, and bilateral, white pharyngeal exudates
    C. A 4-year-old girl with fever, conjunctivitis, cough, and mild throat pain
    D. A teenage girl with exudative pharyngitis, fatigue, fever, and splenomegaly
    E. A 7-year-old boy with fever, throat pain, whitish exudate on the tonsils, and anterior cervical adenopathy

123. A 9-month-old, previously healthy child presents for well-child care. On physical examination, she is found to be pale, though not jaundiced. She has no palpable liver or spleen. A CBC demonstrates a hemoglobin of 6.0 g/dL with an MCV of 63. Her WBC count and platelet count are normal for her age. Her reticulocyte count is 0.5%. Her mother has weaned her from breastfeeding to whole cow's milk. The most likely cause of her anemia is:

    A. Autoimmune hemolytic anemia
    B. Hereditary spherocytosis
    C. Iron-deficiency anemia
    D. Pyruvate kinase deficiency
    E. Glucose-6-phosphate dehydrogenase (G6PD) deficiency

124. A 2-year-old boy presents to the ED with right upper quadrant pain, nausea, bruising, lethargy, and mild jaundice. His mother reports that aside from some vomiting 2 days ago, he has been healthy. There is the possibility that he may have accidentally ingested some tablets 3 days ago, but the mother is not sure. Which of the following medications could the child have ingested to account for this clinical picture?

    A. Clonidine
    B. Acetaminophen
    C. Morphine
    D. Diphenhydramine
    E. Amphetamine

125. A 20-month-old toddler with an 8-hour history of difficulty breathing is brought to the ED at 3 AM by his parents. Previously, the child had been perfectly well. After supper, he began having paroxysmal coughing and wheezing. The cough has now subsided considerably, but the wheezing persists. The child was not febrile at home. He has not had any previous similar episodes. He has no siblings and does not go to day care. He has not slept this evening, and refused a bottle of his favorite juice. At triage, the nurse assessed him as a pale child, with a moderately increased work of breathing. On auscultation, the wheezing is heard only over the right chest. His vitals are temperature 37°C, RR 60, pulse 136. The most likely diagnosis is:

    A. Asthma
    B. Cystic fibrosis (CF)
    C. Pneumonia
    D. Foreign body aspiration
    E. Peanut allergy with anaphylaxis

126. A 12-year-old boy arrives at the ER by ambulance. The boy was hit by a car while riding his bicycle. He was not wearing a helmet. He has an

open fracture of his right humerus, and extensive abrasions on his forehead, trunk, and extremities. He is drowsy and keeps his eyes closed, but will open his eyes when asked to look at the light. However, he asks if the exam light is the sun, and believes that he is still outside. He will wiggle his toes when asked to. His Glasgow Coma Scale score is:

A. 15
B. 14
C. 13
D. 8
E. 4

The response options for items 127 to 129 are the same. You will be required to select one answer for each item in the set.

A. Henoch-Schönlein purpura
B. JRA
C. SLE
D. Sarcoidosis
E. Dermatomyositis
F. Kawasaki disease
G. Reiter syndrome

For each patient description, select the most likely rheumatologic disorder.

127. A 12-year-old female presents with symmetric, proximal muscle weakness and fatigue. The physical examination reveals normal DTRs, a violaceous discoloration of the eyelids, with swelling, and shiny, erythematous, scaly plaques over the extensor surfaces of the metacarpophalangeal (MCP) joints bilaterally. Blood work reveals an elevated CPK and aldolase.

128. A 5-year-old boy presents to the ER with abdominal pain and scrotal edema. The parents report that he had a fever with URI symptoms last week but was feeling better this week. The physical examination reveals a discrete, palpable, purple rash over the legs and buttocks. Scrotal edema is noted, but there is no evidence of testicular pain. The abdomen is diffusely tender and the rectal examination reveals Hemoccult-positive stool.

129. A 10-year-old African-American female presents with a nonproductive cough, fatigue, and a 4-lb weight loss in 4 months. The review of systems reveals constipation and polyuria. Routine labs reveal a calcium of 13.5 mg/dL. A chest x-ray demonstrates hilar adenopathy with disseminated, peribronchial infiltrates and multiple small, nodular lesions bilaterally.

End of Set

130. A 5-month-old boy comes to you for follow-up of his poor weight gain. You note that he is a bright and cheerful child, but with persistently poor weight gain and linear growth. Additionally, you note a mild degree of clubbing of his fingers. When getting ready for today's trip to your clinic, the child became agitated and started to turn blue. His mother strapped him into his car seat to hurry to your office and noted that his color improved and he seemed comfortable again. Which of the following diagnoses best explains his particular symptoms?

A. CF
B. Tetralogy of Fallot
C. Hypoplastic left heart syndrome
D. Hirschsprung disease
E. Breath-holding spells

131. A 1-month-old infant, who is otherwise well and asymptomatic, has been brought in because of a rash. The child has inflammatory scalp scale, which has a combination of greasy, yellow, and erythematous features, as well as inflammation of the neck, axillary, and inguinal creases. The most likely diagnosis is:

A. Atopic dermatitis
B. Seborrheic dermatitis
C. Psoriasis
D. Langerhans cell histiocytosis
E. Candidiasis

132. Your attending is quizzing you on the many theories of childhood development by giving you a description and having you name the theory's creator. One theory of cognitive development is based on the idea that cognition is qualitatively different at different stages of development. Children progress through successive stages of cognition labeled sensorimotor, preoperational, concrete operations, and formal operations. You correctly respond that this theory is attributed to:

A. Freud
B. Erikson
C. Piaget
D. Jung
E. Montessori

133. A 5-year-old boy with a known seizure disorder is brought to the ED for evaluation of prolonged hemiparesis following one of his typical focal, right-sided seizures. He has been sick with a cold for 2 days, but has been able to take his usual medicines for seizure control. On physical examination, he is found to be appropriate but drowsy. His neurologic exam is significant for right-sided weakness and a positive Babinski reflex on the right. Over the next 24 hours, his symptoms completely resolve. The most likely diagnosis is:

A. Stroke
B. Todd's paralysis
C. Cerebral tumor
D. Status epilepticus
E. Postviral encephalitis

134. A 16-year-old male is in your clinic for a routine visit. During your discussion, he admits to regular cocaine use for the past 4 months. The review of symptoms reveals that he has been having intermittent episodes of chest and abdominal pain associated with the drug use. He also complains of a funny, tingling feeling in his chest during these episodes. A careful physical examination yields an elevated BP of 145/95. The abdomen is not tense, firm, or distended. There is a regular cardiac rhythm. Which of the following is the most likely complication he is experiencing as a result of his cocaine use/overdose?

A. Myocardial infarction
B. Stroke
C. Infarcted bowel
D. Aortic dissection
E. Coronary spasm

135. A 5-year-old girl is seen in your office with a 2-day history of fever, headache, sore throat, and rash. On physical examination, you notice a mildly ill appearing child with bilateral, shotty, cervical lymphadenopathy, a fine, diffuse maculopapular rash on her chest and arms, and involvement of the oral mucosa (Figure 3-135). The most likely diagnosis is:

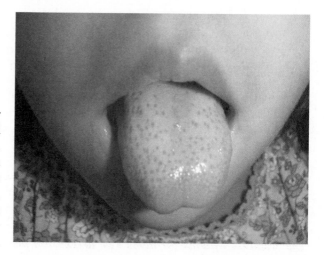

Figure 3-135•Image Courtesy of the Phoenix Children's Hospital, Phoenix, Arizona.

A. Kawasaki disease
B. Roseola
C. Scarlet fever
D. Fifth disease
E. Rubeola (measles)

136. You are asked to counsel a pregnant mother at 32 weeks gestation. The pregnancy has been characterized by poor fetal growth and oligohydramnios. You are most concerned about which of the following?

A. Gastroschisis
B. Neural tube defects
C. Gestational diabetes
D. Renal agenesis and pulmonary hypoplasia
E. Diaphragmatic hernia

137. A 13-year-old female presents to the ER after a syncopal episode. The mother reports that the girl had just gone out to the car and was standing, when she suddenly turned pale and became dizzy. The girl fainted, fell, and sustained a laceration to her forehead. Her parents carried her back into their air-conditioned house and laid her on the couch. She had already regained consciousness by the time they entered the house. Her mother (who is a nurse) noted that her pulse was only 50. When the EMS arrived 10 minutes later, her color was almost back to normal and she was able to walk and talk normally. She had been well prior to the incident. In the ER, her vital signs, physical examination, and ECG are 100% normal. Further questioning

reveals that there is no family history of cardiac sudden death or related problems. Which of the following is the most likely diagnosis?

A. Ventricular tachycardia
B. Vasovagal hypotension
C. Stroke
D. Viral meningitis
E. Attention seeking

138. An 8-year-old girl developed crampy, abdominal pain and loose, watery stools after a Girl Scout camping trip. Several of the other girls are also complaining. On physical examination, she does not appear dehydrated. Her abdomen has very mild, periumbilical tenderness but without guarding or rebound. Examination of the stool is negative for polys and blood. Stool studies are negative for cysts. A duodenal biopsy is performed with the following findings (Figure 3-138). The causative agent for this girl's diarrhea is:

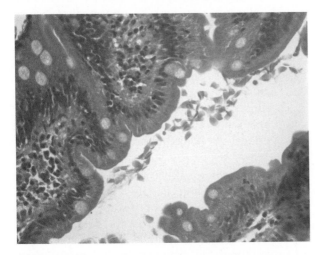

Figure 3-138 • Image Courtesy of the Department of Pathology, Phoenix Children's Hospital, Phoenix, Arizona.

A. Acanthamoeba
B. Amebic dysentery
C. *Vibrio cholera*
D. *Giardia lamblia*
E. *Blastocystis hominis*

139. You are seeing an 11-month-old boy in your clinic. He has been growing and developing normally up to this point, however, his mother is concerned about her child's hand. A picture of the child's hand is shown in Figure 3-139. What is an accurate statement regarding this patient's condition?

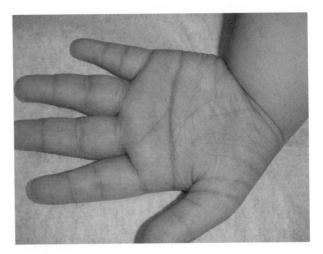

Figure 3-139 • Image Courtesy of the Phoenix Children's Hospital, Phoenix, Arizona.

A. Down syndrome should be suspected
B. Its development occurred during the third trimester
C. A maternal history of cocaine use should be suspected
D. Simple reassurance should be provided
E. A chromosome analysis should be ordered to rule out other chromosomal abnormalities

140. The mother of a 3-month-old girl brings her daughter to your office because of episodes of severe crying that occur at about the same time every day. You suspect that the baby has colic. Which of the following statements about colic is true?

A. It starts at 3 months and peaks at about 6 months of age
B. Almost all cases are due to lactose intolerance
C. The episodes of crying typically occur in the late afternoon or evening
D. Paregoric should generally be prescribed
E. Patients with any degree of abdominal distension should have a CT scan of the abdomen

141. You are the physician for a local high school football team. The coach is about to start summer practices and asks you how to prevent and identify heat stroke. Which of the following statements about heat-related illness is true?

A. Athletes should be offered small amounts of warm fluids to avoid cramps

B. Dehydration is rarely associated with heat stroke

C. Ambient humidity plays no role in the development of heat stroke

D. Heat stroke is usually associated with an altered mental status

E. Antipyretics can minimize body temperature elevations in exercising athletes

142. A 6-month-old African-American infant is in your office for a follow-up visit. His mother is concerned that he may have sickle cell anemia. A previously ordered hemoglobin electrophoresis is available for your review. In interpreting the results, you recall that adult hemoglobin (hemoglobin A) is composed of two α chains and two β chains ($\alpha_2 \beta_2$). Fetal hemoglobin (hemoglobin F) is composed of

A. Four α chains (α_4)

B. Two α chains and two γ chains (α_2, γ_2)

C. Two δ chains and two γ chains (δ_2, γ_2)

D. One α chain and one γ chain

E. One δ chain and one γ chain

143. A 2-year-old boy is seen in your office because of fever, ear pain, and postauricular swelling, erythema, and tenderness. The pinna protrudes out on the involved side. The tympanic membrane is red and bulging, with decreased mobility seen on pneumatic otoscopy. The angle of the jaw is easily palpated and the opening to Stensen's duct appears normal. The patient has never had an MMR vaccine. The most likely diagnosis is

A. Bacterial parotitis

B. Mumps

C. External otitis

D. Acute mastoiditis

E. Chronic mastoiditis

144. A 6-year-old child is being seen in the ER. He has a history of bedwetting for which he has been placed on Imipramine. On physical examination, you notice that he has an irregular heart rate. Which of the following is the most common arrhythmia in tricyclic antidepressant (TCA) toxicity?

A. Ventricular fibrillation

B. Ventricular tachycardia

C. Sinus tachycardia

D. Sinus bradycardia

E. Electrical alternans

The response options for items 145 to 147 are the same. You will be required to select one answer for each item in the set.

A. *H. influenzae*

B. EBV

C. *Bordetella pertussis*

D. Respiratory syncytial virus (RSV)

E. *Streptococcus pyogenes*

For each patient described, select the most likely causative organism.

145. It is January and you are working in the pediatric ED. You are evaluating a 1-month-old female brought in by her mother for cough and poor feeding for 3 days. Her 17-month-old brother has a runny nose and slight fever. She is a full-term baby with no past medical history. On examination, you find she is afebrile and has a pulse oximetry reading of 93% on room air. She is alert and breathing with slight intercostal muscle use. She has obvious nasal congestion and audible upper airway congestion. Her lungs sound diffusely coarse in all lung fields. Her chest x-ray reveals bilateral hyperinflation and perihilar streaking, but no discrete infiltrates.

146. You are seeing a 12-year-old boy in the pediatric ambulatory clinic in late September. He has been complaining of fever, fatigue, poor appetite, and a sore throat for 7 days. Many of his classmates at middle school have similar symptoms. On examination, he appears tired, with a temperature of 38.5°C. His tonsils are bilaterally enlarged with a white exudate and halitosis. The lungs are clear. His abdomen is slightly tender in the LUQ and you feel his spleen 2 cm below the costal margin. His rapid strep test is negative. His CBC reveals an increased WBC count, and the path review note says "reactive lymphocytes present."

147. A 4-month-old Mexican boy is admitted to the hospital for apnea. The parents tell you that he has been sick for 5 days with a slight fever, decreased feeding, and fits of horrible coughing. He will cough out all his air, get red in the face, and stop breathing for 10 to 15 seconds. He often

will vomit a little after one of these spells. He has received no vaccinations. Multiple family members are sick with similar symptoms. On examination, he is found to be afebrile, the oropharynx is normal, and the lungs are clear to auscultation. The chest x-ray has a lot of air in the stomach, but is otherwise normal. The CBC has an increased WBC with an absolute lymphocytosis.

End of Set

148. You are evaluating the developmental progress of an 18-month-old infant in your practice. His mother is concerned that he has only 6 words. Language development occurs most rapidly during which period?

    A. Birth to 6 months
    B. 7 to 12 months
    C. 13 to 18 months
    D. 19 to 24 months
    E. 2 to 5 years

149. A 10-year-old boy is in your office for the evaluation of recurrent headaches. The headaches started 6 months ago and occur about once a month. He is asymptomatic between episodes. Each headache begins with blurry vision and abdominal pain, followed by right-sided, throbbing pain. It lasts about 60 minutes, during which he feels better if he takes some ibuprofen

and rests in a darkened room. The most likely diagnosis is:

    A. Brain tumor
    B. Seizure disorder
    C. Migraine
    D. Todd's paralysis
    E. Heterophoria

150. A 21-month-old boy is admitted to the hospital for evaluation of fever with a limp. The mother has noticed low-grade fevers intermittently for the past 6 weeks. Over this time period, the boy has had progressive pain in the left knee, and is now refusing to walk or bear weight on that leg. On physical examination, you find he is febrile and irritable. The left knee is slightly swollen compared to the right. He refuses to stand unassisted. His total serum WBC count and ESR are elevated. A blood culture drawn during a febrile episode is growing Gram-positive cocci on the Gram stain. Plain radiographs of the left lower extremity reveal periosteal elevation and a subperiosteal fluid collection of the medial, distal left femur. The most likely diagnosis is

    A. Osteomyelitis
    B. Cellulitis
    C. Legg-Calvé-Perthes disease (LCPD)
    D. Osgood-Schlatter disease (OSD)
    E. SCFE

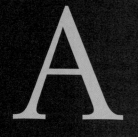

Answers and Explanations

101. D	118. B	135. C
102. D	119. D	136. D
103. D	120. B	137. B
104. D	121. C	138. D
105. C	122. E	139. D
106. D	123. C	140. C
107. C	124. B	141. D
108. D	125. D	142. B
109. B	126. C	143. D
110. D	127. E	144. C
111. E	128. A	145. D
112. C	129. D	146. B
113. D	130. B	147. C
114. D	131. B	148. E
115. B	132. C	149. C
116. D	133. B	150. A
117. B	134. E	

101. **D. The growth delay, pallor, hypertension, nocturia, and evidence of rickets all indicate that this boy suffers from chronic renal insufficiency. An elevated serum BUN and creatinine most assuredly will confirm this diagnosis.**

    A. Measurement of 1,20-dihydrocholecalciferol is generally not necessary in patients with renal osteodystrophy. It is low, but it is also low in other forms of rickets.
    B. Although x-rays will likely show evidence of rickets, they will not distinguish renal rickets (a finding in renal osteodystrophy) from other forms of rickets.
    C. The anemia found on a blood count in chronic renal failure is due to deficiency of erythropoietin. This is usually a normocytic anemia, and it supports the diagnosis of chronic renal disease.
    E. The serum phosphorus will be high and the calcium low in untreated chronic renal failure, but they are also nonspecific. Hypoparathyroidism can cause the same calcium and phosphorus changes.

102. **D. Golf would be the most appropriate choice. Marfan syndrome is a connective tissue disorder with skeletal, ocular, and cardiovascular involvement. 50% of patients have clinically evident cardiovascular disease by age 21. Dilation of the weakened aortic root can lead to aneurysm and dissection, causing sudden death. Activities that involve isometric exercise or heavy straining can increase the likelihood of aortic root dissection. Golf is a low dynamic, low static sport that is relatively safe for Marfan patients.**

    A, E. Contact sports or sports that involve a risk of chest contusion should be avoided.
    B. The tall, long-limbed Marfanoid habitus may seem well suited to basketball, but the risk of contact and excessive strain is too great.
    C. Weight training requires excessive isometric effort, placing undue strain on the weak aorta.

103. **D. This baby is being overfed, with the additional calories coming from the formula feedings. Overfed babies often have symptoms of gastroesophageal reflux, especially after abdominal examination. The baby's weight should even out with only breast feeds. Simply stopping the extra calories and seeing the baby back at the 9-month visit for another weight check is an acceptable course of action.**

    A. A morning cortisol determination looking for cortisol excess would not be necessary at this point without other findings.
    B. CT of the abdomen to evaluate the adrenal glands would not be indicated.
    C. MRI of the brain looking for a pituitary tumor would not be necessary in this infant.
    E. Evaluating the infant for diabetes with an HbA1C value would not fit the clinical findings in this case. Infants with diabetes typically lose weight and have polyuria.

104. **D. Shaken baby syndrome usually includes retinal and intracranial bleeding without, or in excess of, any external signs of injury. Multiple retinal and preretinal hemorrhages scattered throughout the entire back of the eye, many with minute yellow or white centers, are typical.**

    A. A cherry red spot in the center of a pale macula is typical of storage disorders such as Tay-Sach disease.
    B. The low lying, slightly hazy, cotton wool spot found in diabetic and hypertensive retinopathy is an indication of local axonal damage and edema.
    C. Retinitis pigmentosa usually presents in later childhood with progressive loss of peripheral vision and exceedingly poor night vision. The optic nerve becomes pale and atrophic, and the retina outside the macula becomes pigmented with a dark lattice pattern.
    E. The "blood and thunder" changes of CMV retinitis are usually seen in immunocompromised patients and appear as scattered, large white inflammatory lesions of the choroid and retina.

105. **C. The most important source of lead exposure in the pediatric population is lead paint. Water sources may become contaminated from lead pipes, food sources may be contaminated by lead cookware, and soil may become contaminated from residue of deteriorated house paint. Leaded gasoline has historically served as a potential source for lead exposure, although the regulated removal of lead from gasoline has resulted in a dramatic decrease; leaded gasoline may still be employed in the agricultural setting.**

A. Lead poisoning may result in transverse bands of increased density in the metaphyseal regions of bone. These "lead lines" represent lead's toxic effect on bone growth, not the deposition of lead.

B. Neurologic symptoms are frequently seen in lead poisoning. These may include headache, impaired concentration, and irritability, which may lead to poor school performance. In severe poisonings, encephalopathy may even develop. Other more nonspecific signs include anorexia, vomiting, abdominal pain, and constipation.

D. Routine screening for lead poisoning is recommended by the CDC from ages 1 to 2 years.

E. The management of lead poisoning is determined by the actual blood lead level, which will need to be determined in this patient. Blood lead levels between 10 and 45 μg/dL will need continued close clinical monitoring, and education; referral to the department of health for levels greater than 14 μg/dL would also be warranted. Chelation therapy would only be recommended for patients with blood lead levels greater than 45 μg/dL, with immediate hospitalization for those with lead levels of 70 μg/dL or greater.

106. D. Scorpion venom is a neurotoxin that causes prolonged and repetitive action potentials by opening sodium channels. An envenomation may present with signs such as tongue fasciculations, disconjugate eye movements, arching of the back, and hypersalivation. Parents should be aware that scorpions (bark scorpions) can climb up walls and may drop into a child's crib in search of a warm place. The history of a scorpion sting may not be elicited.

A. A necrotic area is more typical of certain spider bites and is not seen after a scorpion sting.

B. Scorpion stings often have minimal physical evidence, such as swelling or bruising, following such a sting.

C. Rigid abdomen, hypertension, and emesis are findings typical of a black widow spider bite, not a scorpion envenomation.

E. Pinpoint pupils and hypoventilation are suggestive of an ingestion, and not a scorpion sting.

107. C. Comprehensive laboratory testing is unnecessary and unhelpful in arriving at a diagnosis.

A. The incidence of obesity is rising in the pediatric population, with estimates of 25% to 30% of the population affected.

B. In a majority of circumstances, the physical examination as well as laboratory evaluation will be normal.

D. A weight reduction program, if properly monitored by a physician-nutritionist medical team, is safe and essential for the management of obesity in the pediatric population.

E. A positive family history, excessive caloric intake, and minimal physical activity are paramount in making the diagnosis.

108. D. Epiphyseal fractures can be classified into five types. A type IV fracture, as depicted in the radiograph, crosses the metaphysis, growth plate, and epiphysis.

A. Type I consists of separation through the growth plate.

B. Type II involves a fracture through the growth plate, and extension through the metaphysis.

C. Type III is defined as a fracture through the growth plate, extending through the epiphysis.

E. A type V fracture involves a crush injury and near obliteration of the growth plate.

109. B. A diagnosis of rheumatic heart disease is made after confirming antecedent rheumatic fever. The modified Jones criteria (revised in 1992) provide guidelines for the diagnosis of rheumatic fever. The Jones criteria require the presence of two major, or one major and two minor, criteria for the diagnosis of rheumatic fever, plus documentation of recent group A streptococcal infection. The major diagnostic criteria include carditis, polyarthritis, chorea, subcutaneous nodules, and erythema marginatum. The minor diagnostic criteria include fever, arthralgia, prolonged PR interval on the ECG, and elevated acute phase reactants, including ESR/CRP.

A. Subcutaneous nodules are a major criteria. ANA titers and thrombocytopenia are not part of the Jones criteria.

C. Arthralgias are a minor criteria, as is an elevated CRP.

D. Polyarthritis is a major criteria and elevated ESR is a minor criteria. Anemia is not in the Jones criteria.

E. Prolonged PR interval and fever are both minor criteria. Leukocytosis is not a criterion.

110. **D.** Dry skin, flexural lichenification, and pruritus are classic features of atopic dermatitis.

    A. The incidence of atopic dermatitis is increasing dramatically.

    B. Dietary proteins are only occasional causes of atopy.

    C. Atopic dermatitis usually improves by age 10 years.

    E. Atopic dermatitis is usually very itchy and can result in areas of superinfection secondary to pruritus.

111. **E.** Adrenal insufficiency is a potentially life-threatening condition; typified by the decreased production of mineralocorticoids, glucocorticoids, and/or adrenal androgens. Adrenal insufficiency can be caused by diseases of the adrenal cortex (primary adrenal insufficiency), the pituitary gland and the secretion of ACTH (secondary adrenal insufficiency), or the hypothalamus and the secretion of corticotropic-releasing hormone (CRH) (tertiary adrenal insufficiency). This patient has autoimmune adrenalitis, which is the most common cause of primary adrenal insufficiency in industrialized countries. It is a result of an autoimmune process that destroys the adrenal cortex. About 50% of patients with autoimmune adrenal insufficiency have one or more other autoimmune endocrine disorders. The combination of autoimmune adrenal insufficiency with other autoimmune endocrine disorders is referred to as the polyglandular autoimmune syndromes type I or II.

    A. Infiltration of the adrenal cortex with disease processes such as HIV, tuberculosis, and histoplasmosis may cause adrenal crisis. However, autoimmune adrenalitis is the most common cause of Addison disease in this age group and thus is the most likely explanation.

    B. Adrenal hemorrhage can certainly cause adrenal insufficiency and crisis. However, it is not the most likely explanation.

    C. Patients with meningococcal sepsis often progress to shock and adrenal crisis. Meningococcemia presents acutely with fever and may have a petechial, purpuric rash progressing rapidly to shock.

    D. Just as adrenal hemorrhage or infiltration of the adrenal gland with infectious diseases can cause adrenal crisis, an adrenal tumor can also produce this disease.

112. **C.** Idiopathic scoliosis is not associated with significant pain, unless a severe curve is present.

    A. Patients with a curve of less than 25 degrees can usually be monitored at 3 to 6 month intervals. If progression of the curve extends to 25 degrees or more, a referral to an orthopedic surgeon is indicated for further management.

    B. The incidence of idiopathic scoliosis is higher in females.

    D. There is often a positive family history of idiopathic scoliosis in 30% of the patients.

    E. Routine radiography is adequate for further evaluation of scoliosis. The routine use of MRI is expensive and unnecessary.

113. **D.** Any time a baby has an elevated direct bilirubin level, it is important to identify the reason as soon as possible. In cases of biliary atresia, jaundice may develop gradually over several weeks. It may also be a continuation of physiologic jaundice with concern raised only when the jaundiced color fails to fade in a few weeks. Patients may have a small or absent gallbladder, noted on abdominal ultrasound. To be effective, the Kasai procedure (designed to relieve biliary obstruction) should be performed early, preferably in the first 2 to 3 months of life.

    A. Prolonged physiologic jaundice is indirect, and is not associated with light-colored stools.

    B. Breast-milk jaundice usually peaks between 10 and 14 days of life and is indirect.

    C. Both biliary atresia and neonatal hepatitis can result in direct hyperbilirubinemia. The differentiation between biliary atresia and neonatal hepatitis may be difficult and hepatobiliary scintigraphy (HIDA scan) or liver biopsy may be needed.

    E. Gilbert syndrome is associated with an elevation in indirect bilirubin related to deficient glucuronyl transferase levels.

114. **D.** Dental caries can be caused by the overgrowth of bacterial organisms that are transmitted from the mother to her baby at 6 to 30 months of age, when the primary teeth are erupting. Prevention of tooth decay in a baby can be accomplished by decreasing the amount of bacteria in the mother's mouth at this critical time of dental bacterial colonization. This can be best achieved by ensuring that the mother maintains good oral hygiene, avoids sugary foods, uses fluoride toothpaste or

rinse, and sees a dentist regularly. Maternal use of xylitol chewing gum has also been shown to reduce the child's caries rate.

A. Even when the water supply contains fluoride levels of less than 0.3 parts per million, fluoride supplements for babies younger than 6 months of age are not recommended.
B. Children who sleep with a bottle or are breastfed throughout the night can develop caries. Breastfeeding is not protective.
C. Soy formula does not decrease the risk of caries.
E. Sharing utensils will expose the baby's teeth to more of the mother's oral bacteria. This may actually increase the chance of developing dental decay.

115. **B. The typical "congenital clubfoot" deformity generally has mild calf atrophy, with tibial and fibular hypoplasia. Congenital clubfoot is also called idiopathic or neurogenic clubfoot.**

A. In 75% of the cases, congenital clubfoot is not associated with other congenital abnormalities. Those clubfeet that are associated with other congenital abnormalities are called "teratologic." They are frequently associated with myelodysplasias, arthrogryposis, and other syndromes.
C. Congenital clubfoot is bilateral in 50% of cases.
D. Clubfoot occurs in about 1 in 1000 newborns, and there is a 2:1 male preponderance. However, there is about a 3% incidence in subsequent siblings, and a 20% to 30% incidence in the offspring of affected parents.
E. The typical deformity in clubfoot shows hindfoot equinus, a varus hindfoot and midfoot, and **adduction** of the forefoot.

116. **D. There are two meiotic cell divisions. In the first meiotic division, the number of chromosomes is reduced to 23; and in the second, each of the 23 are duplicated. Trisomy occurs when a duplicated chromosome in meiosis fails to separate (nondisjunction), resulting in a daughter cell with an extra chromosome.**

A. When a fragment of a chromosome is lost, a "deletion" syndrome may occur in the offspring. Most of these result from an unbalanced translocation.
B. Nondisjunction occurring in mitosis (cell division after meiosis) results in a "mosaic" abnormality in the offspring.

C. When a fragment of one chromosome attaches to another chromosome in meiosis, and is passed on to the offspring, a translocation syndrome occurs.
E. Syndromes associated with three of the same chromosomes result mostly from nondisjunction in meiosis, and not from the formation of an extra chromosome.

117. **B. Pregnancy is a common cause of secondary amenorrhea and needs to be evaluated before an extensive diagnostic workup is undertaken. A urine pregnancy test is sensitive and easily acquired in the office setting.**

A. If the patient had a history of heavy menstrual cycles and you were concerned about anemia or a bleeding disorder, a CBC may be helpful.
C. If the suspicion for pregnancy is high, a serum quantitative hCG can be ordered.
D. LH levels have been used in the past to evaluate for hyperandrogenic states, but are not always useful.
E. Serum testosterone levels are usually mildly elevated with hyperandrogenic states and secondary amenorrhea.

118. **B. In the direct antiglobulin (Coombs) test, an antibody directed against human immunoglobulin (Ig) or complement is used to detect the presence of antibodies on the surface of red cells by agglutination.**

A. The indirect Coombs test detects antibody circulating in serum that is directed against RBC membrane proteins.
C. Hemoglobin electrophoresis detects the percentage of circulating fetal hemoglobin.
D. The percentage of RBCs in the circulation that are less than 1 day old is measured by the reticulocyte count.
E. Although a positive direct Coombs test may be seen as an autoimmune hemolytic manifestation of SLE, a variety of other criteria must be met to confirm the definitive diagnosis of SLE.

119. **D. Shock is defined as a condition in which decreased tissue perfusion results in insufficient delivery of oxygen and substrate to meet the metabolic needs of the tissues and end organs. It can be classified as either compensated (normal blood pressure) or decompensated (hypotension).**

A. Blood pressure can be increased, decreased, or normal when a patient is in shock.

B. Cardiac output can be increased in septic shock, decreased in hypovolemic shock, and normal in distributive shock.

C. The patient can be alert and conversant in compensated shock, but will have some other signs or symptoms of poor tissue perfusion.

E. In high output failure, the patient can be pink and warm with an elevated heart rate.

120. **B. CAH is a common autosomal recessive disease. CAH is caused by an inborn error of steroid biosynthesis. The most common cause (90%) of CAH is 21-hydroxylase enzyme deficiency. Patients with the salt-wasting variety cannot produce adequate amounts of cortisol, and in some cases are also aldosterone deficient. These hormones are essential to glucose metabolism and salt reabsorption. Untreated CAH has serious consequences and can suddenly lead to adrenal insufficiency with dehydration, shock, and even death. Newborn screening for CAH due to 21-hydroxylase deficiency is detected by measuring the 17-hydroxy (OH) progesterone accumulation level. CAH presents with ambiguous genitalia only in females, but males may have excessive scrotal pigmentation.**

A. Patients with CAH secondary to 21-hydroxylase enzyme deficiency may have various levels of 21-hydroxylase enzyme. Therefore, the level would not help confirm the diagnosis in all CAH cases.

C. Karyotype would give the genotypic gender but would not give any information about the steroid biosynthesis.

D. Random cortisol levels fluctuate throughout the day and would not be useful diagnostically in a nonstress situation.

E. Rectal exam may help in evaluating the external and internal genitalia of the child, but will not make the diagnosis of CAH.

121. **C. A vibratory innocent murmur, also called a Still, classically presents as a midsystolic, 2-3/6 murmur with a musical or vibratory sound heard best at the lower left sternal border without any accompanying thrill or ejection click.**

A. The murmur of aortic valve stenosis is usually heard at the upper right sternal border and has a rough, grating quality with an ejection click.

B. Murmurs related to a small VSD can be heard at the left lower sternal border, but are generally high-pitched and blowing in nature.

D. Murmurs of pulmonic valve stenosis are generally heard at the upper left sternal border and are also of a rough grating quality.

E. An ASD is heard best at the upper left sternal border as a systolic ejection murmur with a widely split and fixed S2 sound.

122. **E. Patients with streptococcal pharyngitis often have fever, sore throat, headache, abdominal pain, nausea, and vomiting. Cough, conjunctivitis, rhinorrhea, hoarseness, and diarrhea are more indicative of viral infection. On physical examination, patients with streptococcal pharyngitis can be seen to have pharyngeal exudates and erythema, tender anterior cervical nodes, palatal petechiae, and a scarlet fever "sandpaper" rash.**

A. The presence of cough and coryza, and the absence of adenopathy and tonsillar exudate are more typical of viral infection.

B. Children under 1 to 2 years of age generally do not get streptococcal pharyngitis. At this young age, their pharyngeal cells do not have the bacterial receptor sites necessary for infection.

C. Conjunctivitis and cough are most often associated with viral infection. Adenovirus is a common agent in conjunctivitis.

D. The pattern of exudative pharyngitis, hepatosplenomegaly, cervical adenopathy, and fever in a teenager strongly suggests infectious mononucleosis, most often due to EBV.

123. **C. Iron-deficiency anemia is the most common cause of microcytic anemia in the infant and toddler. In most cases, it is due to poor intake of bioavailable iron. Cow's milk enteropathy may result from the early introduction of milk before 1 year of age and/or excessive milk consumption. The resulting effect may be microscopic intestinal bleeding and manifest as an iron-deficient anemia.**

A. Autoimmune hemolytic anemia causes the breakdown of RBCs, resulting in jaundice, anemia, and an elevated reticulocyte count.

B. Hereditary spherocytosis is a genetic disorder in which the red cell membrane is unstable. This results in RBC destruction in the spleen. Patients develop anemia and jaundice with an elevated reticulocyte count.

D. Pyruvate kinase deficiency is an autosomal recessive disorder with decreased RBC pyruvate kinase levels and activity. This enzyme lacks results in insufficient production of ATP. Ultimately, the RBCs become rigid and RBC lifespan is considerably reduced.

E. G6PD deficiency results in episodes of hemolytic anemia, usually provoked by an inciting factor such as certain infections or drugs. Patients may develop jaundice, and the reticulocyte count will be elevated.

124. **B. This is a classic presentation of delayed acetaminophen toxicity. At 48 to 96 hours after ingestion of a toxic amount of acetaminophen, hepatic toxicity and failure will ensue if left untreated. These patients require treatment with N-acetylcysteine until their coagulopathy or encephalopathy (if present) resolves.**

A. Clonidine toxicity may present with hypertension followed by hypotension, bradycardia, respiratory depression, drowsiness, weakness, and miosis.

C. Morphine toxicity may present with hypotension, bradycardia, bradypnea, stupor, or coma.

D. Diphenhydramine toxicity may present with anticholinergic symptoms of dry skin, tachycardia, arrhythmias, delirium, psychosis, and coma.

E. Fever, mydriasis, tachycardia, seizures, and hypertension may all be manifestations of amphetamine toxicity.

125. **D. The history and focal physical findings are most consistent with foreign-body aspiration. Foreign-body aspiration should be considered in a toddler with unilateral wheezing and refusal to take liquids, such as their favorite juice.**

A. Asthma should produce bilateral wheezes.

B. CF would most likely present with poor growth and multiple episodes of breathing difficulties by this age, not as an acute presentation.

C. Pneumonia is usually associated with fever and persistent cough, as well as the observed signs of respiratory distress in this child.

E. Peanut allergy with anaphylaxis would present more acutely with upper airway edema, shock, and bilateral wheezing.

126. **C. The Glasgow Coma Score (GCS) provides an objective measure of a person's level of consciousness and neurologic status. It is graded on a scale from 3 to 15 and is specifically useful in trauma situations. The patient's score in this scenario is 13, calculated from the data below:**

- Eye opening to verbal stimuli = 3 out of possible 4
- Verbal – confused = 4 out of possible 5
- Motor – follows commands = 6 out of possible 6

GCS scores of less than 8 are concerning and prompt immediate attention to protection of the airway. Remember the adage, "less than 8, intubate."

A, B, D, E. These scores are incorrect. See explanation for C.

127. **E. Juvenile dermatomyositis presents with symmetric weakness of the proximal muscles at onset. Limb-girdle musculature of the lower extremities is the most common group of muscles affected. The etiology is unclear except for chronic inflammation of the skin and striated muscle. Skin changes include the heliotrope discoloration of the eyelids with periorbital swelling. Gottron papules are a scaly rash with erythema and edema over the MCP joints that can be seen with this disease. Abnormal labs include an elevated CPK, aldolase, LDH or AST, all of which are markers of muscle inflammation. An electromyogram (EMG) would demonstrate characteristics of myopathy and denervation**

128. **A. Henoch-Schönlein purpura is a small-vessel vasculitis that typically follows a viral URI. The hallmark of the disease is the rash, beginning as pinkish maculopapules that progress to palpable purpura (nonblanching). The rash characteristically occurs in dependent areas such as the lower extremities and the buttocks. Edema can also be seen in the scrotum, hands, feet, lips, and eyes. The GI tract is frequently involved with the vasculitis, resulting in colicky abdominal pain and occult blood in the stools. Intussusception may occur, resulting in bowel ischemia and currant jelly stools. There are no specific or diagnostic blood tests. A biopsy of the rash reveals a leukocytoclastic angiitis.**

129. D. Sarcoidosis has a variable presentation in the pediatric population. Familial clustering is seen and it is more common in African-American patients than in Caucasian patients. Children usually present with cough, weight loss, fatigue, joint and bone pain, and anemia. Pulmonary involvement can include hilar adenopathy with parenchymal infiltrates, and miliary nodules. Noncaseating granulomas can occur in any organ of the body. Uveitis, iritis, and skin granulomas can also be seen. Children under 4 years of age can have a distinct form of sarcoidosis consisting of a maculopapular, erythematous rash, uveitis, and arthritis but no pulmonary findings. There are no specific diagnostic tests. Hypercalcemia can occur with sarcoid and accounts for the patient's symptoms of constipation and polyuria. An elevated angiotensin-converting enzyme level is common.

    B. JRA is an autoimmune disorder that causes chronic synovial inflammation lasting for at least 6 weeks. The three types of JRA are systemic, pauciarticular, and polyarticular. Those with systemic disease often present with a history of fevers, rash, and arthritis, as well as lymphadenopathy, or hepatosplenomegaly. Pauciarticular JRA is defined as five or fewer joints being affected, whereas those with five or more joints affected are classified as having polyarticular JRA.

    C. SLE is an autoimmune disorder that can result in multiorgan system involvement. Classically, patients present with fever, arthritis, and malar rash, but the clinical presentation is extremely variable. Patients need to have 4 of the following 11 criteria to meet the diagnosis of SLE: malar rash, discoid rash, oral ulcers, photosensitivity, arthritis, any cytopenia, seizures/psychosis, nephritis, pleuritis or pericarditis, positive ANA, and antibodies to double-stranded DNA.

    F. Kawasaki disease or mucocutaneous lymph node syndrome is diagnosed clinically by a 5-day history of fever accompanied by four of the five following criteria: nonexudative bulbar conjunctivitis, polymorphic rash, indurated or edematous hands and feet, unilateral cervical lymphadenopathy measuring greater than 1.5 cm, and oral mucosal involvement, which may include cracking, reddened lips, or strawberry tongue. Children with Kawasaki disease should be treated with high-dose aspirin and IVIG within 10 days of the onset of symptoms to minimize the risk of developing coronary artery dilation and aneurysms.

    G. Reiter syndrome is defined as urethritis, arthritis, and ocular inflammation. The arthritis is typically found to be pauciarticular with a predilection for larger joints. Males are predominantly affected. Although the typical clinical history is found in an adolescent following sexual intercourse and infection with *Neisseria gonorrhea*, it has been reported in children following infections with *Yersinia enterocolitica* and *Shigella*.

130. B. Tetralogy of Fallot is a complex congenital heart disease that includes four distinct abnormalities: VSD, pulmonary stenosis, overriding aorta, and RV hypertrophy. The increase in pulmonary vascular resistance due to crying or agitation increases the right-to-left shunt of blood flow in the heart and causes hypoxemia and cyanosis. This is known as a "Tet spell." Sitting with the knees up toward the chest, as in a car seat or in a squatting position, increases systemic vascular resistance, and reduces the degree of right-to-left shunting, improving oxygenation.

    A. CF is an inheritable defect in sodium transport that causes chronic pulmonary and GI disease. This child's poor growth and the clubbing of his fingers and toes (the result of chronic hypoxemia) are consistent with CF. However, the harsh murmur and the Tet spells are not explained by a diagnosis of CF.

    C. Hypoplastic left heart syndrome is a severe congenital defect in which the left ventricle is small or absent. These children present with congestive heart failure in the first few weeks of life and, if untreated, generally do not survive past 6 weeks.

    D. Hirschsprung disease is a congenital absence of the ganglion cells in the lower intestinal tract causing functional intestinal obstruction. It has no associated cardiac abnormalities.

    E. Breath-holding spells are typically provoked by an upsetting circumstance for the child. They usually present from age 2 to 5 years, and are rare before 6 months of age. They would not be expected to be accompanied by poor weight gain or clubbing on exam.

131. **B. This is a classic description of seborrheic dermatitis.**

   A. Dry skin, pruritus, and flexural lichenification are typical of atopic dermatitis.
   C. Psoriasis is rare at this age. Psoriatic lesions would be dry with a silvery scale.
   D. Patients with Langerhans cell histiocytosis have deep, pruritic, papular, nonconfluent, scarring lesions with lymphadenopathy and hepatosplenomegaly.
   E. Candidiasis is very rarely present on the scalp. It is typically located in the inguinal region and has associated satellite lesions. Axillary lesions are rare in candidiasis.

132. **C. This progression accurately describes Piaget's theory of cognitive development. Piaget's stages of cognitive development include sensorimotor (birth to 2 years), preoperational (2 to 6 years), concrete operations (6 to 12 years), and formal operations (12 years to adulthood).**

   A. The psychosexual theory of development is attributed to Freud.
   B. Erikson espoused the psychosocial theory.
   D. Jung was a Swiss psychologist who studied the psyche, ego, and libido.
   E. Montessori was an Italian pediatrician who developed a new educational system for young children that served as the basis for the development of the Montessori school system.

133. **B. Todd's paralysis is a temporary hemiparesis following a focal seizure and may be confused with a stroke. The symptoms should completely resolve within 24 hours after the seizure.**

   A. Strokes are not transient and would not resolve completely over 24 hours.
   C. A cerebral tumor would likely cause permanent, progressive weakness.
   D. Status epilepticus would not be expected to improve without treatment.
   E. Postviral encephalitis can cause hemiparesis, but would include additional symptoms, including fever, headache, neck pain, photophobia, and personality changes.

134. **E. Cocaine possesses sympathomimetic properties that can cause hypertension, tachycardia, and hyperthermia. Numerous vascular problems including infarction and ischemia or even aortic** dissection have been reported in the setting of cocaine toxicity. Chronic hypertension can occur with repeated use of cocaine, even in young patients. This patient is experiencing symptoms of vascular ischemia related to cocaine-induced vascular spasm. He is at risk of additional and significant health problems and needs immediate intervention to assist him in eliminating his drug dependency.

   A. Myocardial infarction can certainly occur as a complication of cocaine overdose. However, this patient does not have clinical symptoms suggestive of a myocardial infarction. A silent infarction would be extremely unlikely in such a young patient without other health problems.
   B. This young man is not having headaches, weakness, or problems with speech or motor function. Strokes can result from cocaine use, but this patient has not yet experienced one.
   C. A patient with infarcted bowel would most likely be hypotensive, and in severe pain. The abdomen should be exquisitely tender, firm, and guarded and may be distended. Signs of shock are likely.
   D. Aortic dissection is a very serious complication that can occur as a result of cocaine use. Patients experiencing an aortic dissection will be in severe pain and may have a palpable abdominal mass.

135. **C. The patient has a clinical picture consistent with scarlet fever. This disease is caused by group A β-hemolytic *Streptococcus*. The classic presentation includes a fine, sandpapery rash, strawberry tongue (as in Figure 3-135), fever, cervical lymphadenopathy, and pharyngitis. The rash typically starts on the trunk and spreads outward. The treatment is identical to that for streptococcal pharyngitis.**

   A. The diagnosis of Kawasaki disease requires the presence of fever for 5 days or more, and at least four of the five following criteria: (1) bilateral, nonexudative conjunctivitis, (2) oral mucosal changes: red mouth and pharynx, strawberry tongue, and/or cracked lips, (3) exanthema, ranging from morbilliform to maculopapular, (4) edema of the hands and feet, and (5) unilateral cervical lymphadenopathy greater than 1.5 cm.

B. Roseola infantum presents with fever for 3 to 7 days and a blanching, maculopapular rash. It is not associated with a strawberry tongue.

D. Fifth disease, caused by parvovirus B19, usually presents with a lacy, reticular, erythematous rash that may be accompanied by reddened or "slapped" cheeks.

E. The clinical presentation of rubeola, or measles, consists of fever, cough, coryza, conjunctivitis, and a maculopapular, erythematous rash that begins on the head and spreads down to the feet. Koplik's spots are white patches that are seen in the oropharynx, associated with measles.

136. D. Oligohydramnios is associated with abnormalities of the fetal kidneys, as well as pulmonary hypoplasia. The most severe manifestation is Potter syndrome, which is characterized by clubfeet, compressed facies, low-set ears, pulmonary hypoplasia, and renal agenesis; a potentially lethal condition.

A. Gastroschisis is associated with polyhydramnios.

B. Neural tube defects may result in impaired fetal swallowing, which leads to polyhydramnios.

C. Gestational diabetes can be associated with increased or normal amounts of amniotic fluid.

E. Diaphragmatic hernia and other GI abnormalities often result in altered GI fluid absorption leading to polyhydramnios.

137. B. This patient has a typical history for vasovagal syncope, which is more frequent in adolescent females. Some stimuli, such as a sensation of nausea, queasiness, sight of blood, and heat, stimulate the vagus nerve and produce temporary bradycardia. The cardiac output falls and the patient experiences a brief period of hypotension, which often leads to complete syncope. This happens more frequently when the patient changes quickly from a cooler to a warmer environment because there is increased blood flow to the skin. This patient experienced symptoms when she went outside of her air-conditioned house. Standing also accentuates venous pooling.

A. Ventricular tachycardia is uncommon, but if the episodes are repeated, a 24-hour Holter monitor would be useful to rule out the presence of frequent arrhythmias.

C. A stroke would not self-resolve in a matter of minutes.

D. Viral meningitis presents with fever, headache, and vomiting; all of these are absent in this patient.

E. It is unlikely that this episode was attention seeking, because the patient sustained a laceration to her forehead, and the event was also accompanied by relative bradycardia. Vasovagal episodes are common in the adolescent age group.

138. D. This slide demonstrates typical sickle-shaped or ghost-like trophozoites adhering to the villous surface. Clubbing of villi may also be seen on biopsy. *Giardia* may also be diagnosed by testing for stool *Giardia* antigen, or duodenal fluid testing. Stool examination may show typical *Giardia* oval cysts with four nuclei. Symptoms include crampy abdominal pain or bloating, with or without diarrhea, which may persist for weeks or sometimes months to years. Infection with *Giardia* may result from the ingestion of contaminated water sources or person-to-person spread. Treatment with oral Flagyl (metronidazole) is usually successful.

A. Acanthamoeba infections result in encephalitis and are typically seen in chronically ill or immunocompromised patients. Symptoms may be insidious but include HA, stiff neck, and altered mental status. Trophozoites may be identified in the CSF, and cysts can be seen in biopsy specimens. Mortality rates are high.

B. Amebic dysentery is caused by *Entamoeba histolytica*. Infections occur after ingestion of contaminated water or food. Patients may develop abdominal pain and diarrhea, which tends to be bloody. Trophozoites may be seen in stool samples, and amebic serology is also available. Amebic abscesses may develop in the liver.

C. *Vibrio cholera* is a motile, Gram-negative rod with polar flagella. It exists in brackish or coastal saltwater pools, but human infection usually occurs as a result of fecal exposure. Symptoms include severe watery diarrhea that is rapidly progressive.

E. *Blastocystis hominis* is a protozoan that has been more recently noticed. Most patients who carry *Blastocystis* in the GI tract are asymptomatic. A few patients with abdominal pain and diarrhea may benefit from treatment with Flagyl or Iodoquinol.

139. D. Figure 3-139 depicts a simian crease. Simple reassurance should be provided in a normally developing child with a simian crease. Simian creases may be found in approximately 3% of the general population.

   A. Although a simian crease may be seen in Down syndrome, it is not diagnostic. Other clinical signs and symptoms are important to make the diagnosis. Aside from being seen in the general population, simian creases are also associated with a variety of other disorders including trisomy 13, fetal alcohol syndrome, pseudohypoparathyroidism, cri du chat, and others.
   B. Palmar creases develop during the first trimester at the eleventh to twelfth week.
   C. A simian crease can be seen in fetal alcohol syndrome, but is not typically associated with maternal cocaine use.
   E. A chromosome analysis in an otherwise asymptomatic child without any additional abnormal physical findings would not be indicated at this time.

140. C. Colic refers to a symptom complex of paroxysmal abdominal pain and severe crying. The paroxysms may last for several hours. In addition to crying, the baby may draw his legs up to the chest or demonstrate a mildly distended abdomen. Episodes tend to occur late in the afternoon or early evening.

   A. Colic occurs in infants less than 3 months old and will resolve spontaneously.
   B. The cause of colic is not clear. Although a few babies may have food allergies, colic can also be caused by swallowed air, overfeeding, high carbohydrate foods, and temperament issues.
   D. Narcotics, such as paregoric, should be avoided.
   E. Although intussusception, strangulated hernia, ocular foreign body, otitis media, and pyelonephritis should be considered in infants with unexplained crying episodes, patients with a typical history of colic and a normal physical examination do not require radiographic studies, even if mild abdominal distension occurs.

141. D. Heat stroke is the most serious form of heat-related illness. It is generally associated with a body temperature of greater than 40°C and altered mental status. Patients become dehydrated and may have electrolyte abnormalities, seizures, pulmonary edema, renal, liver, and/or cardiac failure, rhabdomyolysis, disseminated intravascular coagulation, and death. Following heat stroke, patients may have permanent and serious neurologic abnormalities. Heat stroke is a medical emergency that requires CPR, rapid cooling, and rehydration with large amounts of IV fluids.

   A, B. Heat-related illness can be prevented by avoiding heavy activity outside in the hottest part of the day, wearing light-colored and lightweight clothing, taking frequent breaks in hot weather, and ensuring adequate hydration. Cold water, which is absorbed better than warm water, should be offered liberally to athletes. Preparticipation screening of athletes should focus on high-risk conditions such as obesity, lack of conditioning, prior heat injury, and drugs/medications known to be associated with heat injury (i.e., amphetamines, alcohol, antihistamines, anticholinergics, diuretics, phenothiazines, and thyroid hormone).
   C. The outside temperature and humidity both play a role in heat stress. In conditions of high humidity, evaporation of sweat is not as effective as a body cooling mechanism.
   E. Antipyretics function in the hypothalamus to lower the body's "thermostat" setting. Although antipyretics are useful in patients with fever, when the body thermostat setting is elevated, antipyretics will not prevent or treat elevated temperature due to heat stress.

142. B. Fetal hemoglobin is composed of two α chains and two γ chains (α_2, γ_2).

   A. Hemoglobin with four α chains (α_4) is hemoglobin Barts.
   C. Embryonic hemoglobin is composed of two δ chains and two γ chains (δ_2, γ_2).
   D, E. These molecules would not exist as hemoglobin. Hemoglobin is a tetramer molecule composed of four different polypeptide chains.

143. D. Acute mastoiditis is caused by extension of infection from otitis media into the mastoid air cells. The presentation usually includes fever, ear pain, postauricular swelling and erythema, and a protruding pinna. The common causative organisms are *Streptococcus pneumonia*, *Streptococcus pyogenes*, and *Staphylococcus aureus*.

A, B. Bacterial parotitis and mumps cause swelling of the parotid gland, which can cause the ear pinna to protrude; however, in these conditions, the enlarged parotid will cover the angle of the jaw and make palpation difficult. The opening of Stensen's duct into the oral cavity may be inflamed and purulent material can sometimes be expressed with parotid massage.

C. External otitis (swimmer's ear) can cause pain with manipulation of the tragus. Unlike mastoiditis, however, this condition does not cause the pinna to protrude out and there is generally no fever.

E. In chronic mastoiditis, fever and postauricular swelling are generally absent. The patient presents with ear pain, hearing loss, and persistent drainage from the ear canal for several weeks.

144. C. The initial manifestations of TCA toxicity include the onset of anticholinergic symptoms, including sinus tachycardia, mucous membrane dryness, dilated pupils, urinary retention, flushing, and even hallucinations. Hypertension may initially be present, but is soon followed by hypotension. Cardiac arrhythmias evident on ECG may occur later, with the most common being widening of the QRS complex.

A, B, E. Ventricular fibrillation, ventricular tachycardia, and electrical alternans would not be expected. See explanation for C.

D. Sinus tachycardia, rather than sinus bradycardia, would be present. See explanation for C.

145. D. RSV is a common cause of bronchiolitis and hospitalization for children during the winter months. The common clinical presentation of cough, congestion, and evidence of respiratory distress with a chest radiograph showing hyperinflation and perihilar streaking would suggest the diagnosis of RSV. Supportive care with pulmonary toilet, hydration, and oxygen are the mainstays of treatment.

146. B. EBV, also commonly referred to as mononucleosis ("mono"), often presents with fever, malaise, sore throat, lymphadenopathy, and hepatosplenomegaly. An atypical or reactive lymphocytosis can be seen on peripheral smear. The clinical spectrum of disease may vary from an acute illness that resolves without problems to fulminant sepsis. EBV has also been linked as a causative organism in X-linked lymphoproliferative disorders, Burkitt lymphoma, and nasopharyngeal carcinoma.

147. C. The history of coughing fits (whooping cough), immunization delay, other sick contacts, and a CBC showing an absolute marked lymphocytosis should suggest the diagnosis of *Bordetella pertussis.* Pertussis begins in the catarrhal phase of mild respiratory symptoms of rhinorrhea and congestion that progresses to the paroxysmal or whooping cough phase, followed by the convalescent phase over weeks to months of chronic cough. Erythromycin is the recommended treatment of choice for pertussis.

A. *H. influenzae* is responsible for a variety of infections ranging from otitis media, conjunctivitis, pneumonia, meningitis, and epiglottitis to overwhelming sepsis. Patients who present with pneumonia typically have an acute infiltrate seen on chest radiograph and appear clinically ill with respiratory distress and hypoxia. The incidence of serious disease from *H. influenzae* has dramatically decreased since the widespread use of the Hib vaccine.

E. *Streptococcus pyogenes*, or group A β-hemolytic *Streptococcus* (GAS), is most commonly associated with acute pharyngitis or "strep throat." Patients may typically present with fever, enlarged tonsils with exudates, lymphadenopathy, and a strawberry tongue. Scarlet fever, which presents as a sandpaper-like rash, possibly in association with these symptoms, is a result of exotoxins produced by GAS. GAS is also responsible for causing superficial and deep skin infections, such as cellulitis and osteomyelitis.

148. E. Language development occurs most rapidly between 2 and 5 years of age. The number of words in a child's vocabulary increases from about 100 to more than 2000 during this time period. Additionally, syntax advances from simple two- and three-word phrases to complete sentences. The child in this scenario has appropriate language development for his age. According to Denver developmental screening, 25% to 75% of children this age will have six words.

A. Language development from birth to 6 months consists of the development of sounds such as cooing, laughing, squealing, and responding to sounds such as a bell or a voice.

B. Infants 7 to 12 months of age will begin to jabber, imitate sounds, and develop a few specific single words.

C. At 13 to 18 months, children begin to add more words, and may point to or name a picture.

D. Children between 19 and 24 months begin to combine words and rapidly add words. Speech becomes more understandable.

149. **C. Migraine headaches are the most common type of headache in pediatrics. There is usually a positive family history. Migraines can be divided into three categories: migraine without aura, migraines with aura, and migraine equivalents with symptoms that cause transient neurologic dysfunction. The child in this scenario is most likely experiencing a migraine with aura. Patients are noted to be asymptomatic between migraine episodes.**

A. The headache caused by a brain tumor is often due to increased intracranial pressure and typically produces morning emesis and pain.

B. A seizure disorder will typically produce some sort of manifestation with convulsions.

D. Todd paralysis occurs when hemiparesis follows a focal seizure. The paralysis resolves within 24 hours.

E. Heterophoria is latent strabismus brought about by fatigue, illness, or stress. It rarely causes transient diplopia (double vision) and headaches.

150. **A. Osteomyelitis is an infectious process involving the bone. Hematogenous spread is the most likely etiology for disease in children less than 10 years of age. The typical radiographic findings of periosteal elevation and/or bony destruction may not be seen on plain films for 7 to 10 days. If the clinical suspicion is high enough in early disease, a bone scan or MRI can be diagnostic.**

B. Cellulitis is an infectious process primarily involving the skin.

C. LCPD is idiopathic osteonecrosis or avascular necrosis of the capital femoral epiphysis.

D. OSD results from microtrauma to the tibial tubercle from repetitive use.

E. SCFE disease develops later in childhood and is not infectious. It typically presents during adolescence in obese or tall, thin individuals following a growth spurt.

BLOCK 4

151. You are educating a class of prepubertal girls on the normal progression of puberty in females. Which of the following best describes this normal progression?

    A. Thelarche, growth spurt, pubarche, menarche
    B. Pubarche, thelarche, menarche, growth spurt
    C. Thelarche, pubarche, growth spurt, menarche
    D. Pubarche, menarche, thelarche, growth spurt

152. A 3-year-old girl is brought to your office because of a URI and rash. The rash was first noted as an intense, erythematous flushing on her face. The rash then spread to the trunk and proximal extremities and developed a lacy, reticulated appearance. The patient is afebrile and not particularly ill appearing. The organism responsible for this child's rash is also known to commonly cause which of the following?

    A. Deafness
    B. Developmental delay
    C. Aplastic crisis in patients with sickle-cell anemia
    D. Renal failure
    E. Severe diarrhea and dehydration

153. An obese 9-year-old girl is brought to your office because of a week-long history of persistent headache and blurred vision. She has been alert and has had no constitutional or focal neurologic symptoms. She has had some mild vomiting, but no fever. On physical examination, you find papilledema. Visual field testing reveals an inferior nasal blind spot. An MRI scan is normal. When you perform a lumbar puncture, the opening pressure is elevated, but the CSF composition is normal. Laboratory tests, including a CBC, comprehensive metabolic panel, and thyroid tests, are all normal. The most likely diagnosis is:

    A. Meningitis
    B. Migraine
    C. Pseudotumor cerebri
    D. Brain tumor
    E. Subdural hematoma

154. You have been following a 3-year-old in your practice since birth. The mother is concerned about speech delay in her 36-month-old daughter. The toddler will babble, inhibits to "No," follows one-step commands, says "Mama" and "Dada" correctly, but only has a 10-word vocabulary. Her developmental speech age is closest to:

    A. 6 months
    B. 12 months
    C. 18 months
    D. 24 months
    E. 36 months

155. A full-term newborn is born vaginally after a pregnancy complicated by gestational diabetes. The diabetes was poorly controlled due to noncompliance with diet and insulin therapy. He has scleral icterus at the time of delivery. Three hours after birth, he is noted to be plethoric, irritable, and cyanotic. Six hours after birth, he develops a generalized seizure. The most likely hematologic abnormality found on his CBC will be:

    A. Anemia
    B. Polycythemia
    C. Neutropenia
    D. Thrombocytopenia
    E. Lymphopenia

156. A healthy 18-month-old boy is brought to your office because his mother is concerned about his "pigeon-toed" gait. You place him in the prone position on the examining table with his knees flexed as shown in Figure 3-156. The most likely diagnosis is:

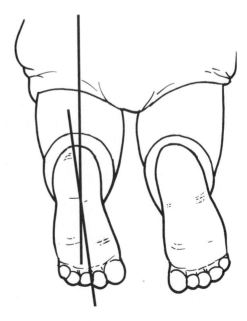

Figure 3-156

A. Metatarsus adductus
B. Internal tibial torsion
C. Internal femoral torsion (anteversion)
D. Genu varum
E. Pes planus

157. You are seeing a 5-day-old, ex-27-week infant who has been having apneic episodes. He has a normal head ultrasound and has clinically been stable on low ventilator settings. The most common type of apnea to be expected in this preterm infant is:

A. Obstructive apnea
B. Central apnea
C. Mixed obstructive and central apnea
D. Apnea secondary to infection
E. Apnea secondary to a metabolic cause

158. A 5-year-old boy gives a history of urinary frequency, day and night. He is constantly drinking and urinating. A urinalysis reveals a specific gravity of 1.005, negative glucose, and negative protein. Which one of the following would be consistent with this patient's central diabetes insipidus?

A. Urine osmolality 100 mOsm/kg, serum sodium 150 mEq/L, urine sodium 5 mEq/L
B. Urine osmolality 350 mOsm/kg, serum sodium 125 mEq/L, urine sodium 5 mEq/L
C. Urine osmolality 100 mOsm/kg, serum sodium 140 mEq/L, urine sodium 70 mEq/L
D. Urine osmolality 600 mOsm/kg, serum sodium 140 mEq/L, urine sodium 5 mEq/L
E. Urine osmolality 600 mOsm/kg, serum sodium 125 mEq/L, urine sodium 50 mEq/L

159. A newborn infant is born with a port-wine nevus, which is well demarcated over the distribution of the right trigeminal area of the face. Which one of the following is most frequently associated with this condition?

A. Hemangiomas of the abdominal viscera
B. Normal mental development
C. Absence seizures
D. Buphthalmos and glaucoma
E. The facial hemangioma may not be apparent for several weeks after birth

160. A 15-month-old female presents to the ER with a history of bloody stool. She was well until this afternoon when she developed episodes of inconsolable crying, as if she is in pain. The parents state that she pulls her legs up and cries for 7 to 8 minutes and then seems to feel better. There has been no history of fever, vomiting, or diarrhea. Just prior to arrival, she passed a maroon-colored, mucousy stool. The baby has a palpable mass in the right upper abdomen. Which of the following is the most likely diagnosis?

A. Viral gastroenteritis
B. *E. coli* 0157-H7 bacterial enteritis
C. Acute cholecystitis
D. Acute appendicitis
E. Intussusception

161. A 16-year-old female presents to the clinic with a complaint of irregular menses. Menarche occurred at 11 years of age. Her periods occur every 2 to 3 months and last for 5 to 7 days with moderate to heavy flow, but she denies any cramping. She complains that she is never able to predict when her menses will occur. She has never been sexually active. On physical examination, you note that her weight is greater than the 95th percentile. She has dark hair on her upper lip and chin, with papulopustular acne scattered on her face. Which of the following is the most likely diagnosis?

A. Polycystic ovary syndrome (PCOS)
B. Pregnancy
C. Immature hypothalamic-pituitary-ovarian axis
D. Cushing syndrome
E. Hypothyroidism

162. A previously healthy, term, 3-month-old male presents to the ER with tachypnea, poor feeding, and pallor over the last 24 hours. The patient is tachycardic, and when the cardiac monitor is placed, the HR is 240 with narrow QRS complexes. Vagal maneuvers are attempted and prove to be unsuccessful. Which of the following drugs should be given?

A. Lidocaine
B. Procainamide
C. Metoprolol
D. Adenosine
E. Magnesium sulfate

163. A mother brings in her 12-month-old infant for a routine well check. At the visit, she expresses concern that her child has only two teeth in each of the upper and lower gums. In which of the following age groups do the primary mandibular first molars typically erupt?

A. 7 months
B. 8 months
C. 9 months
D. 10 to 12 months
E. 12 to 16 months

164. The parents of an 8-year-old girl bring her to your office for a second opinion concerning the management of her attention deficit disorder (ADD). Her primary care physician and school teachers are recommending a trial of stimulant medication. The parents note that her only problem is a lack of attention during school and while doing homework. She is not hyperactive and has never been a real behavior problem, although her school performance is suffering. What should you tell them?

A. Stimulant medication is not indicated, because there is no hyperactivity and no behavior problem
B. A trial of stimulant medication is indicated for inattentive type ADHD
C. TCAs are a better choice for first-line therapy of inattentive type ADHD
D. Stimulant medications are generally no better than placebo for ADD
E. The situation should improve as the child becomes older

165. A 15-year-old boy has been struggling with anorexia for 18 months. His weight has been stable at 80% of his ideal body weight for the past 5 months. Which of the following sets of clinical findings are most consistent with this state?

A. Sinus tachycardia, dehydration, hypotension
B. Hypotension, sinus bradycardia, elevated BUN
C. Low body temperature, metabolic acidosis, elevated BUN
D. Elevated body temperature, sinus bradycardia, hypotension
E. Low body temperature, metabolic alkalosis, and low BUN

166. You are seeing a mother for a prenatal consult. Her last child was born via Cesarean section and underwent an orchiopexy at 13 months for an undescended left testis. She is curious about the risk of this child having the same problem. Which of the following increases the risk of cryptorchidism?

A. Trisomy 21
B. Diabetic mother
C. Prenatal exposure to tobacco
D. Spina bifida
E. Cesarean section

167. You are called emergently to see a 10-year-old patient on the wards for evaluation of sudden tachypnea, hemoptysis, and hypoxia. The patient has been hospitalized for 3 weeks for treatment of invasive osteomyelitis. A chest x-ray has already been ordered. You are concerned about the possibility of a pulmonary embolus (PE). What is the most important risk factor for PE in children?

A. Heart disease
B. Immobility
C. Obesity
D. Central venous catheter
E. Trauma
F. Neoplasia
G. Ventriculoatrial shunt

168. A 3-year-old African-American toddler comes to your office with the chief complaint of coughing. He has had rhinorrhea for 2 days and now he is coughing. The mother notices that this happens every time he gets a cold. Reviewing his chart, you find several office visits a year for "bronchitis." There is no CF in the family, but the father had asthma as a child. Further questioning reveals that he often coughs when he plays actively outside, trying to keep up with his older brother. On physical examination, you occasionally hear an expiratory wheeze. He is afebrile. The most likely explanation for this child's cough is:

A. Viral pneumonia
B. Tuberculosis
C. Gastroesophageal reflux (GER)
D. Milk allergy and lactose intolerance
E. Asthma triggered by viral URIs and exercise

169. While examining a newborn infant in the nursery, you notice that the entire right side of the baby's face is paretic. The right corner of the mouth droops. Review of the mother's chart reveals a history of prolonged labor with a forceps delivery. What is the most likely etiology of this facial palsy?

A. Viral infection
B. Leukemia
C. Lyme disease
D. Compression neuropathy
E. Facial nerve schwannoma

170. A 13-year-old male presents to the clinic with the complaint of intermittent, bloody stools. Over the last several weeks, he has noticed blood mixed in his stools. He denies fever, dysphagia, dyspepsia, rash, arthralgias, oral ulcerations, abdominal pain, diarrhea, or weight loss. A finger stick hemoglobin in the office is 10. The physical examination reveals T 36.6, P 88, R 16, BP 110/60. He appears to be a healthy, young male with a benign abdomen and no hepatosplenomegaly. The rectal examination is negative for hemorrhoids and the scant brown stool is guaiac positive. Which of the following tests is most likely to reveal a diagnosis?

A. UGI
B. Upper endoscopy (EGD)
C. Lower endoscopy (colonoscopy)
D. CT scan of the abdomen
E. Abdominal ultrasound

171. A 15-year-old female with CF comes to your office for a school physical. She has done well in the past and has not been seen at the CF Center for almost 2 years. You hear fine crackles in the posterior, upper lobes during auscultation of her lungs. There is no wheezing. You obtain a sputum culture that grows *Pseudomonas aeruginosa* and a chest radiograph that shows overinflation and increased peribronchial markings most prominent in the upper lung zones. How do you explain these findings to the patient and her family?

A. She probably has GER and is aspirating in her sleep
B. She may have developed asthma
C. This is probably *Mycoplasma pneumoniae* and will go away with clarithromycin
D. This is probably bronchiectasis, representing progression of CF lung disease
E. She has been exposed to tuberculosis

172. In evaluating a 13-year-old girl with short stature, you obtain a bone age and find that the growth plates have fused. You suspect that she has completed her growth spurt. Which of the following hormones is responsible for growth plate fusion?

A. Testosterone
B. Cortisol
C. Aldosterone
D. Estradiol
E. Thyroxine (T_4)

173. Because of splenic dysfunction and an increased risk of bacterial infection, children with sickle-cell anemia should be placed on prophylactic penicillin VK by 4 weeks of age. Children with sickle-cell anemia are particularly susceptible to:

A. Gram-negative rods such as *E. coli*
B. Encapsulated organisms such as *Streptococcus pneumoniae* and *Neisseria meningitis*
C. Fungal infections
D. Viral infections
E. *Staphylcoccus aureus*

174. An 8-year-old female presents to the ER with hematemesis after vomiting for the last 2 days. The emesis has been nonbilious, but today had streaks of bright red blood. Other than mild dehydration, the physical examination is unremarkable. The most likely etiology of the hematemesis is which of the following?

A. Mallory-Weiss tear
B. Gastric ulcer
C. Erosive esophagitis
D. Esophageal varices
E. Nonsteroidal-induced gastritis

175. An 18-year-old male who ingests large quantities of alcohol on a daily basis presents with a hemoglobin of 8.5 g/dL, a mean corpuscular volume of 110 fL, and a reticulocyte count of 0.5%. His most likely diagnosis is:

A. Iron-deficiency anemia
B. Thalassemia minor
C. Lead intoxication
D. Vitamin B_{12} deficiency
E. Anemia of chronic disease

176. In the newborn nursery, you carry out the physical examination of a full-term, 3150-g, Native-American male. Which of the following findings is most consistent with the diagnosis of leukocoria of the left eye?

A. A mucoid discharge is noted from the medial aspect of the left eye, but the conjunctiva is white

B. The corneal light reflex of the right eye is just medial and inferior to midpupil, but that of the left eye is overlying the lateral border of the pupil

C. The retinal reflex is noted to be slightly yellow in hue from both eyes

D. The child refuses to open the left eye for evaluation

E. The retinal reflex is noted to be slightly yellow in hue from the right eye, but is absent in the left eye

177. You are seeing a 13-year-old female in your office for a cough of 6 weeks' duration. As part of your evaluation, you place a PPD to assess whether or not *Mycobacterium tuberculosis* might be the cause of the chronic cough. Which of the following is true about the PPD?

A. The size of the PPD reaction is reported as the sum of the induration plus the erythema

B. The size of the reaction that is considered positive varies according to the patient's risk of having a mycobacterial infection

C. The PPD will be meaningless in this patient, since she had an MMR immunization when she was 15 months old

D. The PPD is not the best way to diagnose *M. tuberculosis* infection; the chest x-ray is more sensitive

E. The PPD may be falsely negative if the patient had a BCG vaccination in early childhood

178. A 13-month-old boy is admitted from the ED with a chief complaint of cough. He has been sick with URI symptoms for 3 days. The mother notes a sharp decline in his energy level and activity. His appetite is diminished and now he has post-tussive emesis. On examination, the most notable findings are diminished heart sounds without any murmurs and wet crackles in the lung fields. He had been well up to this point, and has not had any prior episodes of cyanosis. A chest X-ray is obtained (Figure 3-178). An ECG reveals an ejection fraction of 20%. The most likely diagnosis is:

A. Tetralogy of Fallot
B. Dilated cardiomyopathy
C. Kawasaki syndrome
D. Small VSD
E. Small patent ductus arteriosus (PDA)

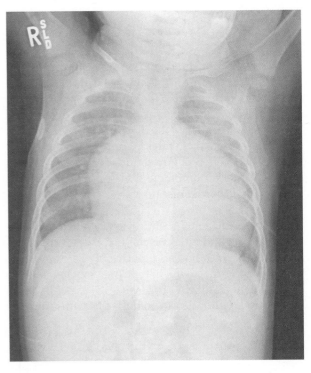

Figure 3-178 • Image Courtesy of the Department of Radiology, Phoenix Children's Hospital, Phoenix, Arizona.

179. A 3-year-old boy presents with petechiae, 2 weeks after experiencing a URI. His mother reports no fever. On physical examination, there is no palpable liver or spleen. His vital signs are normal and he is in no distress. His CBC demonstrates a WCB count of 7000 with an absolute neutrophil count of 2300, a hemoglobin of 13.5 g/dL, and a platelet count of 3000. His most likely diagnosis is:

A. Bernard-Soulier syndrome
B. Gray platelet syndrome
C. Disseminated intravascular coagulation (DIC)
D. HUS
E. Idiopathic thrombocytopenic purpura (ITP)

180. A diagnosis of celiac disease is made by a pediatric gastroenterologist in an 18-month-old Caucasian female with diarrhea and failure to thrive (FTT). The parents received instructions about care, but continue to be confused about the diagnosis. They have researched the topic on the Internet and recently made an appointment with the toddler's pediatrician. Which of the following statements is likely to be supported by the pediatrician?

A. Celiac disease is the result of an improper response to exposure to wheat, barley, and rye

B. The disease is likely a rare complication following childhood immunizations

C. A diet high in gluten, wheat, and rye will help desensitize the toddler

D. Successful treatment is short-lived, and unfortunately, the lifespan will be drastically shortened even with appropriate therapy

E. The altered bowel lumen protects against other autoimmune diseases such as diabetes and thyroid disease

181. Type II diabetes mellitus (DM), which was once rare in children, is on the rise in the U.S. population. In clinical practice, it is important to determine which type of diabetes a given patient is likely to have (e.g., type I versus type II), and then to confirm this with appropri-ate testing. A distinguishing clinical feature of type I DM is that patients tend to:

A. Be obese

B. Exhibit acanthosis nigricans on the neck and in the axillae

C. Have a family history of DM

D. Be of Caucasian (white) race

E. Have high serum insulin and C-peptide levels

182. You are seeing a 6-month-old girl in clinic. This is her first visit since the age of 1 month because her family members are migrant workers. The infant has been breastfed and is just starting solids. Stooling has not been a problem. The mother reveals no intercurrent illnesses or problems. On physical examination, you find the infant is notice-ably thin but the remainder of the examination is normal. Her growth chart is shown in Figures 3-182A and 3-182B. CBC, lead level, urinalysis,

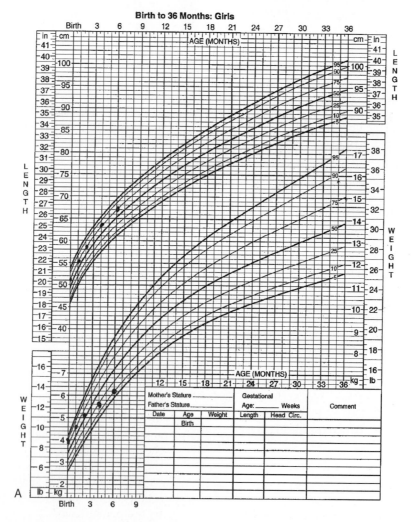

Figure 3-182 • Images Courtesy of the Phoenix Children's Hospital, Phoenix, Arizona.

Birth to 36 Months: Girls

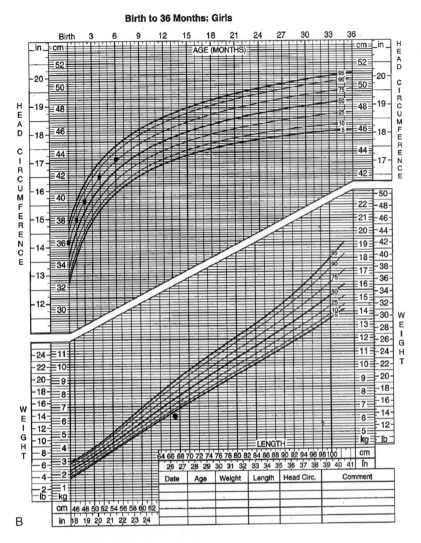

Figure 3-182 • (*Continued*)

CMP, thyroid function, HIV testing, and sweat test are all normal. The most likely diagnosis is:

A. Chronic anemia
B. CF
C. Hypothyroidism
D. Renal tubular acidosis
E. Inadequate caloric intake

183. You are seeing a 10-year-old boy in clinic with a chief complaint of double vision. He and his mother report that he began to complain of double vision in the afternoon. His schoolteacher also noticed the problem and thought he "looked sleepy." On detailed questioning, he reveals that he also tires faster than his classmates in gym class due to muscle fatigue, not respiratory symptoms. On physical examination, his growth and development have been normal. His pupils and visual acuity are normal, but you notice a distinct ptosis. His extraocular muscle exam is also abnormal. The rest of the exam is within normal limits. The most likely diagnosis is

A. Pituitary tumor
B. Amblyopia
C. Myasthenia gravis
D. Botulism
E. Tick paralysis

184. A newborn in the nursery is noted to have frothy secretions from the mouth and nose, and has coughing and cyanosis when given a bottle. The nurse reports that she was unable to pass an NG tube into the stomach. A flat-plate x-ray of the abdomen reveals gaseous dilatation of the stomach. Which of the following is the most likely diagnosis?

A. Tracheoesophageal fistula (TEF)
B. Isolated esophageal atresia
C. Choanal atresia
D. Gastroesophageal reflux disease (GERD)
E. Duodenal atresia

185. A 12-year-old boy is seen because of a progressive visual, hearing, speech, and gait impairment. Although he has done rather well in school through the fifth grade, he is now doing poorly in the sixth grade. Your suspicion is that this boy suffers from some sort of CNS degenerative disease. Basic chemistries reveal a serum sodium of 128 mEq/L, potassium 5.8 mEq/L, chloride 100 mEq/L, and CO_2 18 mEq/L. Your impression is that these chemistries are compatible with adrenal insufficiency. Which one of the following would apply to this patient?

A. This syndrome is sporadic and not likely to occur in a sibling
B. The metabolic defect is an inability to degrade very long chain fatty acids in peroxisomes
C. Addison disease is frequently delayed for years after the CNS manifestations
D. A specific gene mutation has not been identified
E. This disease is not usually associated with a seizure disorder

186. The family of a 2-year-old child with Tay-Sachs disease is interested in having another child. They would like to know the risk of having a second child with Tay-Sachs. What advice would you give?

A. No risk, since Tay-Sachs is caused by a sporadic mutation
B. 100%, since Tay-Sachs is an autosomal-dominant disease
C. 25%, since Tay-Sachs is an autosomal-recessive disease
D. It depends on the sex of the fetus, since Tay-Sachs is X-linked
E. One can determine the risk only by genetic testing after conception

187. A 17-year-old female is seen on a mobile health van for homeless youth. She complains of chronic skin infections of her arms and thighs. She had seen a doctor for the rash in the ER 2 weeks ago. She was given a prescription for cephalexin, which she took for 6 days, but quit because the rash was not getting better. She has a history of drug use by subcutaneous injections (skin-popping). Which of the following statements is likely to be true?

A. Culture of her lesions will show a resistant organism
B. Biopsy of the lesions will show a granulomatous process IV therapy is required
C. Culture of the wounds will show *Mycobacterium marinum*
D. The lesions would improve with warm compresses, and the length of therapy increased to 3 weeks

188. A 2-month-old baby is noted to be cyanotic with a loud heart murmur. His chest radiograph is obtained (Figure 3-188). The most likely reason that this baby is cyanotic is:

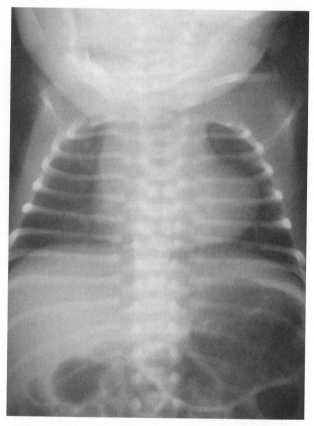

Figure 3-188 • Image Courtesy of the Department of Radiology, Phoenix Children's Hospital, Phoenix, Arizona.

A. Left-to-right shunting through an ASD
B. Right-to-left shunting through a PDA
C. Left-to-right shunting through a VSD
D. Right-to-left shunting through a VSD
E. Mixing of oxygenated and desaturated blood in a persistent truncus arteriosus

189. You are about to see a new patient in your general pediatric clinic. She is a 12-year-old female who needs a routine preventive health care visit. You notice that she plots well above the 95th percentile for weight. You also note that she falls below the 5th percentile for height, and she is hypertensive for her age and height. She denies using any medications or other pills. She does report easy bruising, irregular menses, fatigue, and symptoms of a depressed mood. Her physical examination demonstrates that she is short, exhibits central obesity, and has a mound of fat over her upper thoracic and cervical spine. Her skin examination is remarkable for reddish purple striae over the sides of her trunk, as well as moderate facial acne and facial hair. Laboratory testing confirms your suspicion of an elevated serum cortisol level. Given the above information, what is the best term for this patient's diagnosis?

    A. Addison disease
    B. Klippel-Trenaunay-Weber syndrome
    C. Cushing disease
    D. Cushing syndrome
    E. Multiple endocrine neoplasia (MEN) type 2A

190. You are seeing a 5-year-old African-American boy with a history of sickle-cell anemia. On physical examination, he looks well except for mild tachypnea, an oxygen saturation of 91% on room air, and a temperature of 38.4°C. Which of the following is required to make the diagnosis of acute chest syndrome in this patient?

    A. Supplemental oxygen requirement
    B. Change in appearance of chest radiograph
    C. Increased respiratory rate
    D. Documented bacterial infection
    E. Pain

191. A thin 13-year-old is seen at a primary care office for a preparticipation sports physical. There have been no past medical problems and the adolescent is interested in trying out for the track team. The physician notes a systolic ejection murmur, best heard on the upper left sternal border. The S2 component is widely split and fixed. The ECG shows mild RVH. Which of the following statements is true?

    A. The lesion described is most likely a PDA
    B. The lesion described is most likely an ASD
    C. Spontaneous resolution of this defect is common during the adolescent growth spurt

    D. Cardiac catheterization is the next step in the diagnosis
    E. Pulmonary hypertension is inevitable given the late diagnosis

192. A 5-year-old boy (Figure 3-192) is admitted to the hospital for vomiting, diarrhea, and dehydration. His past medical history is significant for moderate mental retardation. On physical examination, you notice a III/VI harsh, systolic, ejection murmur at the upper left sternal border. His admission electrolytes are Na 135 mmol/L, K 3.2 mmol/L, Cl 101 mmol/L, CO_2 14 mmol/L, BUN 25 mg/dL, Cr 0.5 mg/dL, Ca 12.6 mg/dL. Which of the following likely explains this patient's clinical syndrome?

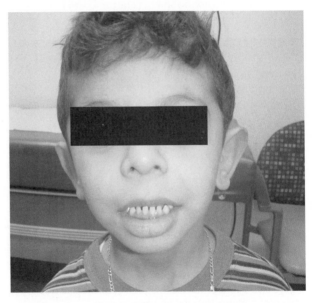

Figure 3-192 • Image Courtesy of the Phoenix Children's Hospital, Phoenix, Arizona.

    A. Down syndrome
    B. Williams syndrome
    C. Prader-Willi syndrome
    D. Angelman syndrome
    E. Velocardial facial syndrome

193. The mother of a 3-month-old boy reports that his eyes are frequently crossed, especially when the child looks to either side. The most important finding that would differentiate pseudostrabismus from strabismus is

A. The corneal light reflex is noted to be just medial to and below the physical center of the cornea in both eyes
B. There is a subtle movement of the right eye outward on covering the left eye
C. With the alternate cover test, the eyes begin to jerk inwardly once uncovered
D. The right eye is deviated significantly toward the nose, but makes no movement with either cover-uncover or alternate cover testing
E. It is noted that the child has broad epicanthal folds

194. A short, 7-year-old boy presents with intermittent, anterior thigh pain and limp. Although he has not had significant fever or hip pain, the physical examination reveals limited hip range of motion and proximal thigh atrophy. Radiographs of the hips are obtained (Figure 3-194). The most likely diagnosis is

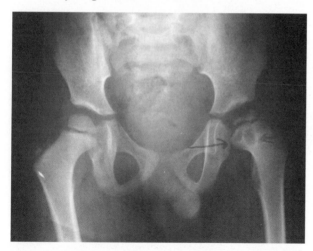

Figure 3-194 • Image Courtesy of the Department of Radiology, Phoenix Children's Hospital, Phoenix, Arizona.

A. Septic arthritis of the hip
B. Osteomyelitis
C. SCFE
D. Legg-Calvé-Perthes disease
E. Transient synovitis

The response options for items 195 to 200 are the same. You will be required to select one answer for each item in the set.

A. Bronchopulmonary dysplasia (BPD)
B. Acute respiratory distress syndrome (ARDS)
C. Pyloric stenosis
D. Diabetic ketoacidosis (DKA)
E. Appropriate mechanical ventilation in a healthy child after orthopedic surgery
F. Narcotic overdose in a patient receiving supplemental O_2 by nasal cannula

195. pH 7.37, pCO_2 44, pO_2 52, HCO_3 24

196. pH 7.20, pCO_2 28, pO_2 93, HCO_3 6

197. pH 7.40, pCO_2 40, pO_2 130, HCO_3 23

198. pH 7.25, pCO_2 60, pO_2 70, HCO_3 24

199. pH 7.50, pCO_2 66, pO_2 92, HCO_3 42

200. pH 7.41, pCO_2 68, pO_2 65, HCO_3 42

End of Set

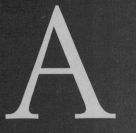

A Answers and Explanations

151. C	168. E	185. B
152. C	169. D	186. C
153. C	170. C	187. A
154. C	171. D	188. D
155. B	172. D	189. D
156. B	173. B	190. B
157. C	174. A	191. B
158. A	175. D	192. B
159. D	176. B	193. A
160. E	177. B	194. D
161. A	178. E	195. B
162. D	179. E	196. D
163. E	180. A	197. E
164. B	181. D	198. F
165. B	182. E	199. C
166. D	183. C	200. A
167. D	184. A	

151. C. The definition of puberty is the onset of secondary sex characteristics, growth spurt, and bone age advancement. This happens in girls between the ages of 8 and 13 years with the onset of menarche by age 16. In boys, puberty starts between the ages of 9 and 14 years. In girls, puberty starts with thelarche (breast development), followed by pubarche (pubic hair development), growth spurt, and then menarche (menstruation).

A, B, D, E. These progressions are incorrect. See explanation for C.

152. C. The organism that causes this rash is parvovirus B19. The clinical findings are consistent with a mild illness called erythema infectiosum or "Fifth disease." Parvovirus B19 may also cause transient aplastic crises in patients with any type of chronic hemolytic anemia such as sickle-cell disease. When the virus affects the bone marrow of a fetus, hydrops fetalis (anemia, cardiac failure) may result. Parvovirus B19 is also associated with arthritis and arthralgia, thrombocytopenia, and aseptic meningitis.

A. Parvovirus is not known to cause deafness.
B. Developmental delay has not been described as a result of parvoviral infection.
D. Renal failure is uncommon in patients with parvovirus infection.
E. Diarrhea is not typically a feature of parvoviral illness.

153. C. This case is typical of pseudotumor cerebri, a clinical syndrome that mimics brain tumors. In this condition, the intracranial pressure (ICP) is increased, but the CSF has a normal cell count, protein, and glucose. The MRI shows normal ventricles and no evidence of bleeding. Pseudotumor cerebri is associated with a wide variety of conditions, including various metabolic disorders, prolonged corticosteroid use, excess or deficiency of vitamin A, obesity, pregnancy, infections (roseola, chronic otitis media), Guillian-Barré syndrome, drugs (tetracycline, accutane, nitrofurantoin), and anemia. Treatment is aimed at the underlying condition. Some patients require serial lumbar punctures to remove CSF to decrease ICP. Acetazolamide and corticosteroids may also be used to decrease ICP.

A. Meningitis is associated with fever, pleocytosis, and elevated CSF protein levels.
B. Migraine is not typically associated with increased ICP or papilledema.
D. E. Both a brain tumor and a subdural hematoma would be evident on an MRI scan.

154. C. This child has a developmental speech age appropriate for an 18-month-old child. The average 18-month-old has a 10-word vocabulary, with a few specific words and can follow one-step commands. The child should have further evaluation for this speech delay.

A. Most babies begin monosyllabic babbling at around 6 months.
B. Infants understand "No" on average by 10 months. The first real words begin at about 12 months of age.
D. By 24 months, the child should be able to put two to three words together in a phrase and know 50 words, with half of those words being understandable to strangers.
E. By 36 months, the child should be able to count to 3, know his or her age and sex, and construct a simple sentence; three-quarters of a 3-year-old's words should be comprehended by a stranger.

155. B. Polycythemia is known to be a complication in the infant of a diabetic mother. The signs and symptoms are irritability, cyanosis, seizures, jaundice, stroke, and headache.

A. An anemic child may exhibit all of the above findings, but will be pale, not plethoric.
C, E. A newborn with neutropenia or lymphopenia will not typically present with seizures.
D. A newborn with thrombocytopenia would more likely have petechiae and ecchymosis.

156. B. Internal tibial torsion is a common cause of in-toeing, which is often seen in the second year of life. This condition is due to normal in-utero positioning of the legs. In internal tibial torsion, the thigh-foot angle (as shown in the diagram) will demonstrate the internal rotation of the foot. Normally, the thigh-foot angle will be slightly externally rotated. Internal tibial torsion generally resolves spontaneously without the need for casting or special shoes or braces.

A. In metatarus adductus, the foot itself is misshapen and is easily diagnosed by examination of the sole of the foot. The lateral border of the foot will have a prominence that corresponds to the base of the fifth metatarsal and a skin crease may be noted on the medial side of the foot.

C. Femoral anteversion is a hip deformity that causes in-toeing. Children with this condition can sit comfortably on the floor with their legs in a "W-position." Most resolve without treatment.

D. Genu varum refers to "bowed legs."

E. Pes planus is the scientific term for "flat feet"; it does not cause a pigeon-toed gait.

157. **C. Apnea refers to the cessation of respiratory air flow, and may occur as the result of many causes. Central apnea occurs when there is no respiratory effort. Obstructive apnea occurs when the respiratory flow is blocked. The most common pattern of apnea in preterm babies has a mixed etiology (in 50% to 75%). Obstructive apnea usually precedes the central apnea, but at times the reverse occurs.**

A. Obstructive apnea can occur due to pharyngeal and upper airway collapse or craniofacial anomalies or during feedings, or it may be positional, but it is not the most common type.

B. Central apnea occurs when there are insufficient CNS stimuli to the respiratory muscles. Premature infants are at a higher risk for central apnea because of the immature development of their respiratory and central nervous systems. Most premature infants have factors that result in a mixed pattern combining central and obstructive apneas.

D. Sepsis is a cause of preterm apnea and must always be considered, but it is not the most frequent cause of apnea.

E. Metabolic causes must also be considered as the source in neonatal apnea. Hypoglycemia, hypocalcemia, hypernatremia, hyperammonemia, organic academia, and hypothermia can all produce apnea in a tiny neonate. However, these are much less common.

158. **A. Central diabetes insipidus is characterized by an inability to concentrate urine, free water loss, and volume depletion, causing increased sodium reabsorption. Therefore, the urine will be dilute (lower than isotonic), resulting in hypernatremia, and there will be very little sodium in the urine. These findings are also consistent with nephrogenic diabetes insipidus.**

B. Diabetes insipidus is never characterized by hyponatremia, and the urine is almost never above isotonic.

C. Very dilute urine would not have this much sodium under any circumstances.

D. Concentrated urine is not compatible with either central or nephrogenic diabetes insipidus.

E. Concentrated urine with hyponatremia and with significant urine sodium concentration is more compatible with SIADH than with diabetes insipidus.

159. **D. This newborn has Sturge-Weber syndrome. The hemangioma or vascular proliferation that is visible on the skin is also associated with vascular proliferation within the eye and brain. Buphthalmos and glaucoma are frequent complications that are secondary to vascular proliferation involving the eye on the ipsilateral side.**

A. Generally, Sturge-Weber syndrome is limited to the face, eye, meninges, and brain on one side. Von Hippel-Lindau syndrome is a different condition, which affects the CNS and abdominal viscera.

B. Mental retardation is common, as are the development of intractable seizures, cerebral atrophy, and hemiplegia. These occur as a result of intracranial and cerebral proliferations of blood vessels.

C. Patients with the Sturge-Weber syndrome frequently present with the early onset of focal or generalized tonic-clonic seizures, not absence-type seizures. On EEG, the seizures are seen to be mostly unilateral, on the contralateral side to the lesion, and can be quite difficult to control. They may become bilateral with time, related to cerebral atrophy.

E. The port-wine stain of Sturge-Weber syndrome is always present at birth.

160. **E. Intussusception is the most common cause of intestinal obstruction in children between 3 months and 6 years of age. It presents with the sudden onset of severe, colicky abdominal pain and lethargy, with resolution between the paroxysms of pain. A currant jelly stool (blood mixed with mucus) is seen about 60% of the time. An air contrast or barium enema is diagnostic and sometimes therapeutic. If the radiologist is unable to reduce the intussusception, immediate surgical intervention is necessary.**

A. Patients with viral enteritis usually present with fever, vomiting, and diarrhea. Stools are usually loose and watery. An abdominal mass would not be present.

B. Bacterial enteritis with *E. coli* 0157-H7 presents with fever, abdominal pain, and diarrhea, which may be bloody. These patients are also at risk for HUS.

C. Acute cholecystitis presents with fever, right upper quadrant pain, and elevated alkaline phosphatase and bilirubin.

D. A patient with acute appendicitis will usually localize pain to the right lower quadrant and have peritoneal signs and fever.

161. **A. This adolescent has chronic menstrual irregularity, with evidence of a hyperandrogenic state (i.e., acne, facial hair, and probable anovulation), which is consistent with polycystic ovarian syndrome (PCOS). For diagnosis, the patient must have clinical and laboratory evidence of increased androgens such as testosterone and dihydroepiandrosterone-sulfate (DHEA-S). Many patients become amenorrheic.**

B. Pregnancy must always be considered in any adolescent with menstrual irregularity, but it does not explain the rest of her symptoms.

C. An immature hypothalamic-pituitary-ovarian axis is the most common cause of menstrual irregularities in adolescents after menarche occurs. Most adolescents will develop normal menstrual cycles within 2 to 3 years of menarche, especially if menarche occurs prior to the age of 13 years.

D. Cushing syndrome can cause weight gain, abdominal striae, and menstrual irregularity, but is much less common than PCOS.

E. Hypothyroidism can also be responsible for menstrual irregularities and weight gain, but would not explain the hirsutism and acne.

162. **D. This infant has supraventricular tachycardia (SVT) and is exhibiting signs of congestive heart failure. Adenosine transiently blocks AV conduction and sinus node pacemaking activity. It is the drug of choice in treating SVT. If adenosine is unavailable, cardioversion of 0.5 J/kg can be attempted.**

A. Lidocaine is helpful with other dysrhythmias, including ventricular tachycardia.

B. Procainamide is used infrequently in children with arrhythmias.

C. Metoprolol, a β-blocker, is not the treatment of choice for SVT; it can cause extreme bradycardia and sometimes hypotension.

E. Magnesium sulfate is used to treat torsades de pointes.

163. **E. This child has experienced eruption of the central maxillary and mandibular incisors. The first mandibular molars may erupt before the mandibular canines between 12 and 16 months. The central mandibular incisors erupt at around 6 months, followed by the lateral mandibular incisors at around 8 months. This child is slightly behind the normal, with delayed eruption of the lateral incisors. However, there is a wide variation in the time of dental eruption.**

A. Primary tooth eruption begins at about age 6 months. The central mandibular incisors are the first to arrive, followed by the central maxillary incisors.

B. C. The lateral maxillary and mandibular incisors will follow the central incisors.

D. All of the eight anterior teeth are usually present by the end of the first year. By age $2\frac{1}{2}$ years, all 20 primary teeth will usually have erupted.

164. **B. A trial of stimulant medication is indicated for inattentive-type ADHD. Hyperactivity is not a necessary component of ADD and is less common in girls. A child with ADHD, predominantly inattentive type, who has severe academic problems at school and with homework may be considered for stimulant treatment, even if peer relationships and family functioning are not otherwise affected. As with any stimulant trial, parent and teacher ratings of behavior at baseline and after initiation of therapy should be obtained. Studies of stimulant medication show an effect on both attention and behavior.**

A. As in the explanation for B, hyperactivity is not necessary to make a diagnosis of ADD. A trial of stimulant medication is indicated in this case.

C. TCAs are indicated as a second-line drug for therapy of ADHD. They are used only after stimulant medications have failed or a suspected coexisting mood disorder is present.

D. Randomized controlled studies have identified a significant benefit from stimulant medication compared to placebo.

E. It is unlikely that the child will "outgrow" these symptoms. Continued observation without further evaluation and treatment would further jeopardize this child's future school performance and other behaviors as well.

165. **B. Hypotension, sinus bradycardia, and an elevated BUN would be expected. Severe anorexia is associated with changes in nearly every organ system. Some of these changes are primary responses and some are due to chronic malnutrition. Hypotension is usually postural. Bradycardia can be severe, with rates as low as 20 beats per minute. BUN can be elevated due to dehydration and increased protein catabolism. Signs consistent with hypothyroidism, including a low body temperature, cold intolerance, and dry skin and hair, are present, although TSH is usually normal.**

   A. Tachycardia is not typically associated with prolonged anorexia.
   C. Metabolic alkalosis is possible, particularly when the patient has been abusing laxatives or diuretics, but metabolic acidosis is uncommon.
   D. Low or normal body temperature would be expected.
   E. Low BUN is not expected, although BUN may remain normal.

166. **D. Several inherited syndromes are associated with cryptorchidism. Neurogenic (e.g., spina bifida) and mechanical anomalies (e.g., arthrogryposis multiplex), hypothalamic dysfunction, and connective tissue disorders may all disrupt testicular descent. Cryptorchidism is also common in infants with abdominal wall defects, such as exomphalos or omphalocele, gastroschisis, and exstrophy of the bladder.**

   A. Trisomy 21 is not associated with an increased risk of cryptorchidism.
   B. Infants of diabetic mothers have no increased risk of cryptorchidism.
   C. Although prematurity is associated with cryptorchidism, prenatal exposure to tobacco by itself is not.
   E. Cesarean section has not been shown to be a risk factor for cryptorchidism.

167. **D. The top risk factors for PE in children, in order of clinical importance, include:**

   1. The presence of a central venous catheter
   2. Immobility
   3. Heart disease
   4. Ventriculoatrial shunt
   5. Trauma
   6. Neoplasia
   7. Operation
   8. Infection
   9. Medical illness
   10. Dehydration
   11. Shock
   12. Obesity

   A, B, C, E, F, G. Heart disease, immobility, obesity, trauma, neoplasia, and ventriculoatrial shunt are all risk factors for PE in children, but, as in the explanation for D, are not the most clinically important.

168. **E. The history of recurrent "bronchitis," coughing with exercise, URIs, and wheezing on exam is supportive of the diagnosis of asthma. To further confirm this diagnosis, the patient can be given a trial of an acute bronchodilator in your office and reevaluated to see if the wheezing improves.**

   A. Viral pneumonia typically presents acutely with fever, cough, and crackles on examination.
   B. Tuberculosis usually presents as a primary pneumonia in this age group.
   C. GERD should be associated with vomiting and should have less relationship to URIs and exercise.
   D. Food allergy can cause wheezing, but also has associated symptoms, such as eczema and diarrhea.

169. **D. Compression of the facial nerve with forceps during a delivery can result in Bell palsy. This will recover spontaneously in a few days or weeks in most cases.**

   A. Most cases of Bell palsy occur about 2 weeks following a viral illness. EBV is the source in 20% of cases.
   B. Leukemic cells can infiltrate the facial nerve and cause paralysis, but other obvious signs of leukemia would be expected to make this diagnosis. This diagnosis is rare in the newborn period.
   C. Lyme disease can cause a prolonged Bell palsy. There is no clinical history or exposure in this case to suggest this disease.
   E. Since most cases of Bell palsy resolve spontaneously, a facial nerve schwannoma is suspected only in cases in which resolution does not occur.

170. **C. This patient most likely has a colonic polyp or an arteriovenous malformation (AVM) as the source of his lower GI blood loss. Colonoscopy will elucidate a colonic polyp, and it can be removed or biopsied at that time.**

A, B. An upper GI source of blood typically presents with melena or black/tarry stools. Upper GI bleeds are evaluated by EGD in most cases.

D. A CT scan of the abdomen with oral contrast may reveal a large polyp in the colon, but it cannot provide a tissue diagnosis.

E. Abdominal ultrasound is not typically helpful in diagnosing lower GI bleeds.

171. **D. Bronchiectasis is the result of longstanding inflammation in the CF lung. It is often more prominent in the upper lung zones. Eighty percent of CF patients in North America have chronic endobronchial infection with *Pseudomonas aeruginosa*. Failure to participate in comprehensive CF care often leads to deterioration. This patient would likely benefit from aggressive airway clearance and antibiotic treatment directed against the *Pseudomonas*.**

A. Although GER is often associated with obstructive lung diseases, bronchiectasis develops only after prolonged chronic aspiration.

B. Uncomplicated asthma usually has a nearly normal chest x-ray and is not associated with *Pseudomonas* lung infection.

C. *Mycoplasma pneumoniae* lung infections are frequent in adolescence. They usually produce symptoms of acute infection such as fever, severe cough, malaise, and chest pain.

E. Tuberculosis infection is always a concern in patients with lung disease, but it usually presents as acute pneumonia in adolescence.

172. **D. Short stature must be evaluated by a thorough history and physical examination. It is important to obtain an annualized growth velocity. Prepubertal growth velocity is about 4 to 6 cm/year, and pubertal annualized growth velocity is about 8 to 10 cm/year. In addition, a child's probable inherited growth potential can be estimated by midparental height percentiles:**

- Boys = (mother's height + 13 cm) + father's height divided by 2; +/− 8 cm
- Girls = mother's height + (father's height— 13 cm) divided by 2; +/− 8 cm

It is important to note the Tanner stage, as pubertal hormones affect linear growth. Estrogens (estradiol) mediate breast growth, leucorrhea, bone growth, and epiphyseal closure while androgens (testosterone) mediate sexual hair, external genitalia growth, bone growth, acne, and body odor.

A. Testosterone is converted to estradiol by the aromatase enzyme in boys. Thus, it is estrogen, not testosterone, that leads to growth plate closure in males.

B, C, E. Cortisol, aldosterone, and thyroxine do not promote growth plate fusion.

173. **B. The child with sickle-cell anemia is vulnerable to life-threatening infection as early as 2 months of age. Splenic dysfunction results from sickling of the red cells within the spleen. The spleen is unable to filter microorganisms from the bloodstream. Splenic dysfunction is followed eventually by splenic infarction, usually by 2 to 4 years of age. As a consequence of this dysfunction, there is an increased risk of infection from encapsulated organisms, such as *S. pneumoniae* and *N. meningitis*. The hallmark of infection is fever. The child with a sickle-cell syndrome who has a temperature greater than 38.5°C must be evaluated immediately by qualified medical providers.**

A. Children with sickle-cell disease can develop infections with any bacteria, but are most at risk from *S. pneumoniae* and *N. meningitis*.

C. Fungal infections are unusual in children with splenic dysfunction.

D. Viral infections can occur commonly in children with sickle cell, but the highest risk is from encapsulated bacteria.

E. *Staphylococcus aureus* can be life-threatening in any child, including children with sickle cell, but *S. pneumoniae* and *N. meningitis* are more common.

174. **A. With a history of recurrent vomiting, a Mallory-Weiss tear is the most likely etiology of the hematemesis. Small tears in the mucosa of the esophagus can result in streaks or flecks of bright red blood in the emesis.**

B. A bleeding gastric ulcer is typically accompanied by significant epigastric or left upper quadrant abdominal pain.

C. Erosive esophagitis is seen in patients with untreated or inadequately treated GERD.

D. Esophageal varices can bleed after vomiting due to increased venous pressure, but this patient has no known history of chronic liver disease.

E. Nonsteroidal medications can induce gastritis and result in hematemesis, but there is no history of NSAID use in this patient.

175. **D.** The patient in this question has a macrocytic anemia with an inappropriately depressed reticulocyte response. Individuals who consume large quantities of alcohol on a daily basis often become deficient in both vitamin B_{12} and folate. Deficiencies of both lead to a macrocytic anemia.

   A, B, C. Iron-deficiency anemia and thalassemia minor are characterized by a microcytic anemia, as is lead intoxication.

   E. Anemia of chronic disease can present as either a microcytic or normocytic anemia.

176. **E.** The direct translation of leukocoria is "white pupil." This can manifest as an absent/abnormal/asymmetric retinal reflex, or as a white tissue occluding the pupil on direct examination. The differential diagnosis for the etiology includes, but is not limited to, toxoplasmosis, toxocara, syphilis, congenital rubella, CMV, fungal endophthalmitis, congenital cataract, retinoblastoma, neuroblastoma, leukemia, retinal detachment, and retinal coloboma.

   A. In the newborn, cautious observation of conjunctivitis neonatorum is necessary. In a baby with eye drainage and a white conjunctiva, the nasolacrimal duct is occluded.

   B. An abnormal corneal light reflex, as in this case of left eye esotropia, can be an indication of blindness. In the absence of a white pupil, leukocoria is not illustrated in this example.

   C. The retinal reflex is given the misnomer "red reflex." This is a Eurocentric term referring to the color of the normal reflex in lightly pigmented eyes. In patients with dark eyes, a yellowish appearance is typical. In people of Asian heritage, a yellow-white reflex is typical. In this example, the fact that the reflection is symmetric suggests normality, or at least the equivalence of the two eyes.

   D. An inadequate examination such as this COULD be brought about because of photophobia and one of the underlying conditions producing leukocoria. However, in this example, the eye could also be perfectly healthy.

177. **B.** The size of the induration of the PPD that qualifies as a positive result depends on the potential risk of *Mycobacterium tuberculosis* infection. An induration greater than 15 mm is positive for children older than 4 years with no known risk or potential TB contact. For children less than 4 years old, or children with certain chronic illnesses (e.g., Hodgkin lymphoma, diabetes mellitus, chronic renal failure, or malnutrition) or increased exposure risk, the PPD is considered positive with an induration greater than 10 mm. An induration of 5 mm or greater is considered positive for children with close contact, suspected active infection, or HIV infection (or other immunosuppressing conditions).

   A. Only the induration is important in the measurement, not the erythema.

   C. The measles vaccine can temporarily suppress the response to the PPD for 4 to 6 weeks, so PPD testing should be deferred (if possible) until 4 to 6 weeks after the MMR vaccination.

   D. Most children are identified as infected by a positive PPD. A chest radiograph is important to identify active versus latent disease in patients with a positive PPD. It would be reasonable to obtain a chest radiograph in this case scenario as part of the evaluation for cough independent of the PPD status.

   E. The BCG can enhance the induration of the PPD, not reduce it. Interpretation of the PPD is generally the same for those who have and those who have not received BCG vaccination.

178. **B.** The combination of cardiomegaly and a very low ejection fraction indicates dilated cardiomyopathy (DCM). All ages can be affected by DCM with an insidious onset. Irritability, poor appetite, cough (caused by pulmonary congestion), and dyspnea with mild exertion are frequent presenting complaints. A history of preceding viral infection indicates some possible role for myocarditis.

   A. Tetralogy of Fallot is a form of cyanotic congenital heart disease and should have presented earlier. The classic x-ray finding is a boot-shaped heart.

   C. Kawasaki syndrome (or mucocutaneous lymph node syndrome) causes coronary artery abnormalities, not cardiomegaly.

   D. A small VSD is usually well tolerated, does not cause cardiomegaly, and should produce a murmur.

   E. A small PDA does not cause cardiomegaly but should produce a continuous "machinery-like" murmur.

179. **E.** ITP is an autoimmune condition in which antiplatelet antibodies are produced. It most commonly presents days to weeks after a viral infection. If a child presents with fever, organomegaly, diffuse lymphadenopathy, or bone pain, other diagnoses must be considered.

A, B. Bernard-Soulier syndrome and gray platelet syndrome are both inherited deficiencies of platelet aggregation. In both syndromes, the platelet count is normal.
C. A child with DIC would be expected to be quite ill and have an accompanying anemia.
D. A child with HUS will also have renal failure and microangiopathic hemolytic anemia.

180. **A.** Celiac disease results from an abnormal immunologic response after exposure to proteins found in wheat, barley, and rye in genetically predisposed persons. This response leads to the many complaints (diarrhea, FTT, constipation, and/or malabsorption) in these individuals.

B. The disease is not linked to immunizations.
C. A gluten-free diet will allow for resolution of the symptoms.
D. If a gluten-free diet is maintained with control of symptoms, lifespan should not be affected.
E. The disease is linked to other autoimmune diseases, such as diabetes.

181. **D.** With the exception of D, all of the answers provided are more characteristic (though not diagnostic) of type II DM. Caucasian race is very common in type I DM (the majority of children with this disorder are white), but less common in type II DM. African-Americans represent the highest proportion of patients with type II DM nationally. Hispanic-American and Native-American ethnicities are also at high risk for developing type II DM.

A. Patients with type II DM tend to be overweight or obese. Obesity also occurs in type I DM, but less commonly.
B. Acanthosis nigricans is associated with a high-insulin or insulin-resistant state, which occurs in type II, but not in type I DM.
C. Family history does not correlate as strongly with the incidence of type I DM as it does with type II DM.
E. Type II DM is associated with high serum insulin and C-peptide levels, whereas type I DM is not.

182. **E.** Because the medical workup is unrevealing, the most likely diagnosis would be FTT secondary to inadequate caloric intake. Inadequate caloric intake affects the weight first, followed by the height, and then the head circumference. The prevalence of FTT in children living in poverty is 5% to 10%, due to inadequate food available.

A. Anemia would have been detected on the CBC.
B. An abnormal sweat test would diagnose CF.
C. Thyroid function would not be normal in hypothyroidism.
D. The urinalysis should reflect the electrolyte abnormalities associated with renal tubular acidosis, as well as a nongap acidosis detected on CMP.

183. **C.** Myasthenia gravis characteristically produces ptosis and diplopia due to extraocular muscle weakness. It is caused by autoimmune receptor blockage of the postsynaptic acetylcholine receptors. It is progressive and typically gets worse throughout the day.

A. A pituitary tumor can cause eye symptoms, but more often causes a homonymous hemianopsia along with endocrine problems.
B. Amblyopia is defined as a reduction in visual acuity in the involved eye; it is often associated with strabismus.
D. Botulism may begin with a prodrome of gastroenteritis before the progressive onset of generalized weakness. Patients are often hypotonic and often present with constipation.
E. Tick paralysis begins with a prodromal illness, followed by progressive neuromuscular dysfunction that does not wax and wane like myasthenia gravis.

184. **A.** The classic presentation of TEF is an infant with feeding difficulties, excessive oral secretions, and the inability to pass an NG tube. There may be a history of polyhydramnios. The most common form of TEF has an esophageal blind pouch with a TEF distally. This blind esophageal pouch is the reason for the inability to pass the NG tube. Only 4% of TEFs present as the H-type; in H-type fistulas there is no esophageal atresia, but simply a fistula between the esophagus and trachea.

B. Since there is air in the stomach, the patient cannot have isolated esophageal atresia.

C. Newborns with choanal atresia have difficulty with mouth breathing and cyanosis occurring during feedings; they do not typically have frothy secretions.

D. GERD causes vomiting associated with feeds.

E. Duodenal atresia presents with bilious emesis in the absence of abdominal distension in the first day of life. Abdominal films will reveal the classic "double bubble" sign.

185. **B. The disease described is consistent with adrenoleukodystrophy. The metabolic defect is the inability to degrade very long chain fatty acids in peroxisomes due to a gene mutation on the X chromosome. It is therefore an X-linked trait occurring only in boys.**

A. Adrenoleukodystrophy is an X-linked disorder occurring only in boys. The chances are that it will occur in half of the male offspring of this carrier mother.

C. Addison disease occurs in about 50% of cases of adrenoleukodystrophy. When present, it generally either precedes or accompanies the onset of the CNS manifestations. Occasionally, Addison disease occurs without the CNS manifestations.

D. The gene has been identified on the X chromosome (at Xq28). More than 100 mutations have been identified.

E. Generalized seizures are common in the early stages of adrenoleukodystrophy.

186. **C. Tay-Sachs disease is an autosomal-recessive disease that results in a deficiency of the lysosomal enzyme B-hexosaminidase. Each parent must carry an abnormal gene, and the fetus must receive the abnormal gene from each parent (homozygous) to be affected. Heterozygotes for Tay-Sachs disease (carriers) are not affected.**

A. A sporadic mutation would have to occur on both sets of genes.

B. Tay-Sachs is not autosomal dominant.

D. Tay-Sachs disease affects boys and girls in equal distribution and is not X-linked.

E. The risk can be stated prior to conception, but confirmation cannot be achieved until after conception.

187. **A. Skin infections are common among drug users. Often with chronic infections, a resistant** organism such as methicillin-resistant *Staphylococcus aureus* develops.

B. Biopsy of the lesions would be expected to show an infectious process with neutrophil proliferation and further signs of inflammation.

C. IV antibiotics are sometimes needed, but sensitivities may reveal an oral antibiotic that will be effective, such as clindamycin.

D. *Mycobacterium marinum* is an organism that is commonly associated with chronic skin infections in people who sustain an injury around water and is often referred to as a "fish tank granuloma."

E. Cephalexin is a useful antibiotic in most skin infections; however, it would not be expected to work in this case.

188. **D. The radiograph is typical of tetralogy of Fallot with a normal heart size, decreased pulmonary markings, and typical boot-shaped heart. This condition classically has four abnormalities: (1) a large VSD, (2) RV outflow obstruction (pulmonic stenosis), (3) RV hypertrophy, and (4) overriding of the aorta. Because of the RV outflow obstruction, blood is shunted from right to left through the large VSD. Since blood on the right side of the heart is desaturated, the patient will appear cyanotic.**

A, B. With both an ASD and PDA, shunting is from left to right and there is no cyanosis.

C. It should be remembered that in a VSD alone, blood shunts from left to right and cyanosis is not seen.

E. In a persistent truncus arteriosus, there are marked cardiomegaly and increased pulmonary markings noted on chest x-ray.

189. **D. Cushing syndrome is a state of glucocorticoid excess, and it is characterized by the clinical features described in the patient in this question. Cushing *disease* describes a specific entity in which there is pituitary hypersecretion of ACTH, which leads to excess cortisol release and the described clinical features. In contrast, Cushing *syndrome* is the end result of whatever physiologic process leads to the clinical manifestations, and is not specific to pituitary hypersecretion of ACTH. The correct answer in this case is therefore D, since the necessary data for diagnosing the etiology of this patient's Cushing syndrome are not provided.**

A. Addison disease is a chronic adrenocorticoid insufficiency, not excess.

B. Klippel-Trenaunay-Weber syndrome involves asymmetric limb hypertrophy and vascular lesions (mainly cutaneous).

C. See explanation for D.

E. MEN type 2A is a disorder characterized by medullary thyroid carcinoma, parathyroid hyperplasia, and pheochromocytoma.

190. B. Acute chest syndrome in a patient with sickle-cell anemia is defined as a fever and change in the chest radiograph compared to previous films. If no previous films are available, any abnormality is considered sufficient. Acute chest syndrome is caused by either vaso-occlusive crisis involving the rib bones or infection of the lungs. It is treated symptomatically with pain medications, empiric antibiotics, and aggressive pulmonary toilet.

A. Supplemental oxygen requirement can be a result of infection or a variety of other etiologies, including acute chest syndrome.

C. An increased respiratory rate is a nonspecific finding that can occur as a result of anxiety, pain, fear, or other etiologies.

D. A documented bacterial infection could be the cause of the findings in this patient; however, findings such as sepsis or osteomyelitis would not correlate with acute chest syndrome.

E. Pain is common in patients with acute chest syndrome but is not a diagnostic criterion.

191. B. ASD is one of the more common congenital heart defects. Usually asymptomatic, these children will have a murmur as described in the vignette. There is a left-to-right shunt that produces increased pulmonary flow and increased work for the right side of the heart. Left untreated, pulmonary hypertension can develop, usually in adult life. At this stage, treatment is effective and the next step is cardiac echo and cardiology referral.

A. Patients with a PDA are usually asymptomatic when the ductus is small. The murmur of a patent ductus is typically a I–III/VI, continuous, machinery-like murmur at the upper left sternal border.

C. Spontaneous closure of this lesion at this point in life would not be expected.

D. Echocardiogram and/or cardiology referral is the next step.

E. Pulmonary hypertension can still be avoided at this point.

192. B. The boy in the picture has Williams syndrome, which is characterized by mild-to-moderate mental retardation (MR), prominent lips, a long philtrum, and cardiovascular anomalies, most often pulmonic stenosis (as described in this scenario) or supravalvular aortic stenosis. Hypercalcemia is also associated with this syndrome.

A. The patient pictured does not have the classic physical findings associated with Down syndrome. The most common associated cardiac anomaly in Down syndrome is an endocardial cushion defect.

C. Prader-Willi syndrome, is characterized by mild-to-moderate MR, obesity, hypotonia in the newborn period, and hypogonadism.

D. Angelman syndrome, or "happy puppet syndrome," is associated with moderate-to-severe MR, an ataxic, puppet-like gait, seizures, and outbursts of laughter.

E. Velocardial facial syndrome is characterized by mild-to-moderate MR, specific craniofacial abnormalities, such as cleft palate, prominent nose, deficient malar area, and elongated facies. The most common associated cardiac defect is a VSD or right aortic arch.

193. A. In a small child, sometimes the only strabismus evaluation they will allow is the corneal light reflex test. In this test, a bright penlight is shown from a few feet away, and its reflection from the corneal surface is noted. When the eyes are straight, the reflection is placed symmetrically on both corneas, usually just a bit below and medial to the center of the pupil.

B. With the cover-uncover test, movement of the noncovered eye indicates that it was misaligned, and not fixing on the target. This is consistent with strabismus.

C. The alternate cover test for strabismus is designed to demonstrate subtle, intermittent, or latent strabismus. Movement on uncovering indicates deviation of the eye under occlusion.

D. Observation, especially using the corneal light reflex test, can show the misalignment of the eyes in cases of poor vision. With amblyopia, or other conditions of poor vision, there is often little attempt of the affected eye to refixate with cover-uncover testing or with alternate cover testing.

E. Broad epicanthal folds give the appearance of crossing or esotropia. This is the more common form of pseudostrabismus. However, in the option for E, no comment is made about any testing done to rule out concurrent strabismus. The two diagnoses are NOT mutually exclusive.

194. D. Legg-Calvé-Perthes disease is an avascular necrosis of the capital femoral epiphysis (CFE). The cause is unknown, but is due to an interruption of the blood supply to the area involved. The condition occurs in boys 80% of the time, and most often presents between 4 and 8 years of age. Most children present with mild or intermittent, anterior thigh pain associated with limp. The Trendelenberg test is abnormal. (When the patient stands on the affected leg, the pelvis on the opposite side drops instead of showing the normal elevation.) Radiographs first demonstrate the CFE to be abnormally small. Later, subchondral fracture, resorption, and fragmentation are seen. Legg-Calvé-Perthes disease is a self-healing disorder. Treatment is aimed at maintenance of hip range of motion, prevention of CFE collapse and dislocation, and ensuring that the femoral head heals in a spherical shape. The CFE must be contained in the acetabulum using casts, orthoses, or surgical means.

A. Children with septic arthritis of the hip usually appear very ill, with associated fever and intense hip pain. Radiographs may show widening of the joint space.

B. Osteomyelitis is usually associated with fever and the indolent onset of bone or joint pain. Plain films may not show periosteal elevation and bone destruction for 10 to 14 days into the infection.

C. In SCFE, the patients are usually older and many are obese. On radiographs, the epiphysis is seen to be displaced from the femoral neck.

E. In transient synovitis, the radiograph is usually normal or may show a small effusion.

195. B. ARDS is a clinical syndrome caused by various etiologies that all produce lung injury and surfactant disruption. This results in alveolar collapse and atelectasis, decreasing available surface area for gas exchange, leading to hypoxia. Ventilation (i.e., CO_2 exchange) is compensated for with tachypnea, which will initially maintain a normal pH and pCO_2. However, oxygenation is affected. This blood gas is consistent with ARDS, with a normal pH and pCO_2, but with significant arterial hypoxia manifested by the decreased pO_2.

196. D. DKA causes a significant metabolic acidosis. The patient with DKA will have effortless, deep respirations with mild tachypnea (Kussmaul breathing), in an attempt to create a compensatory respiratory alkalosis. The second blood gas reflects a significant metabolic acidosis with partial respiratory compensation.

197. E. Appropriate mechanical ventilation should result in a normal pH, pCO_2, and adequate oxygenation, as reflected in the well-oxygenated normal ABG in question 197.

198. F. This blood gas demonstrates an acute respiratory acidosis with marginally acceptable oxygenation. The acidosis is acute, since the serum bicarbonate is normal and has not had a chance to adjust for the respiratory acidosis, reflected by the elevated pCO_2. This clinical picture would be most consistent with narcotic overdose, which causes respiratory depression. Acceptable oxygenation is being provided by the supplemental O_2 delivered via nasal cannula.

199. C. This ABG reflects a significant metabolic alkalosis with a bicarbonate of 42. There is partial respiratory compensation with an elevated pCO_2. This clinical picture is consistent with pyloric stenosis, which results in a hypochloremic metabolic alkalosis.

200. A. A patient with bronchopulmonary dysplasia (BPD) typically has a chronically elevated pCO_2 due to his underlying chronic lung disease. The patient is able to compensate for the chronic respiratory acidosis and normalize his pH by retaining bicarbonate. This clinical scenario is reflected in the blood gas, which demonstrates a normal pH, respiratory acidosis, and compensatory metabolic alkalosis.

Section

4 Psychiatry

BLOCK 1

1. A 45-year-old woman is brought to the ER after being found lying down on the bathroom floor next to an empty bottle of pills. Her vital signs indicate that she is tachycardic and hypotensive and has a low-grade fever. On examination, the patient is found to be confused, with dilated pupils and warm, reddish skin. An ECG demonstrates a prolonged QT interval. Which medication did the patient most likely use to overdose?

   A. Fluoxetine
   B. Valproic acid
   C. Nortriptyline
   D. Sertraline
   E. Paroxetine

2. A 28-year-old taxi driver has been referred by his psychiatrist for assessment of an elevated TSH. The patient is being considered for treatment with lithium. Which of the following is true regarding lithium?

   A. Lithium has a more rapid onset of action against manic symptoms than does valproic acid
   B. Dysequilibrium in sodium regulation is likely a critical element in pathogenesis of bipolar illness
   C. Steady-state levels of lithium are achieved after 3 days
   D. Lithium is contraindicated in patients with less severe bipolar illness, such as cyclothymia or bipolar II disorder
   E. Lithium treatment may prevent future depressive episodes in patients with recurrent unipolar depressions and may be useful as an adjunct to antidepressants

3. A 38-year-old woman with a history of depression is brought to the emergency room by her husband complaining of severe headache, anxiety, diaphoresis, and confusion. The patient's husband states she had been in good health until they had lunch at a French restaurant earlier in the day. The patient herself remembers having only some bread, cheese, and two glasses of wine. On examination, you find the patient's BP is 210/123 and heart rate is 125. Her pupils are dilated bilaterally. Which medication is most likely responsible for the patient's condition?

   A. Sertraline
   B. Lithium
   C. Fluoxetine
   D. Phenelzine
   E. Valproic acid

4. A 43-year-old homeless man presents to the emergency center complaining he does not know his name and can't recall how he ended up in Phoenix. Which of the following types of amnesia is associated with loss of memory for a few hours to a few days?

   A. Localized amnesia
   B. Generalized amnesia
   C. Selective amnesia
   D. Systematized amnesia
   E. Continuous amnesia

The response options for items 5 to 9 are the same. You will be required to select one answer for each item in the set.

A. DEA Control Level I
B. DEA Control Level II
C. DEA Control Level III
D. DEA Control Level IV
E. DEA Control Level V

For each descriptive phrase, select the most likely Drug Enforcement Agency (DEA) regulation for controlled substances.

5. Lowest abuse potential

6. No refills without examination

7. Not for prescription use

8. Lower abuse potential, but prescriptions must be rewritten after 6 months or five refills

9. Moderate physical dependence liability but high psychological dependence liability

End of Set

10. A 68-year-old widow is seen in consultation on the general medical floor for evaluation of confusion. This hospitalization was precipitated by a hip fracture. The patient also has a history of congestive heart failure and type II diabetes. Which one of the following clinical symptoms will help you confirm a diagnosis of delirium and rule out dementia?

    A. Insidious onset
    B. Intact orientation
    C. Chronically progressive
    D. Fluctuating consciousness
    E. Irreversible

11. Preparing for an upcoming rotation on the psychiatric inpatient service, you begin perusing the *Diagnostic and Statistical Manual* (DSM IV). The multiaxial evaluation format used in diagnosing psychiatric patients includes how many axes?

    A. One
    B. Two
    C. Three
    D. Four
    E. Five

12. While assigned to the clinic's diabetes care program you are asked to give the staff a talk on relating to patients. Which of the following physician-patient relationship models do you tell them is most appropriate in the treatment of chronic illnesses?

    A. Active-passive model
    B. Teacher-student model
    C. Mutual participation model
    D. Intimate model
    E. Transference-countertransference model

13. Your faculty supervisor on the inpatient psychiatry service has asked you to read up on the functions of a multidisciplinary team and discuss them with her during rounds tomorrow. Which one of the following do you tell her best describes the inclusion of factors such as metabolic status, motivation, family dynamics, and cultural influences on the patient's illness?

    A. Topographic model
    B. Structural model
    C. Mechanisms of defense
    D. Biopsychosocial model
    E. Global assessment of functioning (GAF)

The next three questions (items 14 to 16) correspond to the following vignette.

Knowing you are interested in a career in psychiatry, your supervising resident in the obstetrics clinic asks you some questions about psychiatric illnesses and pregnancy.

14. You explain that which one of the following best describes psychiatric disorders during pregnancy?

    A. Much is known about the course of psychiatric illnesses during pregnancy
    B. Pregnancy is a time of emotional stability
    C. Pharmacotherapy takes precedence over psychotherapy during pregnancy
    D. The goal of pharmacotherapy during pregnancy is maximum control of the symptoms
    E. Many women experience the onset of psychiatric illness during pregnancy

15. That same obstetrics resident asks you what you know about the safety of psychotropic medications during pregnancy. You respond that which one of the following U.S. FDA-labeled psychotropic medications is safest during pregnancy?

    A. Class A
    B. Class B
    C. Class C
    D. Class D
    E. Class X

16. During obstetrics rounds the next day, you are asked to discharge a 22-year-old woman 2 days postpartum who also has a history of serious mental illness. Your resident now questions you on the use of psychopharmacologic medications in breastfeeding mothers. You reply, correctly, that it should include which of the following?

A. Maximum dosing to ensure control of symptoms
B. Limiting bottle feeding
C. Routine infant serum assays
D. Use of long-acting over short-acting medications
E. Abstaining from prescribing lithium

End of Set

17. The University Hospital's Women's Health Center has decided to screen its patients for emotional and mental symptoms. You are asked to develop a screening tool that the nursing staff can use in assessing new patients. Compared with men, women with bipolar disorder are more likely to

A. Experience fewer dysphoric manias
B. Experience fewer depressions
C. Develop lithium-induced hypothyroidism
D. Cycle less rapidly
E. Have much higher lifetime prevalence

18. A 28-year-old administrative assistant is being seen in the clinic for the first time. She relates that she has little energy, cries frequently, and does not look forward to anything. She adds that she starts feeling this way every year just before the holidays, and she is wondering if she might have seasonal affective disorder (SAD). Which of the following do you tell her is true regarding SAD?

A. Men are more likely to experience SAD
B. Winter SAD is more common in the southern hemisphere
C. SAD becomes severe in one's 20s
D. SAD appears to be primarily psychosocial in origin
E. SAD does not respond to antidepressants

19. Your community psychiatry rotation includes an afternoon each week with the clinical outreach team visiting shelters for the homeless. While on rotation, you learn that which one of the following statements about the prevalence of psychiatric illness among the homeless is true?

A. Homeless adults have a relatively low prevalence of personality disorders
B. Drug abuse is more common than alcohol abuse
C. Sexual assault is less common among homeless women than among the nonhomeless
D. The duration of homelessness is correlated with major psychiatric illness
E. The majority of homeless adults have had a psychiatric hospitalization

The response options for items 20 to 23 are the same. You will be required to select one or more answers for each item in the set.

A. Thiamine
B. Fluoxetine
C. Chlordiazepoxide
D. Oxazepam
E. Folate
F. Lorazepam
G. Chloral hydrate

For each prescribing schedule, select the most appropriate medication to prescribe (based on your knowledge of medication half-lives) to a 53-year-old housepainter with chronic depression admitted with symptoms of impending alcohol withdrawal.

20. Three times a day **(SELECT TWO)**

21. Two times a day **(SELECT ONE)**

22. At bedtime **(SELECT THREE)**

23. Once a day **(SELECT ONE)**

End of Set

24. After examining a 16-year-old girl in the child and adolescent psychiatry clinic, your faculty supervisor asks you to present your findings to him leading to a differential diagnosis. Which one of the following is an Axis I psychiatric disorder per the DSM-IV classification system?

A. Autism
B. Attention deficit hyperactivity disorder (ADHD)
C. Mental retardation
D. Borderline personality disorder
E. Asperger's disorder

25. A 4-year-old boy is brought to the clinic for evaluation of ADHD. Preschool teachers and his parents agree that the boy has been irritable and aggressive, and has a poor attention span. As an astute clinician, you recognize the importance of ruling out potential medical causes for his symptoms. Which test do you order first?

    A. Ceruloplasmin level
    B. Blood lead level
    C. Serum ammonia level
    D. 24-hour urine VMA and metanephrines levels
    E. Head CT

26. During the initial evaluation of a Vietnam War veteran, he expresses frustration regarding a recent magazine article. He claims that the story contained a quite disturbing message that was intended specifically for him, and was planning to sue the editor for "messing with my head." After you suggest it might simply be a coincidence, he looks at you incredulously. What type of delusion might this patient be experiencing?

    A. Delusion of control
    B. Persecutory delusions
    C. Grandiose delusions
    D. Delusions of reference
    E. Thought insertion

The response options for items 27 to 30 are the same. You will be required to select one answer for each item in the set.

    A. Phencyclidine intoxication
    B. Opioid withdrawal
    C. Opioid intoxication
    D. LSD intoxication
    E. Amphetamine intoxication
    F. Amphetamine withdrawal

For each descriptive phrase, select the most likely drug effect causing those symptoms.

27. Drowsiness, euphoria, analgesia, anorexia, and hypoactivity

28. Delusions, belligerence, nystagmus, and numbness

29. Pupillary dilatation, piloerection, sweating, and yawning

30. Heightened perception, panic reaction, and hallucinations

End of Set

31. Your first assignment in the substance abuse treatment clinic is to interview a new admission to the rehabilitation program. The patient is a 36-year-old hairdresser with a longstanding history of cocaine and alcohol use. Of the following screening questionnaires, which one is most appropriate for assessing the level of alcohol use?

    A. YBOCS
    B. CAGE
    C. GAF
    D. MMSE
    E. BPRS

32. A 32-year-old unemployed carpenter is self-referred to the emergency center with an acute exacerbation of his chronic mental illness. The patient has been homeless the past 3 months and has a strong odor of alcohol on his breath. Which of the following is considered a positive symptom of schizophrenia?

    A. Poverty of speech
    B. Social isolation
    C. Impaired attention
    D. Affective flattening
    E. Paranoid delusions

The response options for items 33 to 37 are the same. You will be required to select one answer for each item in the set.

    A. Zolpidem
    B. Fluoxetine
    C. Risperidone
    D. Alprazolam
    E. Valproic acid

For each primary clinical function, select the most appropriate pharmacologic agent.

33. Anxiolytic

34. Antidepressant

35. Antipsychotic

36. Hypnotic

37. Mood stabilizer

End of Set

The response options for items 38 to 42 are the same. You will be required to select one answer for each item in the set.

    A. Bipolar disorder, manic
    B. Schizophrenia, chronic undifferentiated type
    C. Dementia
    D. Major depressive disorder
    E. Attention deficit disorder
    F. Borderline personality disorder
    G. Delirium

For each mental status examination finding, select the most likely diagnosis.

38. Stooped posture, anhedonic, slow speech, alert, and oriented

39. Unkempt appearance, flat affect, auditory hallucinations, ideas of reference, and clang associations

40. Loud voice, elated mood, pressured speech, and flight of ideas

41. Poor grooming, apathetic, uneven speech, concrete thinking, disorientation, and impaired memory

42. Angry affect, threats of suicide, auditory hallucinations, and projective identification

End of Set

43. A 26-year-old single mother of three children has been admitted to the neurology service with complaints of diminished sensation in both legs. Which one of the following psychological defense mechanisms could this patient be suffering from that is associated with a breakdown of consciousness, memory, sensory, or motor behavior?

    A. Denial
    B. Displacement
    C. Dissociation

    D. Projection
    E. Splitting

44. While counseling a nursing supervisor about the struggles he is having with his staff, you get a sense that an intellectual understanding of what seems to be occurring may be helpful. Which one of the following psychological mechanisms best typifies the adaptive response of individuals in subordinate positions?

    A. Suppression
    B. Passive aggression
    C. Reaction formation
    D. Undoing
    E. Devaluation

The response options for items 45 to 50 are the same. You will be required to select one answer for each item in the set.

    A. Scopophilia
    B. Koro
    C. Frottage
    D. Coprolalia
    E. Priapism
    F. Exhibitionism

For each descriptive phrase, select the most likely related sexual disorder.

45. Compulsive use of obscene words

46. Compulsive need to expose one's body

47. Sexual pleasure by rubbing bodies

48. Fear that one's penis is shrinking

49. Compulsive desire to view sex acts

50. Persistent penile erection

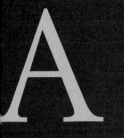

Answers and Explanations

1. C	18. C	35. C
2. E	19. D	36. A
3. D	20. D, F	37. E
4. A	21. C	38. D
5. E	22. A, B, E	39. B
6. B	23. G	40. A
7. A	24. B	41. C
8. D	25. B	42. F
9. C	26. D	43. C
10. D	27. C	44. B
11. E	28. A	45. D
12. C	29. B	46. F
13. D	30. D	47. C
14. E	31. B	48. B
15. A	32. E	49. A
16. E	33. D	50. F
17. C	34. B	

1. **C.** Nortriptyline is a tricyclic antidepressant (TCA). Complications from a tricyclic overdose include anticholinergic-like side effects (warm, red skin, dry mouth, and mydriasis), hypotension, sinus tachycardia, and cardiac arrhythmias (QT prolongation).

   A. Fluoxetine, a selective serotonin reuptake inhibitor (SSRI), does not cause severe anticholinergic side effects or cardiac arrhythmias in overdose.
   B. Valproic acid can cause somnolence, encephalopathy, respiratory depression, and occasionally heart block in overdose, but not the severity of anticholinergic side effects nor the hypotension or sinus tachycardia.
   D. Sertraline would not cause the severe anticholinergic side effects or cardiac arrhythmias.
   E. Paroxetine, like fluoxetine and sertraline, all of which are SSRIs, would not demonstrate the side effects observed with this patient.

2. **E.** Lithium is known to have antidepressant effects as well as mood-stabilizing properties. For a patient who has not been treated successfully with an SSRI or an atypical antidepressant, lithium is a valid treatment option. Lithium may also be effective as an adjunct to antidepressants in patients only partially responsive to treatment.

   A. Lithium has a slower onset of action against manic symptoms than does valproic acid. Because of the delay in efficacy of lithium for the treatment of mania, benzodiazepines and antipsychotics may be required early in treatment to decrease agitation and manage behavior in a patient experiencing acute mania.
   B. Dysequilibrium in calcium regulation, not sodium regulation, is likely to be a critical element in the pathogenesis of bipolar illness. Lithium is thought to work at the level of second messenger systems in a variety of cells throughout the body.
   C. Blood levels of lithium may be checked on the fifth day of dosing, with the steady-state levels achieved after approximately 4 days. Blood work should be obtained 12 hours after the last dose. The therapeutic range for lithium is between 0.6 and 1.2 meq/L.
   D. Lithium may be useful in treating patients with cyclothymia or bipolar II disorder.

3. **D.** Phenelzine is an antidepressant belonging to a class known as MAO inhibitors (MAOIs). Their mechanism of action is the irreversible inhibition of the enzyme monoamine oxidase (MAO), which is found in the central nervous system, the GI tract, and platelets. Inhibition of MAO in the GI tract leads to the increased absorption of tyramine, which can act as a false neurotransmitter and elevate blood pressure. To avoid a hypertensive crisis, patients taking MAOIs must avoid foods containing high amounts of tyramine such as aged cheeses, Chianti wines, and caviar.

   A. Sertraline is an SSRI. SSRIs would not interact with wine or aged cheese to cause a hypertensive crisis.
   B. Lithium is a salt used for mood stabilization for bipolar disorder. Tremor, GI distress, polyuria, polydipsia, and confusion can all be seen with lithium toxicity—but not hypertensive crisis.
   C. Fluoxetine is an SSRI. It would not interact with aged cheese or wine to lead to a hypertensive crisis.
   E. Valproic acid is an anticonvulsant used to treat bipolar disorder. Adverse reactions include nausea, vomiting, dizziness, tremors, and hepatitis—but not hypertensive crisis.

4. **A.** Localized amnesia is the most common type of amnesia and is characterized by loss of memory for events over a short period of time.

   B. Generalized amnesia covers a whole lifetime.
   C, D. Selective and systematized amnesias involve failure to recall some, but not all, events.
   E. Continuous amnesia involves forgetting successive events as they occur despite being alert.

5. **E.** Control level V drugs have the lowest abuse potential of all controlled drugs.

6. **B.** Control level II drugs have high abuse potential and both severe physical and psychological dependence liabilities. Examples include amphetamines, morphine, secobarbital, and glutethimide.

7. **A.** Control level I drugs also have high abuse potential and no accepted use in medical treatment. Examples include LSD, peyote, mescaline, and phencyclidine.

8. **D.** Control level IV drugs have low abuse potential and limited dependence liability. Examples include phenobarbital, meprobamate, and benzodiazepines in most states.

9. C. Control level III drugs also require rewritten prescriptions after 6 months. Examples include nalorphine and compounds containing codeine, hydrocodone, and naltrexone.

10. D. Fluctuating consciousness is a hallmark symptom differentiating delirium from dementia.

 A. Delirium typically has a rapid onset whereas dementia is insidious.

 B. The patient with delirium is always disoriented in some fashion, but this may not be the case in early dementia.

 C. Dementia is expectedly progressive over time whereas delirium should resolve when the cause is corrected.

 E. Although the majority of deliriums are reversible, such is not with case with dementia.

11. E. Five. The five axes include: Axis I (clinical disorders); Axis II (personality disorders and mental retardation); Axis III (general medical conditions); Axis IV (psychosocial and environmental problems); and Axis V (global assessment of functioning scale).

 A, B, C, D. These are incorrect.

12. C. The mutual participation model fosters input from both the physician and the patient and is best for chronic conditions such as diabetes and renal failure.

 A. The active-passive model is more appropriate for the delirious patient or someone with an extremely passive personality.

 B. The teacher-student model works best in an acute care situation.

 D. The intimate model often represents the psychological needs of the physician and is generally considered dysfunctional or unethical.

 E. Transference and countertransference are considered to occur to some degree in all physician-patient relationships.

13. D. The three-pronged biopsychosocial approach to assessment and treatment involves a variety of factors. These include anatomic, physiologic, infectious, medication, and other biologic influences; psychodynamic and personality factors; and environmental influences.

 A. The topographic model is a psychoanalytic concept of the mind including the unconscious, preconscious, and conscious.

 B. The structural model is another psychoanalytic concept that includes the id, ego, and superego.

 C. Psychological defense mechanisms dampen conflicts arising from the unconscious between the id, ego, and superego.

 E. GAF is the numeric (0 to 100) description of a psychiatric patient's highest level of adaptive functioning at the time of assessment.

14. E. The childbearing years are also the most frequent age for the onset of psychiatric disorders in women.

 A. Little is known or predictable about the influence of pregnancy on the course of psychiatric illness.

 B. Contrary to traditional thought, pregnancy can be a time of emotional instability.

 C, D. In an effort to minimize harm to the mother or fetus, psychosocial treatments and symptom reduction, rather than control, may be more prudent.

15. A. Controlled studies of Class A medications show no risk.

 B. Despite adverse findings in animals, there is no evidence that Class B medications have risk in humans, implying a possible but remote likelihood of harm.

 C. Risk cannot be ruled out for Class C medications, but the potential benefits may outweigh potential risks.

 D. Class D medications show positive evidence of risk.

 E. Class X medications are contraindicated in pregnancy.

16. E. The American Academy of Pediatrics contraindicates the use of lithium for nursing mothers. Adverse effects include cardiotoxicity; the risk of lithium accumulation in the infant is high.

 A. Dosing is of concern, especially if the infant is premature.

 B. Bottle feeding would necessarily limit breast feeding and potentially harmful exposure.

 C. The primary role of serum assays would be reassurance.

 D. Shorter-acting medications are more rapidly metabolized.

17. C. Women are more likely to develop lithium-induced hypothyroidism.

A. Women experience more dysphoric manic episodes.

B. Whereas women experience more depressions, men experience more manic episodes.

D. Women are more likely to be rapid cyclers.

E. The disorder essentially occurs equally in men and women, but there are several differences in its course and manifestation.

18. **C. SAD tends to start during adolescence and becomes more severe during the third decade.**

A. SAD occurs more frequently in women.

B. SAD is experienced more often by those living in the northern climes.

D. SAD runs in families and clearly appears to be biological.

E. SAD responds well to antidepressants as well as light exposure.

19. **D. The presence of major psychiatric illness such as schizophrenia or mania is highly correlated with the duration of homelessness.**

A. Homeless adults have a high prevalence of personality disorders; antisocial personality disorder is common.

B. Alcohol abuse is much more common than drug abuse among homeless adults.

C. Sexual assault is 20 times more common among homeless women.

E. Approximately one-quarter of homeless adults have had psychiatric hospitalization.

20. **D, F. Oxazepam and lorazepam are relatively short-acting benzodiazepines given orally to minimize alcohol withdrawal.**

21. **C. Chlordiazepoxide is a moderate-acting benzodiazepine typically given twice a day for alcohol withdrawal.**

22. **A, B, E. Thiamine deficiency is common in chronic alcohol dependence and thiamine should be replenished quickly to prevent Wernicke's encephalopathy. Typically 100 mg is prescribed once daily for several days. Fluoxetine is an SSRI antidepressant with a long half-life, so prescribed daily. Folate deficiency is also common in chronic alcoholics, and folate can be replenished by a 1-mg per day oral dose over a prolonged period.**

23. **G. Chloral hydrate is a potent sedative hypnotic and expectedly prescribed at bedtime.**

24. **B. Attention deficit hyperactivity disorder is the only Axis I disorder listed.**

A, C, D, and E are all considered Axis II disorders.

25. **B. Lead poisoning in children may mimic ADHD and may result in chronic irreversible cognitive defects. Screening for lead poisoning is an important part of preventative care, particularly if exposure is expected.**

A. A ceruloplasmin deficiency would suggest Wilson's disease, which can cause psychiatric symptoms resembling schizophrenia or bipolar disorder. However, clinical manifestations of Wilson's disease are almost never seen before age 5 years.

C. Hyperammonemia would cause lethargy and twitching, but would not look like ADHD.

D. Evaluation for pheochromocytoma might be appropriate if he had intermittent hypertension, tachycardia, tachypnea, flushing, and clammy skin.

E. A head CT would not be an appropriate first test to order in this case.

26. **D. Delusions of reference are characterized by insignificant events or messages to which a patient assigns a special and personal meaning. This commonly involves print media, radio, or television.**

A. Delusions of control occur when the patient believes that an outside force or person is controlling his behaviors or feelings.

B. Persecutory delusions are characterized by thoughts that others are conspiring against or spying on the patient.

C. Grandiose delusions usually consist of the belief that one has special powers or aptitudes that are clearly unrealistic.

E. Thought insertion involves the belief that others are able to put thoughts into one's head or that thoughts are not one's own.

27. **C. Opioids can be ingested (methadone), inhaled (opium), and injected (heroin). Opioid overdose can be lethal.**

28. **A. Phencyclidine, or PCP, is a dissociative anesthetic. The degree of intoxication is typically dose dependent and symptoms may emerge up to a week after use, probably due to PCP's fat solubility.**

29. B. Opioid withdrawal is associated with long-term use. There is often a flu-like syndrome of gastrointestinal distress, muscle aches, rhinorrhea, and diarrhea.

30. D. LSD can cause misperceived sensory stimuli, intense anxiety ("a bad trip"), and cartoonlike visual hallucinations. It does not cause the numbness associated with PCP.

31. B. The CAGE questions consist of four questions relating to alcohol use: Have you felt the need to cut back on your drinking? Do you get annoyed with others who criticize your drinking? Do you feel guilty about your drinking? Do you ever have an eye-opener in the morning to get rid of a hangover?

    A. YBOCS, or Yale-Brown Obsessive-Compulsive Scale, is used to monitor symptoms of OCD.
    C. GAF, or Global Assessment of Functioning, is a subjective scale from 0 to 100, which rates a patient's overall wellbeing. Clinicians assign the number to Axis V of the psychiatric diagnoses.
    D. MMSE, or Mini-Mental State Exam, is a structured interview designed to assess cognitive functioning in multiple areas. It is scored on a 30-point scale.
    E. BPRS, or Brief Psychiatric Rating Scale, is used to assess a wide range of psychiatric symptoms, and would not be as specific as CAGE in assessing alcohol use.

32. E. Paranoid delusions are considered part of the positive symptom cluster seen in schizophrenia. The positive symptoms classically include delusions, hallucinations, and disordered thinking.

    A. Poverty of speech is classified under alogia, which is a negative symptom of schizophrenia. The negative symptoms are characterized by a deficit in normal mental functioning.
    B. Social isolation, another negative symptom, is part of the asocial component commonly seen in schizophrenia.
    C. Impaired attention is considered a negative symptom because it reflects a loss of normal function.
    D. Flat affect is also considered a negative symptom because it reflects a loss of normal functioning.

33. D. Alprazolam is a potent, short-acting benzodiazepine with a dosage range of 0.75–4 mg per day.

34. B. Fluoxetine is an SSRI used to treat depression and obsessive-compulsive disorder (OCD). Its dosage range is 20–60 mg per day.

35. C. Risperidone is an atypical antipsychotic with a dosage range of 2–6 mg per day.

36. A. Zolpidem is a hypnotic with a dosage range of 5–10 mg at bedtime.

37. E. Valproic acid is an anticonvulsant and mood stabilizer with a typical dosage range of 750–4000 mg per day, depending on the patient's weight and subsequent blood levels targeting a therapeutic range.

38. D. Mood disorders are often manifest as energy disturbances with slowness associated with depression. Anhedonia, the inability to experience pleasure, in a patient with an intact sensorium and orientation suggests a major depressive disorder.

39. B. Schizophrenia often evolves into a chronic condition with impaired social skills, affective deficits, and persistent thought content and thought process abnormalities.

40. A. Manic episodes are typically manifest with heightened energy and more rapid thinking and speech. Stimulants can produce a similar set of symptoms.

41. C. Dementia is a condition of gradual losses—of activities of daily living, interests, thought production and speech, the ability to abstract, memory, cognition, and intellectual functioning.

42. F. People with a borderline personality disorder typically have an angry or hostile affect, a history of impulsive and destructive behaviors, and a propensity for brief psychotic episodes. The primitive defense mechanisms of projective identification and splitting are associated with this personality disorder.

43. C. Dissociation can include disturbances in consciousness, memory, and sensory and motor behaviors and is the defense mechanism used in the clinical syndromes of hysteria, conversion disorder, and amnesia.

A. Denial implies a refusal to acknowledge some painful aspect of reality.

B. Displacement involves transferring a feeling to a less threatening object.

D. Projection typically involves a potentially threatening object, as seen in paranoia.

E. Splitting involves compartmentalizing opposing emotional states.

44. **B. Passive aggression typically is manifest as overt compliance by subordinates masking covert resistance or hostility.**

A. Suppression involves the intentional avoidance of disturbing problems.

C. Reaction formation involves substituting unacceptable feelings with opposite behaviors.

D. Undoing allows negating unacceptable thoughts.

E. Devaluation involves attributing exaggerated negative feelings to others.

45. **D. Coprolalia is the compulsive use of obscene words.**

46. **F. Exhibitionism is typically the exposure of the genitals and almost always occurs in men.**

47. **C. Frottage is almost always done by men rubbing against females in crowded places such as subways and elevators.**

48. **B. Koro is an acute anxiety state seen primarily in Asian men.**

49. **A. Scopophilia is also known as voyeurism.**

50. **F. Priapism is a persistent erection, which can result in severe pain and is a medical emergency. Untreated priapism can result in thrombosis and gangrene.**

BLOCK 2

51. A 33-year-old lawyer has a chief complaint of obsessive counting and ritualistic handwashing for 3 years. Which one of the following antidepressant treatments would be the most effective for treating his obsessive-compulsive disorder (OCD)?

    A. Tricyclic antidepressants (TCAs)
    B. Selective 5-HT reuptake inhibitors
    C. MAOIs
    D. 5-HT$_{1A}$ agonists
    E. Electroconvulsive therapy (ECT)

52. A 16-year-old high school student shares with her PCP that over the past several weeks she has experienced symptoms of extreme anxiety every time she places her family's garbage container in the back alley for pick-up the next morning. The symptoms first appeared when she saw a snake in the alley. What parasympathetic nervous system response to fear is she experiencing?

    A. Increased heart rate
    B. Increased blood pressure
    C. Slowed digestion
    D. Increased blood flow
    E. Increased adrenaline

53. A 28-year-old woman expresses concern that her 6-year-old son is obsessed with dinosaurs. Her concern stems from her experiences with the boy's father and his preoccupation with unrealistic physical ailments and hoarding old newspapers. Which of the following statements regarding the heritability of OCD do you tell her is most correct?

    A. Concordances in dizygotic and monozygotic twins are equal
    B. Concordance is greater in monozygotic twins
    C. Inheritance is greater in male offspring
    D. Heritability is infrequent
    E. Concordance with parents is very high

The response options for items 54 to 56 are the same. You will be required to select one answer for each item in the set.

    A. Seasonal pattern specifier
    B. Atypical features specifier
    C. Catatonic features specifier
    D. Melancholic features specifier
    E. Rapid cycling specifier
    F. Postpartum ooset

For each constellation of symptoms, select the most accurate mood disorder specifier.

54. Mood reactivity, increased appetite, and hypersomnia

55. Cataplexy, negativism, and posturing

56. Anhedonia, diurnal variation, and early morning awaking

End of Set

57. A 26-year-old recently divorced graduate student presents with a 10-year history of OCD and recurrent panic attacks over the past few months. Which one of the following is the most effective pharmacologic treatment for her coincidental conditions?

    A. Buproprion
    B. Imipramine
    C. Phenelzine
    D. Fluoxetine
    E. Risperidone

The response options for items 58 to 60 are the same. You will be required to select one answer for each item in the set.

    A. Olanzapine
    B. Paroxetine
    C. Valproic acid
    D. Lorazepam
    E. Zolpidem
    F. Modafinil

For each general drug description, select the most commonly prescribed psychotropic medication.

58. Sedative-hypnotic

59. Antidepressant

60. Antipsychotic

End of Set

61. A group of third-year medical students on their psychiatry clerkship ask you if schizophrenia is a functional or organic illness. Regarding the neurologic basis of schizophrenia, which one of the following do you tell them is true?

A. The cerebral cortex volume is increased
B. The cerebral cortex demonstrates impaired activation during cognitive tasks
C. The volume of the thalamus is increased
D. The volume of the thalamus is increased in relatives of patients with schizophrenia
E. There is a loss of neurons in the cerebral cortex

62. A young couple has been referred by their 6-year-old son's pediatrician. The boy has been developmentally delayed, showing signs of autism. The boy's mother is 4 months pregnant. Which one of the following statements about autism do you tell them is true?

    A. The rate of reported autistic disorders in the United States leveled off in the 1990s
    B. The rate of autistic disorders is higher in children who received the measles, mumps, and rubella (MMR) vaccine
    C. Autism is associated with exposure to thimerosal-containing vaccines
    D. Autism is associated with rapid brain growth
    E. Genetic studies suggest an abnormality on the Y chromosome

The next two questions (items 63 and 64) correspond to the following vignette.

During rounds on the geriatric psychiatry inpatient service, one of the medical students asks you to comment on the genetics of senile dementia.

63. Regarding the genetic risks for Alzheimer's disease (AD), which one of the following statements is correct?

    A. The apolipoprotein E gene (APOE) 3 allele increases the risk for AD
    B. The APOE gene 4 allele increases the risk for AD
    C. APOE alleles are located on chromosome 15
    D. APOE genes are dominant genes
    E. The APOE gene is related to early-onset AD

64. As a follow-up to your discussion with the medical students about genetic influences and dementia, one student asks you to explain the mechanism causing neuritic plaques. Regarding the pathophysiology of AD, the APOE gene 4 allele appears to do which one of the following?

    A. Increase the clearance of A-β 42 amyloid
    B. Decrease the clearance of A-β 42 amyloid

C. Increase production of A-β 42 amyloid
D. Decrease production of A-β 42 amyloid
E. Account for the majority of early-onset cases

End of Set

65. While you are examining an older man in the outpatient clinic, he comments on someone he sat across from in the waiting room who jerked his arms up suddenly and was making barking noises. You tell him that the symptom complex of motor tics and vocal tics he witnessed is referred to as which one of the following syndromes?

    A. Tardive dyskinesia
    B. Gilles de la Tourette
    C. Akathisia
    D. Trichotillomania
    E. Parkinson's disease

66. A 30-year-old male being seen as an outpatient becomes upset when his psychiatrist receives a call regarding an emergency. In therapy, the patient has discussed his feelings of rejection regarding his relationship with his father who was a highly successful businessman and CEO of a large company. When the psychiatrist apologizes for the interruption, the patient replies, "Go ahead. It's not as if my problems are important." The patient's reply is an example of a phenomenon that occurs during psychotherapy as well as in ordinary physician-patient relationships which is called

    A. Reaction formation
    B. Identification
    C. Projection
    D. Transference
    E. Countertransference

The response options for items 67 to 74 are the same. You will be required to select one answer for each item in the set.

    A. Hallucination
    B. Delusion
    C. Illusion
    D. Ideas of reference
    E. Obsession
    F. Compulsion
    G. Flight of ideas
    H. Circumstantiality

For each patient quote, select the psychiatric symptoms that would most likely apply.

67. "That man in the commercial just told me I need to fight the devil."

68. When asked why she came to the emergency room, the patient says, "I'm sick and I need medication. Speaking of medication, I went to the drug store and there was a nice lady behind the counter, she looked just like my aunt who lives in California. Have you ever been to California? It's a wonderful place to visit. I remember when I was at Disneyland as a kid . . ."

69. "When I walk down the street I can tell I'm being watched. I'm telling you, the CIA is after me!"

70. "There are rats on the ceiling!" yells a distraught patient in the ICU.

71. When a patient was asked where he lived, he responded, "I grew up in a small town in Idaho. My father was a banker there and we had a lovely house. In fact, I went back there this summer and it was just as I recalled. My mother, bless her soul, was a schoolteacher and I can tell you it's hard to get out of line when you know your mother is just two doors down the hall from your classroom. You know, there's a schoolhouse right next to where I live now, on 24th and Roosevelt."

72. "A man was staring at me from the window last night," relates a patient, pointing to the mirror in his hospital room.

73. "I feel horrible about this, doctor, but I keep thinking about throwing my baby over the railing of our staircase. I don't know why, I just can't get that image out of my head, even though I would never do anything to harm my baby!"

74. "Every day before I leave for work I have to go back and check my front door nine times. It's gotten so bad that I'm often late for work."

End of Set

75. A family physician has been asked by his patient if he would be willing to prescribe psychiatric medications for his longstanding but stable bipolar disorder. When prescribing lithium, it is important to consider that the blood level of lithium may be decreased by which of the following medications?

    A. Thiazide diuretics
    B. Nonstreroidal antiinflammatory drugs (NSAIDs)
    C. Furosemide
    D. Valproic acid
    E. Theophylline

76. Your multispecialty group practice has many subspecialty clinics. After opening a program for patients with treatment-resistant schizophrenia, referrals from psychiatry to endocrinology increased. In particular, there has been a marked increase in patients with sedation, increased appetite, tachycardia, and hyperlipidemia. These are common side effects of which one of the following medications?

    A. Clozapine
    B. Fluoxetine
    C. Methylphenidate
    D. Clonazepam
    E. Haloperidol

The next two questions (items 77 and 78) correspond to the following vignette.

Knowing you are a psychiatrist, one of your neighbors casually asks you about OCD.

77. Which one of the following do you say is true about OCD?

    A. The prevalence of OCD is very rare
    B. First-line treatments for OCD include medication and behavior therapy
    C. Few patients with OCD respond favorably to treatment
    D. Compulsions are repetitive, unwanted, extreme, or nonsensical thoughts
    E. Functional imaging studies of OCD implicate abnormalities in the cerebellum

78. This same neighbor also wonders what you know about the new drugs she hears teenagers are using. In particular, she is curious about gamma hydroxybutyric acid (GHB). You tell her that GHB has become a popular drug of abuse. Which of the following statements regarding GHB do you tell her is correct?

A. GHB is a CNS stimulant
B. GHB decreases growth hormone
C. GHB overdose results in tachycardia
D. GHB is not addictive
E. GHB is used to treat narcolepsy

End of Set

79. In preparation for a rotation at a community mental health center with an elderly patient population, you have decided to become more knowledgeable about geropsychiatry. Regarding dementia with Lewy bodies (DLB), which one of the following statements is correct?

A. DLB accounts for one-fifth of all dementias in the elderly
B. Few patients with DLB experience extrapyramidal symptoms (EPSs)
C. DLB patients have pronounced hippocampal atrophy
D. DLB does not respond to acetylcholinesterase inhibitors
E. Parkinson's disease (PD) and DLB do not share an underlying disease process

The response options for items 80 to 83 are the same. You will be required to select one answer for each item in the set.

A. Bipolar disorder
B. Cyclothymic disorder
C. Dysthymic disorder
D. Major depressive episode
E. Manic episode

For each constellation of symptoms, select the most accurate diagnosis.

80. Two weeks of anhedonia, sleep disturbance, and low energy

81. Two years of hypomanic episodes and mild depressions

82. Irritability, decreased need for sleep, pressured speech, and grandiosity

83. Hypomanic episodes interspersed with severe depressions

End of Set

The response options for items 84 to 86 are the same. You will be required to select one answer for each item in the set.

A. Medial temporal region
B. Orbitofrontal cortex
C. Substantia nigra
D. Cerebellum
E. Prefrontal cortex

For each mental function, select the matching region of the brain.

84. Storage and consolidation of new memories

85. Ambiguous learning situations

86. Working memory

End of Set

The response options for items 87 to 92 are the same. You will be required to select one answer for each item in the set.

A. Drug-based theory
B. Global-based theory
C. Classical conditioning
D. Operant conditioning
E. Social learning theory
F. Biological theory

For each descriptive phrase, select the most appropriate disease theory of substance abuse.

87. Genetics

88. Drugs as reinforcers

89. Often plays a major role in relapse

90. Variant of normal behavior

91. Inherent biochemical effects

92. Group dynamics

End of Set

The response options for items 93 to 97 are the same. An answer may be used once, more than once, or not at all.

A. SSRI
B. MAOIs
C. TCAs
D. Mirtazapine
E. Bupropion

For each neurophysiologic effect of long-term administration of 5-HT neurotransmission, select the most appropriate antidepressant medication.

93. No significant effect on 5-HT$_{1A}$ somatodendritic autoreceptors

94. Decreased function of terminal 5-HT$_{1B}$ autoreceptors

95. Increased responsiveness of postsynaptic 5-HT$_{1A}$ receptors

96. Decreased responsiveness of postsynaptic 5-HT$_{1A}$ receptors

97. No significant effect on the function of terminal 5-HT$_{1B}$ autoreceptors

End of Set

98. A 56-year-old divorced woman has been referred by her cardiologist 4 weeks after suffering her second myocardial infarction. Since leaving the hospital, she has been weepy, isolative, and more easily fatigued than her cardiologist feels is warranted. When you question the patient about her psychological state before her most recent heart attack, she admits to frequent bouts of anxiety and irritability since her divorce. Which one of the following statements about the relationship of stress and anger to human physiology is true?

    A. Platelet aggregation is increased
    B. Production of cytokines is reduced

C. The sympathetic nervous system (SNS) is suppressed
D. The parasympathetic nervous system (PNS) is activated
E. Hostility is a stress-related Type B personality trait associated with increased heart disease

The next two questions (items 99 and 100) correspond to the following vignette.

A sexually active 16-year-old girl is referred by her high school counselor for psychotherapy. As you interview the patient, she relates that she has been HIV-positive since infancy, presumably related to her mother's drug abuse.

99. Which one of the following is presently the most common method of becoming HIV positive among teenagers in the United States?

    A. Unprotected sexual behavior
    B. Drug use
    C. Skin piercing
    D. Vertical transmission
    E. In utero transmission

100. Regarding the psychosocial issues of HIV and AIDS in youth, which one of the following statements is true?

    A. The number of HIV-positive teens is declining
    B. Youths in psychiatric care are at lower risk than their peers
    C. Girls are especially vulnerable to HIV infection
    D. Knowledge about the causes of HIV transmission has led to changes in sexual risk taking among youths
    E. Achievement motivation and sexual activity are not linked

End of Set

A

Answers and Explanations

51. B	68. G	85. B
52. C	69. B	86. E
53. B	70. A	87. F
54. B	71. H	88. D
55. C	72. C	89. C
56. D	73. E	90. B
57. D	74. F	91. A
58. E	75. E	92. E
59. B	76. A	93. C
60. A	77. B	94. A
61. B	78. E	95. C
62. D	79. A	96. B
63. B	80. D	97. D
64. B	81. B	98. A
65. B	82. E	99. A
66. D	83. A	100. C
67. D	84. A	

51. **B. Selective 5-HT reuptake inhibitors are effective in treating depression and OCD.**

    A. TCAs are effective in treating depression but, with the exception of chlorimipramine with its potent 5-HT reuptake blocking property, are not useful in OCD.
    C. MAOIs are effective in depression but not particularly in OCD.
    D. 5-HT$_{1A}$ agonists are helpful in treating depression but not OCD.
    E. ECT is an efficacious treatment for severe depression but not OCD.

52. **C. The PNS response to fear includes slowed digestion.**

    A. Increased heart rate is an SNS response to fear.
    B. Increased blood pressure is also an SNS response to fear.
    D. Increased blood flow is another SNS response to fear.
    E. Fear results in increased adrenaline (an SNS response), which may be relevant to memory formation to better encode the threatening situation.

53. **B. Monozygotic concordance rates for OCD are in the 50% to 80% range.**

    A. Dizygotic concordance rates for OCD are in the 30% to 40% range.
    C. The risk of OCD among male and female offspring is equal and generally 10% to 12%.
    D. Heritability for OCD is in the 40% to 50% range.
    E. 20% of parents of those with OCD may have evidence of the illness.

54. **B. Atypical features of a major depressive episode can also include significant weight gain and long-standing interpersonal rejection sensitivity.**

55. **C. Catatonic feature specifiers can apply to depressive and manic episodes.**

56. **D. The depressed patient with melancholia has a distinct quality. Besides the pronounced anhedonia, diurnal variation to symptoms and early morning awakening, there is frequently psychomotor agitation or retardation, significant anorexia, and excessive guilt.**

57. **D. Fluoxetine is a potent selective 5-HT reuptake inhibitor and is an effective treatment for both OCD and panic disorder.**

    A. Buproprion is primarily a dopaminergic antidepressant and not an effective treatment for either OCD or panic episodes.
    B. Imipramine, a TCA, is also effective for panic disorder but not for OCD.
    C. Phenelzine is an MAOI and effective in treating depression and panic disorder but not OCD.
    E. Risperidone is primarily used to treat psychosis.

58. **E. Zolpidem is a sedative-hypnotic indicated for the short-term treatment of insomnia.**

59. **B. Paroxetine is an SSRI antidepressant.**

60. **A. Olanzapine is an atypical antipsychotic indicated for the treatment of schizophrenia and acute mania.**

61. **B. Individuals with schizophrenia demonstrate impaired activation of the cerebral cortex during cognitive tasks.**

    A. The cerebral cortex volume is decreased in schizophrenia.
    C. The volume of the thalamus, especially the mediodorsal nucleus, is decreased in schizophrenia.
    D. Relatives of patients with schizophrenia also demonstrate decreased volume of the thalamus.
    E. Despite a decreased volume, there is no loss of neurons in the cerebral cortex in individuals with schizophrenia.

62. **D. A new study does suggest that one causative factor in autism is too much brain growth too soon. The growth spurt occurs during the first year of life.**

    A. The rate of reported autistic disorders increased in the United States in the 1990s, rising from 3 in 10,000 in 1991 to 52 in 10,000 in 2001. This increased reporting is related to greater awareness, better standardized screening tests, and the inclusion of education and treatment of autistic children in the 1990 Disabilities Education Act.

B. Recent studies have not shown an increase in the rate of autism in children receiving the MMR vaccine.

C. Recent studies have also shown no increased rate of autism in children receiving vaccines with the mercury-containing preservative thimerosal.

E. Although relatively rare, the genetic variant of autism is associated with a component of the X chromosome regulating protein synthesis required for the construction of synapses. This X chromosome linkage explains the higher rates of autism in boys, in that girls have a second "protective" X chromosome.

63. **B. The APOE gene 4 allele does increase the risk for AD.**

A. The APOE gene 3 allele does not increase the risk for AD.

C. APOE alleles are located on chromosome 19.

D. APOE genes are recessive genes.

E. The APOE gene 4 allele is related to later-onset AD.

64. **B. The APOE-4 allele appears to decrease the clearance of A-β 42 amyloid, resulting in its accumulation in neuritic plaques.**

A. Clearance of amyloid decreases in AD.

C. The amyloid precursor protein gene rather than APOE increases production of A-β 42 amyloid.

D. The APOE gene is involved in clearance rather than production of amyloid.

E. Early-onset AD is related to Presenilin 1 gene.

65. **B. Gilles de la Tourette, or Tourette's syndrome, is the correct answer. It is manifest by motor and vocal tics, which wax and wane and have an age of onset of around 7 years old.**

A. Tardive dyskinesia is manifest as abnormal motoric movements alone and is typically associated with prolonged exposure to antipsychotic medications.

C. Akathisia is an inner restlessness associated with more acute exposure to antipsychotic medications.

D. Trichotillomania is compulsive hair pulling, often associated with other OCD symptoms.

E. Parkinson's disease is a neurologic illness related to dopamine depletion, typically manifest with bradykinesia and tremors.

66. **D. Transference is the unconscious reexperiencing of feelings about parents or important figures in the patient's life in his or her current relationship with the therapist. This can be quite useful in therapy, as it can provide a way for the therapist to better understand the patient's problems. The therapist can then assist the patient in stepping back to observe this pattern to increase the patient's insight and self-understanding.**

A. Reaction formation is a specific defense mechanism that entails adopting opposite attitudes to avoid unacceptable emotions, such that the individual uses unconscious hypocrisy. An example would be a person who is fascinated by fires deciding to become a firefighter.

B. Identification is a specific defense mechanism in which a person patterns his or her behavior after that of someone more powerful. This may be positive or negative. An example is a mother who was verbally abused in childhood by a parent saying demeaning things to her own children.

C. Projection is a specific defense mechanism involving attributing one's unacceptable feelings to others. This defense mechanism is associated with paranoid symptoms and ordinary prejudice.

E. Countertransference is the unconscious reexperiencing of feelings about parents or other important figures in the therapist's life in his or her current relationship with the patient.

67. **D. An idea of reference is a symptom of psychosis in which there is a false belief that one is the subject of attention from other people or the media.**

68. **G. Flight of ideas is a rapid, obliquely related string of thoughts. It is typically seen in mania.**

69. **B. A delusion is a symptom of psychosis that is a false, fixed, typically bizarre or improbable belief from which a person cannot be dissuaded. These beliefs can take various forms, such as grandiose, nihilistic, somatic, and paranoid.**

70. **A. Hallucinations are sensations without basis in reality. Any of the five senses may be involved—sight, hearing, smell, taste, and touch.**

71. H. Circumstantiality is a thought process marked by the introduction into the conversation of details only distantly related or entirely unrelated to the main subject of the conversation, eventually getting to the sought after point in a roundabout manner.

72. C. An illusion is a misperception of an actual sensory stimulus. While hallucinations are associated with psychotic illnesses, illusions are more likely associated with organic disorders or the vivid imagination of childhood.

73. E. An obsession is an unwanted, intrusive thought or image of which an affected person is well aware and can be quite distressed. Thus, obsessions are ego-dystonic.

74. F. A compulsion is a repetitive, irresistible behavior unconsciously designed to ward off or alleviate anxiety. These behaviors impair social or occupational functioning because of their excessiveness or lack of any realistic connection with the object of anxiety.

75. E. Theophylline will increase the renal clearance and result in a lower Li level.

   A. Thiazide diuretics can significantly raise the level of Li, and thus Li levels should be closely monitored in a patient on both of these medications.
   B. Some NSAIDs, such as indomethacin, may increase the plasma level of Li. Because of the ubiquitous use of NSAIDs, patients being started on Li should specifically be told to avoid them.
   C. Furosemide, as a diuretic, tends to elevate Li levels as well and may lead to toxicity.
   D. Valproic acid is an anticonvulsant with mood-stabilizing properties. It does not affect Li levels.

76. A. Clozapine is an atypical antipsychotic medication approved for schizophrenia. Because of its serious adverse effects, it is reserved for refractory cases. Other side effects are sialorrhea and agranulocytosis, which can be fatal and occurs in 1% of patients taking the medication. A weekly CBC is required to monitor for any drops in WBCs.

   B. Fluoxetine is an SSRI antidepressant that is more likely to cause insomnia. It does not

commonly cause tachycardia or hyperlipidemia.
   C. Methylphenidate is a stimulant commonly used to treat ADHD and as such is not sedating. Although it might cause tachycardia, it usually decreases appetite.
   D. Clonazepam is a benzodiazepine anxiolytic that can be sedating. It does not cause tachycardia or lipid abnormalities.
   E. Haloperidol is an antipsychotic medication that can cause sedation and increased appetite. It may also cause hyperlipidemia in some patients. Although it can cause arrhythmias in rare cases, it does not commonly cause tachycardia.

77. B. First-line treatments for OCD include both medication and behavior therapy. The serotonergic medications are most helpful.

   A. The worldwide prevalence of OCD is 1% to 3%.
   C. 60% to 80% of patients with OCD respond favorably to treatment.
   D. Obsessions are thoughts; compulsions are behaviors.
   E. Imaging studies implicate abnormalities in the orbitofrontal cortex, cingulate cortex, and caudate.

78. E. The only accepted use for GHB in the United States is to treat narcolepsy. It is used as an anesthetic in Europe.

   A. GHB is a CNS depressant.
   B. GHB increases growth hormone and therefore is of interest to body builders.
   C. Overdose of GHB results in bradycardia.
   D. After prolonged use of GHB, withdrawal can result in anxiety, insomnia, paranoia, and hallucinations.

79. A. DLB does account for 15% to 20% of dementias in the elderly.

   B. 75% of patients with DLB experience EPSs.
   C. DLB patients demonstrate occipital hypoperfusion on neuroimaging; hippocampal atrophy is associated with AD.
   D. Acetylcholinesterase inhibitors can substantially improve DLB.
   E. PD and DLB are both associated with a profound loss of nigrostriatal dopaminergic innervation.

80. D Major depressive episodes also include depressed mood nearly every day, feelings of worthlessness and guilt, trouble concentrating, and often thoughts of death and suicide.

81. B. Cyclothymia implies a persistent fluctuating course of hypomania and mild depressions with no relief for longer than 2 months.

82. E. A patient with mania may experience an elevated, expansive, or irritable mood. Other symptoms of mania include flight of ideas, distractibility, increased activity, and reckless behaviors.

83. A. Bipolar II disorder is a variant of bipolar or manic-depressive illness, marked by hypomanic episodes and severe depressions. The latter are what typically prompt the patient to seek treatment.

84. A. The medial temporal region of the brain processes information to establish and maintain new and longer lasting memories.

85. B. The orbitofrontal cortex of the brain is involved in ambiguous learning situations such as gambling.

86. E. The prefrontal cortex is involved in working memory, which allows one to keep several ideas in the mind at once.

87. F. The biologic theory of substance abuse implies that genetics cause some individuals to be more sensitive to drugs.

88. D. Operant conditioning implies that drugs themselves serve as reinforcers to increase frequency.

89. C. Classical conditioning identifies the effects of drugs as associated stimuli promoting relapse.

90. B. The global-based theory categorizes substance abuse as a variant of normal behavior subject to the same factors that control other behaviors (e.g., eating, exercise) in everyone.

91. A. The drug-based theory implies that abused drugs have a biochemical effect that results in continued use.

92. E. Social learning theories focus on cultural aspects of drug abuse, group and peer dynamics, and learned expectations.

93. C. TCAs have no significant long-term effect on somatodendritic or terminal autoreceptors.

94. A. SSRIs cause downregulation of terminal 5-HT$_{1B}$ autoreceptors after long-term administration.

95. C. TCAs increase responsiveness of postsynaptic 5-HT$_{1A}$ receptors.

96. B. MAOIs are associated with decreased responsiveness of 5-HT$_{1A}$ receptors.

97. D. Mirtazapine seems to have a net increased effect on 5-HT neurotransmission over time, but no significant effect on either terminal 5-HT$_{1B}$ autoreceptors or postsynaptic 5-HT$_{1A}$ receptors.

98. A. Platelet aggregation is increased under stress. This protective mechanism to slow down bleeding and heal wounds can also cause heart attacks and strokes.
    B. Stress activates cytokines, which can cause inflammation in the heart.
    C. Hostility activates the SNS, causing a rise in blood pressure.
    D. Hostility is associated with suppression of the PNS offsetting the normal balance with the SNS.
    E. Type A personality traits such as impatience and hostility are associated with increased heart disease. Individuals with Type B personality traits are more phlegmatic.

99. A. Unprotected sexual behavior is the most common method of acquiring HIV among youth.
    B. Drug use is a less common method of transmitting HIV infection through direct intravenous exposure and impaired ability to make safe decisions.
    C. Skin piercing and tattooing are much less common methods for acquiring HIV.
    D. The number of new cases of vertically transmitted HIV has decreased significantly in the United States, although those infected as infants are surviving into adolescence and becoming sexually active.
    E. In utero transmission is an example of vertical transmission.

100. C. Girls are especially vulnerable to HIV infection from sexual activity, presumably because of the immaturity of the cervical mucosa and hormonal changes.

  A. The number of HIV-positive teens is increasing dramatically. Young people account for 50% of new infections annually in the United States.

  B. Youths in psychiatric care are at elevated risk in that they engage in the same risky behaviors as their peers but at higher rates.

  D. Knowledge about the causes of HIV infection has not appreciably changed risk-taking behavior in adolescents.

  E. Increased risk is linked to low achievement motivation; high achievement motivation is linked to delayed sexual activity.

BLOCK 3

101. A 28-year-old elementary school teacher with a longstanding history of dysthymic disorder and generalized anxiety has recently been diagnosed with irritable bowel syndrome (IBS). Her gastroenterologist plans to start her on the antispasmodic dicyclomine but consults with you first as her psychiatrist regarding drug-drug interactions. Which one of the following is the most troublesome side effect the patient is likely to encounter by combining an SSRI and an antispasmodic?

A. Sedation
B. Seizures
C. Constipation
D. Respiratory arrest
E. Prolactin elevation

The response options for items 102 to 105 are the same. You will be required to select one answer for each item in the set.

A. Clozapine
B. Olanzapine
C. Ziprasidone
D. Haloperidol

For each side effect descriptive phrase, select the most relevant antipsychotic medication.

102. Hyperprolactinemia

103. Weight neutral

104. Agranulocytosis

105. Insulin resistance and elevated lipid levels

End of Set

106. A 53-year-old unemployed single man with a 35-year history of paranoid schizophrenia has been referred by his retiring psychiatrist. Except for persistent delusions and occasional auditory hallucinations, the patient has done reasonably well on haloperidol the past 20 years. When asked how he has tolerated the haloperidol, the patient denies any symptoms of drug-induced parkinsonism or dyskinesia. Which one of the following statements regarding tardive dyskinesia (TD) is true?

A. Younger age is a risk factor
B. Positive symptoms of schizophrenia are a risk factor

C. Affective disorders are a risk factor
D. The incidence of TD is increasing
E. TD is ameliorated by anticholinergic medications

107. As you are finishing what appeared to be a routine annual physical examination, your middle-aged patient says, "There is one other thing, Doc . . . I'm impotent." He wants to know more about pharmacologic treatments. Which of the following do you tell him best describes the mechanism of action of sildenafil citrate?

A. Postsynaptic dopamine receptor blockade
B. Selective serotonin reuptake inhibition
C. Inhibition of phosphodiesterase
D. GABA enhancement
E. Inhibition of aldehyde dehydrogenase

The response options for items 108 to 112 are the same. You will be required to select one answer for each item in the set.

A. Non-REM sleep
B. REM sleep
C. Stage 1 sleep
D. Stage 2 sleep
E. Stages 3 and 4 sleep

For each descriptive phrase, select the correct phase of normal sleep architecture.

108. Heart rate and respiration speed up

109. Comprises sleep stages 1–4

110. Deep sleep

111. 50% reduction in activity from wakefulness

112. Heart rate and body temperature begin to decrease

End of Set

113. While rotating as a medical student on the hospital's toxicology service, you are taken aback that so many of the referrals from the Poison Control Center are purposeful overdoses. Regarding the demographics of suicide in the United States, which one of the following is true?

A. Most suicides in the United States are women
B. Whites are twice as prone to suicide as African-Americans and Hispanics
C. Married men are more prone to suicide than single men
D. Few suicides in the United States are by gunshot
E. The risk of suicide decreases with age

114. Your upcoming psychiatry clerkship experience will include attending a support group at the veteran's hospital. To prepare, you read up on posttraumatic stress disorder (PTSD). Which one of the following statements about PTSD is correct?

    A. Comorbid psychiatric conditions are the exception
    B. Women have a higher lifetime prevalence of PTSD than men
    C. Benzodiazepines are a first-line treatment for chronic PTSD
    D. The trauma most often associated with PTSD in women is combat exposure
    E. Aging tends to mask PTSD symptoms

115. A 32-year-old musician presents to the emergency center after a 3-day binge of snorting cocaine. This is his third presentation in a similar state within the past 4 weeks. On each previous occasion he has left against medical advice, but today he is seeking admission. Which one of the following do you expect as a symptom of his cocaine withdrawal?

    A. Euphoric mood
    B. Increased energy
    C. Increased appetite
    D. Nausea
    E. Slurred speech

116. As the psychiatric consultant to the hospital's affiliated outpatient clinic, you have been asked to establish a mood disorders program. Which of the following has the highest correlation to suicidal ideation in bipolar patients?

    A. Family history of suicide
    B. Bipolar first-degree relative
    C. Psychotic index episode
    D. History of suicide attempts
    E. Alcohol abuse

117. The hospital has also asked if you will provide psychiatric consultation and medication management to the patients in the substance abuse aftercare program. Many of the patients in the program have a history of episodic alcohol abuse. Which one of the following is the mechanism of action of the alcohol deterrent disulfiram?

    A. SSRI
    B. Dopamine antagonist
    C. MAOI
    D. Acetaldehyde metabolism inhibitor
    E. Norepinephrine reuptake inhibitor

The next three questions (items 118 to 120) correspond to the following vignette.

A 35-year-old man presents to his community mental health clinic complaining of neck spasms and difficulty keeping still, adding, "I feel like I have ants in my pants." On physical exam, he is found to have moderate cogwheel rigidity.

118. Which one of the following medications is most likely causing these symptoms?

    A. Ambien
    B. Amantadine
    C. Amitriptyline
    D. Bromocriptine
    E. Fluphenazine

119. Which one of the following medications is the best acute treatment of pseudoparkinsonism?

    A. Carbamazepine
    B. Ibuprofen
    C. Fluoxetine
    D. Benztropine
    E. Diazepam

120. Which group of side effects is associated with the correct medication choice for the previous question?

    A. Dilated pupils, dry mouth, and constipation
    B. Leukopenia, thrombocytopenia, and aplastic anemia
    C. Renal impairment
    D. Nausea, sexual dysfunction, and vivid dreams
    E. Ataxia, respiratory depression, and dependence

End of Set

The response options for items 121 to 125 are the same. You will be required to select one answer for each set. You may use an option once, more than once, or not at all.

    A. Increased effect
    B. Decreased effect
    C. No significant effect

For each pharmacologic combination, select the appropriate effect caused by the interaction of the prescribed agent with a self-medicated substance.

121. Digoxin plus St. John's wort

122. Warfarin plus ginseng

123. Acetylsalicylic acid (ASA) plus gingko biloba

124. Nefazodone plus triazolam

125. Lithium plus NSAIDs

End of Set

126. Your upcoming psychiatry clerkship includes a day-long field trip with your classmates to the mental health annex of the county jail. Your faculty supervisor encourages you to read about a variety of clinical syndromes, including personality disorders, in preparation for the field trip. Which of the following is true regarding antisocial personality disorder?

    A. There must be evidence of conduct disorder before the age of 18
    B. The most common comorbid condition found in antisocial individuals is substance-related disorder
    C. The majority of individuals diagnosed with conduct disorder develop antisocial personality disorder
    D. Individuals with antisocial personality disorder most commonly use the defense mechanisms of avoidance, regression, and intellectualization
    E. Typically, individuals with antisocial personality disorder perform behaviors that are ego-dystonic

The response options for items 127 to 134 are the same. You will be required to select one answer for each item in the set.

    A. Psychotic disorder
    B. Mood disorder
    C. Anxiety disorder
    D. Somatoform disorder
    E. Dissociative disorder
    F. Cognitive disorder
    G. Paraphilia
    H. Factitious disorder

For each patient profile, select the most appropriate diagnostic class.

127. A 67-year-old man is brought to the emergency room by nursing home staff who say that his behavior has been markedly changed over the past 48 hours. He has had a change in his sleep-wake cycle and has been disoriented. He has no previous psychiatric history and was transferred to the nursing home after surgery for a fractured hip.

128. A 25-year-old housewife is seen in the emergency room complaining of sudden loss of vision after she witnessed her son being hit by a car outside their home.

129. A 32-year-old woman comes into the emergency room accompanied by her husband. She has recurrent thoughts and images of drowning her 3-month-old baby in the bathtub. She denies having auditory hallucinations commanding her to do this, and is very distressed by these thoughts. Because of these thoughts and images, she excessively checks on her baby "to make sure he is safe."

130. A 19-year-old soldier is triaged from the battlefield for emergency care. He is distraught that he cannot remember the events of a battle in which most of his squad were killed.

131. A woman comes into the emergency room complaining of fever that has persisted despite multiple trials of oral antibiotics. Her medical record reveals she has an extensive history of hospitalizations and procedures. One of the medicine residents who treated the patient during past hospital stays confides that there had been suspicions that the woman was inducing these fevers by covert means for the sole purpose of obtaining medical attention.

132. A man is brought into the emergency room by the police for treatment of various cuts and abrasions after he was assaulted by a neighbor for spying on the neighbor's wife as she undressed. The patient has had two previous brief incarcerations for similar infractions.

133. A 51-year-old man is brought into the emergency room by a close friend. For longer than a month, he has claimed that the CIA is spying on him. He believes that his house is bugged and that the CIA has started to dig underground tunnels to be able to enter and leave his house at will. He denies having auditory or visual hallucinations, and his friend denies that the gentleman has shown any bizarre behavior.

134. A man brings his wife to the emergency room complaining that she is "out of control." She has rapid speech and has completely disrobed. She talks about a plan to write the "greatest novel ever written," sell it to the largest publishing houses, and make a million dollars. Her husband denies that she has ever used illicit drugs.

End of Set

135. During your assignment to the university's student health clinic, you will spend some time in the gynecology clinic. Which of the following psychotropic medications is most likely to be helpful for premenstrual dysphoric disorder (PMDD)?

A. Diazepam
B. Fluoxetine
C. Risperidone
D. Molindone
E. Naltrexone

136. A 48-year-old man with longstanding psychotic delusions has been referred to you for medication management. He has recently been hospitalized with a heart condition. Which one of the following antipsychotics has the highest risk for QT cardiac conduction prolongation?

A. Ziprasidone
B. Risperidone
C. Thiothixene
D. Aripazole
E. Fluphenazine

The response options for items 137 to 141 are the same. You will be required to select one answer for each item in the set.

A. Sleep latency
B. Sleep quality
C. Non-REM sleep
D. REM sleep
E. Insomnia
F. Primary insomnia
G. Sleep efficiency
H. Wake after sleep onset
I. Restless leg syndrome

For each descriptive phrase, select the correct terminology.

137. Minutes awake after falling asleep

138. Percentage of time asleep

139. Not attributable to medical, psychiatric, or environmental causes

140. Changes in physiological states

141. Time it takes to fall asleep

End of Set

142. A 43-year-old Vietnamese immigrant has been hospitalized on the psychiatric inpatient service. He is experiencing command hallucinations to harm himself. Which one of the following treatments would be the most efficacious for his major depressive disorder with psychotic features?

A. Fluoxetine
B. Imipramine and haloperidol together
C. ECT
D. Haloperidol
E. Fluoxetine and lorazepam together

The response options for items 143 to 149 are the same. You will be required to select one answer for each item in the set.

A. Alprazolam
B. Sertraline
C. Venlafaxine
D. Amantadine
E. Haloperidol
F. Chloral hydrate
G. Trihexyphenidyl

H. Disulfiram
I. Fluoxetine
J. Paroxetine
K. Fluvoxamine
L. Donepezil

For each pharmacologic mechanism of action, select the most relevant medication.

143. Inhibits both serotonin and norepinephrine reuptake

144. Enhances the effect of gamma-aminobutyric acid (GABA)

145. Releases dopamine

146. Nonspecific CNS depressant

147. Inhibits acetylcholinesterase

148. Postsynaptic blockade of dopamine receptors

149. Anticholinergic

End of Set

150. A 19-year-old Cambodian college student is seen in the campus behavioral health center. She was asked to be guest speaker for a movie night on campus that featured a movie about the Killing Fields. She had lived through Pol Pot's regime, and although she was reluctant to share her experiences, she believed it was important that others know about the atrocities that occurred. Since the movie night 10 days ago, she has had recurrent nightmares of the times she was beaten for attempting to escape a children's forced labor camp. She also has intrusive thoughts of her escape to a refugee camp that required crossing a river at night "with dead bodies floating by." She has recurrent memories of her baby brother's death. When the infant became ill and died, she remembers a soldier burying him by "throwing him into a hole as if he were a dog." After being reunited with her family in a refugee camp, she was surprised by her sense of detachment and numbness. She still finds it difficult to become close to others. For the past 10 days she has been unable to do homework and feels increasingly irritable. She has started to avoid areas of construction where she may see digging going on. She is easily alarmed. Which of the following is true regarding PTSD?

A. Sertraline is a first-line pharmaceutical agent for PTSD
B. To meet criteria for PTSD, a person must experience at least one reexperiencing symptom, one avoidance behavior, and one hyperarousal symptom
C. The duration of the disturbance must be more than 2 months for a diagnosis of PTSD
D. The disorder is specified as "acute" if duration of symptoms is less than 6 months
E. The disorder is specified "with delayed onset" if onset of symptoms is at least 12 months after the stressor

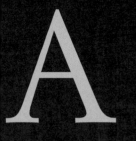

A Answers and Explanations

101. A	118. E	135. B
102. D	119. D	136. A
103. C	120. A	137. H
104. A	121. B	138. G
105. B	122. B	139. F
106. C	123. A	140. D
107. C	124. A	141. A
108. B	125. A	142. C
109. A	126. B	143. C
110. E	127. F	144. A
111. C	128. D	145. D
112. D	129. C	146. F
113. B	130. E	147. L
114. B	131. H	148. E
115. C	132. G	149. G
116. D	133. A	150. A
117. D	134. B	

101. A. Increased sedation is a common side effect when combining most psychotropic and antispasmodic medications.
    B. Neither SSRIs nor antispasmodics are particularly associated with seizures.
    C. Constipation is not a typical (but not unheard of) side effect of SSRIs; loose stools are more common.
    D. Respiratory arrest would not be expected from either medication at prescribed doses.
    E. Prolactin elevation is associated with dopamine-blocking agents.

102. D. The typical antipsychotic haloperidol is a potent dopamine-blocking agent and can cause elevated prolactin levels.

103. C. Ziprasidone is a relatively weight-neutral antidepressant.

104. A. Approximately 1% of patients taking clozapine develop agranulocytosis, a potentially life-threatening condition.

105. B. The atypical antipsychotic olanzapine is associated with elevated lipids, diabetes, and weight gain.

106. C. Affective disordered patients are at an increased risk to develop TD when exposed to antipsychotic medications.
    A. Older age is a risk factor for TD.
    B. Negative symptoms of schizophrenia are a risk factor for TD.
    D. The advent of atypical antipsychotics has decreased the number of new cases of TD by as much as tenfold
    E. Anticholinergics worsen symptoms of TD.

107. C. Sildenafil citrate was the first effective pharmacologic treatment for erectile dysfunction. It acts by inhibiting phosphodiesterase type 5, an enzyme found in the corpus cavernosum. This results in relaxation of smooth muscle with concomitant increased blood flow to the penis, leading to an erection.
    A. Postsynaptic dopamine receptor blockade is a primary mechanism of action of typical antipsychotics.
    B. Serotonin reuptake inhibition is associated with a variety of antidepressants.

    D. GABA enhancement is associated with the benzodiazepine anxiolytics.
    E. The alcohol deterrent disulfiram inhibits the enzyme aldehyde dehydrogenase.

108. B. REM sleep is distinguishable from non-REM sleep by changes in physiologic states, including increased heart rate and respirations and characteristic rapid eye movement.

109. A. Non-REM sleep comprises stages 1 to 4.

110. E. Stages 3 and 4 are deep sleep stages, also known as slow-wave or delta sleep.

111. C. Polysomnography shows a 50% reduction in activity between wakefulness and stage 1 sleep.

112. D. Stage 2 sleep is a period of light sleep during which polysomnographic readings show intermittent peaks and valleys, indicating spontaneous periods of muscle tone mixed with periods of muscle relaxation. As the heart rate and body temperature decrease, the body prepares to enter the deep sleep of stages 3 and 4.

113. B. Whites have double the rate of suicide of African-Americans and Hispanics.
    A. 80% of suicides in the United States are men.
    C. Single men are twice as prone to suicide as married men.
    D. 60% of suicides in the United States are by gunshot.
    E. The risk of suicide rises with age because of one group—white men over 50.

114. B. Overall, women have a significantly higher lifetime prevalence of PTSD.
    A. Comorbid psychiatric conditions are the rule rather than the exception with PTSD.
    C. SSRIs are the first-line pharmacologic treatment for chronic PTSD. There is no consistent evidence that benzodiazepines are efficacious for the treatment of chronic PTSD.
    D. Combat exposure is the most common trauma associated with PTSD in men; for women, it is sexual assault.
    E. Aging tends to contribute to the emergence of PTSD symptoms seemingly related to the onset of physical illness and losses of family and occupational activities.

115. C. Increased appetite is a manifestation of cocaine withdrawal, typically occurring within a few hours or days after abstaining.

    A. Dysphoric mood such as irritability and depression is typical during cocaine withdrawal. Euphoria is seen during cocaine intoxication.
    B. Fatigue is experienced during cocaine withdrawal; increased energy occurs during intoxication.
    D. Nausea is not a typical symptom of cocaine withdrawal, but is seen during alcohol intoxication and withdrawal.
    E. Slurred speech is associated with alcohol and sedative-hypnotic intoxication.

116. D. A history of suicide attempts has the highest correlation to current suicidal ideation. The correlation is 60%.

    A. There is an 11% correlation to suicidal ideation when there is a family history of suicide.
    B. There is a 50% correlation to suicidal ideation when there is a bipolar first-degree relative.
    C. There is a 35% correlation to suicidal ideation when there is a psychotic index episode for bipolar patients.
    E. There is a 46% correlation to suicidal ideation with alcohol abuse and dependence.

117. D. Disulfiram inhibits the metabolism of acetaldehyde, a toxic substance that results from the metabolism of alcohol.

    A. SSRIs are a particular class of antidepressants.
    B. Antipsychotics commonly have dopamine antagonist properties.
    C. MAOIs are another class of antidepressants.
    E. Norepinephrine reuptake inhibitors are also antidepressants; an example is the TCA desipramine.

118. E. Fluphenazine is an antipsychotic with a mechanism of action of postsynaptic blockade of dopamine receptors. Common side effects include dystonia, pseudoparkinsonism, and akathisia.

    A. Ambien is a sedative hypnotic and does not affect dopamine.
    B. Amantadine is an antiparkinsonian agent and could relieve this patient's symptoms.
    C. Amitriptyline is an antidepressant and does not affect dopamine.

    D. Bromocriptine also activates dopaminergic receptors and is used to treat Parkinson's disease.

119. D. Benztropine is an anticholinergic agent that can be given orally or parenterally. A typical dosage is 1 or 2 mg.

    A. Carbamazepine is an anticonvulsant used to treat seizures and bipolar disorder.
    B. Ibuprofen is an anti-inflammatory agent.
    C. Fluoxetine is an SSRI antidepressant.
    E. Diazepam is a GABA-enhancing benzodiazepine; although it is not specifically used for parkinsonism, it is a muscle relaxant and can also be helpful in treating akathisia.

120. A. Mild to moderate anticholinergic side effects include dilated pupils, dry mouth, constipation, and urinary retention.

    B. Blood dyscrasias are uncommon but potentially life-threatening side effects associated with carbamazepine.
    C. Renal impairment is associated with prolonged use of the NSAID ibuprofen.
    D. Serotonergic agents such as fluoxetine frequently cause mild gastrointestinal distress, sexual dysfunctions for both men and women, and vivid dreams.
    E. At higher doses, benzodiazepines such as diazepam can cause CNS and respiratory depression and physical dependence.

121. B. St. John's wort, often taken for depression, reduces digoxin levels by 20%.

122. B. Ginseng, used to enhance sexual performance, decreases the response to the anticoagulant warfarin.

123. A. Gingko biloba, used to remedy memory decline, increases the bleeding potential of ASA.

124. A. The antidepressant nefazodone is a potent P450 3A4 inhibitor and can markedly increase the concentration of the hypnotic triazolam.

125. A. NSAIDs reduce the renal clearance of Li, increasing its levels and the risk for toxicity.

126. B. Although anxiety and depression are frequent comorbid diagnoses of antisocial personality disorder, the most common comorbidity is substance abuse.

A. There must be evidence of conduct disorder before the age of 15. A personality disorder may be diagnosed once an individual is at least 18 years of age.
C. Approximately 30% of individuals with conduct disorder develop antisocial personality disorder.
D. The most common defense mechanisms used by individuals with antisocial traits are denial, rationalization, acting out, minimization, splitting, and hypochondriasis.
E. Typically, these individuals perform behaviors that are ego-syntonic. In other words, their behaviors are in harmony with their sense of self (ego) and its standards, despite the fact that their behaviors are not in keeping with societal standards.

127. F. Delirium is a type of cognitive disorder. Features of cognitive disorders are defects in memory, orientation, judgment, or mental function.

128. D. This individual suffers from conversion disorder, which is a type of somatoform disorder. The somatoform disorders consist of hypochondriasis, conversion disorder, body dysmorphic disorder, somatization disorder, and somatoform disorder not otherwise specified.

129. C. OCD is an anxiety disorder in which patients experience recurrent, intrusive, unwanted feelings, thoughts, and images (obsessions) that cause anxiety that is relieved, to an extent, by performing repetitive actions (compulsions). The five major DSM-IV classifications of anxiety disorders are panic disorder, phobias, OCD, generalized anxiety disorder, and PTSD.

130. E. The hallmarks of dissociative disorders are a sudden but temporary loss of memory or identity or extreme feelings of detachment due to emotional factors. The four major DSM-IV classifications are dissociative amnesia (as in this individual), dissociative fugue, dissociative identity disorder, and depersonalization disorder or derealization.

131. H. Factitious disorder is also known as Munchausen syndrome. Unlike patients with somatoform disorder (who truly believe that they are ill), patients with factitious disorder are pretending to have a mental or physical illness to obtain medical attention. In factitious disorder by proxy, an adult, typically a parent, feigns or induces illness in a child to obtain medical treatment.

132. G. This individual exhibits a disorder called voyeurism, in which a person obtains sexual pleasure from secretly watching people (often with binoculars) undressing or engaging in sexual activity. Voyeurism is a type of paraphilia. Paraphilias are characterized by the preferential use of unusual objects of sexual desire or engagement in unusual sexual activity over a period of at least 6 months, causing impairment in occupational or social functioning. Unless they are recurrent or intense, paraphilic fantasies are not paraphilias but simply normal components of human sexuality. Other types of paraphilias include fetishism, frotteurism, pedophilia, or exhibitionism.

133. A. Delusional disorder is a type of psychotic disorder characterized by a nonbizarre, fixed delusional system. The delusional thinking is circumscribed, not affecting other aspects of the patient's life. Subtypes of delusional disorder are erotomanic, grandiose, jealous, persecutory, somatic, and mixed types. The patient has to have a delusion lasting at least 1 month for the diagnosis to be made. Unlike in schizophrenia, prominent hallucinations and bizarre behavior are absent.

134. B. This patient is likely in an acute manic episode due to bipolar disorder, which is a type of mood disorder. Other types of mood disorders are major depressive disorder, dysthymia, and cyclothymia.

135. B. The SSRIs such as fluoxetine, paroxetine, sertraline, and citalopram have demonstrated effectiveness for the treatment of PMDD.

A. Antianxiety agents such as diazepam are not particularly effective as a treatment for PMDD.
C. Risperidone is an antipsychotic and is not indicated for PMDD.
D. Molindone is also an antipsychotic and is not indicated for PMDD.
E. Naltrexone is an opioid antagonist used in the treatment of alcohol and opioid dependence.

136. A. Ziprasidone has a moderate to high risk for QTc cardiac conduction prolongation, which can lead to arrhythmias.

   B. Risperidone is an atypical antipsychotic with low to moderate risk for QTc prolongation.
   C. Thiothixene is a typical antipsychotic with low to moderate risk for QTc prolongation.
   D. Aripazole is an atypical antipsychotic with minimal risk for QTc prolongation.
   E. Fluphenazine is a typical antipsychotic with minimal risk for QTc prolongation.

137. H. Wake after sleep onset (WASO) is the total number of minutes during the night that a person is awake after falling asleep.

138. G. Sleep efficiency is the percentage of time spent asleep compared to time spent in bed.

139. F. Primary insomnia is a syndrome not mainly attributable to medical, psychiatric, or environmental causes that is characterized by difficulty initiating or maintaining sleep or nonrestorative sleep.

140. D. REM sleep is distinguishable from non-REM sleep by changes in physiologic states including characteristic rapid eye movement.

141. A. Sleep latency is the number of minutes it takes a person to get to sleep.

142. C. ECT is the most effective treatment for psychotic depression, often achieving remission rates of more than 80% within 3 weeks.

   A. The antidepressant fluoxetine alone is typically not adequate to treat psychotic depression, with only a 30% to 40% success rate.
   B. The antidepressant imipramine plus the antipsychotic haloperidol may achieve a 50% to 60% success rate for psychotic depression; this can be maximized with TCA blood levels.
   D. An antipsychotic alone would not likely address the underlying mood disorder.
   E. An antidepressant plus anxiolytic such as lorazepam would not be much more efficacious than an antidepressant alone in treating a psychotic depression.

143. C. Venlafaxine is an antidepressant with both selective serotonin and norepinephrine reuptake properties.

144. A. Alprazolam is a potent benzodiazepine. Its anxiolytic effect is produced by enhancing GABA, which blocks cortical and limbic arousal.

145. D. Amantadine is an antiparkinsonian agent thought to cause the release of dopamine in the substantia nigra.

146. F. Chloral hydrate is a sedative-hypnotic with nonspecific CNS depressant properties similar to barbiturates.

147. L. Donepezil is an acetylcholinesterase inhibitor used for patients with mild dementia.

148. E. Haloperidol is a typical antipsychotic whose primary mechanism of action is to block postsynaptic dopamine receptors.

149. G. Trihexyphenidyl is an anticholinergic agent used to treat primary and medication-induced parkinsonism.

150. A. SSRIs such as sertraline are first-line agents for treating PTSD.

   B. To meet criteria for PTSD, a person must experience at least one reexperiencing symptom (nightmares, recollections, and flashbacks), three avoidance behaviors or numbing of general responsiveness, and two hyperarousal disturbances (criteria B, C, and D in DSM IV). A 1:1:1 pattern of disturbance after a traumatic event would be more in keeping with an acute stress disorder.
   C. The duration of the disturbance must be greater than 1 month for a diagnosis of PTSD.
   D. The disorder is specified as "acute" if the duration of symptoms is less than 3 months, and "chronic" if the duration of symptoms is 3 months or more.
   E. The disorder is specified as "with delayed onset" if onset of symptoms is at least 6 months after the stressor.

BLOCK 4

The response options for items 151 to 154 are the same. You will be required to select one answer for each item in the set.

A. A
B. B
C. C
D. D

For each description of the longitudinal course for depressive disorders, select the most accurate diagrammatic representation in Figure 4-151. The horizontal lines represent a euthymic state.

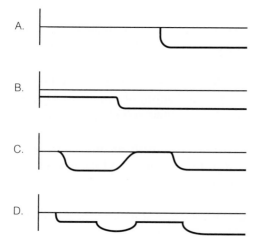

A.

B.

C.

D.

Figure 4-151

151. Recurrent depressions without full interepisode recovery superimposed on dysthymia

152. Single depressive episode superimposed on dysthymic disorder

153. Single depressive episode with no dysthymia

154. Recurrent depressions with full interepisode recovery and no dysthymia

End of Set

155. During rounds on the geropsychiatric unit, a 73-year-old retired surgeon with hypertension, mild congestive heart failure, hypothyroidism, and memory complaints is interviewed. Following your interview, your suspected diagnosis is depression, but you must rule out a differential diagnosis of dementia. Which one of the following is true and will help differentiate depression from dementia?

A. Decline in mental functioning is more rapid with dementia than with depression
B. People with dementia and depression are both usually disoriented
C. In depression, writing, speaking, and motor skills are not usually impaired
D. People with depression have problems with short-term memory whereas those with dementia have trouble concentrating
E. Depressed people may seem indifferent to their memory problems

156. An 18-year-old male was brought in to a doctor's office by his mother. She says that his mood, energy level, interest, and motivation are all decreased and asks you to evaluate him for depression. On physical exam, you find he is unkempt with a normal neurologic exam. A HEENT exam is significant for dry oral mucosa and injected conjunctivae. Suspecting acute intoxication, you presume his urine drug screen will be positive for which drug?

A. Cocaine
B. Methamphetamine
C. PCP
D. Marijuana
E. MDMA (ecstasy)

157. A 38-year-old obese caucasian female is being treated for schizophrenia, paranoid type. Which of the following is true regarding her antipsychotic treatment options?

A. Traditional antipsychotics are better at treating the negative symptoms of schizophrenia than the atypical antipsychotics
B. Olanzapine is not known to cause weight gain, hyperlipidemia, or diabetes
C. Hyperprolactinemia may occur at all dosages of risperidone and at higher levels of olanzapine
D. Haloperidol and chlorpromazine are potent 5-hydroxytryptamine receptor-blocking agents
E. Quetiapine is considered to be problematic because of its anticholinergic side effects

The response options for items 158 to 165 are the same. You will be required to select one answer for each item in the set.

A. Basic trust versus mistrust
B. Autonomy versus shame and doubt
C. Initiative versus guilt
D. Industry versus inferiority
E. Identity versus identity confusion
F. Intimacy versus isolation
G. Generatively versus stagnation
H. Integrity versus despair and disgust

For each human value or ego strength, select the appropriate developmental crisis from Erikson's eight stages of psychosexual development.

158. Purpose

159. Fidelity

160. Care

161. Hope

162. Will

163. Competence

164. Love

165. Wisdom

End of Set

166. A 26-year-old psychology intern has been referred by her PCP for evaluation and treatment of symptoms of depression. Her PCP has tried a variety of antidepressants, but each trial has resulted in severe orthostatic blood pressure changes, weight gain, or sedation. Which one of the following antidepressant medications would be the best to try next to minimize these side effects?

    A. Imipramine
    B. Phenelzine
    C. Fluoxetine
    D. Desipramine
    E. Parnate

167. A 28-year-old attorney is considering becoming pregnant. She was diagnosed with ADHD at age 9 years. She seeks consultation in your outpatient practice about the heritability of ADHD. To simplify your response to her, you relate that a heritability of 0 means there is no

genetic input and a heritability of 1 means the disorder is completely determined by genetics. Which one of the following has the highest heritability?

    A. Depression
    B. Generalized anxiety disorder
    C. Breast cancer
    D. ADHD
    E. Identical twins reared in the same environment

The response options for items 168 to 171 are the same. You will be required to select one answer for each item in the set.

    A. Serotonin (HT)
    B. GABA
    C. Norepinephrine (NE)
    D. Substance P
    E. Dopamine (DA)
    F. Corticotropin releasing factor (CRF)

For each anatomic structure or pathway, select the most appropriate neurotransmitter affecting mood.

168. The hypothalamic-pituitary-adrenal (HPA) axis

169. Lateral tegmental area and locus coerulus

170. Dorsal and caudal raphe nuclei

171. Mesolimbic-mesocortical pathway

End of Set

The response options for items 172 to 175 are the same. You will be required to select one or more answers for each item in the set.

A 20-year-old gravid female with a history of bipolar disorder is diagnosed as being HIV positive. She was admitted to the hospital for new-onset seizures, and a biopsy revealed cerebral toxoplasmosis. She complains of depression and not wanting to live. The chart reveals that she has been started on phenytoin as well as diazepam as needed for anxiety. She is not currently on a mood stabilizer.

    A. Valproate
    B. Lithium
    C. Diazepam
    D. Carbamazepine
    E. Phenytoin

For each syndrome, select the most likely teratogenic pharmacologic agent.

172. Neonatal withdrawal syndrome **(SELECT ONE)**

173. Spina bifida **(SELECT TWO)**

174. Ebstein's anomaly **(SELECT ONE)**

175. Growth deficiency, microcephaly, and mental deficiency **(SELECT ONE)**

End of Set

The response options for items 176 to 180 are the same. You will be required to select one answer for each item in the set.

A 46-year-old waitress with a 20-year history of mood symptoms is seeking consultation regarding her intolerance of antidepressant medications and recurrent symptoms of anhedonia, insomnia, and loss of appetite.

    A. Histamine blockade
    B. Dopamine reuptake inhibition
    C. Serotonin blockade
    D. Serotonin reuptake inhibition
    E. Norepinephrine reuptake inhibition
    F. α1-adrenergic blockade
    G. α2-adrenergic blockade
    H. Acetylcholine blockade

For each clinical effect, select the causative antidepressant neurotransmitter action.

176. Reduces depression and anxiety, causes tremors and tachycardia

177. Causes sedation, hypotension, and weight gain

178. Reduces depression, suicidal behavior, and psychosis

179. Causes hypotension and reflex tachycardia

180. Reduces depression and has antiparkinsonian effects

End of Set

The response options for items 181 to 185 are the same. You will be required to select one answer for each item in the set.

    A. D_2 (dopamine) receptors in the nigrostriatum
    B. D_2 receptors in the tuberoinfundibular system
    C. 5-HT_3 and 5-HT_4 receptors
    D. 5-HT_2 receptors
    E. α-adrenergic receptors
    F. Histaminic receptors
    G. Muscarinic receptors
    H. Nicotinic receptors

For each side effect profile, select the most likely neurotransmitter receptor being regulated.

181. Nausea, vomiting, and diarrhea

182. Parkinsonian syndrome and extrapyramidal side effects

183. Weight gain and hyperprolactinemia

184. Hypotension and dizziness

185. Acute agitation, anxiety, noctural myoclonus, and sexual dysfunction

End of Set

The response options for items 186 to 190 are the same. You will be required to select one or more answers for each item in the set.

    A. Lorazepam
    B. Amitriptyline
    C. Naltrexone
    D. Valproic acid
    E. Lithium carbonate
    F. Bupropion
    G. Olanzapine
    H. Disulfuram
    I. Carbamazepine
    J. Tramadol

For each clinical scenario, select the appropriate drug(s).

186. A 27-year-old female with a history of bipolar disorder is admitted to the hospital in a manic state. She is 4 weeks pregnant and refuses to take any medication associated with birth deformities in humans. Which medication is appropriate? **(SELECT ONE)**

187. A 36-year-old male has been enrolled in a methadone maintenance program continuously for 1 year and has been compliant with

treatment. Which medications would be CONTRAINDICATED due to increased risk of respiratory depression? **(SELECT FIVE)**

188. In the same patient above, which medications would be CONTRAINDICATED due to precipitation of opiate withdrawal? **(SELECT TWO)**

189. A 42-year-old male is currently taking fluoxetine for depression, buspirone for anxiety, and trazodone for insomnia. You are concerned about potential drug interactions and recognize that the addition of this medication may result in cardiac death. **(SELECT ONE)**

190. In the same patient as above, you also recognize that adding any of these four medications would put him at high risk for a serotonin syndrome. **(SELECT FOUR)**

End of Set

The response options for items 191 to 196 are the same. You will be required to select one answer for each item in the set.

    A. 2 weeks
    B. 1 month
    C. Less than 1 month
    D. 2 years
    E. Less than 1 day
    F. 1 year
    G. 1 week
    H. 4 days
    I. 6 months

For each diagnosis, select the required duration of symptoms.

191. Manic episode

192. Schizophreniform disorder

193. Hypomanic episode

194. Dysthymia

195. Major depressive episode

196. Brief psychotic episode

End of Set

The response options for items 197 to 200 are the same. You will be required to select one answer for each item in the set.

    A. A
    B. B
    C. C
    D. D

For each description of the longitudinal course for bipolar I disorder, select the most accurate diagrammatic representation in Figure 4-197. The horizontal lines represent a euthymic state.

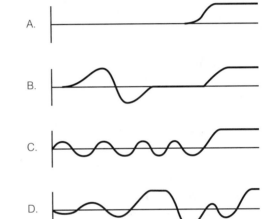

Figure 4-197

197. Recurrent bipolar I disorder without full interepisode recovery superimposed on cyclothymic disorder

198. Single episode of bipolar I disorder with no cyclothymic disorder

199. Recurrent bipolar I episodes with full interepisode recovery and no cyclothymic disorder

200. Single bipolar I episode superimposed on cyclothymic disorder

End of Set

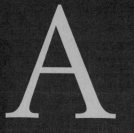

A Answers and Explanations

151. D	168. F	185. D
152. B	169. C	186. G
153. A	170. A	187. A, B, F, G, J
154. C	171. E	188. C, I
155. C	172. C	189. B
156. D	173. A, D	190. B, E, F, J
157. C	174. B	191. G
158. C	175. E	192. B
159. E	176. E	193. H
160. G	177. A	194. D
161. A	178. C	195. A
162. B	179. F	196. C
163. D	180. B	197. D
164. F	181. C	198. A
165. H	182. A	199. B
166. C	183. B	200. C
167. E	184. E	

151. D. The combination of major depressive episodes and dysthymia is referred to as a double depression.

152. B. A lingering dysthymia after improvement of the more pronounced major depressive symptoms may imply incomplete treatment of the later condition.

153. A. A single depressive episode without a history of dysthymia does not typically require prolonged treatment after the presenting symptoms have been in remission for 6 months.

154. C. Fifty percent of individuals experiencing a depressive episode will have a recurrence.

155. C. Skills such as writing, speaking, and motor skills tend to remain intact with depression but are lost as a dementia progresses.

   A. Decline in mental functioning tends to be more rapid with depression than with dementia.
   B. Depressed people are usually not disoriented, unlike dementia patients.
   D. Depressed people have trouble concentrating and those affected by dementia have short-term memory problems.
   E. Dementia patients may seem indifferent to their memory problems whereas depressed people typically comment about such changes.

156. D. This patient is displaying the amotivational syndrome associated with marijuana use. Other signs of intoxication with marijuana are injected conjunctivae, dry mouth, and tachycardia.

   A. Cocaine is a stimulant, and intoxication is characterized by agitation, irritability, and pupillary dilation.
   B. Methamphetamine is another stimulant, and intoxication would look similar to cocaine intoxication.
   C. PCP intoxication has the behavioral effects of a stimulant, and neurologic findings might include nystagmus, hypertension, tachycardia, muscle rigidity, and seizures.
   E. MDMA (ecstasy) is an amphetamine analog that causes restlessness, diaphoresis, tremor, and piloerection. It is not known to cause conjunctival injection.

157. C. Hyperprolactinemia may occur at all doses of risperidone and at higher levels of olanzapine. Dopamine inhibits prolactin production. Because antipsychotics block postsynaptic dopamine receptors, there is decreased inhibition of prolactin production, and thus increased prolactin levels. Male and female patients started on antipsychotics should be warned about the risk of side effects from hyperprolactinemia, such as galactorrhea, gynecomastia, and sexual dysfunction (e.g., loss of libido or erectile dysfunction).

   A. Atypical antipsychotics are better at treating the negative symptoms of schizophrenia than traditional antipsychotics.
   B. Drug-induced weight gain is a common complaint of patients taking a variety of antipsychotics, including olanzapine. Like many antipsychotics, olanzapine may affect appetite by targeting dopaminergic pathways in the tuberoinfundibular system (pituitary and hypothalamus). This female, who is obese, is also vulnerable to iatrogenic diabetes mellitus due to antipsychotic treatment. Schizophrenia is associated with a two- to threefold increase of diabetes even without antipsychotic treatment. Overweight individuals or those with a family history of high cholesterol or triglycerides are particularly vulnerable to antipsychotic-induced hyperlipidemia. Serious hyperlipidemia is particularly a concern with olanzapine.
   D. Unlike traditional antipsychotics, such as haloperidol and chlorpromazine, the newer atypical antipsychotics are potent $5-HT_2$ receptor-blocking agents in addition to being dopamine blockers.
   E. Although quetiapine may cause oversedation, it does so via its antihistaminic properties. The anticholinergic properties of quetiapine are considered very low relative to others in this class.

158. C. Purpose is the ego strength fostered during the psychosocial crisis of initiative versus guilt experienced during play age.

159. E. Fidelity is the ego strength fostered during the psychosocial crisis of lientity versus identity confusion experienced during adolescence.

160. G. Care is the ego strength fostered during the psychosocial crisis of generativity versus stagnation experienced during adulthood.

161. A. Hope is the ego strength fostered during the earliest psychosocial crisis of basic trust versus basic mistrust experienced during infancy.

162. B. Will is the ego strength developed during the second psychosocial crisis of autonomy versus shame and doubt experienced during early childhood.

163. D. Competence is the ego strength fostered during the school-age psychosocial crisis of industry versus inferiority.

164. F. Love is the ego strength fostered during young adulthood while transgressing through the psychosocial crisis of intimacy versus isolation.

165. H. Wisdom is the ego strength associated with old age gained during the psychosocial crisis of integrity versus despair.

Late in his career, Erik Erikson amplified his stages of development by highlighting the "dystonic" element first (i.e., basic mistrust versus trust) in considering the coping skills (in this case, hope) required to deal with very old age. Erikson's epigenetic model of development includes biologic, psychologic, and social determinants.

166. C. The SSRI fluoxetine would be the best next choice, in that it is typically not associated with orthostasis, weight gain, or sedation.

   A. Imipramine is a TCA with frequent side effects of orthostasis, weight gain, and sedation.
   B. Phenelzine is an MAOI antidepressant with frequent orthostasis and weight gain side effects.
   D. Desipramine is another TCA with orthostasis and weight gain side effects; sedation is less common.
   E. Parnate is another MAOI with side effects similar to those of phenelzine.

167. E. 1.0 is the expected heritability of identical twins reared in the same environment.

   A. The heritability of depression is approximately 0.39, which means 39% of the etiologic contribution is genetic.
   B. The heritability of generalized anxiety disorder is approximately 0.32.
   C. The heritability of breast cancer is approximately 0.27.
   D. The heritability of ADHD is 0.75, making it one of the most highly inherited common psychiatric syndromes.

168. F. The HPA is frequently overactive in depression because of elevated CRF, which may be caused by stress.

169. C. NE cell bodies originate in the brainstem in both the lateral tegmental area and the locus ceruleus. These cell bodies are also very responsive to stress.

170. A. Serotonergic cell bodies are concentrated in the dorsal and caudate raphe nuclei, and their projections extend to the hypothalamus, amygdala, cortex, hypocampus, basal ganglia, and brainstem—all believed associated with symptoms of depression.

171. E. Dopaminergic neurons comprise three main pathways: mesolimbic-mesocortical, nigrostriatal, and tuberoinfundibular.

172. C. Diazepam, a benzodiazepine, has been known to cause neonatal withdrawal syndrome. Gradual tapering of a benzodiazepine before delivery is recommended to minimize neonatal withdrawal phenomena. This has also been reported with several other benzodiazepines, such as alprazolam and triazolam. If a benzodiazepine is required, lorazepam may be a better option because of its possible lower accumulation in fetal tissue. There is also a weak positive relationship between diazepam exposure and oral clefts. Avoidance of diazepam is recommended until after the tenth week of gestation, to decrease the risk of oral defects.

173. A, D. In fetuses exposed to valproate in the first trimester, 1% to 2% have developed neural tube defects and 1% spina bifida. Therefore, women of childbearing age who are on valproate should take folate supplementation. Carbamazepine also has the risk of causing congenital malformations, including spina bifida. Interestingly, since the three most commonly used mood stabilizers are all teratogenic, the least risk may be with Li (0.1%

compared to 5% to 5% for valproate and 1% to 3% for carbamazepine). Furthermore, consideration of these risks must be balanced with up to a 50% risk of relapse of mood symptoms. According to the FDA's teratogenicity ratings, Li, carbamazepine, and valproate are all category D drugs, indicating that there is positive evidence of risk to the fetus. Nevertheless, the potential benefits may outweigh the risks.

174. B. Li should be discontinued during pregnancy and nursing, when clinically possible. The greatest concern regarding Li as a teratogenic agent is the possibility of cardiac malformations; more specifically, Ebstein's anomaly, a tricuspid valve malformation, may occur when a fetus is exposed to Li during the first trimester. The relative risk for this anomaly in children with fetal exposure to Li may be 20 times higher than the risk to unexposed children, although the absolute risk remains low (1 in 1000 births). "Floppy baby" syndrome, resulting in infants with hypotonicity and cyanosis, is the most recognized adverse event in infants exposed to Li. Neonatal hypothyroidism and nephrogenic diabetes insipidus have also been reported.

175. E. The risk of congenital malformations in fetuses exposed to phenytoin include cleft lip and palate, heart malformations, and fetal hydantoin syndrome. Fetal hydantoin syndrome consists of prenatal growth deficiency, microcephaly, and mental deficiency. This syndrome can also be seen in children born to mothers who have received barbiturates, alcohol, or trimethadione.

176. E. Norepinephrine reuptake inhibitors such as desipramine and mapratoline are effective antidepressants and, when coupled with serotonergic agents, can relieve anxiety. The side effects of tremors and rapid heart rate are common with noradrenergic agents.

177. A. The antihistamine properties of TCAs frequently cause sedation, hypotension, and weight gain. At lower doses, the sedating side effects may be useful as a soporific.

178. C. Serotonin blockade not only helps depression presumably related to an eventual upregulation of receptor sites, but also dampens psychotic symptoms. Several of the newer atypical antipsychotics rely on these actions. Low serotonin metabolite levels have been correlated with suicidal behavior.

179. F. The side effect profile of $\alpha 1$ blockade includes postural hypotension, dizziness, and reflex tachycardia and is seen most frequently with TCAs.

180. B. Dopaminergic neurons activate areas of the brain associated with behavioral functions altered in depression such as the cortex, limbic region, and pituitary gland as well as the nigrostriatal pathway affecting motor functions. There is a high degree of comorbidity between depression and Parkinson's disease.

181. C. Chemoreceptors in the brainstem can mediate vomiting through activation of 5-HT_3 receptors. Peripheral 5-HT_3 and 5-HT_4 receptors in the gastrointestinal tract may also be responsible for GI cramping and diarrhea associated with SSRI treatment.

182. A. Dopaminergic pathways in the nigrostriatum are likely involved in the extrapyramidal side effects and parkinsonian syndrome seen with antipsychotic treatment.

183. B. Dopaminergic pathways in the tuberoinfundibular system (pituitary and hypothalamus) may result in hyperprolactinemia and increased appetite, which may be associated with antipsychotic treatment.

184. E. TCAs possess an α-adrenergic portion that inserts into α-adrenergic receptors, possibly resulting in side effects such as dizziness, hypotension, and drowsiness.

185. D. Serotonin receptors that exist in the brain, spinal cord, and gastrointestinal tract may help explain various side effects of SSRIs. Acute stimulation of 5-HT_{2A} and 5-HT_{2C} receptors in raphe projections to the limbic cortex may result in acute mental agitation and anxiety, especially when treatment is started. Thus, in patients with agitated depression, one should start with a low dose and increase slowly to a therapeutic dose. Stimulation of 5-HT_{2A} receptors in the basal ganglia can lead to restlessness,

psychomotor retardation, or even mild parkinsonism and dystonic movements. Stimulation of 5-HT$_{2A}$ receptors in the brainstem sleep centers may cause nocturnal myoclonus and may also disrupt slow-wave sleep and result in insomnia. Stimulation of 5-HT$_{2A}$ receptors in the spinal cord may inhibit the spinal reflexes of orgasm and ejaculation and cause sexual dysfunction. Stimulation of 5-HT$_{2A}$ receptors in pleasure centers of the mesocortex may decrease dopamine activity there and cause apathy or decreased libido.

186. G. Olanzapine is an atypical antipsychotic medication that is approved for short-term treatment of bipolar mania. Its use during pregnancy is very limited, although it has not been associated with human fetal deformities. Current birth registry data are inconclusive for this pregnancy category C drug. Lithium carbonate is established as an effective therapy for management of bipolar disorder, but it is a pregnancy category D drug. It is associated with an increased risk of Ebstein's anomaly, in addition to other cardiac defects and neonatal goiters. The highest risk is in the first trimester. Valproic acid is also effective for bipolar disorder, but it is also a category D drug. Human data have associated valproic acid with neural tube defects such as spina bifida. Although carbamazepine is not an FDA-approved treatment for bipolar disorder, it is sometimes used off-label. Data from a study of exposure to carbamazepine in the first trimester suggest that the risk of spina bifida is roughly 1%. This is also a category D drug. Lorazepam may be used for temporary symptom management in manic patients, although it is also a category D agent and exposure to benzodiazepines in the first trimester has been linked to cleft palate.

187. A, B, F, G, J. Methadone is an opiate agonist, which interacts with many other drugs, potentially leading to dangerous CNS depression. Lorazepam is a benzodiazepine that may cause synergistic sedation when combined with methadone. Amitriptyline and olanzapine both have anticholinergic effects that may cause additive CNS depression when used in combination with methadone. Bupropion is an inhibitor of cytochrome P450 (CYP) 2D6 isoenzyme, which

is responsible for methadone clearance. Adding this drug to someone at steady state on methadone may result in elevated methadone levels and CNS depression.

188. C, I. Naltrexone is an opiate antagonist, which would be very dangerous in this patient because it may precipitate acute opiate withdrawal. Carbamazepine induces CYP3A4 (also responsible for methadone metabolism) and may increase the rate of methadone clearance, resulting in withdrawal symptoms over time.

189. B. Amitriptyline is a tertiary amine TCA that is metabolized by CYP2D6 to an active metabolite (nortriptyline). Combination with fluoxetine, a CYP2D6 inhibitor, would result in toxic and potentially fatal levels of both amitriptyline and nortriptyline.

190. B, E, F, J. This patient is already taking three serotonergic medications. Serotonin syndrome is characterized by altered mental status, restlessness, myoclonus, fever, diaphoresis, tremor, and seizures. The risk of this potentially fatal condition is increased in patients taking multiple serotonergic medications. Lithium carbonate and amitriptyline can both enhance serotonergic transmission, which would put this patient at higher risk for serotonin syndrome. Bupropion is a CYP2D6 inhibitor that may increase fluoxetine and norfluoxetine levels and also increase this patient's risk factors. Tramadol is an analgesic that may also precipitate serotonin syndrome through an unknown mechanism.

191. G. A manic episode is a distinct period of abnormally and persistently elevated, expansive or irritable mood, lasting at least 1 week, or any duration if hospitalization is necessary.

192. B. Schizophreniform disorder may be diagnosed if two or more criteria A symptoms (delusions, hallucinations, disorganized speech, disorganized behavior, or negative symptoms) are present for at least 1 month but less than 6 months.

193. H. A hypomanic episode is a period of persistently elevated, expansive, or irritable mood, lasting throughout at least 4 days, that is clearly different from the usual nondepressed mood.

194. D. Dysthymia is defined as depressed mood for most of the day, for more days than not, as indicated either by subjective account or observation by others, for at least 2 years.

195. A. A major depressive episode may be diagnosed if symptoms are present most of the day nearly every day during a 2-week period and represent a change from previous functioning.

196. C. A brief psychotic disorder is diagnosed if an individual exhibits one or more of the following symptoms: delusions, hallucinations, disorganized speech, or grossly disorganized or catatonic behavior, with the disturbance lasting at least 1 day but less than 1 month, with eventual full return to premorbid functioning.

197. D. Recurrent bipolar I episodes superimposed on cyclothymia implies either inadequate treatment or no treatment at all.

198. A. Bipolar disorder is typically a recurrent disorder, so with time other episodes would be expected to occur. Treatment often attenuates the severity and frequency of subsequent episodes.

199. B. Recurrent episodes are the usual longitudinal course for bipolar I disorder.

200. C. Cyclothymic patients tend not to seek treatment for their less severe symptoms but present when acutely manic or severely depressed.

5 Surgery

BLOCK 1

The next four questions (items 1 to 4) correspond to the following vignette.

A 57-year-old female is referred to your office because of an abnormality on her annual mammogram. This is the first mammogram she has had in several years. The patient denies any recent weight loss or nipple discharge. The patient reports that her sister had breast cancer that required a mastectomy. On physical examination, you palpate a 3-cm, mobile, nontender mass. You observe the following mammogram (Figure 5-1A).

1. Which of the following is the appropriate next step in the workup of this patient?

    A. CT scan
    B. BRCA1 genetics
    C. Biopsy
    D. Chest x-ray
    E. Follow-up in 2 weeks

2. The patient is eventually diagnosed with invasive ductal adenocarcinoma. Which of the following is most important factor in the staging of this patient's cancer?

    A. Age
    B. Tumor size
    C. Histologic grade
    D. Estrogen receptor and progesterone receptor status
    E. Lymph node involvement

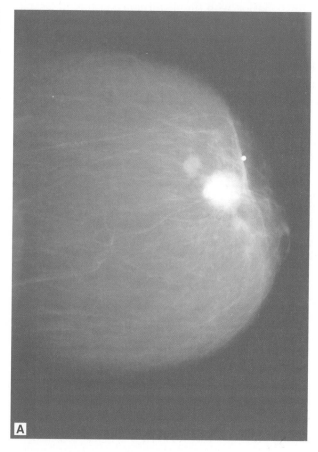

Figure 5-1A • Image Courtesy of the University of Utah School of Medicine, Salt Lake City, Utah.

3. The patient desires breast conservation therapy. In addition to a lumpectomy, what other procedure(s) will always be required?

A. Full-beam external radiation
B. Supraclavicular node dissection
C. Intrathecal chemotherapy
D. Local radiation therapy and axillary node dissection
E. Lumpectomy only

4. Which of the following is a definite risk factor for breast cancer in women?

A. Multiparity
B. Strong family history of colon cancer
C. History of previously treated breast cancer
D. An aunt with breast cancer
E. High fat diet

End of Set

5. A healthy 35-year-old female complains of bloody discharge from her right nipple that occurred spontaneously while she was showering. The patient has never been hospitalized, denies any previous surgeries, and is not taking any medications. The following images (Figure 5-5A and B) are of an ultrasound and a galactogram of the involved breast. What is the most likely diagnosis?

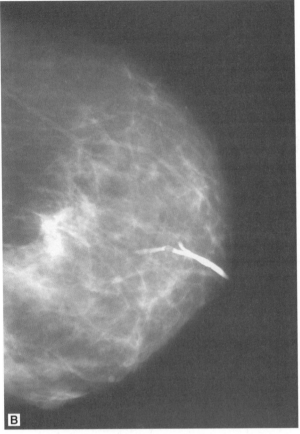

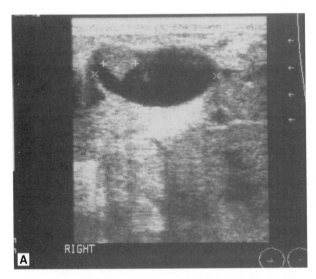

Figure 5-5A • Image Courtesy of the University of Utah School of Medicine, Salt Lake City, Utah.

Figure 5-5B • Image Courtesy of the University of Utah School of Medicine, Salt Lake City, Utah.

A. Intraductal papilloma
B. Duct ectasia
C. Fibroadenoma
D. Lactocele
E. Paget's disease

6. A new mother presents to your office with a painful right breast. The patient states that she has been breastfeeding without difficulty up until 2 days ago. Examination reveals a cracked, erythematous breast, which is extremely tender to touch around the areola. An ultrasound of the breast is negative. Being an astute physician, you diagnose mastitis. Which is the most appropriate next step?

A. Instruct the woman to stop breastfeeding
B. Explain to the patient that she can continue breastfeeding, but only if she uses the other breast
C. Take her emergently to the operating room for incision and debridement
D. Inform her that she may continue breastfeeding and give her a prescription for dicloxacillin
E. No action is needed; this will resolve on its own

The next two questions (items 7 and 8) correspond to the following vignette.

A 50-year-old female was sent to you for a large upper inner quadrant mass seen on her initial mammogram. The mammogram was done under a federally funded program. The patient had felt a vague fullness of her right breast, but she did not seek medical help until getting the results of the mammogram in the mail. The patient and her family have been without insurance for close to 3 years since her husband lost his job. The patient is the main source of income for the family and works as a waitress. You have performed a right modified radical mastectomy, and the pathology shows a 4.2 cm, moderately differentiated, infiltrating ductal carcinoma, ER/PR negative, Her-2 neu 3+, with 4 of 15 positive nodes. A preoperative chest X-ray was negative, and all her labs are normal. The patient returns to your clinic for her first postoperative discharge visit, and she seems to be doing well except for protrusion of the right scapula.

7. Which nerve was damaged during the operative procedure?

   A. Thoracodorsal nerve
   B. Long thoracic nerve
   C. Intercostobrachiales nerve
   D. Subscapular nerve
   E. Axillary nerve
   F. Phrenic nerve

8. Which nerve, if damaged during an axillary dissection, will result in only a sensory deficit?

   A. Medial pectoral nerve
   B. Intercostobrachial nerve
   C. Thoracodorsal nerve
   D. Axillary nerve
   E. Long thoracic nerve
   F. Radial nerve

End of Set

The next two questions (items 9 and 10) correspond to the following vignette.

A 45-year-old female presents to your office with intermittent right upper quadrant pain. The patient states that it has been occurring on and off for the past 2 years, usually begins after eating a meal, and subsides after several hours. On physical exam, you find the patient is overweight and demonstrates no abdominal pain to palpation. You suspect biliary colic.

9. Which is the most appropriate next step in the workup of this patient?

A. Serum cholesterol
B. Abdominal CT scan
C. Abdominal ultrasound
D. ERCP
E. No further workup is necessary at this time

10. On further workup, you diagnose the patient with symptomatic cholelithiasis. The treatment of choice is

   A. Waiting until more substantial symptoms develop
   B. Exercise and low-cholesterol diet
   C. Chenodeoxycholic acid
   D. Laparoscopic cholecystectomy
   E. ERCP

End of Set

The response options for items 11 to 14 are the same. You will be required to select one answer for each item in the set.

   A. Tamoxifen
   B. Vinblastine
   C. Cyclophosphamide
   D. Bleomycin

For each description, select the most appropriate chemotherapeutic agent.

11. The metabolic product of this drug is known to cause hemorrhagic cystitis.

12. This drug inhibits the polymerization of microtubules, thus halting mitosis.

13. This drug may cause pulmonary fibrosis.

14. This antiestrogen drug is used to treat breast cancer.

End of Set

The next three questions (items 15 to 17) correspond to the following vignette.

A 60-year-old male presents to the ED with a 2-day history of fever and chills. The patient states he has been unable to eat anything at home due to nausea and vomiting. The vital signs in the ED are T 39.3°C, HR 98, BP 115/75, and an SaO_2 of 98 % on room air. On physical exam, you note the patient appears ill, but nontoxic. The patient has scleral icterus, dry mucous membranes, and his abdomen is tender to palpation in the right upper quadrant. The following labs are obtained: WBC 18,000, total bilirubin 4.0 mg/dL, alkaline phosphatase 450 U/L.

15. What is the most likely cause of this disease?

A. Tumor of the pancreatic head
B. Choledocholithiasis
C. Duodenal ulcer
D. Acute viral gastritis
E. Acute pneumonia

16. Which organism is most likely to be isolated in this patient's disease?

A. *Escherichia coli*
B. *Bacteroides fragilis*
C. *Enterococcus*
D. *Klebsiella pneumonia*
E. *Pseudomonas aeruginosa*

17. Which of the following is the most appropriate treatment?

A. ERCP with sphincterotomy
B. Pancreaticoduodenectomy
C. Percutaneous cholecystostomy
D. Antibiotics only
E. Oral bile salts to dissolve the stone

End of Set

18. A 59-year-old male presents to the ED with complaints of recurrent UTIs. On further questioning, it sounds to you as if the patient is also experiencing pneumaturia. What is the most likely underlying cause for this patient's symptoms?

A. Prostatitis
B. Diverticulitis
C. UTI caused by anaerobic organisms
D. Bladder cancer
E. Colon ureteral fistula

19. A 45-year-old Hispanic female is referred to your office for abdominal pain. The patient was seen previously in the ED with complaints of epigastric and right upper abdominal pain after meals. The pain originally began 30 to 60 minutes after meals and lasted for 2 to 3 hours. There was also associated nausea without emesis. An abdominal ultrasound demonstrated multiple gallstones without cholecystic wall thickening or surrounding fluid. The

common bile duct was visualized and within normal limits for size. The patient has no other health conditions, takes no medications, and has had no prior surgery. Physical exam reveals a mildly obese female in no apparent distress. Vital signs and the physical exam are unremarkable. Laboratory values are as follows: WBC 7,000, HCT 25%, PLTS 130,000, total bilirubin 1.0 mg/dL, AST 25 U/L, ALT 22 U/L, amylase 22 U/L, lipase 13 U/L. A diagnosis of symptomatic cholelithiasis is made and the patient decides to undergo an elective laparoscopic cholecystectomy the following week. During the dissection, what commonly found structure would you expect within the triangle of Calot?

A. Right hepatic duct
B. Common bile duct
C. Gastroduodenal artery
D. Cystic artery
E. Foramen of Winslow
F. Right gastroepiploic artery
G. Ducts of Lushka
H. Coronary vein

20. You are consulted by the medicine service to see a 73-year-old female with nausea, vomiting, and abdominal distention. The patient states that these symptoms began 2 days ago and she also complains of obstipation. The patient is afebrile, with slight tachycardia, and her abdomen is distended without peritoneal signs. You obtain an abdominal CT (Figure 5-20A). What is the most likely cause of this patient's bowel obstruction?

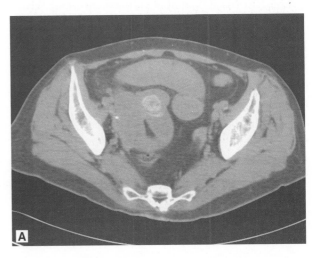

Figure 5-20A • Image Courtesy of the University of Utah School of Medicine, Salt Lake City, Utah.

A. Cancer
B. Adhesions
C. Gallstone ileus
D. Intussusception
E. Ileus

The next two questions (items 21 and 22) correspond to the following vignette.

A critically ill intubated patient on vasopressors with a history of a recent myocardial infarction and a long ICU course begins having fevers. In your workup, you obtain labs with the following results: WBC 19,000, AST 100 U/L, ALT 45 U/L, ALK Phos 345 U/L, total bilirubin 3.0 mg/dL, direct bilirubin 2.8 mg/dL, and lipase 33 U/L. Suspecting gallbladder disease, you obtain an abdominal ultrasound (Figure 5-21A).

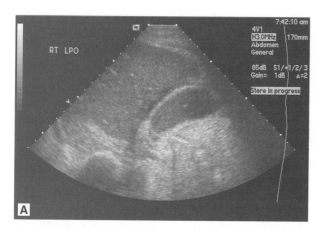

Figure 5-21A • Image Courtesy of the University of Utah School of Medicine, Salt Lake City, Utah.

21. Which of the following is the most likely diagnosis?

    A. Acute calculous cholecystitis
    B. Acute pancreatitis
    C. Acute cholangitis
    D. Acute acalculous cholecystitis
    E. Acute hepatitis

22. What is the most appropriate next step given the patient's condition?

    A. Emergency open cholecystectomy
    B. Elective laparoscopic cholecystectomy
    C. Percutaneous cholecystostomy
    D. Emergency laparoscopic cholecystectomy
    E. No treatment

End of Set

The response options for items 23 to 26 are the same. You will be required to select one answer for each item in the set.

For each clinical scenario, select the most appropriate findings from the pulmonary artery catheter (refer to Table 5-23).

23. An 18-year-old male restrained driver with tachycardia, hypotension, and a rigid abdomen on physical exam.

24. An 80-year-old nursing home resident, febrile, unresponsive, hypotensive, with Gram-negative rods cultured from their urine.

25. A 16-year-old male victim of a motor vehicle crash with hypotension, bradycardia, and the inability to move or feel both lower extremities.

26. A 67-year-old male in the medical ICU, on 15 L of oxygen by facemask, hypotension, and crackles in the bases of both lungs.

End of Set

The next two questions (items 27 and 28) correspond to the following vignette.

■ TABLE 5-23 Pulmonary Artery Catheter Findings

	Cardiac Output	Central Venous Pressure	Pulmonary Wedge Pressure	Systemic Vascular Resistance
A	Decreased	Decreased	Decreased	Increased
B	Increased	Decreased	Decreased	Decreased
C	Decreased	Increased	Increased	Increased
D	Decreased	Decreased	Decreased	Decreased

You are called to evaluate a 41-year-old male in the ER for hemorrhoids and to help arrange follow-up. The patient is otherwise very healthy and takes no medications, but you note that his BP in the ER is 178/86. On follow-up in your clinic, his BP is 192/82 and the following week it is 184/78.

27. The most likely cause of this patient's elevated blood pressure is
    A. Pheochromocytoma
    B. Conn's syndrome
    C. Renal artery stenosis
    D. Essential hypertension
    E. Cushing's syndrome

28. During this patient's follow-up visits, further questioning of the patient reveals that he has complaints of anxiety, occasional palpitations, and tremulousness. These findings suggest which etiology?
    A. Pheochromocytoma
    B. Conn's syndrome
    C. Renal artery stenosis
    D. Essential hypertension
    E. Cushing's syndrome

End of Set

29. A 37-year-old female presents to your office to be evaluated for possible surgical hypertension. Essential hypertension has been excluded by her primary care physician. The patient's BP in your office is 188/92, pulse is 88, and temperature is 37.2°C. A CT scan shows an adrenal mass. You suspect the refractory hypertension is due to Cushing's syndrome. Which of the following would you expect to see?
    A. Peripheral obesity
    B. Hypopigmentation
    C. Muscle weakness in all extremities
    D. Reddish striae
    E. Hyperkalemia
    F. Cachectic face

The next three questions (items 30 to 32) correspond to the following vignette.

A 49-year-old female undergoes a total abdominal colectomy with ileoanal anastomosis for ulcerative colitis. On pathologic examination of the colon, an adenocarcinoma is found in the proximal colon that invades through the muscularis propria to the serosa. The patient is taken back to the operating room for further lymph node dissection, and H&E staining shows evidence of tumor in 1 of 17 lymph nodes.

30. The pathologic stage of the tumor by Duke's staging is
    A. A2
    B. B1
    C. B2
    D. C1
    E. C2

31. What, if any, further therapy is recommended for this patient?
    A. No adjuvant therapy
    B. Radiation only
    C. 5 fluorouracil only
    D. 5 fluorouracil/leucovorin
    E. 5 fluorouracil/leucovorin + radiation

32. Which of the following best describes the issue of survival of this patient with Duke's C2-staged colon cancer?
    A. Survival is directly related to length of symptoms
    B. Right colon lesions have a worse survival
    C. Left colon lesions have a worse survival
    D. Survival is improved if laparoscopic resection is used
    E. A patient with a Duke's C2 lesion has a 20% to 30% 5-year survival rate
    F. Survival is inversely related to the preoperative CEA level

End of Set

33. A 52-year-old female presents to the ED with a 5-day history of increasing left lower quadrant pain, nausea, vomiting, and being febrile. The patient reports two prior episodes of similar pain that were treated successfully with antibiotics but she never followed up as instructed. On your exam, you find the patient is tachycardic and has left lower quadrant pain with diffuse peritoneal signs. A CT scan of the abdomen is performed (Figure 5-33A). What is the next most appropriate therapy?

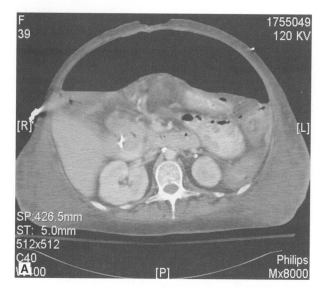

Figure 5-33A • Image Courtesy of the University of Utah School of Medicine, Salt Lake City, Utah.

A. Admit for IV fluids and IV antibiotics
B. Admit for IV fluids, IV antibiotics, and elective resection of the sigmoid colon
C. Percutaneous drainage of the abscess, followed by IV fluids and IV antibiotics
D. Proceed directly to the operating room for resection of the sigmoid colon with diverting colostomy
E. Proceed directly to the operating room for resection of the sigmoid colon with primary anastomosis

34. A 40-year-old female has been referred to you for a recent ER and hospital admission, from which she was given a diagnosis of acute diverticulitis. Treatment at that time consisted of antibiotics, bowel rest, and IV fluids. The patient reports to you that she has also recently been diagnosed with arthritis and takes ibuprofen three times a day. The patient also tells you that the left lower quadrant pain is improved but still present. The WBC today, 2 days after completion of the course of antibiotics she was given in the ER, is 9000. You've scheduled her for abdominal pelvic CT scan. Which of the following choices would be the most appropriate for performing an elective surgery for diverticulitis in this patient?

A. A family history
B. A second episode
C. A continued low-grade leukocytosis
D. Continued left lower quadrant abdominal pain

E. Evidence of an abscess
F. Hematemesis

35. A 19-year-old male presents to clinic with complaints of abdominal pain for the last 3 months. The patient states it is diffuse without any distinguishable inciting events. At times it is accompanied by a low-grade fever and multiple bouts of diarrhea. There are intervals without any of these symptoms. For the last week he states the pain has become more persistent and the frequency of stools has increased. The patient takes ibuprofen for the pain and denies allergies to any medications, and he has never been hospitalized or undergone prior surgery. Vital signs are within normal limits. On physical exam, the patient is found to be thin and in no apparent distress. The abdomen is scaphoid and diffusely tender to palpation, but it is soft without any peritoneal signs. Routine laboratory values obtained are all normal. You suspect this patient has inflammatory bowel disease and schedule a colonoscopy for the following week. Which of the following, if present, is more characteristic of Crohn's disease?

A. Pseudopolyps
B. Mucosal and submucosal involvement only
C. Small bowel strictures
D. Confluent disease
E. Rectal involvement
F. Depletion of goblet cell mucin
G. Granular, flat mucosa

36. A 27-year-old male comes to the ED with complaints of severe right lower quadrant abdominal and testicular pain that began 5 hours ago. The pain is the worst he has ever experienced and it is associated with nausea but not vomiting. The patient is writhing in pain and cannot seem to sit still while you are speaking with him. The patient is afebrile and has a WBC of 10,300, with no left shift. What is the next most appropriate study to obtain?

A. Amylase and lipase
B. Upper GI series
C. HIDA scan
D. Liver function tests
E. Urinalysis

37. While on a general surgery service at the Veterans Administration Hospital you are consulted to see a 75-year-old male. The patient tells you that over the last 2 months he has become more fatigued

and complains of dyspnea on exertion and often feels lightheaded during ambulation. The patient also claims to have lost 30 lbs unintentionally over the last 6 months. The cardiology team did a full workup on the patient and has effectively ruled out his heart as the likely source. During the cardiac workup, he was found to be anemic with a hematocrit of 30%, at which time he underwent a colonoscopy by the GI team. A 4-cm villous polyp was found near the hepatic flexure. Regarding polyps found within the GI system, which type is associated with the greatest likelihood of carcinoma in situ or invasive cancer?

A. Hamartomatous polyps
B. Tubular polyps
C. Tubulovillous polyps
D. Villous polyps
E. Juvenile polyps
F. Inflammatory polyps

38. You are called to see an 80-year-old female in the ED. The patient was transferred by ground from a local nursing home. Presently, she is coherent and reports to you that she began vomiting approximately 10 hours ago and has vomited five times throughout the day. It has been thick and brown in appearance. The patient also is complaining of severe abdominal pain that started last evening and has progressively gotten worse. The patient also tells you that she has not had a bowel movement or had any flatus throughout the day. Medical-surgical history does not include any previous surgery, and 1 month ago she underwent a colonoscopy to evaluate a history of chronic constipation, which was reported as normal. Vital signs are BP 106/68, HR 77, and T 36.6°C. Labs are WBC of 13.3 and HCT of 36.8%. You suspect she may have a large bowel obstruction. What is the most likely cause of a large bowel obstruction in this 80-year-old female?

A. Adhesions
B. Ascending colon mass
C. Sigmoid volvulus
D. Diverticular stricture
E. Intussusception
F. Incarcerated inguinal hernia

39. A 72-year-old female with von Hippel-Lindau disease has been in the hospital for the last 3 days with dehydration from severe gastroenteritis. Over the last 6 months the patient has had a substantial weight loss of 35 lbs. The patient's urinalysis shows gross hematuria and her hematocrit is 27%. What is the likely cause of this patient's symptoms?

A. Renal cell carcinoma
B. Nephrolithiasis
C. UTIs
D. Bladder trauma
E. Colon cancer

The next two questions (items 40 and 41) correspond to the following vignette.

A 20-month-old female is referred to your office by the child's pediatrician for evaluation of a urinary tract infection (UTI). This is the third infection in the last 6 months. The patient has been treated with sulfa each time and the infection has resolved. It recurs typically 6 months later. The child's development has been otherwise normal. Currently, she is getting amoxicillin and her symptoms have resolved. You suspect she may have vesicoureteral reflux, leading to her recurrent infections. You appropriately obtain a voiding cystourethrogram, which confirms your suspicion.

40. In a child with vesicoureteral reflux, which of the following is an indication for surgery?

A. UTI prior to age 1 year
B. Horseshoe kidney
C. BUN:creatinine ratio greater than 15:1
D. Noncompliance with medical management
E. Electrolyte abnormalities

41. Complications that may result from this patient's vesicoureteral reflux include which of the following?

A. Decreased sodium clearance
B. Pyelonephritis
C. Decreased transmitted pressures to the kidneys
D. Increased potassium clearance
E. Increased renin-angiotensin activity

End of Set

The next two questions (items 42 and 43) correspond to the following vignette.

A 42-year-old female presents to your office for a routine physical exam. The patient has not been to a physician for the last 6 years. In that time, she has been very healthy. The patient is 5'6" tall and weighs 50 kg.

42. What is this patient's calculated total body water (TBW)?

A. 15 kg
B. 20 kg
C. 25 kg
D. 30 kg
E. 35 kg

43. The amount of fluid in this patient that is estimated to be intracellular is

A. 66% TBW
B. 33% TBW
C. 25% TBW
D. 75% TBW
E. 15% TBW

End of Set

The next three questions (items 44 to 46) correspond to the following vignette.

A diabetic male patient on your surgical service recently underwent a Billroth II for peptic ulcer disease. The patient recently began eating, but is not being adequately covered by his insulin doses. The patient's recent blood glucoses have been consistently high. This morning, you note the sodium to be 134 mmol/L in addition to the glucose being 500 mg/dL.

44. What is the corrected sodium level?

A. 136
B. 138
C. 140
D. 142
E. 144

45. The remainder of this patient's chemistry panel shows Na 134 mmol/L, K 4.4 mmol/L, Cl 102 mmol/L, CO_2 23 mmol/L, BUN 28 mg/dL, and creatinine 1.3 mg/dL. The calculated plasma osmolality is

A. 278 mmol/kg
B. 306 mmol/kg
C. 334 mmol/kg
D. 368 mmol/kg
E. 404 mmol/kg

46. An osmolar gap is present if the measured osmolality and calculated osmolality differ by how much?

A. 8 mOsm/kg
B. 10 mOsm/kg
C. 12 mOsm/kg
D. 15 mOsm/kg
E. 18 mOsm/kg

End of Set

47. A 32-year-old female is admitted for alcoholic pancreatitis. The patient's initial fluid resuscitation requires a total of 9 L of lactated Ringer's. Morning labs show a Na 129 mmol/L, K 3.8 mmol/L, Cl 99 mmol/L, BUN 12 mg/dL, creatinine 0.7 mg/dL, and glucose of 131 mg/dL. Which of the following is the cause of the patient's hyponatremia?

A. Increased total body sodium
B. Decreased total body sodium
C. Increased total body water
D. Decreased total body water
E. Increased aldosterone production

The next three questions (items 48 to 50) correspond to the following vignette.

Renin is released from the juxtaglomerular cells of afferent arterioles in response to changes in arterial pressure, increases in β-adrenergic activity, increases in cellular cAMP, and changes in sodium delivery to the macula densa.

48. Renin is an enzyme that catalyzes the conversion of angiotensinogen to angiotensin I in which location in the body?

A. Liver
B. Lungs
C. Plasma
D. Kidneys
E. Bone marrow

49. Angiotensin I is then converted to angiotensin II by angiotensin converting enzymes. The actions of angiotensin II include which of the following?

A. Decreases vascular tone
B. Stimulates catecholamine release from the adrenal medulla
C. Increases renal plasma flow, which increases sodium reabsorption
D. Suppresses release of aldosterone from the adrenal cortex
E. Decreases systemic blood pressure

50. Aldosterone has multiple effects within the body. Which of the following is true regarding the actions of aldosterone?

A. Decreases renal tubular reabsorption of sodium
B. Acts directly on the distal collecting tubules
C. Decreases the Na/K ATPase activity
D. Is regulated by renin from the pituitary gland
E. Increases potassium reabsorption

End of Set

Answers and Explanations

1. C	18. B	35. C
2. E	19. D	36. E
3. D	20. C	37. D
4. C	21. D	38. C
5. A	22. C	39. A
6. D	23. A	40. D
7. B	24. B	41. B
8. B	25. D	42. C
9. C	26. C	43. A
10. D	27. D	44. C
11. C	28. A	45. B
12. B	29. D	46. D
13. D	30. E	47. C
14. A	31. D	48. C
15. B	32. E	49. B
16. A	33. D	50. B
17. A	34. B	

1. C. Approximately one in eight women will develop breast cancer. Therefore, the workup of a breast mass is common and extremely important. Mammograms are used as a screening tool to view possible breast pathology that is not palpable. The mammogram shows (note the arrow on Figure 5-1B) an obvious dense, spiculated mass diagnostic of breast cancer. Although FNA would also be considered, obtaining tissue via a biopsy is the most appropriate of the choices given.

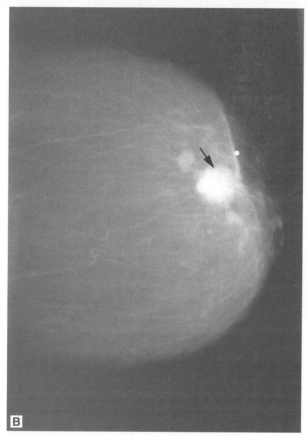

Figure 5-1B • Image Courtesy of the University of Utah School of Medicine, Salt Lake City, Utah.

A, D. A CT scan and chest x-ray will be helpful in determining metastatic disease, but they are not the initial step required in workup.

B. Only 5% to 10% of breast cancer is inherited and, because of that, the *BRCA1* gene would be most appropriate after the diagnosis is made if a genetic predisposition is suspected.

E. Any woman with a complaint of a new breast mass should have a thorough physical exam and a mammogram, and undergo a biopsy of the suspected mass in a timely manner. One of the most common causes of malpractice in the United States is failure to diagnose breast cancer.

2. E. This patient was diagnosed with invasive ductal carcinoma, which is responsible for 90% of breast cancers. Staging of the cancer is important in ascertaining the prognosis as well as determining the best method of treatment. The pathologic status of the lymph nodes is important in staging because it indicates the probability of systemic disease that may require chemotherapy.

A, B, C, D. Although tumor size, histologic grade, and receptor status contribute to the overall prognosis of this disease, lymph node involvement is the most important factor in staging.

3. D. Breast conservation therapy is important in the treatment of breast cancer. It involves lumpectomy and radiation therapy to the breast to treat local disease, as well as an axillary node dissection for staging purposes. If lymph nodes are found to be involved, the patient may be placed on a chemotherapy protocol for systemic treatment. A modified radical mastectomy includes removal of the breast, axillary nodes, and nipple areolar complex. Selective sampling of lymph nodes, termed sentinel lymph node biopsy, to determine lymph node staging in breast cancer is being studied in large clinical trials. The National Surgical Adjuvant Bowel and Breast Project (NSABP) B-32 trial (A Randomized, Phase III Clinical Trial to Compare Sentinel Node Resection to Conventional Axillary Dissection in Clinically Node-Negative Breast Cancer Patients) as well as the American College of Surgeons Oncology Group (ACOSOG) Z0010 trial (A Prognostic Study of Sentinel Node and Bone Marrow Micrometastases in Women with Clinical T1 or T2 N0 M0 Breast Cancer) have recently completed enrollment, and the data analyses will provide practitioners with guidelines for use of this new method in the surgical treatment of breast cancer.

A. Radiation therapy with full-beam external therapy is usually not needed after this procedure.

B. A supraclavicular lymph node dissection is not necessary in breast conservation therapy.

C. Intrathecal chemotherapy is reserved for metastatic disease that may involve the spinal cord.

E. Although lumpectomy with negative margins may remove the tumor, an axillary lymph node dissection is required for staging.

4. C. Factors that place an individual at higher risk of developing breast cancer include the following:

- A previous personal history of breast cancer.
- Family history of breast cancer, including a first-degree relative (mother or sister, not an aunt) with a malignancy under the age of 40 years, history of bilateral breast cancer, or history of ovarian cancer.
- *BRCA1* positivity: The *BRCA1* gene is associated with 5% of all breast cancers. This gene is transmitted in an autosomal-dominant pattern and is linked to chromosome 17. Approximately 1 in 200 women is a carrier. *BRCA1* is also linked to ovarian cancer. Carriers have an 85% lifetime risk of developing cancer.
- History of previous breast biopsy, regardless of pathology.
- Nulliparity.
- Early menarche, late menopause.
- Ductal carcinoma in situ (DCIS).

A. Nulliparity, not multiparity, increases the risk of breast cancer.

B. A strong family history of colon cancer is more concerning for an increased risk of colon cancer.

D. Although any family history increases a woman's risk of breast cancer, a clinically important risk is associated with the presence of breast cancer in a first-degree relative.

E. Only weak or nonexistent associations have been made in human studies between a high-fat diet and breast cancer.

5. A. Nipple discharge in females is common. It is considered pathologic when it is unilateral and spontaneous. The most common cause of bloody nipple discharge in a young woman is an intraductal papilloma. The papillomas are located in the major ducts under the areola and are usually only 3 to 4 mm in size. Therefore, they are rarely palpable. They can, however, be visualized by ultrasound. Galactograms are useful but painful for the patient, and not always obtained. Surgical treatment involves excision of the draining duct containing the papilloma. The ultrasound shown in Figure 5-5C shows the papilloma within a dilated duct with an arrow in the galactogram. Figure 5-5D shows a corresponding filling defect consistent with an intraductal papilloma.

C, E. Fibroadenomas and Paget's disease do not usually cause bloody nipple discharge.

B, D. Although nipple discharge is associated with a lactocele and duct ectasia, the most common cause is an intraductal papilloma.

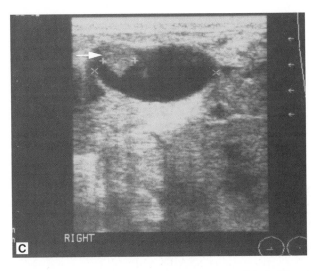

Figure 5-5C • Images Courtesy of the University of Utah School of Medicine, Salt Lake City, Utah.

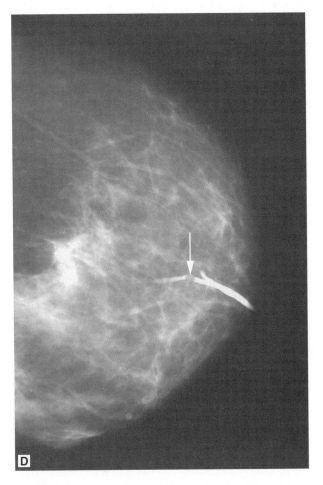

Figure 5-5D • Images Courtesy of the University of Utah School of Medicine, Salt Lake City, Utah.

6. **D.** Mastitis is a superficial infection of the breast. It usually occurs in a woman who is breastfeeding, with the most likely pathogen being *Staphylococcus aureus*. This should be differentiated from inflammatory breast cancer that can have a similar appearance. The main difference between the two is pain, since mastitis is very painful and inflammatory breast cancer may not be particularly painful. A negative ultrasound will help rule out a breast abscess that would require surgical drainage.

A, B, C. Treatment for mastitis does not involve surgery or discontinuation of breastfeeding from the affected side. The patient should be prescribed antibiotics and use warm compresses and NSAIDs, judiciously, for analgesia.

E. If no action is taken toward resolving this problem, it could develop into a breast abscess requiring surgical debridement.

7. **B.** The thoracodorsal and long thoracic nerves are two critical motor nerves. The thoracodorsal nerve provides motor function to the latissimus dorsi, and damage to this nerve results in weakness with shoulder abduction. The long thoracic nerve provides motor function to the serratus anterior, and damage causes a winged scapula. The subscapular nerve provides innervation to the subscapularis muscle.

A. Injury to the thoracodorsal nerve would result in weakness on adduction and internal rotation of the shoulder.

C. If the intercostobrachial nerve is damaged, decreased sensation to the axilla and medial brachium occurs.

D. The subscapular nerves innervate the subscapular muscle, which also assists in adduction of the shoulder.

E. Decreased ability to abduct the shoulder as well as numbness on the lateral shoulder would occur, should the axillary nerve sustain damage.

F. The phrenic nerve arises from the third, fourth, and fifth cervical nerve roots. It supplies the muscle of the diaphragm, and damage to this could result in respiratory compromise. It does not have anything to do with the motor function of the scapula.

8. **B.** Multiple nerves are at risk when an axillary dissection is performed, including the intercostobrachial nerve, thoracodorsal nerve, and long thoracic nerve. The intercostobrachial nerve accounts for the sensation on the medial brachium. There is no motor component of this nerve.

A. The medial pectoral nerve contributes motor innervation to the pectoral muscles.

C. The thoracodorsal nerve innervates the latissimus dorsi muscle.

D. The axillary nerve innervates the deltoid and teres major muscle.

E. The long thoracic nerve innervates the serratus anterior muscle.

F. The radial nerve is one of the terminal branches of the brachial plexus. The radial nerve and its branches supply all extensors in the arm. The injury that you typically see with damage to this nerve is the "Saturday night" or crutch palsy, affecting extensor muscles in the arm, forearm, and wrist (wrist drop). Damage to this nerve during an axillary dissection is unlikely.

9. **C.** This patient demonstrates a history of biliary colic, or symptomatic gallstones. Gallstones develop in approximately 10% of the U.S. population. Risk factors are commonly remembered by the politically incorrect mnemonic "fat, forty, female, and fertile." Other factors include oral contraceptives, Native American and Hispanic heritage, and chronic hemolysis. Seventy-five percent of stones are cholesterol. Biliary colic occurs when gallbladder contractions cause intermittent obstruction by the stone at the gallbladder-cystic duct junction. This is characterized clinically by right upper quadrant pain 30 to 60 minutes after a meal. Nausea and vomiting usually accompany this pain, and symptoms resolve within hours. In contrast, acute cholecystitis is caused by impaction of a gallstone in the cystic duct with persistent right upper quadrant pain, fever, and leukocytosis. If biliary colic is suspected, an abdominal ultrasound should be obtained. The arrow in Figure 5-9 demonstrates a gallbladder containing a rather large stone with posterior shadowing.

A. Serum cholesterol is worth checking, but it is not related to this problem.

B. Compared to an ultrasound, a CT scan exposes the patient to radiation and is more expensive, and therefore it is not an initial screening test.

D. An ERCP will assist in diagnosing conditions involving the common bile duct and pancreatic duct, but it is not used for initial evaluation of biliary colic.

E. No further workup is an inappropriate choice.

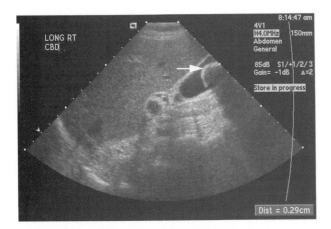

Figure 5-9 • Image Courtesy of the University of Utah School of Medicine, Salt Lake City, Utah.

10. **D.** Unless otherwise medically contraindicated, the treatment of biliary colic is laparoscopic cholecystectomy because of the increased risk of complications, mainly acute cholecystitis, pancreatitis, and choledocholithiasis.

   A, B. Waiting, exercise, and a low cholesterol diet, though they will not resolve this problem, might be the choice of some patients for whom very careful follow-up can be absolutely guaranteed.

   C. Dissolution therapy with chenodeoxycholic acid is a prolonged and marginally effective therapy with a high rate of recurrence of biliary colic, as well as multiple side effects from the treatment itself.

   E. An ERCP is obtained for conditions of the common bile duct and does not treat the source of the gallstones.

11. **C.** Cyclophosphamide (Cytoxan) is an alkylating agent that leads to DNA strand breakage. The metabolite of this drug, acrolein, leads to hemorrhagic cystitis. This can be prevented by concomitantly treating the patient with Mesna.

12. **B.** Vinblastine is a vinca alkaloid that prevents polymerization of microtubules, thus inhibiting mitosis. The primary side effect is myelosuppression.

13. **D.** Bleomycin creates oxygen free radicals that cause damage to the DNA chain. Ten percent of patients taking this drug suffer from a dose-related pulmonary fibrosis.

14. **A.** Surgical oncology patients are commonly on chemotherapeutic drugs. Therefore, it is important to know the mechanism and important side effects associated with each drug. Tamoxifen is a nonsteroidal antiestrogen used for the treatment of breast cancer, and it causes menopausal-type symptoms.

15. **B.** Acute cholangitis is caused by bacterial infection of the biliary tree due to obstruction, most commonly by choledocholithiasis. Patients are typically ill and present with fever and/or chills, right upper quadrant pain, and jaundice, also known as Charcot's triad. Patients who are septic from cholangitis demonstrate Charcot's triad as well as altered mental status and shock, known as Reynolds' pentad. Associated lab values are leukocytosis, increased total and direct bilirubin, and increased alkaline phosphatase. While the other answers may be included on the differential, choledocholithiasis is the most likely answer for this clinical setting.

   A. Pancreatic cancer can cause jaundice and weight loss, but rarely biliary sepsis.

   C. Duodenal ulcers can cause pain, bleeding, obstruction, or peritonitis from perforation, none of which is suggested here.

   D. Viral gastritis would not result in jaundice and the laboratory picture presented here.

   E. Pneumonia can cause right upper quadrant referred pain, but it is not consistent with the rest of the findings presented.

16. **A.** The most common bacteria involved are Gram-negative organisms (*Escherichia coli, Klebsiella, pseudomonas Enterobacter, Proteus,* and *Serratia*), with *E. coli* being the most common.

   B, C, D, E. These organisms may also cause cholangitis, but *E. coli* is the most commonly found inciting agent.

17. **A.** The treatment of choice is IV hydration, IV antibiotics, and common duct decompression with ERCP. Figure 5-17 is an ERCP for cholangitis. Notice the arrows pointing to the enlarged common bile duct, containing a stone in the distal portion.

   B. A Whipple procedure would be more appropriate in obstruction caused by cancer of the pancreatic head.

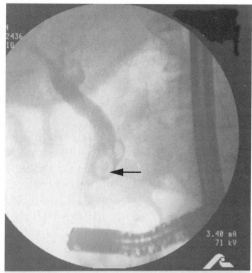

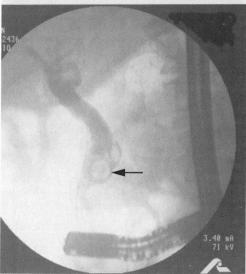

Figure 5-17 • Image Courtesy of the University of Utah School of Medicine, Salt Lake City, Utah.

C. A percutaneous cholecystostomy may decompress the common bile duct via the gallbladder, however, it will not resolve the cause of the distal common duct obstruction.

D. As with any contained infection, drainage is the most important action, not antibiotics alone.

E. Oral bile salts are inappropriate because of the need for immediate treatment of biliary sepsis. Using this type of treatment is inefficient and likely poorly tolerated as an oral medication.

18. B. Any communication between the bladder and the bowel will lead to pneumaturia. This phenomenon is by far most commonly seen as a complication of diverticulitis. The inflammatory process in the left lower quadrant allows for the formation of a fistula between the bladder and the colon.

A, C, D. Prostatitis, UTIs, and bladder cancer would not routinely lead to pneumaturia, but to hematuria.

E. Although a coloureteral fistula could theoretically create the same problem, this would be exceedingly rare.

19. D. The triangle of Calot is an important landmark in biliary surgery. The boundaries include the liver superiorly, the cystic duct laterally, and the common hepatic duct medially. Within this triangle are found Calot's node, the cystic artery, and the right hepatic artery. The proper identification and dissection of these structures is key to achieving an uncomplicated laparoscopic cholecystectomy.

A. The right hepatic duct is found proximal to the common hepatic duct.

B. The common bile duct is found distal to the cystic duct within the hepatoduodenal ligament.

C. The gastroduodenal artery is a branch of the common hepatic artery and is usually found posterior to the first portion of the duodenum.

E. The foramen of Winslow is the opening that connects the lesser and greater sacs of the abdominal cavity. It is found at the lateral border of the hepatoduodenal ligament.

F. The right gastroepiploic artery is usually a branch off of the proper hepatic artery. It supplies blood to the greater curvature of the stomach.

G. The ducts of Lushka describe a variant of the right hepatic ducts that drain directly into the gallbladder. These are divided during the removal of the gallbladder from the liver bed and can result in a postoperative biloma if they are not properly observed and ligated.

H. The vein that drains the lesser curvature of the stomach is the coronary vein.

20. C. Gallstone ileus is an uncommon cause of small bowel obstruction (SBO). It occurs when inflammation leads to a cholecystenteric (gallbladder-to-bowel) fistula releasing a large (greater than 2.5 cm) gallstone into the small intestine. Unable to pass through the ileocecal valve, the stone causes an obstruction. It is most commonly seen in women over 70 years of age and presents with signs and

symptoms of an SBO. A plain abdominal film may demonstrate small bowel distention with air fluid levels, pneumobilia (air in the biliary tree), and a radioopaque stone in the right lower quadrant. Surgical management includes an enterotomy with removal of the stone, cholecystectomy, and fistula repair.

A, B, D. Although tumors, adhesions from previous surgeries, and intussusception can lead to symptoms of an SBO, a gallstone is clearly seen on the CT scan obstructing the ileocecal valve. The CT shown in Figure 5-20B demonstrates a large stone (note arrow) within the dilated small bowel.

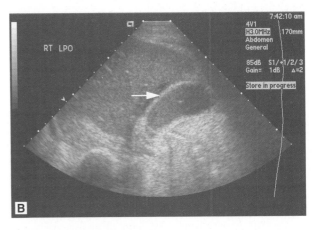

Figure 5-21B • Image Courtesy of the University of Utah School of Medicine, Salt Lake City, Utah.

A. Acute calculous cholecystitis is incorrect because no stones are seen in the ultrasound.
B. Acute pancreatitis is unlikely with a low normal lipase.
C. Acute cholangitis is possible, but not consistent with the ultrasound reading.
E. Acute hepatitis is unlikely, especially with the ultrasound reading.

22. C. The treatment of choice is a cholecystectomy; however, in an unstable patient such as this, a cholecystostomy tube may be placed to decompress the gallbladder until the patient is stable enough to undergo surgery.

A, B, D. Currently, this patient is unstable and should be treated with decompression, followed by an elective cholecystectomy when stable. Cholecystectomy, either laparoscopic or open, may eventually be necessary, depending on the course of the condition after decompression. Multiple other factors will determine whether to proceed with an open or laparoscopic surgery over time.
E. No treatment may lead to a gangrenous gallbladder requiring an emergent operation in a very poor surgical candidate.

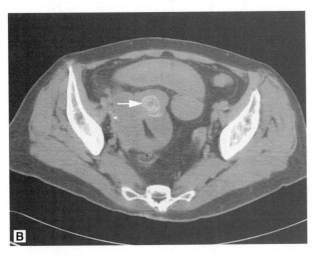

Figure 5-20B • Image Courtesy of the University of Utah School of Medicine, Salt Lake City, Utah.

E. Ileus is often confused with true SBO, but it is not consistent with the clinical setting presented or the CT findings.

21. D. Acute acalculous cholecystitis is acute cholecystitis without evidence of gallstones. It is more commonly seen in critically ill patients who have had prolonged periods of fasting or parenteral nutrition. It can also be seen in patients who have had multiple transfusions and in trauma patients. Fever, leukocytosis, and right upper quadrant pain with increased total and direct bilirubin are usually noted. An abdominal ultrasound (Figure 5-21B) is shown here with an arrow that points to the thickened gallbladder wall with surrounding fluid. No stones are identified. Acute acalculous cholecystitis is thought to be due to biliary sludge secondary to inactivity of the biliary tree.

23. A. Shock is commonly seen in the surgical patient. Four types of shock exist: hypovolemic, cardiogenic, neurogenic, and distributive. With the invention of the Swan-Ganz catheter, the cardiac parameters of each specific type of shock can be more readily identified. The most common type of shock is hypovolemic shock resulting from decreased intravascular volume from hemorrhage, dehydration,

or third spacing of fluids. Hemodynamically, it is characterized by a decrease in cardiac output (CO) due to decreased filling pressures, central venous pressure (CVP), and pulmonary capillary wedge pressure (PCWP), with a compensatory increase in systemic vascular resistance (SVR).

24. B. Distributive shock is seen in sepsis or anaphylaxis. It is caused by an inflammatory response with massive cytokine release. The peripheral vessels are subsequently dilated due to histamine and prostaglandins, resulting in decreased CVP, PCWP, and SVR, with a compensatory increase in CO. This is typically seen in early sepsis. In late sepsis, the compensatory mechanism of the heart fails, resulting in a decrease in CO along with an increase in SVR and PCWP.

25. D. Neurogenic shock is seen in patients with spinal cord injuries, not head injuries. It is caused by a decrease in sympathetic output and is accompanied by decreased CO (bradycardia), as well as decreased CVP, PCWP, and SVR.

26. C. Cardiogenic shock is often seen in patients with acute myocardial infarctions in respiratory distress and is characterized by a decrease in CO, with subsequent increase in PCWP leading to respiratory embarrassment. On physical exam, an increase in the CVP is demonstrated by jugular venous distention. In an attempt to maintain blood pressure, the SVR increases.

27. D. Although there are many causes of surgical hypertension, the most common cause of hypertension remains essential hypertension (more than 90%). This gentleman should be managed medically, and if his hypertension is refractory to medical therapy, other possible causes should be considered.

   A. Hypertension in pheochromocytoma is caused by an increased production of epinephrine and norepinephrine, which could potentially be treated with surgery.
   B. Hypertension in Conn's syndrome is caused by increased production of aldosterone, which could potentially be treated with surgery.
   C. Hypertension in renal artery stenosis is caused by an increase in the renin-angiotensin system, which could potentially be treated with surgery.
   E. Hypertension in Cushing's syndrome is caused by increased production of corticosteroids, which could potentially be treated with surgery.

28. A. Symptoms of a pheochromocytoma are caused by an elevated level of circulating catecholamines. Symptoms include anxiety, palpitations, tremulousness, and headache. The diagnosis is made by measuring 24-hour urine catecholamine and catecholamine metabolite levels (epinephrine, norepinephrine, metanephrine, and vanillylmandelic acid). Pheochromocytomas are associated with MEN IIA and IIB syndrome.

   B. Conn's syndrome is hypertension secondary to hyperaldosteronism from an adrenal tumor or adrenal hyperplasia. Serum potassium is a good screening test for this syndrome. A marked hypokalemia will be seen if Conn's syndrome is present.
   C. Renal artery stenosis causes hypertension through activation of the renin-angiotensin system secondary to decreased perfusion of the affected kidney. Patients typically have an elevated renal vein renin level. A renal vein renin ratio of greater than or equal to 1.5 confirms the diagnosis of a hemodynamically significant stenosis.
   D. While there are many causes of surgical hypertension, the most common cause of hypertension remains essential hypertension (more than 90%). It is not, however, associated with anxiety and tremulousness.
   E. Cushing's syndrome is likewise associated with refractory hypertension due to elevated cortisol levels. The diagnosis is confirmed by elevated cortisol levels, which cannot be suppressed with low-dose steroids (dexamethasone suppression test).

29. D. Cushing's syndrome is associated with refractory hypertension due to elevated cortisol levels. Other clinical findings include central obesity, hyperpigmentation, proximal muscle weakness, hypokalemia (not hyperkalemia), reddish abdominal striae, plethora, moon facies, and hirsutism. The diagnosis is confirmed by elevated cortisol levels, which cannot be suppressed by low-dose steroids (dexamethasone suppression test).

   A. Cushing's syndrome is associated with central obesity, not peripheral obesity.
   B. Hyperpigmentation, not hypopigmentation, is frequently seen with Cushing's syndrome.
   C. Proximal muscle weakness is commonly seen rather than weakness in all extremities.
   E. Hypokalemia, not hyperkalemia, is a common finding as potassium is wasted with increased resorption of sodium in Cushing's syndrome.

F. Moon facies, not cachexia, is a common finding with Cushing's syndrome.

30. E. This patient has a Duke's C2 tumor, progressing through the muscularis propria (designated as "II"), and the presence of a positive node (making the tumor a "C"). Table 5-30A is used for determining Duke's staging for colon cancer. Table 5-30B is the TNM staging for colon cancer, which is now the accepted staging system.

A, B, C, D. See explanation for E.

■ TABLE 5-30A Duke's Staging (Astler-Coller Modification)	
A	Limited to the mucosa (above the lymphatic channels)
B1	Into the muscularis propria
B2	Through the muscularis propria
C1	Into the muscularis propria with (+) nodes
C2	Through the muscularis propria with (+) nodes
D	Metastases or unresectable

31. D. This patient has a Duke's C2 tumor (T3N1M0), as determined in the previous question, therefore 5 fluorouracil and leucovorin are the appropriate treatment choice because of improved survival.

A. To give no adjuvant therapy is an incorrect choice, as adjuvant therapy has been shown to improve survival in advanced colon cancer.

B. Radiation therapy has no routine role in the management of colon cancer, but radiation therapy has been shown to decrease local recurrence rates for rectal cancer.

C. Patients with Duke's C tumors should receive 5 fluorouracil and leucovorin or levamisole. The efficacy of combined therapy is greater than that of 5 fluorouracil alone.

E. As in the explanation for B, radiation therapy has no role in the management of colon cancer.

32. E. The most important variable for prognosis and survival in colon cancer is the stage of the disease, as determined by pathologic status of the lymph nodes. The estimated 5-year survival based on Duke's staging is as follows: Stage A is greater than 90%, Stage B1 is 70% to 85%, Stage B2 is 55% to 65%, Stage C1 is 45% to 55%, Stage C2 is 20% to 30%, and Stage D is less than 1%.

■ TABLE 5-30B TNM Staging for Colon Cancer	
Primary tumor (T)	TX - Primary tumor cannot be assessed
	T0 - No evidence of primary tumor
	Tis - Carcinoma in situ: intraepithelial or invasion of lamina propria
	T1 - Tumor invades submucosa
	T2 - Tumor invades muscularis propria
	T3 - Tumor invades through the muscularis propria into the subserosa, or into nonperitonealized pericolic or perirectal tissues
	T4 - Tumor directly invades other organs or structures, and/or perforates visceral peritoneum
Regional lymph nodes (N)	NX - Regional lymph nodes cannot be assessed
	N0 - No regional lymph node metastasis
	N1 - Metastasis in 1 to 3 regional lymph nodes
	N2 - Metastasis in 4 or more regional lymph nodes
Distant metastasis (M)	MX - Distant metastasis cannot be assessed
	M0 - No distant metastasis
	M1 - Distant metastasis

A. The duration of symptoms has nothing to do with survival from colon cancer. The best indicator of survival is the pathologic status of the lymph nodes, or staging. Long-term survival for node-positive patients is half of that of node-negative patients.

B. Right colon lesions may be detected later in their course because of location, and as such may have a worse survival rate, but taken alone this does not best describe the survival of a Duke's C2 tumor.

C. The statement that left colon lesions have a worse survival rate is incorrect; the staging, not the location, is the most important factor.

D. To state that survival is improved with laparoscopic resection is completely false.

F. The CEA level is the most familiar marker for cancer of the large bowel. An elevated serum CEA is not specifically associated with colorectal cancer, because elevated levels are found in conjunction with a variety of benign diseases. Less than half of patients with localized disease are CEA positive, which makes CEA an inaccurate screening tool. Following the CEA level is most useful in detecting recurrence after a curative surgical resection. If the preoperative elevated CEA returns to normal after surgery and then rises over the follow-up, the likelihood of recurrence is high.

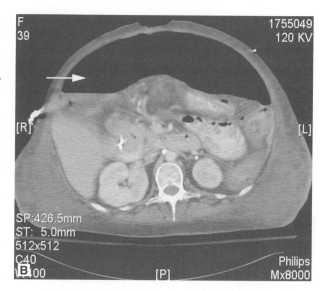

Figure 5-33B • Image Courtesy of the University of Utah School of Medicine, Salt Lake City, Utah.

to undergo an appropriate bowel prep. This usually occurs after medical management of a perforated diverticulum with antibiotics and placement of a percutaneous drain if an abscess exists. A primary anastomosis should not be performed in the face of gross contamination because of the high likelihood of an anastomotic leak.

33. D. The patient has a perforated diverticulum, which is now a surgical emergency because of the evidence of free air on her CT scan (note the arrow in Figure 5-33B). A two-stage operation must be performed, consisting of resection of the diseased colon with creation of a Hartman's pouch and end colostomy, followed by a colostomy takedown at a later time.

A. Admitting the patient for IV fluids and antibiotics is partially correct in that this patient needs IV antibiotics and IV fluids; but with free air in the abdomen, the patient also needs emergent exploration for peritonitis.

B. With free air in the abdomen, the patient needs emergent surgical exploration, not an elective resection.

C. If this was a contained perforation into an abscess, IV antibiotics and percutaneous drainage would be an option. Free air in the abdomen necessitates an emergent surgical exploration.

E. A primary anastomosis is performed only in a controlled operation in which there has been time

34. B. Patients diagnosed with diverticulitis at a young age are likely to have subsequent attacks and suffer complications from them. It would be considered appropriate to electively operate on a young person with a second episode of diverticulitis. Other relative indications for elective surgery include the inability to exclude colon carcinoma endoscopically, and two or more attacks of diverticulitis due to an increased risk of complications.

A. A family history would not be an indication for an elective surgery.

C. A continued low-grade leukocytosis should be evaluated since this could be the failure of nonoperative therapy and require urgent surgery, or it could be unrelated to the diverticulitis.

D. Continued pain should be evaluated further, since it may also be as a result of failure of nonoperative therapy requiring urgent rather than elective surgery.

E. An abscess is an absolute indication for urgent surgery.

F. Hematemesis is not related to diverticulitis and may indicate an upper GI process, which should be evaluated and treated.

35. C. Crohn's disease is a form of inflammatory bowel disease that is associated with transmural inflammation in a segmental fashion along any part of the GI tract. Due to the transmural inflammation associated with Crohn's disease, the development of small bowel strictures leading to obstructive symptoms is common. Figure 5-35 is a small bowel contrast study with an obvious stricture (note arrow) due to Crohn's disease.

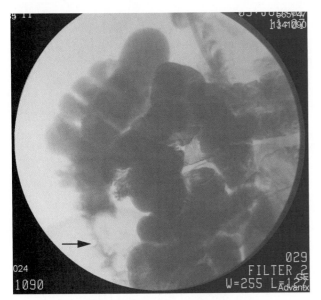

Figure 5-35 • Image Courtesy of the University of Utah School of Medicine, Salt Lake City, Utah.

A, B, D, E, F, G. Pseudopolyps, mucosal and submucosal involvement, confluent disease, rectal involvement, depletion of goblet cell mucin, and granular flat mucosa are all seen in inflammatory bowel disease and are all characteristics of ulcerative colitis. Complications seen with Crohn's disease include bowel obstruction, abscess formation, fistula formation, anorectal lesions, and an increased risk of carcinoma, but less than that of ulcerative colitis.

36. E. Although this patient presents with a story that is concerning for appendicitis, he does not exhibit the classic peritoneal signs. A patient with peritonitis is unlikely to "writhe in pain," as any movement exacerbates the peritoneal irritation. A patient with a kidney stone classically has difficulty getting comfortable, and frequently will be found twisting and turning, as in agony, in bed. Management of a kidney stone is typically nonoperative, and obtaining a urinalysis is routine for all patients who present with right lower quadrant pain.

A. An amylase and lipase would be helpful only if you suspected pancreatitis, which typically presents as midepigastric pain radiating to the back.

B. An upper GI would not be helpful in this scenario, since the pain is clearly located distally from the upper GI tract.

C, D. LFTs and a HIDA scan are helpful in diagnosing hepatobiliary causes of abdominal pain, which usually present as pain in the right upper quadrant.

37. D. Adenomatous polyps are divided into tubular, villous, and tubulovillous types. Villous polyps account for 10% of all polyps, with a 25% incidence of carcinoma. The risk of carcinoma increases for all subtypes with increasing polyp size.

A. Hamartomas are found in adults, and have no malignant potential. They are associated with Peutz-Jeghers syndrome.

B. Tubular polyps are the most common (65%) and have the lowest incidence of malignancy (10%).

C. Tubulovillous polyps account for 20% of polyps and 20% harbor malignancy.

E. Juvenile polyps have no malignant potential and are most commonly hamartomas.

F. Inflammatory polyps are often seen in inflammatory bowel disease.

38. C. This elderly, chronically constipated woman is the classic presentation of a patient with a sigmoid volvulus, and the contrast study shown demonstrates a classically described "bird's beak" sign at the retrosigmoid junction (note the arrow in Figure 5-38). Large bowel obstructions account for only 15% of intestinal obstructions. They are most commonly caused by colorectal cancer (65%) or diverticulitis (20%), neither of which was noted on previous colonoscopy. Volvulus (10%) and miscellaneous causes (10%) make up the remainder of causes for colonic obstruction. Complete large bowel obstruction is considered a surgical emergency, as it is a closed loop obstruction with a functional ileocecal valve with the risk for bowel ischemia and necrosis.

A. Adhesions are by far the most common cause of a small bowel obstruction in someone with previous abdominal surgery. They are significantly less likely to be the cause of a colonic obstruction.

B. As in the explanation for C, colorectal cancer is the most common cause of a colonic obstruction, and since the colonoscopy 1 month prior was normal, an obstructing mass would be extremely unlikely.

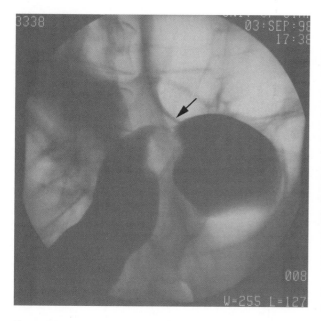

Figure 5-38 • Image Courtesy of the University of Utah School of Medicine, Salt Lake City, Utah.

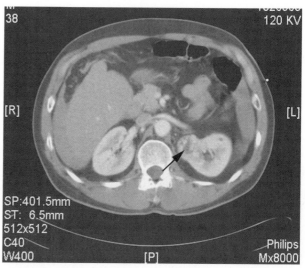

Figure 5-39 • Image Courtesy of the University of Utah School of Medicine, Salt Lake City, Utah.

D. A diverticular stricture is a complication of diverticulitis and likewise would have been seen at the time of colonoscopy.

E. Intussusception is a common cause of colonic obstruction but is less frequently seen than volvulus.

F. An incarcerated inguinal hernia is a common cause of a small bowel obstruction. It is very unlikely this would cause a large bowel obstruction.

39. A. In a patient with hematuria, weight loss, and anemia, one must be very concerned about renal cell carcinoma. The abdominal CT in Figure 5-39 shows a left renal cell cancer (note the arrow). Ninety percent of solid renal tumors are renal cell carcinomas. Other presenting symptoms include pain, presence of a flank mass, and hypertension. Renal cell carcinoma is found in conjunction with von Hippel-Lindau disease linked to chromosome 3.

B, C, D. Although nephrolithiasis, UTIs, and bladder trauma can cause hematuria, they would not account for the substantial weight loss and significant anemia.

E. Colon cancer is usually not associated with hematuria unless a fistula has developed from an advanced tumor.

40. D. Vesicoureteral reflux denotes retrograde passage of urine from the bladder into the ureter. Indications for surgery include recurrent UTIs, progressive renal injury, noncompliance with medical therapy, and severe reflux.

A. UTIs alone are not an indication for surgery, but progressive scarring or pyelonephritis despite medical therapy is an indication.

B. Horseshoe kidneys are not an indication for surgery, although they present a higher risk of developing renal stones and UTIs.

C. A BUN: creatinine ratio of greater than 15:1 is diagnostic of dehydration and not an indication for surgery.

E. Electrolyte abnormalities are not an indication for surgery.

41. B. Vesicoureteral reflux is most commonly seen in females, and common complications include recurrent UTIs and pyelonephritis.

A, D, E. The renin-angiotensin activity and electrolyte clearance are not affected by vesicoureteral reflux.

C. These complications may lead to renal failure due to increased transmitted pressures to the kidney.

42. C. TBW is relatively constant for any given person and depends on the amount of fat present within the body. Fat contains little water. Estimated TBW is 60% of the body weight (BW) in men and 50% of BW in women. Therefore, in our 50-kg female, the TBW is 25 kg (50% × 50 kg).

A, B, D, E. These calculations are incorrect. See explanation for C.

43. **A.** TBW is made up of intracellular fluid (ICF) and extracellular fluid (ECF). ICF equals 66% (2/3) the TBW or 40% of the BW. ECF consists of 33% (1/3) of the TBW or 20% of the BW. ECF includes fluid in intravascular and interstitial spaces. Intravascular space contains approximately 25% of ECF and interstitial space contains 75% of ECF, or 25% TBW.

B, C, D, E. These calculations are incorrect. See explanation for A.

44. **C.** The corrected sodium (Na) accounts for the hyponatremia caused by the shift of water from the intracellular fluid to the extracellular fluid in hyperglycemic states. When calculating the corrected Na level, for every 100 mg/dL increase in blood glucose (from normal at 100), the serum Na increases 1.6 mEq/L (Na + [glucose − 100] × 1.6/100). Thus, 134 + [(500 − 100) × 1.6/100] = 140.

A, B, D, E. These calculations are incorrect. See explanation for C.

45. **B.** Plasma osmolality is calculated by (2 × Na) + (glucose/18) + (BUN/2.8), thus giving (2 × 134) + (500/18) + (28/2.8) − 306 mmol/kg.

A, C, D, E. These calculations are incorrect. See explanation for B.

46. **D.** If the difference between the calculated plasma osmolality and the measured osmolality is greater than 15 mOsm/kg, then there is an osmolar gap. An osmolar gap can be caused by mannitol, ethanol, ethylene glycol, myeloma proteins, or hypertriglyceridemia. The average osmolality is 289 mOsm/kg water.

A, B, C, E. These calculations are incorrect. See explanation for D.

47. **C.** Because total body sodium and potassium remain constant over time, changes in the TBW will be reflected in the extracellular compartment and will affect the serum sodium level.

A. Because of the large fluid resuscitation, the TBW dilutes the serum sodium level, rather than increasing it.
B. Decreased serum sodium, not decreased body sodium, reflects an increase in TBW content.
D. Decreased total body water would result in an increased serum sodium.

E. Because TBW is increased, aldosterone production would be decreased, not increased.

48. **C.** The renin-angiotensin-aldosterone system is a slow hormonal mechanism, which our body uses in long-term blood pressure regulation by adjusting blood volume. Renin is an enzyme that is released from the juxtaglomerular cells of the afferent arterioles and is essential in the conversion of angiotensinogen to angiotensin I in the plasma. Angiotensin I is physiologically inactive. Angiotensin-converting enzyme then converts angiotensin I to angiotensin II, primarily in the lungs.

A. Renin-angiotensin system is not associated with the liver.
B. Conversion of angiotensin I to II occurs in the lungs.
D. Renin is produced from the juxtaglomerular cells of the kidneys.
E. Bone marrow is unrelated to the renin-angiotensin conversion pathway.

49. **B.** Although angiotensin I is physiologically inactive, angiotensin II is physiologically active and will increase vascular tone, stimulate catecholamine release from the adrenal medulla, and decrease renal plasma flow, which increases sodium reabsorption and stimulates release of aldosterone from the adrenal cortex. All of these actions will maintain, not decrease, systemic blood pressure.

A, C, D, E. These are all incorrect answers. See explanation for B.

50. **B.** Aldosterone acts primarily on the distal collecting tubules to increase sodium reabsorption, potassium secretion, and proton secretion by increasing the Na/K ATPase activity. It is a mineralocorticoid produced within the zona glomerulosa of the adrenal cortex and is regulated by renin from the kidney. The primary regulator of aldosterone secretion is angiotensin II, as well as increased potassium, ACTA, and prostaglandins.

A. Sodium reabsorption is increased, not decreased.
C. Na/K ATPase activity is increased, not decreased.
D. Renin from the kidneys, not the pituitary, regulates the system.
E. Potassium secretion is increased.

BLOCK 2

The next two questions (items 51 and 52) correspond to the following vignette.

A 55-year-old obese male visits your office with a 20-year history of heartburn. The patient states he usually experiences it most often at night and uses Tums for relief. The patient has an unremarkable physical exam. You schedule him for esophagoscopy the next day. During endoscopy, you notice the lower esophagus has an uncharacteristic, salmon pink color. Biopsy demonstrates high-grade columnar dysplasia consistent with Barrett's esophagus.

51. Which of the following is the most appropriate treatment?

    A. Esophageal resection of the involved area
    B. Elevation of the head of the bed while sleeping
    C. H₂ blocking agents
    D. Proton pump inhibitors
    E. Antireflux procedure

52. Which of the following, if true, is a risk factor in this patient for adenocarcinoma of the esophagus?

    A. African-American race
    B. Tobacco use
    C. Consumption of alcohol
    D. Columnar metaplasia
    E. Achalasia

End of Set

The next two questions (items 53 and 54) correspond to the following vignette.

A 67-year-old male visits your office after being referred to you by his primary care physician for complaints of regurgitating undigested pieces of food. Past medical history includes a 5-year history of hypertension treated with hydrochlorothiazide. The patient has no allergies to medications and denies any previous surgeries. On physical exam, the patient appears healthy; the exam was normal except for halitosis and a vague left-sided neck mass.

53. The most likely diagnosis for this man's condition is

    A. Pharyngobulbar dysfunction
    B. Zenker's diverticulum

C. Gastroesophageal reflux
D. Achalasia
E. Type I hiatal hernia

54. What is the most important part of the surgical correction of this process?

    A. Myotomy of the cricopharyngeus muscle
    B. Repair of hiatal hernia
    C. Diverticulectomy
    D. Recreation of lower esophageal sphincter
    E. Surgical management is not necessary

End of Set

55. A 6-year-old female with an esophageal stricture has undergone a balloon dilatation procedure today. The patient is brought to the ED 6 hours later because the child has been running a temperature, has been breathing irregularly, and "doesn't look right" according to her mother. To you, the patient appears mottled and pale; she is also tachypneic (RR 40) and somnolent. The following chest x-ray is obtained (Figure 5-55A). What is the most important next step in the management of this child?

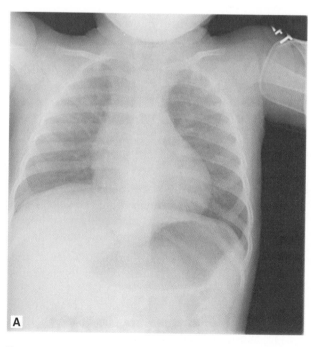

A

Figure 5-55A • Image Courtesy of the University of Utah School of Medicine, Salt Lake City, Utah.

A. Endotracheal intubation
B. CT scan
C. Chest tube placement
D. Broad-spectrum antibiotics
E. IV fluid resuscitation

56. You are on call in the surgical intensive care unit (SICU). A critically ill polytrauma patient has been in the unit for the last 3 weeks. The 38-year-old female patient arrived with multiple orthopedic injuries, including a severe pelvic fracture with retroperitoneal bleeding requiring massive fluid resuscitation. You receive the following arterial blood gas and basic metabolic panel results: pH 7.22, PCO_2 42, PO_2 71, lactate 1.0 mmol/L, Na 137 mmol/L, K 4.5 mmol/L, Cl 110 mmol/L, HCO_3 18 mEq/L, BUN 77 mg/dL, Cr 3.4 mg/dL, glucose 185 mg/dL. Which of the following results in a nonanion gap metabolic acidosis?

A. Salicylate poisoning
B. Ethylene glycol intoxication
C. Diarrhea
D. Uremia
E. Lactic acidosis
F. Methanol intoxication
G. Paraldehyde poisoning
H. Ketone acidosis

The next two questions (items 57 and 58) correspond to the following vignette.

A 26-year-old female is brought to the ED by EMS. The patient was found unconscious behind a dumpster. There is no evidence of obvious trauma, and although the patient is somnolent, she awakens to stimuli. Physical exam is unrevealing. The patient is given naloxone, dextrose, and IV fluid without effect. The following labs are obtained: WBC 12,000, HCT 50%, Plts 460,000, Na 146 mmol/L, K 5.0 mmol/L, Cl 108 mmol/L, HCO_3 12 mmol/L, BUN 25 mg/dL, Cr

1.2 mg/dL, glucose 550 mg/dL, ABG: pH 7.28, PCO_2 26, PO_2 75, BE -5.0, and urine ketones present on UA.

57. The most appropriate immediate treatment for this patient includes?

A. IV antibiotics
B. Insulin drip with IV fluid hydration
C. Exploratory laparotomy
D. Hemodialysis
E. Vasopressin

58. This patient's lab values are most consistent with which of the following conditions?

A. Uncompensated respiratory acidosis
B. Uncompensated metabolic acidosis
C. Compensated respiratory acidosis
D. Compensated metabolic acidosis
E. Mixed acid base disorder

End of Set

The next two questions (items 59 and 60) correspond to the following vignette.

A 67-year-old hospitalized male with multiple previous abdominal surgeries undergoes a difficult open cholecystectomy for resolved acute cholecystitis. On postoperative day 2, his heart rate acutely increases to 150 beats per minute. The patient remains alert with some substernal discomfort. The BP is 155/70 and the following ECG strip is attached to his bedside chart (Figure 5-59). The patient is placed on oxygen, transported to telemetry, and labs are obtained.

59. What is the most appropriate initial management?

A. Nitroglycerin drip
B. Morphine sulfate
C. β-antagonist drip
D. IV fluids
E. Place arterial line

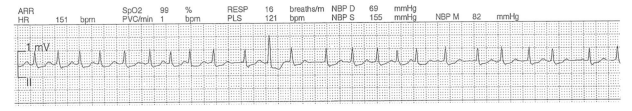

Figure 5-59 • Image Courtesy of the University of Utah School of Medicine, Salt Lake City, Utah.

60. After the initial therapy is implemented, a 12-lead ECG is obtained. Your chief resident describes the ECG as "tachycardia with tombstone waves in V3-5 leads." What is the most likely cause of this ECG finding?

    A. Volume overload
    B. Pain
    C. Myocardial infarction
    D. Hypovolemia
    E. Hypoxia

End of Set

The next two questions (items 61 and 62) correspond to the following vignette.

You are the resident in a busy SICU. You are rounding on a 60-year-old male who is 12 hours postop from an emergency repair of a ruptured AAA. The patient is mechanically ventilated, and you observe the following arterial blood gas results (obtained while on pressure ventilator settings with a FiO_2 of 0.65 and PEEP of 5 cm H_2O): pH 7.27, PCO_2 63, PO_2 50. A chemistry panel is as follows: Na 142 mmol/L, K 4 mmol/L, Cl 115 mmol/L, HCO_3 25 mmol/L, BUN 16 mg/dL, and Cr 1.0 mg/dL.

61. You quickly change the ventilator settings to help resolve the observed problem. Which initial intervention is most appropriate?

    A. Decreasing tidal volume
    B. Decreasing respiratory rate
    C. Decreasing PEEP
    D. Increasing tidal volume
    E. Increasing PEEP

62. What ventilator changes may be used to improve this patient's oxygenation?

    A. Increasing PEEP
    B. Increasing respiratory rate
    C. Increasing tidal volume
    D. Decreasing FiO_2
    E. Decreasing PEEP

End of Set

The next two questions (items 63 and 64) correspond to the following vignette.

A 35-year-old female is seen in clinic for a routine physical. The patient complains of nervousness and diarrhea for the last 4 months, as well as an unintentional loss of 10 lbs and an irregular menstrual cycle. Vital signs demonstrate T 97.2°F, HR 103, BP 125/75, and SaO_2 98% on room air. On physical exam, you notice protrusion of both eyes and a slight tremor in both hands.

63. Which of the following test results are most consistent with this patient's presentation?

    A. Decreased TSH, decreased free T_4
    B. Decreased TSH, increased free T_4
    C. Increased TSH, increased free T_4
    D. Increased TSH, decreased free T_4
    E. Normal TSH, normal free T_4

64. What is the most serious complication following surgical treatment for this patient's disease?

    A. Superior laryngeal nerve damage
    B. Temporary hypoparathyroidism
    C. Recurrent nerve damage
    D. Hypothyroidism
    E. Wound infection

End of Set

65. A 70-year-old female comes to your office complaining of a recent weight gain of 15 lbs over the last 3 months, with no obvious change in intake and constipation that is requiring OTC medications. On initial evaluation, you find the patient's BP is 112/60 with a resting HR of 54. Given her history, you suspect hypothyroidism. Which of the following would most likely explain this diagnosis?

    A. Graves' disease
    B. Toxic multinodular goiter
    C. Thyroid adenoma
    D. Levothyroxyl overdose
    E. Iodine deficiency

66. A 56-year-old male has undergone a total thyroidectomy for suspected papillary adenocarcinoma. During your postoperative checkup, he complains of abdominal cramping as well as numbness and tingling around his mouth. On examination, you notice spasm of the facial muscles while performing a preauricular tap. Which of the following is the most appropriate initial treatment?

A. Administer IV fluids
B. Obtain a basic metabolic panel
C. Start patient on levothyroxine
D. Administer IV calcium gluconate
E. This is normal after surgery so no action is needed

67. A 45-year-old female visits your clinic for the first time. The patient has no allergies, denies any current health issues, and has not had a physical exam in over 5 years. There is a history of depression, but currently the patient is not taking any medications. The only surgery she has had are a tonsillectomy and adenectomy at a young age. Vital signs are as follows: T 37.8°C, HR 72, BP 135/68, RR 15, and SaO$_2$ of 95% on room air. The patient appears to be in excellent condition. The physical exam is remarkable only for a 2-cm, mobile mass in the right lobe of her thyroid gland. What is the most appropriate next step in the workup of this patient?

A. CT scan of the neck
B. Fine-needle aspiration of the mass
C. Radionuclide thyroid scanning
D. Direct laryngoscopy
E. Thyroid antibody assay

68. A 70-year-old female presents to you with a palpable right neck mass. The patient is clinically euthyroid; a fine-needle aspirate of the mass is suspicious for papillary cancer. During the operative neck exploration, you discover thyroid tissue extending superiorly. Based on the embryologic origins of the thyroid, what is the superior extension of the thyroid tissue most likely to be?

A. Isthmus
B. Foramen cecum
C. Pyramidal lobe
D. Ultimobranchial body
E. Tubercle of Zuckerkandl

69. A 56-year-old female with prolonged course in the ICU becomes acutely hypotensive. Initial fluid boluses are unsuccessful in correcting the hypotension, and she is started on an epinephrine drip. This also fails to raise the blood pressure. IV hydrocortisone is administered because of suspected adrenal insufficiency, and this aids in raising the blood pressure back to normal levels. The adrenal gland plays a pivotal role in the stress response produced by the body. The adrenal

cortex consists of three layers, each of which produces certain hormones that contribute to this response. Which in the following list of layers is the primary site of dehydroepiandrosterone (DHEA) production as well as a site of glucocorticoid production?

A. Zona glomerulosa
B. Zona fasciculata
C. Zona reticularis
D. Zona articulata
E. Zona marginatum
F. Zona cavularum
G. Zona primum

The next two questions (items 70 and 71) correspond to the following vignette.

A 42-year-old male visits your office for the first time with complaints of headaches and a racing heart for the last 3 months. The patient states that these usually occur as anxiety attacks that wake him up at night and are often associated with profuse sweating. Vital signs are T 37.8°C, HR 89, BP 180/95, RR 20, and SaO$_2$ of 97% on room air. The patient's physical exam is unrevealing.

70. Which test will be most helpful in obtaining a diagnosis?

A. CBC
B. Total and ionized calcium
C. Urinary catecholamine levels
D. Liver function tests
E. Serum calcitonin

71. After performing the appropriate test, you arrive at the suspected diagnosis. Which of the following imaging exams is most specific in localizing the lesion?

A. CT scan
B. Metaiodobenzylguanidine scan (MIBG)
C. MRI
D. Sestamibi scan
E. Angiography

End of Set

72. A 42-year-old female victim of a motor vehicle crash has been in the ICU for the last 2 weeks. Although she has been hemodynamically stable, she continues to require mechanical ventilation for acute respiratory distress syndrome (ARDS).

You are called to see her for acute hypotension, with arterial line pressures measuring in the 80s/40s. Your physical examination is unrevealing and a chest x-ray (Figure 5-72) is obtained, along with the following labs: WBC 9000, HCT 33%, Plts 330,000, Na 130 mmol/L, K 5.3 mmol/L, Cl 110 mmol/L, HCO_3 24 mmol/L, BUN 16 mg/dL, glucose 93 mg/dL, and Ca 9.5 mg/dL. You initially give the patient 2 L of crystalloid, but the vital signs are unchanged. A norepinephrine drip is started, and the blood pressures remain in the 80s/40s. What is the most likely cause of this patient's hypotension?

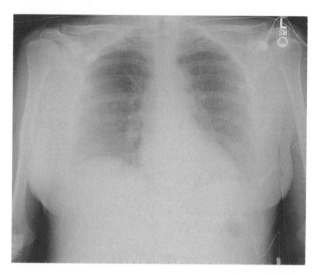

Figure 5-72 • Image Courtesy of the University of Utah School of Medicine, Salt Lake City, Utah.

A. Acute adrenal insufficiency
B. Cardiac tamponade
C. Pneumothorax
D. Sepsis
E. Dehydration

73. A 32-year-old active male presents to clinic complaining of right knee pain. The patient states it has been present for a day and a half. The patient denies any recent trauma, states he is taking only acetaminophen for the pain, is healthy otherwise, and has no known medical allergies. On examination, the knee is found to be swollen, erythematous, and warm to the touch. The patient has decreased ability to extend the knee when asked to do so. Which of the following is the most appropriate action?

A. MRI of the knee
B. Physical therapy sessions
C. Oral antibiotics for 1 week
D. NSAIDs with a follow-up appointment in 2 weeks
E. Needle aspiration of the joint

74. A 7-year-old male fell approximately 12 feet from a tree while vacationing with his family. According to the parents, he fell onto his right side and complained of immediate forearm pain, but he had no obvious deformity. The child was taken to the nearest local clinic where the arm was put in a splint and he was given an ice pack and ibuprofen for pain. The family elected to drive home and see their own physician. During the ride home, the child complained of progressively increasing pain, especially with movement. You see the child approximately 8 hours after the injury, and you suspect a supracondylar humerus fracture. Based on this diagnosis, what complication could this child develop that would be the most debilitating?

A. Musculocutaneous nerve entrapment
B. Radial head dislocation
C. Dupuytren's contracture
D. Charcot's joint
E. Volkmann's contracture

75. You are called to see a 52-year-old male who fell while bike riding. The patient denies any loss of consciousness and his Glasgow Coma Scale score is 15. The patient has a small laceration on his left thigh and a contusion on the right flank. The patient complains of right upper arm pain and supports his right arm with his left hand. On physical exam, you notice swelling and a mass in the mid-right brachium with point tenderness. The sensation is decreased on the dorsum of the right hand and he is unable to extend his right wrist. You observe the following x-ray (Figure 5-75A). What artery is intimately associated with the involved nerve at the level of the fracture?

A. Brachial artery
B. Ulnar artery
C. Axillary artery
D. Brachial profunda artery
E. Recurrent radial artery

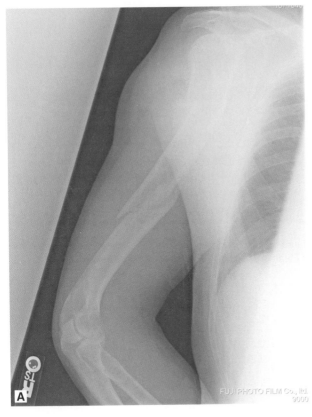

Figure 5-75A • Image Courtesy of the University of Utah School of Medicine, Salt Lake City, Utah.

76. A 24-year-old male presents to your office and reports a family history of dysplastic nevi syndrome. The patient has noticed a couple of new lesions on his arm and is interested in having you evaluate them. Which of the following is true regarding dysplastic nevi?

   A. Patients with a family history of dysplastic nevi have an increased risk for developing squamous cell carcinoma
   B. Dysplastic nevi usually have smooth borders
   C. All dysplastic nevi should be biopsied
   D. All dysplastic nevi should be excised following biopsy
   E. Dysplastic nevi generally measure less than 5 mm in diameter

The next three questions (items 77 to 79) correspond to the following vignette.

A 35-year-old male presents to the ED for severe hematemesis. The patient has recently returned from a weekend vacation with his college football friends, during which time he admits to a significant amount of entertaining and drinking. The patient denies a long history of alcohol intake, although he admits to binge drinking with friends at least once a month. The night before he came to the ED, the patient tells you he felt nauseated immediately after dinner, returned to his motel and proceeded to experience severe vomiting followed by retching with progressive and now significant hematemesis this morning. The labs are HCT 38%, K 3.0 mmol/L, Cr 1.1 mg/dL, glucose 73 mg/dL. Vital signs are T 37.5°C, HR 122, RR 16, and standing BP 118/70, lying BP 138/76. The abdominal exam is unremarkable, except for the patient's continued complaints of nausea.

77. What is the most likely cause of this man's upper GI bleed?

   A. Duodenal ulcer
   B. Esophageal varices
   C. Angiodysplasia
   D. Gastritis
   E. Mallory-Weiss tear
   F. Perforated peptic ulcer

78. What is the proper initial management of this patient's continuous GI bleed?

   A. NG tube placement with gastric lavage and gastric decompression
   B. Endoscopy with electrocautery
   C. Balloon compression of the bleeding site
   D. Urgent exploratory laparoscopy
   E. Urgent exploratory laparotomy

79. Based on your diagnosis, which portion of the upper GI tract would you expect to be involved?

   A. Upper esophagus
   B. Lower esophagus above the lower esophageal sphincter
   C. Proximal stomach near the GE junction
   D. Distal stomach near the pylorus
   E. First portion of the duodenum

End of Set

The next three questions (items 80 to 82) correspond to the following vignette.

A 67-year-old female presents to the ER with the chief complaint of "my skin is turning yellow." The patient denies any associated abdominal pain and reports that she has lost 30 lbs over the last 2 months. On physical exam, you note significant scleral icterus and a nontender right upper quadrant mass.

80. Which of the following is the most established risk factor for this patient's suspected cancer?

    A. Heavy alcohol consumption
    B. Diabetes mellitus
    C. Chronic pancreatitis
    D. Cigarette smoking
    E. Exposure to benzidine and β-naphthylamine

81. What is the most common histopathologic type of the suspected tumor in this patient's case?

    A. Adenocarcinoma
    B. Mucinous cystadenocarcinoma
    C. Adenosquamous carcinoma
    D. Giant-cell carcinoma
    E. Mucinous carcinoma
    F. Papillary-cystic tumor

82. What is the best initial radiographic study to evaluate this patient?

    A. Right upper quadrant ultrasound to rule out cholelithiasis
    B. Upper GI with small bowel followthrough
    C. CT scan with oral and IV contrast
    D. MRI of the abdomen
    E. Endoscopic retrograde cholangiopancreatography (ERCP)

End of Set

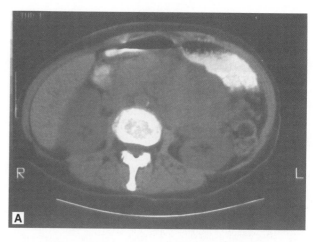

Figure 5-83A • Image Courtesy of the University of Utah School of Medicine, Salt Lake City, Utah.

    C. Plasma glucagon greater than 150 pg/mL
    D. Fasting gastrin level
    E. Fasting glucose greater than 140 mg/dL

End of Set

The next two questions (items 83 and 84) correspond to the following vignette.

A 42-year-old female is referred to your office for evaluation of malnutrition and weight loss. The patient has recently been diagnosed with a mild form of diabetes and necrolytic migratory dermatitis. This CT (Figure 5-83A) scan of the abdomen obtained by her primary care physician shows an intraabdominal mass.

83. What neoplastic cell type accounts for this patient's syndrome?

    A. α cells
    B. β cells
    C. D cells
    D. PP cells
    E. Gamma cells

84. What laboratory test and value will confirm your diagnosis?

    A. Elevated insulin levels with a prolonged fast
    B. Secretin stimulation test

85. A 52-year-old male initially presents to the ED with a 3-hour history of severe abdominal pain radiating to his back. The patient reported having been on a drinking binge over the last 5 days after losing his job. On your initial ED physical exam, the vital signs showed a BP 115/70, HR 125, and RR 18, and his abdomen was diffusely tender. A panel of labs was sent and the WBC was 18,000, HCT 53%, LDH 430 U/L, AST 366 U/L, glucose 242 mg/dL, and amylase 556 U/L. The patient has since then been admitted to the hospital and today, 2 days later, is found to have an HCT of 45%, BUN increase from 25 to 28 mg/dL, serum calcium 8.2 mg/dL, PaO_2 of 72 on 6 L by face mask, and base excess of −3, and has made only 1700 mL of urine in the last 2 days despite 16 L of crystalloid fluid. Ranson's criteria are used on admission and again 48 hours after admission as prognostic indicators in acute pancreatitis. How many criteria does this patient meet?

    A. 2
    B. 4
    C. 6
    D. 8
    E. 11

86. A 66-year-old female has fallen down the stairs and is brought to the ER with a suspected hip fracture. The patient's leg is internally rotated and there is posterior fullness at the hip joint. After obtaining this x-ray (Figure 5-86A), you diagnose her with a posterior hip dislocation. You must immediately reduce the dislocation to prevent what complication?

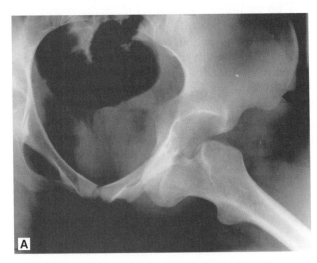

Figure 5-86A • Image Courtesy of the University of Utah School of Medicine, Salt Lake City, Utah.

A. Fat emboli
B. Joint calcification
C. Sciatic nerve injury
D. Avascular necrosis
E. Osteomyelitis

The next two questions (items 87 and 88) correspond to the following vignette.

A 36-year-old Hispanic female is referred to your clinic by her primary care physician. Through her interpreter she tells you she has been referred because she was found to have a calcium level of 12.9 mg/dL. The patient has not told you anything else about her history with the exception that, since the discovery of the elevated calcium, a parathyroid hormone level was obtained and it is 66 mEq/mL. You have a physician assistant training in your office and you instruct him to evaluate the patient and provide you with a complete history and plan for evaluating the newly discovered hypercalcemia. After he is finished with the patient, you ask him the following question.

87. Which of the following is the most likely presentation for a patient with hypercalcemia due to primary hyperparathyroidism?

A. Prolonged QT on ECG
B. Diarrhea
C. Anxiety
D. Hypotension
E. Depression
F. No symptoms

88. What imaging study must you obtain before taking this patient to the operating room to remove her parathyroid glands?

A. Ultrasound
B. Thallium-technetium scan
C. Sestamibi scan
D. CT scan
E. No imaging studies are needed

End of Set

89. A 31-year-old male presents to your office for evaluation of a right groin mass, which he first noticed 2 days after he had completed a 50-mile hiking trip. Over the last 8 hours, the mass has become increasingly tender and he is no longer able to "push it back in." You attempt to reduce the hernia but are unable to do so, after which you diagnose an incarcerated inguinal hernia and decide to take him to the operating room. Which of the following best describes incarcerated inguinal hernias?

A. They occur most often on the left
B. Ten percent of the time, hernias present with incarceration
C. Groin hernias can spontaneously resolve
D. Groin hernias are more common in African-Americans than in Caucasians
E. Women and men are at equal risk for groin hernias

The response options for items 90 to 94 are the same. You will be required to select one answer for each item in the set.

A. Pantaloon hernia
B. Lumbar hernia
C. Hiatal hernia
D. Sliding hernia
E. Internal hernia

For each definition, select the most appropriate hernia.

90. Hernia sac partially formed by the wall of a viscus

91. Hernia through Petit's triangle

92. Hernia into or involving an intra-abdominal structure

93. Both a direct and indirect hernia

94. Hernia parallel to the esophagus

End of Set

95. A 45-year-old male is referred to your office because he has a mole in the middle of his lower back, along the waistline, that his wife noticed has changed in color and size. The lesion is the size of the dime, has dried blood over it, and is raised. The patient tells you that he has noticed blood on his shirts, but he attributed the bleeding to the lesion rubbing on his pants and belt. The patient has numerous moles, especially over his chest and back. A biopsy that was performed by a dermatologist prior to seeing you was read as malignant melanoma. You schedule the patient for a wide excision, lymphoscintigraphy, and sentinel node procedure. Based on Breslow thickness, what general guidelines should be followed regarding surgical procedures used in the diagnosis and treatment of melanomas?

    A. Larger than 3-cm margins are needed for melanomas deeper than 1 mm
    B. Punch or incisional biopsies are appropriate to diagnosis larger lesions
    C. Cryosurgery is appropriate for melanomas in situ
    D. Melanomas 1mm or less in thickness require regional lymphadenotomy
    E. Frozen sections are helpful in establishing the initial diagnosis

The next two questions (items 96 and 97) correspond to the following vignette:

A 31-year-old male who has been diagnosed with GERD by his primary care physician is referred to your office for evaluation for a Nissen fundoplication. The patient has been on medical therapy and continues to have symptoms despite medical management. As part of your preoperative workup, you want to rule out achalasia.

96. What diagnostic study will confirm the absence of this diagnosis?

    A. Enteroclysis
    B. CT scan of chest and abdomen
    C. Esophageal pH probe
    D. Esophageal manometry
    E. Chest x-ray

97. As part of your workup, you refer this patient for an upper endoscopy. The gastroenterologist reports to you that he found tonguelike extensions of epithelium extending up into the distal esophagus from the GE junction. This information is concerning for what diagnosis?

    A. Esophageal stricture
    B. Barrett's esophagus
    C. *Candida* esophagitis
    D. Esophageal carcinoma
    E. Mallory-Weiss tear

End of Set

The next two questions (items 98 and 99) correspond to the following vignette.

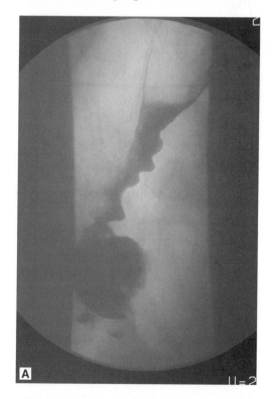

Figure 5-99A • Image Courtesy of the University of Utah School of Medicine, Salt Lake City, Utah.

A 54-year-old male presents to the emergency department with angina-like chest pain, which is usually associated with stress and is relieved by nitrates. The patient is worked up for a myocardial infarction but is found to have a normal ECG and a troponin level of less than 0.06 ng/mL.

98. Which of the following esophageal disorders most likely explains this patient's symptoms?

A. Achalasia
B. Esophageal perforation
C. Diffuse esophageal spasm
D. Esophageal cancer
E. Zenker's diverticulum

99. You order a barium esophagogram (Figure 5-99A) to evaluate the esophagus. What is the typical radiologic finding associated with this patient's condition?

A. Corkscrew esophagus
B. Bird's beak sign
C. Double bubble sign
D. Lower esophageal outpouching
E. Normal esophagogram

End of Set

100. A 5-year-old female is brought to the ED because her parents found her in the cleaning closet and they believe she drank some liquid drain opener (liquid alkali). There are no obvious findings on examination of the patient's oral cavity. An upper endoscopy is performed and shows irritation and some ulceration of the lower esophagus. What potential complication of this injury must you be very concerned about?

A. Perforation
B. Hemorrhage
C. Infection
D. Stricture
E. Nutcracker esophagus

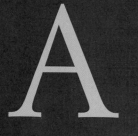

Answers and Explanations

51. A	68. C	85. C
52. D	69. C	86. D
53. B	70. C	87. F
54. A	71. B	88. E
55. A	72. A	89. B
56. C	73. E	90. D
57. B	74. E	91. B
58. D	75. D	92. E
59. C	76. C	93. A
60. C	77. E	94. C
61. D	78. A	95. B
62. A	79. C	96. D
63. B	80. D	97. B
64. C	81. A	98. C
65. E	82. C	99. A
66. D	83. A	100. D
67. B	84. C	

51. **A.** Esophageal resection of the involved area, Barrett's esophagus is the most appropriate treatment. Barrett's esophagus increases the risk of adenocarcinoma of the esophagus to 40 times that of the general population. Therefore, the area of metaplastic change must be routinely surveyed with endoscopic biopsies to look for areas of dysplasia. High-grade dysplasia carries the highest risk of cancer and warrants surgical resection.

    B. This is a lifestyle change often used in an attempt to relieve gastroesophageal reflux. Other changes include losing weight, eating small frequent meals, and smoking cessation. These actions will not change the natural progression of Barrett's esophagus with dysplastic change.

    C. H_2 blocking agents will decrease acid reflux; these drugs will not change the natural progression of Barrett's esophagus with dysplastic change.

    D. Proton pump inhibitors are used to decrease acid reflux, and will not change the natural progression of Barrett's esophagus with dysplastic change.

    E. An antireflux surgical procedure is a reasonable treatment in the case of low-grade dysplastic Barrett's esophagus. Classically, the literature has stated that there is no regression of low-grade dysplastic Barrett's esophagus after an antireflux procedure; however, recent studies have documented otherwise.

52. **D.** Along with Barrett's esophagus (columnar metaplasia), other risk factors for esophageal adenocarcinoma include GERD and Caucasian race.

    A, B, C, E. African-American race, tobacco use, consumption of alcohol, and achalasia are all risk factors for esophageal squamous cell carcinoma. Additional risk factors for esophageal squamous cell cancer include male sex, Plummer-Vinson syndrome, scleroderma, lye stricture, nitrosamine ingestion, and living in China or Iran.

53. **B.** This is a classic presentation for Zenker's diverticulum, which is an outpouching of the esophageal mucosa posteriorly between the inferior pharyngeal constrictor and the cricopharyngeus muscles. The most common symptoms are dysphagia, reflux of undigested food, and halitosis. Diagnosis can be confirmed with a barium swallow (Figure 5-53) or endoscopy.

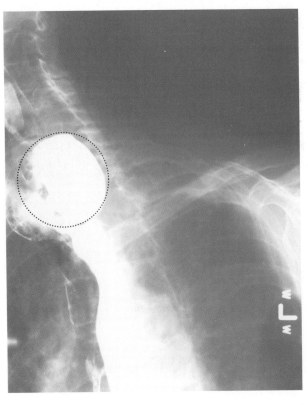

Figure 5-53 • Image Courtesy of the University of Utah School of Medicine, Salt Lake City, Utah.

    A. Dysphagia occurs with pharyngobulbar dysfunction, and it is usually the result of a neurologic problem such as ALS, previous CVA, or Parkinson's disease.

    C. Long-standing GER can result in distal esophageal stricture with dysplasia and a sensation of food sticking in the lower esophagus.

    D. Achalasia usually presents with dysphagia of both solids and liquids. Regurgitation of undigested food particles may occur, but it is not associated with a left-sided neck mass.

    E. A type I hiatal hernia most often is asymptomatic or presents with symptoms of acid reflux.

54. **A.** Treatment of Zenker's involves removal of the diverticulum (seen clearly in Figure 5-54) and myotomy of the cricopharyngeus muscle. The most important part is the myotomy, because the diverticulum results from increased spasticity of this muscle, causing increased luminal pressures and protrusion of the mucosa and esophageal adventitia at Kilian's triangle. Many physicians would argue that only a myotomy of the cricopharyngeus muscle is needed, thus eliminating the increased luminal pressures.

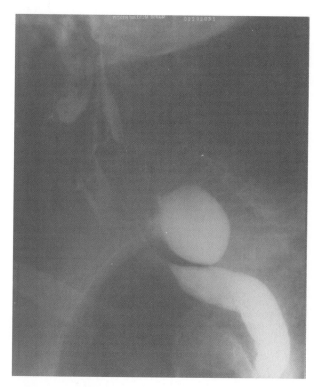

Figure 5-54 • Image Courtesy of the University of Utah School of Medicine, Salt Lake City, Utah.

B. Hiatal hernia is not present in this patient, and is not the cause of this patient's dysphagia.

C. Although a diverticulectomy is advocated, it will not solve the underlying problem that led to the formation of the diverticulum.

D. The cricopharyngeus, not the lower esophageal sphincter, is involved in Zenker's formation.

E. Surgery is the only current therapy for this disorder.

55. A. It is important to be able to identify an acutely ill patient. In the patient presented, there are multiple red flags, mainly, the tachypnea, somnolence, and ill appearance. After the initial assessment in the ED, the ABCs (airway, breathing, and circulation) should always be assessed. In this case, emergent intubation is needed to obtain a secure airway. Once this has been established, further workup may begin. The child most likely suffers from an iatrogenic esophageal perforation after balloon dilatation of an esophageal stricture. The initial x-ray (Figure 5-55B) is suspicious, with mediastinal widening (see arrow), and the x-ray obtained after intubation (Figure 5-55C) and chest tube placement clearly depicts the mediastinal air (see arrows). This is a known complication to balloon dilatation procedures. Every effort should be made to surgically repair the perforation within 24 hours, and the procedure should consist of closure of the perforation and external drainage. Perforations discovered after 24 hours usually require debridement, cervical esophagostomy, wide drainage, and construction of a feeding jejunostomy.

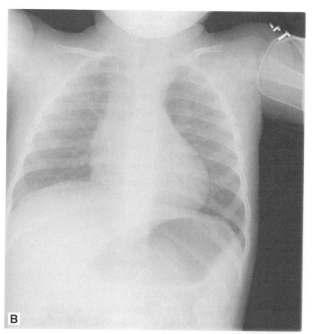

B

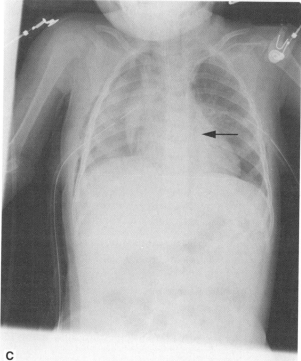

C

Figure 5-55 B and C • Images Courtesy of the University of Utah School of Medicine, Salt Lake City, Utah.

B. Obtaining a CT scan is not an appropriate choice before intubation and airway control because of the patient's instability.

C. Chest tube placement will most likely be needed, but obtaining control of the airway always takes precedence.

D. Patients suspected to have esophageal perforation should be started on antibiotics, but securing an airway always comes first.

E. The rate of fluid accumulation within the chest can be as high as 1 L/hour, so IV fluid resuscitation is important, but airway always comes before circulation.

56. C. Nonanion gap metabolic acidosis is caused by the loss of HCO_3 from the digestive tract, as with diarrhea, or from failure of the kidneys to reabsorb HCO_3. This is usually seen in high-output GI loss (i.e., enterocutaneous fistulas, diarrhea) or renal tubular acidosis. To distinguish between anion and nonanion gap, a urine anion gap can be obtained. This is calculated $U_{Na} - (UCl + UK)$. If a negative value is obtained, the kidneys are working appropriately and the cause is loss from the digestive tract. If positive, the acidosis is due to inadequate renal reabsorption of HCO_3.

A, B, D, E, F, G, H. All have abnormal anions contributing to making up the anion gap and metabolic acidosis. The anion gap is calculated by obtaining the following serum electrolytes: $Na - (Cl + HCO_3)$. An anion gap exists when the calculation is greater than 12. A mnemonic used to help remember causes of this type of acidosis is "MUDPILES," which stands for methanol, uremic acidosis, DKA, paraldehyde, idiopathic acidosis, lactic acidosis, ethylene glycol, and salicylate toxicity.

57. B. This patient suffers from diabetic ketoacidosis (DKA), as demonstrated by the anion gap (26), acidosis, hyperglycemia, and urine ketones, and requires an insulin drip with hydration. These patients are critically ill and should be treated promptly. The hyperglycemia should be treated with an IV insulin drip. Patients in DKA are very often severely dehydrated from osmotic diuresis and require aggressive rehydration. They should be hydrated with normal saline until their glucose reaches close to 300 mg/dL, at which time dextrose should be added to avoid cerebral swelling. Treatment continues until the increased anion gap resolves to normal. Closely monitored repletion of electrolytes is necessary because of the likelihood of hypokalemia and hypophosphatemia.

A. IV antibiotics are indicated if an infection is the underlying cause of the DKA, but this is secondary in terms of priority.

C. There is no indication for surgery at this time.

D. This patient's renal function appears to be intact.

E. Vasopressin is used in diabetes insipidus, not DKA.

58. D. Disorders of the acid-base system are common in critically ill patients. It is very important to be able to distinguish the different types of disorders. Table 5-58 is a summary of the lab values found with each disorder. This patient has an increased anion gap of 26. The pH and HCO_3 are decreased, indicating a metabolic acidosis. The patient is hyperventilating and blowing off CO_2, thus compensating for the acidosis and increasing the serum pH.

■ TABLE 5-58 Metabolic Disorder Lab Values

Disorder	pH	HCO_3	$PaCO_2$
Metabolic acidosis	↓	↓	↓
Metabolic alkalosis	↑	↑	↑
Respiratory acidosis	↓	↑	↑
Respiratory alkalosis	↑	↓	↓

A. An increased PCO_2 and normal HCO_3 would be seen in an uncompensated respiratory acidosis.

B. An uncompensated metabolic acidosis would present with an inappropriately high or normal CO_2 leading to a worsened acidosis. The expected $PaCO_2 = 1.5 \times [HCO_3] + 8 \pm 2$. In this case, $1.5 \times [12] + 8 = 26$; thus she is appropriately compensated.

C. In a compensated respiratory acidosis, both the PCO_2 and HCO_3 would be elevated.

E. When a patient does not adequately compensate for the acid-base disorder, a mixed disorder occurs. This is not the case in this clinical situation.

59. C. A common cause of postoperative tachyarrhythmias is atrial fibrillation with rapid ventricular response, and it is managed with a beta-agonist drip. Atrial fibrillation is verified by an ECG tracing noting a rapid rate, usually in the 130 to 150 range, with an irregularly irregular rhythm and absence of p waves. The initial treatment is rate control. If the patient is hemodynamically unstable, cardioversion should be performed. In a hemodynamically stable patient, there are multiple pharmacologic agents that can be used, including β-blockers, calcium-channel blockers, digoxin, and amiodarone.

   A. Nitroglycerin is a venous and arterial dilator and would most likely lower blood pressure, but not control heart rate.
   B. Morphine would be a good choice if the cause of the tachycardia was pain, such as severe angina during a myocardial infarction (MI).
   D. Although IV fluids would be a good initial treatment for tachycardia, in this case the patient is normotensive, which likely eliminates hypovolemia as the cause of tachycardia.
   E. Placing an arterial line is not the initial step, although it may be needed later, particularly if the tachycardia persists or hypotension ensues.

60. C. MI should always be included in the differential diagnosis of causes of tachyarrhythmias, especially if seen acutely in any patient that had been recovering normally from surgery. In the early stages of an MI, an ECG can be normal or near normal. Less than half of patients with an acute MI have clear diagnostic changes on their first ECG. In practice, ST elevation is often the earliest sign of an MI, and is often evident within hours of the initial onset of symptoms. The term "tombstone" elevation is defined as fusion of the QRS complex, the ST segment, and the T wave into a single monophasic deflection, which looks like a giant R wave or a tombstone. This ST elevation is classic for an MI. It is also an indication for immediate intervention, either thrombolytics or percutaneous transcoronary angioplasty. In surgical patients, thrombolytics are usually contraindicated because of the risk of bleeding. The patient should therefore go emergently to cardiac catheterization for angioplasty and possible coronary stenting. Serial cardiac markers (CPK - MB, troponin I) along with serial ECGs should be evaluated, to help determine the cause of the arrhythmia.

   A. Volume overload can often be seen with atrial fibrillation in patients with heart disease caused by the increased stretch on atrial fibers. Diuretics may help in this scenario. Volume overload alone would not cause tombstone elevation of the ST segment.
   B. Pain can often present as tachycardia, but it will not cause ST segment elevation.
   D. Hypovolemia is also a cause of tachycardia, often seen in postoperative patients, but hypovolemia alone will not cause this type of ECG finding.
   E. Hypoxia is also a cause of tachycardia, especially in postoperative abdominal surgery patients. Respiratory support in postoperative surgery patients is critical, and in acute events such as in this scenario, hypoxemia should be ruled out. Hypoxia alone will not cause this ECG finding.

61. D. Ventilation deals with the exchange of CO_2 and is determined by the minute ventilation calculated as V_E = respiratory rate (RR) multiplied by tidal volume (V_T). CO_2 is retained by decreasing the V_E, which leads to respiratory acidosis. Conversely, CO_2 is blown off by increasing the V_E and results in respiratory alkalosis. This patient's labs reflect a respiratory acidosis, for which the minute ventilation should be increased by increasing the tidal volume.

   A. Decreasing the tidal volume would decrease the minute ventilation and worsen the acidosis.
   B. Decreasing the respiratory rate would decrease the minute ventilation and worsen the acidosis.
   C. Decreasing the PEEP level would not help this patient's respiratory acidosis.
   E. Increasing the PEEP may improve the oxygenation, but it would not address ventilation.

62. A. Oxygenation of patients on a ventilator can be manipulated by adjusting positive end expiratory pressure (PEEP) and the FiO_2 (fraction of inspired oxygen). Increasing the amount of oxygen the patient receives (increasing the FiO_2), or increasing the surface area and amount of time oxygen can diffuse into the pulmonary capillaries (increasing PEEP) can result in improved oxygenation. Adjusting PEEP levels is often used to decrease the FiO_2 to levels at which oxygen toxicity will not occur, usually below 0.6. Therefore, to increase oxygenation, one can increase the levels of either the FiO_2 or the PEEP.

B. Increasing the respiratory rate will increase the minute ventilation and decrease $PaCO_2$.

C. Increasing the tidal volume will increase minute ventilation and decrease the $PaCO_2$.

D. Decreasing the FiO_2 will worsen the oxygenation.

E. Decreasing the PEEP in this case will worsen the oxygenation.

63. **B. Hyperthyroidism is secondary to hyperfunction of the thyroid gland. Clinical features include restlessness, tremor, heat intolerance, tachycardia, muscle wasting and weight loss, diarrhea, and menstrual abnormalities. The most common cause is Graves' disease, which is an autoimmune disease caused by antibodies stimulating the TSH receptors. It mainly affects women between the ages of 30 and 50 years. The thyroid is usually diffusely enlarged and patients with Graves' disease may have exophthalmos (infiltrative ophthalmopathy) and pretibial edema. Diagnosis is confirmed by an increased free T_4 with decreased TSH. Treatment may consist of antithyroid drugs (PTU, methimazole), radioiodine, or subtotal thyroidectomy.**

A. These results describe secondary hypothyroidism.

C. These results describe secondary hyperthyroidism.

D. These results describe a hypothyroid state.

E. This describes the euthyroid state.

64. **C. This surgical complication, recurrent nerve damage, occurs less than 2% of the time in experienced hands. The nerve runs through the tracheoesophageal groove and is most vulnerable at the level of the two upper tracheal rings. It supplies all of the muscles of the larynx except the cricothyroid muscle. Injury results in an abductor laryngeal paralysis with the affected cord assuming the midline. Unilateral injury results in hoarseness. Bilateral injury may lead to airway obstruction.**

A. The superior laryngeal nerve supplies the cricothyroid muscle and may also be damaged. Damage to this nerve is not as serious and results in the lowering of one's voice.

B. Temporary hypoparathyroidism usually results from minor injury to the parathyroid blood supply during surgery. It is manifested

postoperatively by hypocalcemia and it is usually transient.

D. Hypothyroidism is also a common occurrence, and its severity depends on the extent of thyroid tissue removed. It is easily treated with hormone replacement.

E. Wound infection is a very rare complication in elective thyroid surgery and is treated by local wound care.

65. **E. Although this is now a rare cause of hypothyroidism in the United States, it is the only choice given that would cause hypothyroidism. Other causes include thyroiditis, Hashimoto's, viral, Reidel's, prior I^{131} treatment, thyroidectomy, thyroid hormone resistance, and colloid goiter. Hashimoto's thyroiditis is the leading cause of hypothyroidism in the United States. It is an autoimmune disorder that most commonly affects women. Clinical signs and symptoms include cold intolerance, weight gain, mental and physical slowness, menorrhagia, constipation, hair loss, dry skin, myxedema, and increase in relaxation phase of deep tendon reflexes. Treatment consists of hormone replacement with levothyroxine.**

A, B, C, D. Graves' disease, toxic multinodular goiter, thyroid adenoma, and levothyroxyl overdose are all are causes of hyperthyroidism.

66. **D. This man suffers from postoperative hypoparathyroidism, resulting in symptomatic hypocalcemia, and needs IV calcium gluconate. Signs and symptoms usually occur within the first few hours or days after surgery and are usually temporary. Hypoparathyroidism, post-total thyroidectomy, is usually due to an impaired blood supply to all four parathyroid glands, a condition that is rarely (less than 1%) irreversible. The signs and symptoms include perioral numbness, tingling of the fingers, anxiety, and involuntary spasms. Testing can be done by eliciting the Chvostek's sign, which is an ipsilateral facial muscle contraction when the facial nerve is tapped as in this patient, or the Trousseau's sign, which is seen as carpal spasm after occlusion of the brachial artery for 3 minutes. Treatment involves calcium replacement such as IV calcium gluconate. Oral calcium supplemented with vitamin D may also be used.**

A. Administering IV fluids will not help resolve the ongoing hypocalcemia.

B. Obtaining a basic metabolic panel will confirm the serum level of calcium but, clinically, the diagnosis has already been made.

C. Although hormonal replacement with levothyroxine needs to be initiated, this will not resolve the presenting condition of hypocalcemia.

E. Symptomatic hypocalcemia is not a normal expectation, but it should always be monitored for.

67. **B. A fast, inexpensive initial diagnostic tool in the workup of a thyroid nodule is an FNA in the office setting. Papillary, medullary, and anaplastic carcinomas can be diagnosed with this method. Certain findings may also suggest malignancy, such as atypia. An FNA is limited in its interpretation of follicular tumors and is not able to distinguish between a malignant and benign lesion.**

A. A CT scan of the neck may be needed to help stage a patient with malignant disease, but it is not the first step in diagnosis.

C. A radionucleotide thyroid scan is usually used to distinguish between hot (functioning) and cold (nonfunctional) lesions. Tissue will need to be obtained despite the determination of the lesion's functionality.

D. Performing direct laryngoscopy is inappropriate as an initial exam.

E. A thyroid antibody assay is more useful in the workup of hypo- or hyperthyroid states, neither of which is suggested here.

68. **C. Embryologically, the thyroid originates from an evagination of the primitive pharynx between the first and second pharyngeal pouches, called the thyroid diverticulum. As the embryo grows, it descends as a hollow tube in the neck. It remains connected to the tongue for a short period of time as the thyroglossal duct. It eventually fills in to become the thyroid gland. The proximal portion of this gland persists as the foramen cecum. Approximately 50% of people have the distal aspect of this duct, known as the pyramidal lobe. It extends superiorly into the neck from the isthmus.**

A. The isthmus is the portion of the thyroid that connects the right and left lobes.

B. As in the explanation for C, the foramen cecum is the proximal portion of the duct and is found in most individuals.

D. The ultimobranchial body is not part of the thyroglossal duct. It is derived from the ventral portion of the fourth pharyngeal pouch and thought to give rise to the parafollicular cells.

E. The tubercle of Zuckerkandl is not part of the thyroglossal duct; it is the superior pole of either lobe of the thyroid gland.

69. **C. The adrenal cortex is composed of three layers: the zona glomerulosa, the zona fasciculate, and the zona reticularis. The zona glomerulosa is responsible for the production of aldosterone in response to the renin-angiotensin-aldosterone axis. The zona fasciculata and zona reticularis both produce glucocorticoids and androgen steroids; however, the zona fasciculata primarily produces glucocorticoids, whereas the zona reticularis primarily produces sex steroids such as DHEA. They are regulated by the hypothalamic-pituitary-adrenal axis.**

A. The zona glomerulosa produces aldosterone.

B. Although DHEA can come from the zona fasciculata, this layer primarily produces glucocorticoids.

D, E, F G. The zona articulata, zona marginatum, zona cavularum, and zona primum are not true layers of the adrenal cortex.

70. **C. A pheochromocytoma is the cause of hypertension in about 0.1% of hypertensive patients in the United States. A tumor of the adrenal medulla, it produces catecholamines, mainly norepinephrine. It is classically described as hypertension associated with flushing, intermittent palpitations, headaches, and diaphoresis. The diagnostic test of choice when pheochromocytoma is suspected is a urinary screen of catecholamine levels, mainly metanephrine and vanillylmandelic acid (VMA). It is associated with both MEN IIa and MEN IIb syndromes and follows the general rule of "10s," in that 10% are malignant, 10% are bilateral, 10% occur in children, 10% have multiple tumors, and 10% are extraadrenal. The treatment is surgical resection, but patients must be pretreated with fluid resuscitation and α-antagonists to decrease vasoconstriction. Calcium-channel blockers are useful to treat hypertensive crises and α blockade for inoperable disease.**

A. Obtaining a CBC will not help further confirm the diagnosis of pheochromocytoma.

B. Calcium levels (total and ionized) are not important in the initial workup of the patient.

D. Liver function tests will not help further confirm the diagnosis of pheochromocytoma.

E. Serum calcitonin level is used to screen for medullary thyroid cancer.

71. **B. I^{131}-MIBG is a norepinephrine analog that will localize in pheochromocytomas. It is the most specific study available to localize this type of tumor. This scan is most often used when searching for extraadrenal, multiple, or malignant pheochromocytomas.**

A. A CT scan will localize the majority of pheochromocytomas. It is more sensitive, yet less specific, than the MIBG scan. It is less expensive but exposes the patient to radiation.

C. An MRI is also helpful in localizing these tumors, but it is less specific and more expensive than the MIBG scan.

D. A sestamibi scan is used to localize parathyroid adenomas.

E. Angiography is contraindicated in the localization of pheochromocytomas because it may precipitate a hypertensive crisis.

72. **A. Also known as an addisonian crisis, this should be considered in any patient with unexplained hypotension that does not respond to fluids and pressors. It occurs when the normal stress response of glucocorticoid release is impaired, and most often in individuals on long-term steroids experiencing the stress of illness or surgery. A chemistry panel may demonstrate decreased sodium and increased potassium due to decreased aldosterone production. Treatment consists of IV fluid hydration and IV hydrocortisone.**

B. The physical exam should demonstrate Beck's triad, which consists of muffled heart sounds, jugular venous distention, and hypotension with cardiac tamponade.

C. Pneumothorax would be evident on the chest x-ray.

D. Hypotension in sepsis is caused by decreased systemic vascular resistance. Pressors, such as levophed, should result in an increase in blood pressure.

E. The hypotension in this case is unresponsive to fluid challenges and therefore is not related to dehydration.

73. **E. Septic arthritis is the inflammation of a joint, which will eventually lead to the destruction of articular cartilage if untreated. The most common cause is *Staphylococcus aureus*. A notable exception to this cause is *Gonococcus*, seen in sexually active patients. Physical findings include joint pain with swelling, warmth to the touch, and decreased motion of the joint. Needle aspiration of the joint is the diagnostic test of choice. Aspirated contents should be observed for pus, and a culture and Gram stain obtained. Treatment consists of joint decompression and IV antibiotics.**

A. MRIs are expensive and time consuming when a needle aspiration is both diagnostic and therapeutic.

B. Physical therapy is inappropriate and would ultimately lead to irreparable damage to the joint.

C. One-week therapy with oral antibiotics is not sufficient treatment and the joint should be drained as well.

D. Treatment with NSAIDs alone is inappropriate for septic arthritis and would result in irreparable damage to the joint.

74. **E. Volkmann's contracture is a disastrous complication that is secondary to ischemic injury to the deep flexors of the forearm sustained during a supracondylar fracture of the humerus. The contracture results from insufficient arterial perfusion due to swelling and venous stasis followed by ischemic injury to the muscle. Irreversible muscle necrosis begins after 4 to 6 hours of compromised circulation. The necrotic muscle is replaced by scar tissue and causes contraction of the digits and wrist. Testing the compartment pressure will confirm the diagnosis early in the course. Delayed diagnosis or treatment can lead to this severely disabling condition. Other injuries that Volkmann's contracture is seen with are elbow fractures, burns, bleeding disorders, animal bites, and injections of medications into the forearm. Children are the classic group for this problem.**

A. Musculocutaneous nerve entrapment would lead to weakness of the biceps brachii muscle and loss of sensation on the lateral volar component of the forearm.

B. Radial head dislocation, also known as "nursemaid's" elbow, is most commonly seen in infants and young children after an adult pulls upward on their forearm. The child usually will not use the arm and holds it in a pronated position. Treatment consists of supination and extension of the elbow while applying firm pressure to the radial head.

C. A Dupuytren's contracture is not associated with a fracture. It is thickening and contracture of the palmar fascia.

D. Charcot's joint is usually due to peripheral neuropathy.

75. **D. The patient's x-ray demonstrates a humeral fracture and the clinical exam is consistent with radial nerve damage, as demonstrated by decreased sensation on the dorsum of the hand and an inability to extend the wrist. The radial nerve and brachial profunda artery (deep brachial artery) travel posterior to the humerus in the radial grove, and both may be damaged in a midhumeral shaft fracture. Physical findings suggesting vascular insufficiency due to injury include the 6 "Ps," pulselessness, pallor, pain, poikilothermia, paresthesia, and paralysis. Figure 5-75B represents a fracture of the humerus and a probable fracture of the greater tuberosity.**

A. The brachial artery is found medial to the humerus and usually is not involved in a midshaft fracture.

B. The ulnar artery is an artery of the forearm.

C. The axillary artery is too proximal to be involved.

E. The recurrent radial artery is a branch from the radial artery and is found lateral in the distal brachium. Although the artery courses with the radial nerve, this injury is more proximal in the brachium.

76. **C. All dysplastic nevi need to be biopsied because of an increased risk of developing melanoma.**

A. Patients with a family history of dysplastic nevi are at increased risk for melanoma, not squamous cell carcinoma.

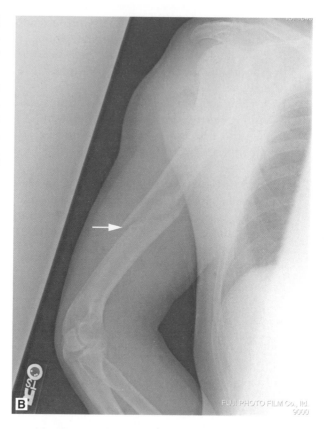

Figure 5-75B • Image Courtesy of the University of Utah School of Medicine, Salt Lake City, Utah.

B. Dysplastic nevi are variegated and usually have fuzzy borders.

D. Although all dysplastic nevi should be biopsied, it is not necessary to excise them all.

E. Dysplastic nevi are generally greater than 5 mm in diameter.

77. **E. Mallory-Weiss tears are upper GI hemorrhages that occur after retching or vomiting, resulting in longitudinal tears through the mucosa and submucosa near the GE junction. Fifty percent of cases are associated with alcohol consumption.**

A. Peptic ulcer disease is the most common cause of upper GI bleeding. This includes both duodenal and gastric ulcers. The history presented here is more consistent with a Mallory-Weiss tear.

B. Esophageal varices are a common cause of upper GI bleeding in patients with cirrhosis and portal hypertension. Bleeding from varices usually occurs spontaneous, not after, severe retching.

C. Angiodysplasias, also known as arteriovenous malformations, are vascular ectasias in the colonic mucosa that develop with aging. They are a common cause of lower GI bleeds, not upper GI bleeds.

D. Gastritis is a common cause of upper GI bleeds in many hospitalized patients. It is associated with painless upper GI bleeds and most are superficial, nonulcerating erosions.

F. A perforated peptic ulcer is unlikely in this scenario. At this point, the patient would most likely have a positive abdominal exam for peritoneal irritation. Significant abdominal pain would be the classic symptom in this case.

78. A. After ensuring that a patient is hemodynamically stable, as this patient is, proper initial diagnosis and management of an upper GI bleed includes placement of a nasogastric (NG) tube for gastric decompression and gastric lavage. In 90% of patients, bleeding stops and rebleeding is rare. In patients with continued bleeding, endoscopic electrocautery can be attempted. Surgery may be required in patients who continue to bleed or who are hemodynamically unstable.

B. Endoscopy with electrocautery is a valuable tool in diagnosis and management of an upper GI bleed; however, it is not the first step in management.

C. Sometimes used in esophageal variceal bleeds, balloon compression of the GE junction is contraindicated because it will propagate the tear.

D. An urgent procedure for bleeding should not be performed by laparoscopy, which would only visualize the external stomach.

E. In a life-threatening upper GI bleed, surgery may be indicated, but placement of an NG tube is the first step, followed by endoscopy if the patient is stable, to localize the source of the bleed before going to the operating room.

79. C. Seventy-five percent of Mallory-Weiss tears are located in the stomach near the GE junction.

A. A Mallory-Weiss tear does not occur in the upper esophagus. This is an injury involving the GE junction.

B. The majority of the remaining tears occurs in the distal esophagus at the GE junction.

D. Tears do not occur in the distal stomach, which is a common site for gastritis or ulcers.

E. Duodenal ulcers, not Mallory-Weiss tears, would be located in the first part of the duodenum.

80. D. Although multiple risk factors are associated with the development of pancreatic cancer, the most established risk factor is smoking. There is a two- to fivefold increased relative risk with heavy smoking. The triad of weight loss, icterus, and a palpable, nontender gallbladder, termed Courvoisier's sign, is classic for pancreatic head tumors.

A, B, C, E. Heavy alcohol consumption, diabetes mellitus, chronic pancreatitis, and exposure to benzidine and β-naphthylamine are suggested, but not proven, risk factors of pancreatic cancer.

81. A. Adenocarcinoma accounts for approximately 75% to 80% of all pancreatic cancers. Mucinous cystadenocarcinoma is the least common type of pancreatic tumor, occurring less than 1% of the time.

B. Mucinous cystadenocarcinoma accounts for fewer than 1% of pancreatic cancers.

C. Adenosquamous carcinoma accounts for 3%.

D. Giant-cell carcinoma accounts for 9%.

E. Mucinous carcinoma accounts for 2%.

F. Papillary cystic neoplasm of the pancreas is uncommon and occurs almost exclusively in young women in the first three decades. The incidence is also less than 1%. Frequently found incidentally, the tumor is most often large, and local invasion and metastases are uncommon. Surgical resection is the treatment of choice.

82. C. A CT scan of the abdomen with oral and IV contrast with a pancreatic phase scan, meaning a thin cut (3 to 5 mm) scan with no contrast phase, arterial phase, or venous phase scan is the best initial radiographic study. It can document the presence of the mass in the pancreas as well as help determine the extent of the disease and its resectability (see arrows in Figure 5-82).

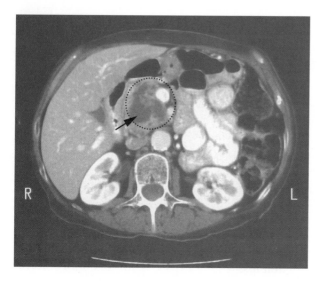

Figure 5-82 • Image Courtesy of the University of Utah School of Medicine, Salt Lake City, Utah.

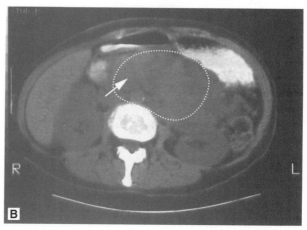

Figure 5-83B • Image Courtesy of the University of Utah School of Medicine, Salt Lake City, Utah.

A. Right upper quadrant ultrasound for jaundice and weight loss is much less specific in a patient who would require a CT eventually.

B. An upper GI might show duodenal involvement with tumor but is much less diagnostic for pancreatic masses.

D. MRI may be helpful at times but is not indicated as the initial study.

E. ERCP is useful for placement of a stent and tissue biopsy of a lesion in the head of the pancreas; however, it is not the initial study of choice.

83. **A.** This patient has findings consistent with a glucagonoma. The triad of findings are necrolytic migratory dermatitis, diabetes mellitus, and weight loss. They constitute 1% of all islet cell tumors. This tumor arises from the α cells of the pancreas. The mass is noted by the arrow in Figure 5-83B.

B. Insulinomas arise from β cells.

C. Somatostatinomas arise from D cells.

D. Vipomas arise from PP cells.

E. Gamma cells are not associated with APUD tumors.

84. **C.** An elevated plasma glucagon greater than 150 pg/mL is diagnostic of a glucagonoma. Many patients will have values in excess of 1000 pg/mL.

A. Elevated insulin levels after a prolonged fast are consistent with an insulinoma.

B. Secretin stimulation test is useful in diagnosiing a gastrinoma.

D. Fasting gastrin level is likewise useful in diagnosing a gastrinoma.

E. Fasting glucose level of greater than 126 mg/dL is diagnostic of diabetes

85. **C.** This patient has acute pancreatitis. Ranson's criteria are a set of specific values that are used as prognostic indicators (Table 5-85). Collected in the first 24 and 48 hours, they help to determine the severity of injury to the pancreas. There are five criteria obtained at admission and six others at 48 hours after admission. This patient has 6 of the 11 criteria, consistent with a 50% predicted mortality rate:

■ TABLE 5-85 Ranson Criteria	
On Admission	**During Initial 48 Hours**
Age >55	↓ Hematocrit >10 percentage points
WBC >16,000	↑ BUN >5 mg/dL
Blood glucose >200 mg/dL	↓ Calcium <8 mg/dL
Serum LDH >350 IU/L	Arterial PO$_2$ <60 mmHg
AST >250 IU/L	Base deficit >4 mEq/L
	Fluid sequestration >6 L

0–2 criteria = 0% mortality
3–4 criteria = 15% mortality
5–6 criteria = 50% mortality
>7 criteria = 100% mortality

A, B, D, E. These are all incorrect. See explanation for C.

86. D. Posterior hip dislocations are the most common type of hip dislocations. If no associated fracture exists, the leg will be internally rotated and there can be a palpable posterior fullness. Initial treatment consists of emergent closed reduction to avoid posterior avascular necrosis that occurs with 15% of posterior dislocations. Note the arrow in Figure 5-86B.

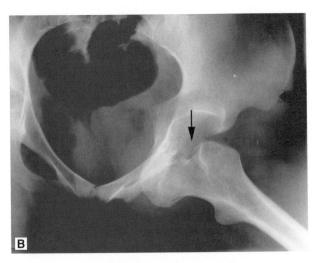

Figure 5-86B • Image Courtesy of the University of Utah School of Medicine, Salt Lake City, Utah.

A. Fat emboli are usually seen with long bone fractures.
B. Joint calcification is not an acute event.
C. Sciatic nerve injury may also occur, but usually at the time of dislocation.
E. Osteomyelitis is not a concern in this particular setting.

87. F. The majority, or over two-thirds, of patients with hyperparathyroidism and hypercalcemia are detected during routine screening. Previously thought to be rare, primary hyperparathyroidism is now found in 0.1% to 0.3% of the general population, and it is the most common cause of hypercalcemia in unselected patients. Peak incidence occurs between the third and fifth decades, and it is two to three times more common in women. When patients do present with symptoms they can be numerous, including kidney stones, ulcers, pancreatitis, cholelithiasis, constipation, hypertension, shortened QT, decreased heart rate, weakness, fatigue, and depression. A very careful history should be taken to review vague symptomatology. After successful surgical treatment, patients who thought that they were asymptomatic become aware of generalized improvement in symptoms such as fatigue, constipation, and joint pain.

A. Shortened, not prolonged, QT on ECG can be associated with this condition.
B. Constipation, rather than diarrhea, can be seen in this condition.
C. Fatigue and weakness are sometimes seen with this condition, not anxiety.
D. Hypertension, not hypotension, can be seen with this condition.
E. Depression is sometimes seen in hyperparathyroidism, but most often there are no presenting symptoms.

88. E. The issue of localization of the parathyroid gland before going to the operating room is controversial. Localization is not thought to increase the success of surgery if an experienced surgeon takes the time to achieve adequate exposure and visualization of the glands.

A, B, C, D. All of the listed studies are ways of localizing the parathyroid glands, with the Sestamibi scan being the most frequently used. Controversy remains as to whether any localization studies before surgery are needed; therefore, none of the studies listed must be obtained.

89. B. Groin hernias, such as in this scenario, present with incarceration in approximately 10% of cases.

A, D, E. Groin hernias are more common in men and in Caucasians, and they occur most frequently on the right side.
C. Hernias will not get better on their own; rather, they will get larger with time. Complications such as bowel obstruction, incarceration, and strangulation may occur.

90. D. A sliding hernia occurs when the hernia sac is partially formed by the wall of a viscus.

91. B. A lumbar hernia is a hernia through either Petit's triangle or the Grynfeltt-Lesshaft triangle.

92. E. An internal hernia involves an intraabdominal structure.

93. A. A pantaloon hernia occurs when the hernia sac is both a direct and an indirect hernia, straddling the inferior epigastric vessels.

94. C. A hiatal hernia is a hernia through the esophageal hiatus.

95. B. The Breslow thickness is the principal prognostic factor associated with a melanotic lesion. The Breslow thickness of a malignant melanoma is used to estimate prognosis. It is measured from the surface to the deepest point of invasion. Table 5-95 lists the guidelines for the required margin of resection for various depths of melanoma. Punch or incisional biopsies are used to establish the diagnosis in large lesions prior to definitive resection. Overall, the requirement of extremely wide margins in skin grafts or flap closures has become more conservative based on lack of benefit.

■ TABLE 5-95 Surgical Margin Guidelines	
Primary Tumor Thickness	Margin
In situ	0.5 cm
≤1 mm	1 cm
>1 to ≤4 mm	2 cm
>4 mm	2 to 3 cm

A. This is incorrect based on the current guidelines.
C. Cryosurgery or electrodissection should never be used in suspected melanomas.
D. The need for regional lymphadenectomy is determined by results of sentinel node biopsies, not depth of invasion.
E. Frozen sections are inappropriate in establishing melanoma depth.

96. D. Manometry is used to diagnose achalasia. As the recording catheter is withdrawn from the stomach into the esophagus, in achalasia the lower esophageal sphincter (LES) fails to completely relax with swallow and esophageal peristalsis is absent. Note the manometry tracing in Figure 5-96A; the LES pressure never returns to baseline on the lowest tracing and esophageal peristalsis is absent because there is high pressure with swallow at the upper, mid, and distal esophagus. Also note the barium swallow seen in Figure 5-96B, with the classic "bird's beak" finding. Performing a Nissen fundoplication in a patient with achalasia will make the stricture worse.

A. Enteroclysis is used to localize obstructions or other lesions of the small bowel.
B. A CT of the chest and abdomen would not be helpful in this situation.
C. Esophageal pH probe monitoring is helpful in diagnosing GER, but not achalasia.
E. A chest x-ray would not be helpful in ruling out achalasia.

97. B. Tongue-like extensions of epithelium, extending from the stomach into the distal esophagus, are suggestive of Barrett's esophagus. Barrett's esophagus is a premalignant lesion, which results in metaplasia of the esophageal mucosa with chronical exposure to gastric acid. Management starts with H_2 blockers or proton pump inhibitors, with surgical intervention if medical therapy fails.

A. Esophageal stricture is seen as a narrowing in the distal esophagus distinct from mucosal surface change.
C. *Candida* esophagitis usually involves more than the distal esophagus, with white plaques that can be extensive in the proximal esophagus.
D. Esophageal carcinoma presents as a mass or stricture at the distal esophagus and is diagnosed by a tissue biopsy.
E. Mallory-Weiss tears appear as discrete lacerations just below the GE junction, which cause hematemesis after severe vomiting or retching.

98. C. Diffuse esophageal spasm is strong nonperistaltic contractions of the esophagus resulting in anginalike pain, which is relieved by nitrates. It is usually just as severe with solids as with liquids. Sphincter tone and function are normal in 75% of patients.

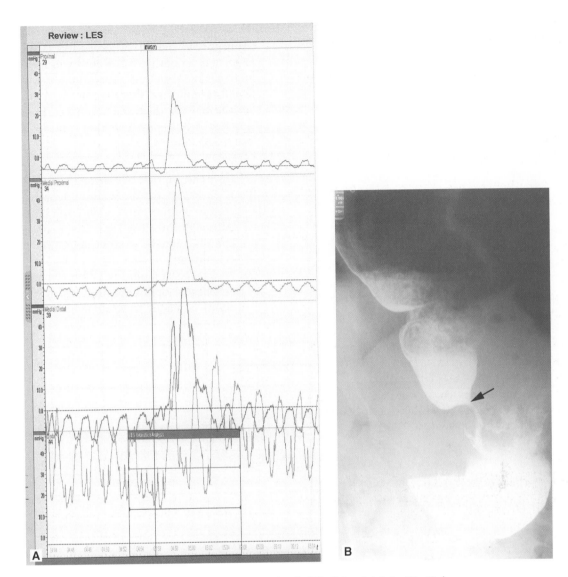

Figure 5-96 A-B • Images Courtesy of the University of Utah School of Medicine, Salt Lake City, Utah.

A. Achalasia presents with dysphagia and effortless regurgitation after a meal, not spasmlike chest pain.

B. Esophageal perforation, or Boerhaave syndrome, is a distal esophageal perforation due to barotrauma from violent retching.

D. Esophageal cancer often presents with dysphagia and is not relieved by nitrates.

E. Zenker's diverticulum is defined as a cervical esophageal diverticulum, which may lead to dysphagia, regurgitation of food, and severe halitosis.

99. A. Barium esophagram of a diffuse esophageal spasm classically shows a "corkscrew esophagus," with muscular hypertrophy sometimes noted on a double contrast study. Note the arrows in Figure 5-99B.

B. A bird's beak sign on X-ray is seen in achalasia.

C. A double bubble sign is seen on X-ray in duodenal atresia.

D. Esophageal outpouching is consistent with an esophageal diverticulum.

E. Normal esophagram would help rule out diffuse esophageal spasm.

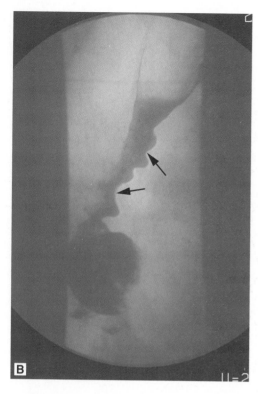

Figure 5-99B • Image Courtesy of the University of Utah School of Medicine, Salt Lake City, Utah.

100. **D. Ingestion of liquid alkali usually does not damage the mouth or oropharynx; therefore, ingestion cannot be ruled out by evaluating the oral cavity. Vomiting should not be induced. Esophagraphy and EGD are necessary to evaluate the injury to the distal esophagus. Esophageal stricture is the most common sequela of alkali esophageal injury.**

A. Perforation is possible, but uncommon, in the consumption of caustic materials.

B. Hemorrhage is likewise not the primary concern in consumption of an alkali liquid.

C. Although infection is always a concern, the complication of a stricture is much more concerning.

E. Nutcracker esophagus is similar to diffuse esophageal spasm, a motility problem in adults unrelated to alkali ingestion as a child.

BLOCK 3

The next three questions (items 101 to 103) correspond to the following vignette.

A 17-year-old male presents to the ED with a 14-hour history of abdominal pain. The patient says the pain began periumbilically as a dull ache, but has since migrated to the right lower quadrant becoming a sharp, constant pain. The patient is anorexic and the pain is associated with emesis. On exam, he feels warm to touch, is ill appearing, and tachycardic. There is localized rebound tenderness in the right lower quadrant, and a positive Rovsing's sign. A CBC demonstrates a leukocytosis of 11,000.

101. The most appropriate next step in the management of this patient is
    A. CT scan of the abdomen
    B. IV hydration and observation
    C. Surgical exploration
    D. Abdominal ultrasound
    E. Oral antibiotics and follow-up in 2 days

102. Overall, the most common etiology of the disease seen in this patient is luminal occlusion secondary to
    A. Fecalith
    B. Lymphoid hyperplasia
    C. Foreign body
    D. Tumor
    E. Parasites

103. If a 1.5-cm carcinoid tumor is found at the distal appendiceal tip, what further treatment should be implemented in this patient?
    A. Right hemicolectomy
    B. Radiation therapy
    C. Chemotherapy
    D. Octreotide infusion
    E. No further treatment is necessary

End of Set

The next two questions (items 104 and 105) correspond to the following vignette.

You are called to see a 30-year-old male in the ED complaining of anal pain. On examination, the patient states the pain began yesterday afternoon and is worse with defecation; he also denies fever, chills, constipation, or any traumatic injury to the area. The patient is otherwise healthy, denies allergies, and is not taking any medication. On physical examination, you find an indurated, erythematous area lateral to the anus that is extremely tender to touch and fluctuant.

104. The next best step in management is
    A. CT scan of the abdomen and pelvis
    B. IV antibiotics and observation
    C. Incision and drainage
    D. Warm sitz baths
    E. Oral antibiotics and observation

105. The important surgical landmark in the anus where embryologic ectoderm has fused with embryologic endoderm is known as the
    A. Columns of Morgagni
    B. Valves of Houston
    C. Anal crypts
    D. Dentate line
    E. Ischiorectal fossa

End of Set

The next three questions (items 106 to 108) correspond to the following vignette.

A 58-year-old male with a history of alcoholic cirrhosis is admitted to the hospital with fevers and abdominal pain. Labs are as follows: WBC 15,500, total bilirubin 1.9 mg/dL, PT 18 seconds, serum albumin 2.4 g/dL. The patient does not have encephalopathy.

106. Which of the following signs of portal hypertension is rarely a cause of secondary complications?
    A. Caput medusae
    B. Hemorrhoids
    C. Esophageal varices
    D. Splenic vein thrombosis
    E. Ascites

107. While in the hospital, the patient develops an upper GI bleed. An endoscopy is performed and the bleeding vessels are sclerosed. If this patient continues to have problems with upper GI bleeds, operative intervention will be required. Which of the following is considered a selective shunt with a lower rate of encephalopathy?
    A. Transjugular intrahepatic portal systemic shunt
    B. Mesocaval shunt "H" graft
    C. Warren distal splenorenal shunt
    D. Side-to-side portocaval shunt
    E. Pett "T" shunt

108. Based on this patient's Child's class, the operative mortality for placement of a portacaval shunt is what percentage?

   A. Less than 5%
   B. 10%
   C. 25%
   D. 50%
   E. 80%

End of Set

The next two questions (items 109 and 110) correspond to the following vignette.

A 67-year-old male returns to the ER 2 weeks after having undergone a Whipple resection for a pancreatic head mass. The patient is somnolent and confused. Vital signs are as follows: T 102.6°F, HR 115, BP 87/45, RR 25, and SaO_2 94% on RA. On exam, his abdomen is found to be distended and tender in the right upper quadrant. A CBC reveals a WBC of 18,000. The patient is transported to the ICU, where aggressive fluid resuscitation is initiated, and after receiving 4 L of crystalloid, his BP remains 88/47.

109. What is the most likely cause of this patient's hypotension?

   A. Hypovolemia
   B. Depressed cardiac function
   C. Decreased autonomic innervation
   D. Loss of systemic vascular resistance

110. What is the most appropriate diagnostic step?

   A. Exploratory laparotomy
   B. Abdominal CT scan
   C. ERCP
   D. Percutaneous transhepatic cholangiogram
   E. Abdominal ultrasound

End of Set

The next two questions (items 111 and 112) correspond to the following vignette.

A 45-year-old man presents to the ER with a 3-day history of crampy abdominal pain associated with nausea and vomiting. The patient denies fever or chills, and states he has not had a bowel movement for 3 days and has passed little gas over the last day. The medical history is significant for exploratory laparotomy following a gunshot wound to the abdomen 3 years ago. On exam, his abdomen is found to be distended and tender to palpation, and there are no peritoneal signs. There is a well-healed midline scar without an underlying hernia, and no groin hernias are appreciated. Vital signs include T 37.5(C, HR 105, and BP 124/73. WBC is 7000 and lactate is 1.0 mmol/L. The following abdominal films are obtained (Figure 5-111A and B).

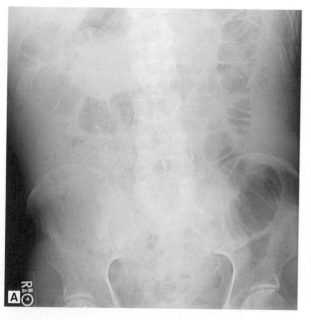
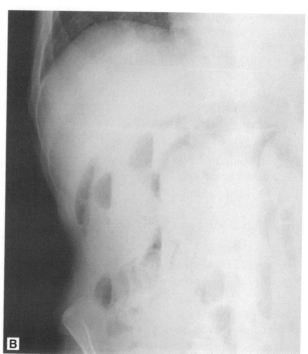

Figure 5-111A and B • Image Courtesy of the University of Utah School of Medicine, Salt Lake City, Utah.

111. Which of the following would be the most appropriate next step in management?

    A. Barium enema
    B. Admission, NG tube decompression, IV hydration, electrolyte repletion
    C. Abdominal paracentesis and lavage
    D. Oral cathartics and enemas until clear
    E. UGI series with barium

112. In order of decreasing frequency, which of the following are the most common causes of this patient's clinical problem?

    A. Cancer, hernias, adhesions
    B. Adhesions, hernias, cancer
    C. Hernias, cancer, adhesions
    D. Adhesions, cancer, hernias
    E. Cancer, adhesions, hernias

End of Set

The next two questions (items 113 and 114) correspond to the following vignette.

You are asked to evaluate a 12-hour-old female, born to a 35-year-old G_4P_4 mother. The pregnancy was complicated by polyhydramnios and the infant is 2 weeks premature. The infant began having bilious vomiting shortly after the first feeding. An abdominal plain film demonstrated a dilated, air-filled stomach and first portion of the duodenum. No air is noted within the colon.

113. The most likely diagnosis is:

    A. Pyloric stenosis
    B. Esophageal atresia
    C. Duodenal atresia
    D. Meconium ileus
    E. Intestinal malrotation

114. Preoperatively, it is imperative which of the following should be done?

    A. Mechanical and chemical bowel preparation
    B. Bronchoscopy
    C. Thorough search for other congenital anomalies, especially cardiac malformations
    D. Gastrografin enemas
    E. Abdominal CT scan

End of Set

115. A 26-year-old male is brought to the trauma bay after being ejected from an all-terrain vehicle (ATV). The patient is intact mentally and answers questions appropriately. Primary survey reveals an intact airway, bilateral clear breath sounds, palpable femoral pulses, and an inability to feel or move any extremity. The patient states he has no sensation below his clavicles. Vital signs are: T 37.3°C, HR 55, and BP 84/42. Fluid resuscitation with crystalloid is initiated. Secondary survey reveals cervical spine tenderness. The abdomen is soft, nondistended, and nontender, and the FAST exam is negative. Two liters of crystalloid are infused without improvement in blood pressure. The most likely cause of this patient's persistent hypotension is

    A. Depressed cardiac function
    B. Decreased autonomic innervation
    C. Septic shock due to multiple trauma
    D. Hypovolemia

The next two questions (items 116 and 117) correspond to the following vignette.

A 27-year-old female presents to the ED with a 24-hour history of intense lower abdominal pain. The patient states the pain actually began 2 weeks ago, starting in the left lower quadrant, with rapid progression over the last 24 hours. The patient states she has been febrile, without nausea or vomiting, and has had multiple loose stools and a burning sensation with urination. There has been no vaginal discharge and her last menstrual period was 10 days prior. The patient has been sexually active with three partners within the past year. The patient reports that she is not currently taking any medications and denies allergies. Physical exam reveals a toxic-appearing patient with diffuse tenderness in the lower abdomen. There are no peritoneal signs and the rectal exam is normal. Pelvic exam reveals discharge from the cervical os. The following CT scan is obtained (Figure 5-116A).

116. What is the most likely diagnosis?

    A. Acute appendicitis
    B. Acute diverticulitis
    C. Ruptured ovarian cyst
    D. Tuboovarian abscess (TOA)
    E. Ectopic pregnancy

117. What organism is most likely responsible for this patient's disease process?

    A. *Staphylococcus saprophyticus*
    B. *Escherichia coli*
    C. *Pseudomonas aeruginosa*
    D. *Neisseria gonorrhoeae*
    E. *Clostridium difficile*

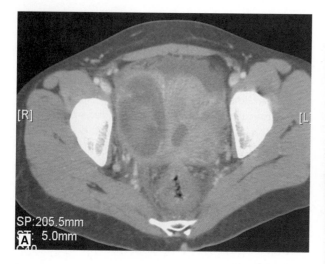

Figure 5-116A • Image Courtesy of the University of Utah School of Medicine, Salt Lake City, Utah.

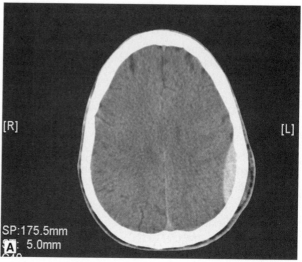

Figure 5-118A • Image Courtesy of the University of Utah School of Medicine, Salt Lake City, Utah.

End of Set

The next two questions (items 118 and 119) correspond to the following vignette.

A 55-year-old male is brought to the ER by ambulance after falling 12 feet onto his head from a roof while placing Christmas lights. According to the patient's family, when they found the patient outside the house he was cooperative but appeared dazed. After he came inside and participated in his usual activities he began slurring his speech and having difficulty walking. Paramedics were called and at the time of their arrival the patient's GCS was 14. By arrival to the ED, the patient has become lethargic and difficult to awaken. The ER staff has intubated the patient to protect his airway. After completing the primary assessment, the secondary survey is remarkable for a fixed, dilated right pupil as well as a bruise over the right temporal area. The patient is taken to radiology for a CT scan (Figure 5-118A).

118. What is the etiology of this patient's current condition?

    A. Rupture of lenticulostriate arteries
    B. Disruption of the middle meningeal artery
    C. Transection of the cerebral veins
    D. Rupture of a cerebral aneurysm

119. What is the most appropriate management option for this patient?

    A. Evacuation of the hematoma
    B. Angiographic embolization
    C. Ventriculostomy
    D. Mannitol and hyperventilation
    E. No treatment is necessary

End of Set

120. A 46-year-old woman is postoperative day 1 after undergoing an exploratory laparotomy with lysis of adhesions for an acute small bowel obstruction. The nurse is calling you because the patient has spiked a fever of 38.6°C. What is the most likely source of the patient's fever?

    A. UTI
    B. Pneumonia
    C. Wound infection
    D. Atelectasis
    E. Intraabdominal abscess

The next two questions (items 121 and 122) correspond to the following vignette.

You are asked by the hematology service to evaluate a 33-year-old female recently (6 weeks ago) diagnosed with idiopathic thrombocytopenic purpura (ITP) after presenting with ecchymoses and a platelet count of 25,000. Since diagnosis, she has been treated with corticosteroids and IVIG, but she continues to require high-dose steroids and daily platelet transfusion to maintain a platelet count above 20,000. After you discuss the options with the patient, she elects to undergo a laparoscopic splenectomy.

121. The splenic artery is a direct branch of which of the following?

    A. Gastroduodenal artery
    B. Superior mesenteric artery
    C. Inferior mesenteric artery
    D. Inferior phrenic artery
    E. Celiac axis

122. After splenectomy, this patient will be more susceptible to infection by which organisms?

    A. *Pseudomonas aeruginosa, Escherichia coli, Klebsiella pneumonia*
    B. *Clostridium difficile, Listeria monocytogenes*
    C. *Streptococcus pneumoniae, Hemophilus influenzae, Meningococcus*
    D. *Entameba histolytica, Echinoccocus granulosum*
    E. *Staphylococcus aureus, Staphylococcus epidermidis*

End of Set

123. One of your splenectomy patients returns to the ED on postoperative day 10 with dull abdominal pain and fever. The patient complains of abdominal distention, denies any nausea and vomiting, but she has been able to eat and is having normal bowel movements. On laboratory examination, the liver transaminases are mildly elevated. The results of an abdominal CT are shown in Figure 5-123A. What is the most appropriate step in management?

    A. Anticoagulation
    B. Antibiotics
    C. Exploratory laparotomy
    D. Bowel rest, IV hydration, and observation
    E. No treatment is necessary

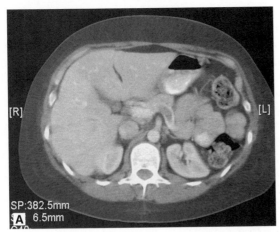

Figure 5-123A • Image Courtesy of the University of Utah School of Medicine, Salt Lake City, Utah.

124. Another of your patients who has been on TPN for several days suddenly develops glucose intolerance, requiring increasing insulin support to maintain blood glucose levels within a reasonable range. What is the most likely cause?

    A. Pharmacy error
    B. Short gut syndrome
    C. Infection
    D. Pancreatitis
    E. Occult diabetes mellitus

The next three questions (items 125 to 127) correspond to the following vignette.

A 31-year-old male sets himself on fire after breaking up with his girlfriend, sustaining a 63% total body surface area burn. The patient is transferred to your facility where he undergoes standard burn fluid resuscitation with Ringer's lactate and albumin. Expecting a long complicated hospital recovery, you place a feeding tube on hospital day 2.

125. How much protein do you anticipate this patient will require?

    A. 0.5 to 0.8 g/kg/day
    B. 0.8 to 1.0 g/kg/day
    C. 1.0 to 1.5 g/kg/day
    D. 1.5 to 2.5 g/kg/day
    E. 2.5 to 3.5 g/kg/day

126. Secondary to enteral feeding intolerance and a prolonged ileus, the patient is started on total parenteral nutrition (TPN). After 2 weeks, the patient is having multiple loose stools and you notice generalized dermatitis and alopecia. Which mineral is the patient most likely deficient in?

    A. Selenium
    B. Zinc
    C. Copper
    D. Manganese
    E. Chromium

127. Three weeks later, you are struggling to wean the patient from the ventilator. The following laboratory results are obtained: Na 143 mmol/L, K 4.2 mmol/L, Cl 103 mmol/L, HCO_3 30 mmol/L, BUN 12 mg/dL, Cr 1.0 mg/dL, glucose 145 mg/dL, Ca 8.5 mg/dL, Mg 2.3 mmol/L, and PO_4 3.0 mg/dL. The most recent morning chest x-ray shows no acute pulmonary process. What complication related to TPN use may be contributing to the patient's respiratory failure?

A. Hyperglycemia
B. Increased CO_2 production
C. Hypophosphatemia
D. Pancreatitis
E. Respiratory alkalosis

End of Set

The next three questions (items 128 and 130) correspond to the following vignette.

A 48-year-old male is brought to your ED by air transport after being stabbed multiple times in the abdomen. The patient is hemodynamically stable as you take him to the operating room for an exploratory laparotomy. The patient is found to have injuries to the spleen, stomach, left kidney, jejunum, and descending colon. There is gross spillage of bowel contents into the abdomen. You irrigate the abdomen until it is clear before closing, but you are still concerned about the possibility of a wound infection.

128. Which injury places this patient at highest risk for a wound infection?

A. Spleen
B. Stomach
C. Jejunum
D. Descending colon
E. Kidney

129. Of the following, which combination of factors is most important in the choice of either primary repair of the colon injury or temporary colostomy?

A. Age and history of diabetes mellitus
B. Steroid use and prolonged time in surgery
C. Poor nutritional status and smoking
D. Degree of contamination and time between injury and repair
E. History of cancer and previous chemotherapy

130. On postoperative day 10 your patient develops a fever of 39.2°C and is complaining of increasing abdominal tenderness. What is the most likely cause of the patient's fever?

A. UTI
B. Pneumonia
C. Intraabdominal abscess
D. Deep venous thrombosis
E. Atelectasis

End of Set

The next two questions (items 131 and 132) correspond to the following vignette.

A 75-year-old male is 3 days postsurgical resection of a ruptured abdominal aortic aneurysm. You are called emergently to the surgical ICU because the patient has become progressively hypotensive. The patient's BP is 84/56, which is down from 136/76 an hour ago. While giving the patient a fluid bolus, you insert a pulmonary artery catheter and obtain the following pulmonary artery values: a cardiac index of 2.0 L/minute/M^2, a CVP of 15 mmHg, a PCWP of 18 mmHg, and an SVR of 1400 dynes∗second/cm^5.

131. Which type of shock is the patient experiencing?

A. Hypovolemic shock
B. Neurogenic shock
C. Septic shock
D. Cardiogenic shock
E. Obstructive shock

132. What is the most appropriate next step in the treatment of this patient?

A. IV fluids
B. Blood transfusion
C. Dobutamine drip
D. Norepinephrine drip
E. Nitroprusside drip

End of Set

The next two questions (items 133 and 134) correspond to the following vignette.

A 65-year-old female with resolving necrotizing pancreatitis has had a prolonged ICU stay. Most recently, a 21-day course of antibiotics for pneumonia complicated by *Pseudomonas aeruginosa* was completed. The patient has a tracheostomy button in place, is on nasal cannula, is ambulating with assistance from physical therapy, and is receiving nutritional support via a jejunostomy tube. Over the last 3 days, the patient has had voluminous, foul-smelling diarrhea. Earlier in the day a temperature of 38.8°C was recorded and the morning CBC reveals a leukocytosis of 18,000.

133. What would be the first most appropriate test to obtain the likely diagnosis?

A. Serum antibody titer
B. CT scan
C. Stool toxin assay
D. Colonoscopy
E. Stool culture

134. What is the most appropriate choice of therapy?

    A. Loperamide
    B. Oral metronidazole
    C. IV vancomycin
    D. Cefazolin
    E. Piperacillin-tazobactam

End of Set

The next three questions (items 135 to 137) correspond to the following vignette.

A 25-year-old female, while riding her bike, is struck by a truck traveling at 40 mph. On her arrival in the ED, the paramedic reports that her blood pressure has been falling over the last 5 minutes; currently it is 62/36 with an HR of 145. The patient tells you that her abdomen and chest are hurting and you notice left-sided rib retraction with inspiration.

135. What is the first step in managing this seriously injured patient?

    A. IV fluid bolus for hypotension
    B. Blood transfusion for hypotension
    C. Chest x-ray
    D. Airway management
    E. Placement of a central line

136. The physical findings of this patient's chest exam are concerning for what injury?

    A. Hemothorax
    B. Pneumothorax
    C. Open pneumothorax
    D. Tension pneumothorax
    E. Flail chest

137. You determine the patient needs a left thoracostomy tube. On placement of the chest tube, 1600 mL of gross blood is evacuated from the pleural space. What is the most likely cause of the bleeding?

    A. Pulmonary laceration
    B. Esophageal perforation
    C. Intercostal artery tear
    D. Aortic transection
    E. Cardiac rupture

End of Set

The next three questions (items 138 to 140) correspond to the following vignette.

A 17-year-old male is brought in to the ER after the horse he was riding fell and rolled over onto him. The patient is hypotensive, difficult to rouse, with obvious bruising on his distended upper abdomen. An open fracture of his right lower leg has soaked the dressing with blood.

138. What is the first step in management of this patient?

    A. Apply direct pressure to the bleeding from his leg
    B. Perform emergent laparotomy
    C. Transfuse 2 units packed RBCs
    D. Intubate the patient
    E. Infuse 2 L crystalloid solution

139. After the patient is stabilized in the trauma bay, he is taken to the CT scanner; Figure 5-139A shows the scan obtained. What injury are you most concerned about after seeing this scan?

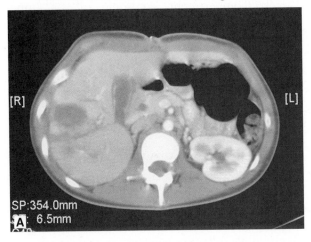

Figure 5-139A • Image Courtesy of the University of Utah School of Medicine, Salt Lake City, Utah.

    A. Liver laceration
    B. Splenic laceration
    C. Intraperitoneal bladder rupture
    D. Left renal devascularization
    E. Internal iliac artery injury

140. Despite a transfusion of 5 units of RBCs and 6 L of crystalloid in the first 2 hours, the patient remains in shock. What is the best management of this patient's condition?

    A. Angiographic embolization
    B. Exploratory laparotomy
    C. Suprapubic catheter placement
    D. Observation

End of Set

The next two questions (items 141 and 142) correspond to the following vignette.

A 28-year-old male is rescued by firefighters from his burning home. The patient has sustained minor burns to his face, neck, and upper extremities and is brought to the ER by ambulance. Initial evaluation reveals that the burns are estimated to be 8% total body surface area (TBSA), and the patient is speaking and coherent, with the following vital signs: BP 145/82, HR 122, RR 24, and SaO_2 of 100% on 2 L nasal cannula.

141. What are you most concerned about in this patient?

   A. Rhabdomyolysis
   B. Infection of burns
   C. Fluid losses from his burn wounds
   D. Inhalation injury
   E. Compartment syndrome of his upper extremities

142. What is the best method to evaluate the severity of this patient's injury?

   A. Central venous pressure monitoring
   B. Urine myoglobin
   C. Sputum Gram stain and cultures
   D. Bronchoscopy
   E. Evaluation of compartment pressures in his upper extremities

End of Set

The next two questions (items 143 and 144) correspond to the following vignette.

A 66-year-old previously healthy male presents to your office for evaluation of a gastric carcinoma, which was found after the patient underwent an upper endoscopy during a workup for anemia. The patient reports that he has had frequent emesis over the last 3 months and a 20-lb weight loss. The tumor is located in the gastric antrum and a CT, which was also done, shows some enlarged perigastric lymph nodes, but no evidence of distant metastasis.

143. Where are the most common locations for tumors in the stomach to occur?

   A. One-quarter in the antrum, one-quarter in the body, and one-half in the cardia

B. One-half in the antrum, one-quarter in the body, and one-quarter in the cardia
   C. One-third in the antrum, one-third in the body, and one-third in the cardia
   D. One-third in the antrum, two-thirds in the body, and none in the cardia
   E. One-quarter in the antrum, one-half in the body, and one-quarter in the cardia
   F. None in the antrum, one-half in the body, and one-half in the cardia

144. The patient undergoes a partial gastrectomy with a relatively uncomplicated postoperative course. At the second follow-up clinic visit, the patient complains of nausea, vomiting, and abdominal cramping occurring 20 to 30 minutes after eating meals. Further questioning reveals that these symptoms are accompanied by lightheadedness and palpitations. What is the most likely cause of these symptoms?

   A. Rapid emptying of stomach
   B. Hypoglycemia
   C. Pancreatitis
   D. Acute cholecystitis
   E. Gastric outlet obstruction

End of Set

The next two questions (items 145 and 146) correspond to the following vignette.

You reevaluate a 44-year-old woman complaining of severe epigastric pain radiating to her back. The patient has recently been consuming at least a quart of hard liquor a day. The patient is unable to tolerate a diet because of persistent nausea and vomiting. A CBC and BMP are normal, and her lipase is 3545 U/L. Repeat CT scan reveals only pancreatic edema with good pancreatic perfusion. The patient is admitted to the hospital for acute pancreatitis. During the first 24 hours of hospitalization, her urine output begins to decrease. Blood pressure gradually drops to 80s/40s and she becomes tachycardic in the 120s.

145. What is the most likely cause of her hypotension?

   A. Neurogenic shock
   B. Obstructive shock
   C. Hypovolemic shock
   D. Cardiogenic shock
   E. Septic shock

146. The patient is transferred to the ICU and a pulmonary artery (PA) catheter and an arterial catheter are placed. Which of the following PA calculations are most consistent with this type of shock?

$$CVP = mmHg, PCWP = mmHg, CI = L/minute/M^2, SVR = dynes*second/cm^5$$

   A. CVP 3, PCWP 8, CI 1.9, SVR 1600
   B. CVP 4, PCWP 12, CI 2.5, SVR 1000
   C. CVP 3, PCWP 9, CI 1.5, SVR 500
   D. CVP 16, PCWP 22, CI 1.5, SVR 1500
   E. CVP 3, PCWP 10, CI 4.3, SVR 430

End of Set

The next four questions (items 147 to 150) correspond to the following vignette.

A 68-year-old female comes to the ED with a 4-day history of fevers, left lower quadrant pain, decreased appetite, and frequent nausea and vomiting. The patient's bowel function has been relatively normal with occasional diarrhea. Medications taken include Lisinopril for hypertension, atorvastatin for hypercholesterolemia, and phenytoin for a seizure history. There is no significant surgical history. The patient's WBC is 16,000 and she is hyponatremic. A CT scan of the abdomen and pelvis shows inflammatory changes consistent with diverticulitis and a possible abscess. The patient is admitted to the hospital for dehydration and IV antibiotics.

147. At what level of hyponatremia would you expect a patient to begin having symptoms?

   A. 115 mEq/L
   B. 120 mEq/L
   C. 125 mEq/L
   D. 130 mEq/L
   E. 135 mEq/L

148. What devastating neurologic condition may develop if sodium is corrected too rapidly?

   A. Spinal cord edema
   B. Cerebral edema
   C. Central pontine myelinolysis
   D. Grand mal seizure
   E. Permanent peripheral neuropathy

149. In addition to admitting this patient and treating for acute diverticulitis, you need to correct the sodium level. Knowing the neurologic effects that may occur from correcting the sodium too rapidly, you are careful in your choice of fluid replacement. Which of the following choices raises the risk for developing the devastating neurologic changes?

   A. Smoking history
   B. Malnutrition
   C. Correcting sodium greater than 1.5 mEq/L/hour
   D. Seizure history
   E. Correcting sodium greater than 10 mEq/L/day

150. If the patient's sodium is 168 mEq/L, what devastating injury may occur with too rapid correction of the sodium?

   A. Spinal cord edema
   B. Cerebral edema
   C. Central pontine myelinolysis
   D. Grand mal seizure
   E. Permanent peripheral neuropathy

End of Set

A

Answers and Explanations

101. C	118. B	135. D
102. B	119. A	136. E
103. E	120. D	137. C
104. C	121. E	138. D
105. D	122. C	139. A
106. A	123. A	140. B
107. C	124. C	141. D
108. B	125. D	142. D
109. D	126. B	143. C
110. B	127. B	144. A
111. B	128. D	145. C
112. B	129. D	146. A
113. C	130. C	147. B
114. C	131. D	148. C
115. B	132. C	149. B
116. D	133. C	150. B
117. D	134. B	

101. C. Acute appendicitis is a common surgical emergency, and it is the most common surgical emergency in children and adolescents. Clinical findings include abdominal pain that usually begins periumbilically and localizes to the right lower quadrant within several hours. This pain is classically accompanied by anorexia with nausea and vomiting. Ninety percent of patients will have a leukocyte count greater than 10,000. The arrow in Figure 5-101 points to a cross-section of an acutely inflamed, fluid-filled appendix. Thickened walls with a diameter greater than 6 mm and periappendiceal fat stranding are usually observed. Acute appendicitis is managed surgically, and this patient warrants a surgical exploration. An appendectomy can be performed using a laparoscopic or open technique.

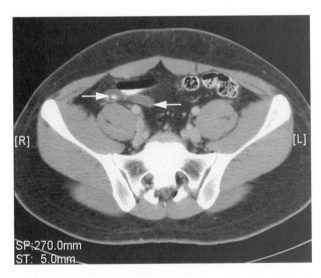

Figure 5-101 • Image Courtesy of the University of Utah School of Medicine, Salt Lake City, Utah.

  A. The clinical presentation, physical exam, and laboratory findings are highly suspicious for appendicitis and this patient should proceed to the operating room. A CT scan of the pelvis with rectal contrast is becoming an important tool in diagnosing acute appendicitis in those patients with atypical symptoms, but it is not needed for this classic case. A CT scan of the abdomen may be helpful in patients with atypical or nonspecific findings.
  B. Although IV hydration is required, the natural progression of acute appendicitis is on to perforation, which greatly increases the risk of morbidity and mortality, making observation an unreasonable choice.
  D. Abdominal ultrasound is especially helpful in diagnosing lower abdominal pain in women of reproductive age and in children. The procedure is user dependent and is not as reliable as a CT scan.
  E. Acute appendicitis is a surgical emergency; consequently, oral antibiotics with follow-up is an inappropriate course of care.

102. B. Luminal obstruction of the appendix is the most common cause of appendicitis in children and results in vascular congestion, ischemic necrosis, and subsequent infection. Sixty percent of cases are caused by lymphoid hyperplasia, with peak incidence during the teen years.

  A. Inspissated stool, termed fecalith, is identified in 20% to 30% of appendicitis cases. Fecaliths can sometimes be seen in the right lower quadrant on abdominal films or CT scans.
  C. Foreign bodies can result in luminal obstruction leading to appendicitis, but this is rarely seen.
  D. Tumors such as an appendiceal carcinoid can also result in appendicitis. The majority of carcinoid tumors found within the appendix are located at the tip of the appendix.
  E. Parasitic infections are reported, but it is an extremely rare cause of appendicitis.

103. E. Carcinoid tumors are the most common tumors of the appendix and are most often detected during the pathologic analysis of the appendix removed for appendicitis. The likelihood for metastasis from a tumor less than 2 cm in size is small, but the risk increases dramatically for tumors greater than 2 cm. Therefore, in this patient, no further treatment is necessary.

  A. Right hemicolectomy is recommended for patients with appendiceal carcinoid tumors greater than 1.5 cm in size.
  B, C. Radiation therapy and chemotherapy have no role in the treatment of localized carcinoid tumors.
  D. Octreotide infusion is often used to treat symptoms of carcinoid syndrome, which this patient does not currently have.

104. **C.** Anorectal abscesses most often arise from obstruction of an anal gland that subsequently becomes infected and overgrown with bacteria. These glands are located between the internal and external anal sphincters. If the infection tracts down this space toward the skin, an anorectal abscess occurs. The patient usually presents with severe anal pain that is worse with straining and defecation. A palpable mass with overlying erythema is also commonly observed. Treatment consists of incision and drainage of the mass. This is best done in the operating room, where adequate evaluation under anesthesia can be obtained to fully explore the extent of the abscess.

  A. CT scan of the abdomen and pelvis is reserved for evaluation of complex or recurrent disease, especially if a supralevator abscess is suspected.

  B, E. Abscesses should be drained surgically. Antibiotics (IV or oral) are used if significant cellulitis is present or if the patient is immunocompromised. Observation alone should not be employed in the treatment of this disease.

  D. Warm sitz baths alone will not adequately treat this type of infection. They may be employed postoperatively to assist with hygiene of the drained area.

105. **D.** The upper third of the anus originates from the endoderm, with the lower two-thirds originating from the ectoderm. The dentate line marks this transition point. This is an important surgical landmark as the blood supply, innervation, and lymphatic drainage differ in relation to the dentate line (Table 5-105).

  A. Columns of Morgagni are mucosal columns extending approximately 1 cm cranially from the dentate line.

  B. The valves of Houston are folds within the rectum often seen on endoscopy.

  C. The anal crypts are found between the columns of Morgagni, at the dentate line. They are the opening of the anal glands. Approximately 6 to 14 anal glands lie in the plane between the internal and external anal sphincters. They produce mucus and lubrication to protect the anus during defecation. Infection of these glands may tract into four potential spaces, creating four types of abscess: intersphincteric, perianal, supralevator, and ischiorectal.

  E. The ischiorectal fossa is the space found within the subcutaneum, lateral to the external anal sphincters, between the pelvic diaphragm and the skin. Abscesses found here are further away from the anus and may be horseshoe shaped, if the entire space is involved.

106. **A.** Portal hypertension is a common finding in patients with cirrhosis of the liver. Portal pressures greater than 18 mmHg are consistent with portal hypertension. Signs of portal hypertension include caput medusae, hemorrhoids, esophageal varices, ascites, splenomegaly, and thrombosis of the splenic vein. Although caput medusae can also be seen, they are rarely more than a physical finding. The increased pressure from the liver is transmitted to collateral venous channels, which appear as dilated venous collaterals. Classically, the distended and engorged umbilical veins radiate from the umbilicus across the abdomen, resembling snakes. The term caput medusae (Medusa's head) refers to the Greek and Roman myth of Medusa, whose hair was turned into snakes by Minerva.

■ TABLE 5-105 Dentate Line Differentiation		
	Above Dentate Line	**Below Dentate Line**
Innervation	Autonomic	Somatic
Arterial blood supply	Superior rectal artery from the inferior mesenteric artery	Middle rectal and inferior rectal arteries from the internal iliac artery
Venous blood supply	Superior rectal vein into the inferior mesenteric vein	Middle rectal vein and inferior rectal veins into the internal iliac vein
Lymphatic drainage	Internal iliac and periaortic nodes	Inguinal nodes
Mucosa	Simple columnar epithelium	Nonkeratinized stratified squamous epithelium

B, C, D, E. Caput medusae, hemorrhoids, esophageal varices, and ascites can all cause secondary complications or clinical issues requiring treatment.

107. C. Multiple measures are used to decompress varices including selective and nonselective shunts. Nonselective shunts also typically have a lower failure rate, although they do not offer a survival benefit. There is a higher rate of postoperative encephalopathy after nonselective shunts. A Warren distal splenorenal shunt is a traditional selective shunt designed to create two separate drainage systems within the portal venous network. This shunt is designed to maintain portal flow to the liver and thereby decrease the risk of encephalopathy.

   A. TIPSS is a surgical shunt that is very successful for decompressing varices and preventing recurrent bleeding.
   B. Mesocaval H shunts are traditional partial nonselective surgical shunts, which are meant to maintain hepatopetal flow while decompressing the high pressures in the portal system.
   D. Portocaval side-to-side shunts are traditional nonselective surgical shunts, which lower the portal pressures and are highly effective in treating esophageal varices.
   E. There is no such thing as a Pett T shunt.

108. B. This patient is a Child's B class. This patient will have 2 points for ascites, 0 points for encephalopathy, 3 points for albumin, 1 point for bilirubin, and 2 points for PT, for a total of 8 points (Table 5-108). This scale was developed to estimate operative mortality for cirrhotics undergoing shunt surgery. Class A: 5 to 6 points (1% mortality), Class B: 7 to 9 points (10% mortality), Class C: 10 to 15 points (50% mortality).

A, C, D, E. These calculations are all incorrect based on the patient's Child's class. See explanation for B.

109. D. This patient has clinical signs consistent with septic shock (fever, hypotension, leukocytosis), most likely attributed to an intraabdominal process following his original surgery. Sepsis disrupts the microvascular endothelium, resulting in massive third spacing and dehydration. Circulating cytokines, part of the inflammatory response cascade, can cause fever, leukocytosis, and the loss of systemic vascular resistance, resulting in hypotension, which can be refractory to fluid resuscitation.

   A. Although septic patients are dehydrated and require aggressive fluid resuscitation, often this alone will not correct the hypotension caused by the loss of systemic vascular tone.
   B. Cardiogenic shock results from depressed cardiac function. This may occur secondary to an MI, arrhythmias, cardiac tamponade, pneumothorax, or toxic doses of medications. In severe sepsis, circulating plasma factors may cause myocardial depression.
   C. Damage to the cervical spinal cord may result in a loss of autonomic innervation, causing not only depressed myocardial function, but the loss of vascular tone as well. This is usually treated with fluid resuscitation and dopamine.

110. B. An abdominal CT scan would be the most appropriate diagnostic test to obtain on a patient who has recently undergone an abdominal operative procedure who returns with increasing pain, fevers, and other signs that suggest an intraabdominal abscess. A CT scan is the most efficient test, since it can also be used to rule out other intraabdominal processes, as well as being a therapeutic tool for potential abscess drainage.

■ TABLE 5-108 Child's Class Points			
Points	1	2	3
Ascites	none	slight	tense
Encephalopathy	none	grade I, II	grade III, IV
Albumin	>3.5	3.0 to 3.5	<3.0
Bilirubin	<2.0	2.0 to 3.0	>3.0
PT (seconds above normal)	<4.0	4.0 to 6.0	>6.0

A. An exploratory laparotomy may be needed, but not without a workup via CT, the best initial test.

C. An ERCP would be impossible after a Whipple resection, which includes the pancreatic head and proximal ductal system.

D. A PTC may be helpful, but only after an initial screening with a CT.

E. An abdominal ultrasound would be limited in sensitivity and specificity. Bowel gas would be a limiting factor.

111. B. Small bowel obstruction (SBO) is a common problem seen by general surgeons. Most patients present with abdominal distention, persistent nausea, and vomiting of less than 24-hour duration. The abdominal pain is usually described as diffuse and colicky. Of utmost importance is the differentiation of complete versus partial bowel obstruction. Complete obstruction is accompanied by obstipation, or the failure to pass gas or stool within the last 12 hours. Abdominal films usually demonstrate a paucity of gas within the colon and rectum. Complete obstruction is an absolute indication for surgery. On the other hand, partial obstruction is accompanied by flatus or diarrhea as well as colonic or rectal gas on abdominal plain films. In both cases, plain abdominal films will demonstrate multiple air-fluid levels and dilated loops of small bowel (see Figure 5-111A and B). Partial SBOs are usually seen in patients with previous abdominal surgery and are initially managed with a trial of conservative therapy. This entails admission, NPO status, NG tube decompression, IV hydration, electrolyte repletion, and close observation. Failure to resolve the obstruction within 48 hours or any change in stability or abdominal exam warrants surgical intervention.

A. A barium enema would be of minimal use in a classic case of SBO such as this.

C. An abdominal paracentesis and lavage would not be helpful, and is potentially dangerous with an abdomen containing distended bowel.

D. Cathartics are contraindicated and would most likely exacerbate the symptoms of SBO. Enemas are not helpful with SBOs.

E. A UGI with barium should not be used to identify the site of obstruction because the barium will solidify, and, if leaked into the abdomen at surgery, it would add to the risks

of infection and recurrent obstruction post-operatively.

112. B. In the United States, adhesions are the most common cause of mechanical SBO, with a 50% to 70% incidence. Most adhesions are acquired from previous abdominal operations, as is the case in this patient. The second most common cause of SBO is incarceration of a femoral, inguinal, or ventral hernia. Although a hernia is usually apparent, it may be overlooked in an obese patient. Cancerous tumors are the third most common cause of SBO and result in occlusion of the bowel lumen or intussusception of the bowel if the tumor is intrinsic. Extrinsic tumors may act like adhesions, leading to twisting or entrapment of the small bowel.

A, C, D, E. These are all causes of SBOs, however, not in the proper order of decreasing frequency.

113. C. Duodenal atresia (DA) originates from recanalization failure of the embryonic duodenum during the eighth to tenth gestational weeks. This failure results in a duodenal obstruction. Bilious vomiting is usually noted during the first day of life. Plain abdominal films demonstrate the classic "double bubble" sign, which is described as a dilated air-filled stomach and duodenal bulb. Absence of air in the distal small bowel and colon signifies a complete obstruction.

A. Hypertrophic pyloric stenosis is a disease of newborns and usually presents between the third and eighth weeks of life. It is seen most often in firstborn males and has a genetic predisposition. Symptoms include nonbilious vomiting, inconsolable hunger, dehydration, and weight loss. The hypertrophied pylorus is usually palpable on exam, and patients usually present with a hypokalemic, hypochloremic, metabolic alkalosis. Treatment includes fluid resuscitation with electrolyte correction followed by a surgical pyloromyotomy.

B. In esophageal atresia, the esophagus ends in a blind pouch. Although there are numerous types, type C is the most common, involving an esophageal atresia with a distal tracheoesophageal fistula. Infants usually present with excessive salivation and repeated episodes of coughing, choking, and cyanosis. Surgical treatment consists of ligation of the fistula with repair of the atresia.

D. Meconium ileus results in obstruction from inspissated meconium within the ileum. Abdominal films demonstrate the "soap bubble" sign, which is air mixed with the meconium. Treatment consists of Gastrografin enemas, which draw water into the bowel and thereby break up the meconium plugs.

E. Intestinal malrotation may result in intestinal obstruction with vascular compromise. Infants usually present with bilious vomiting and abdominal distention. On plain abdominal films, the small bowel, is usually visualized on the right side of the abdomen. Surgical treatment involves exploring the abdomen, untwisting the bowel, and lysing adhesions, also referred to as Ladd's procedure.

114. **C. Duodenal atresia is a result of a defect in embryogenesis and is associated with other congenital anomalies such as Down syndrome, malrotation, congenital heart disease, esophageal atresia, urinary tract malformation, and anorectal malformations. A complete search for other anomalies should be done, with particular attention taken to rule out cardiac malformations.**

A. Mechanical and chemical bowel preparations are usually reserved for procedures involving the colon.

B. Bronchoscopy is an important test to perform on infants who have esophageal atresia. This can help diagnose a tracheoesophageal fistula as well.

D. Gastrografin enemas are used to aid in the diagnosis of Hirschsprung's disease.

E. An abdominal CT scan will be of little benefit in this patient's initial workup.

115. **B. Injury or disruption of the spinal cord at the cervical or high thoracic level can result in decreased or complete loss of autonomic innervation, leading to loss of arterial tone and myocardial depression with bradycardia and hypotension. Management employs Trendelenburg positioning, fluid resuscitation, and a range of vasoconstrictors, such as dopamine.**

A. Depressed cardiac function is usually the result of a cardiac injury, such as MI or cardiac tamponade.

C. Hypotension from a loss of systemic vascular resistance is usually seen in sepsis, but there is no reason to suspect sepsis in this situation.

D. Hypotension from hypovolemia is likely responsive to fluid resuscitation. This can occur with any illness that causes third spacing, such as an SBO or pancreatitis. Hypovolemia also occurs with hemorrhage.

116. **D. In women, pelvic inflammatory disease (PID) often mimics appendicitis. It is most often seen in women less than 35 years old and risk factors may include multiple sexual partners, previous PID, and IUD use. TOAs can develop in up to 15% of women with PID. Treatment usually involves surgical drainage and prolonged hospitalization with IV antibiotics. Abscess rupture may result in septic shock, which is considered a surgical emergency. Long-term complications of PID can include infertility. The CT scan in Figure 5-116B demonstrates a large TOA.**

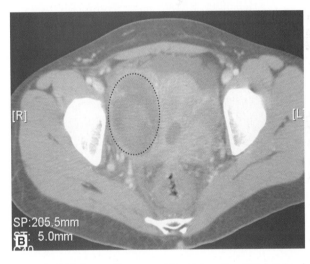

Figure 5-116B • Image Courtesy of the University of Utah School of Medicine, Salt Lake City, Utah.

A. Acute appendicitis usually has a shorter time course and a thickened, fluid-filled appendix would be seen on a CT scan.

B. Acute diverticulitis would be an unusual diagnosis in a patient this age. A CT scan would most likely reveal multiple diverticula with pericolonic fat stranding in the area of concern if the patient has diverticulitis. An abscess or contained extraluminal air may also be present.

C. Ruptured ovarian cyst is also high on the differential in a woman of reproductive age. The CT scan shown demonstrates bilateral pelvic abscesses most consistent with TOA. A ruptured cyst would most likely have a normal pelvic CT with free pelvic fluid.

E. Ectopic pregnancy is always a concern in a female of reproductive age who presents with lower abdominal pain. An ectopic pregnancy diagnosis can be determined by obtaining a serum β-hCG test and a pelvic ultrasound. The CT shown is not consistent with an ectopic pregnancy.

117. **D. The Gram-negative intracellular diplococcus, *Neisseria gonorrhoeae*, is the most common cause of PID. Treatment includes IV cefoxitin plus doxycycline.**

A. *Staphylococcus saprophyticus* is a Gram-positive coccus, and this organism is the second most common cause of urinary tract infections in females of reproductive age.

B. The organism *E. coli* (termed a coliform bacillus) is the most commonly isolated organism in the laboratory and is the most common cause of both community- and hospital-acquired UTIs.

C. *Pseudomonas aeruginosa* is a Gram-negative aerobic rod that is commonly referred to as the most opportunistic pathogen seen in hospital settings. It may be cultured from the sputum, blood, urine, or wound. Aggressive treatment should be undertaken to eliminate this deadly infection.

E. *Clostridium difficile* is an anaerobic spore-forming bacillus found in the normal intestinal flora and is the cause of pseudomembranous colitis, seen in patients who have been treated with antibiotics. Patients with pseudomembranous colitis complain of voluminous, foul-smelling diarrhea and treatment consists of metronidazole and fluid replacement, if needed.

118. **B. Epidural hematomas usually occur as a result of a blunt trauma to the head and are often associated with a temporal skull fracture. Classically, the patient experiences a transient loss of consciousness, followed by a lucid phase, and then neurologic deterioration. The head CT scan (Figure 5-118B) demonstrates a convex hematoma with or without a mass effect. Disruption of the middle meningeal artery is the most common cause.**

A. Ruptures of lenticulostriate arteries are the usual cause of hemorrhagic cerebral vascu-

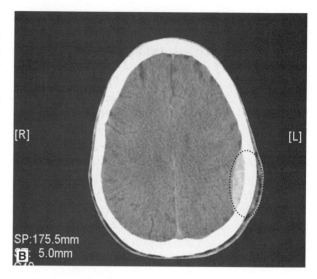

Figure 5-118B • Image Courtesy of the University of Utah School of Medicine, Salt Lake City, Utah.

lar accidents as a complication of hypertension.

C. Transection of the cerebral veins as they enter the superior sagittal sinus is the most common cause of a traumatic subdural hematoma.

D. Rupture of a cerebral aneurysm results in a subarachnoid hemorrhage.

119. **A. Since patients with an epidural hematoma can deteriorate rapidly, any change in consciousness or alteration in the patient's neurologic function requires an emergent surgical evacuation of the hematoma.**

B. Angiographic embolization is not appropriate because it will not relieve the mass effect caused by the expanding hematoma.

C. Placement of a ventriculostomy may be indicated for monitoring the intracranial pressure (ICP), but this procedure is not curative for the epidural hematoma.

D. Mannitol administration and hyperventilation are often used to assist in reducing ICP, but they will not halt the progression of an epidural hematoma.

E. Observation is sometimes appropriate in the case of small hematomas without neurologic deficits. In this patient, surgical intervention is clearly warranted by the deteriorating neurologic status.

120. D. Over 25% of patients who undergo abdominal surgery have some degree of pulmonary collapse, or atelectasis. This results primarily from shallow breathing and failure to periodically hyperinflate the lungs. Atelectasis is responsible for over 90% of febrile episodes within the first 48 hours postoperatively and can ultimately result in pneumonia. It is best prevented by early ambulation, frequent changes in position, coughing, and incentive spirometry.

A. UTIs are the most frequently acquired nosocomial infections. They usually occur after postoperative day 3 and are often accompanied by dysuria and low-grade fever. Diagnosis can be made with a urinalysis and confirmed by cultures. Discontinuation of the urinary catheter and antibiotic therapy are usually sufficient treatment.

B. Pneumonia is commonly seen in patients requiring prolonged ventilatory support or with peritoneal infection. It is usually seen after postoperative day 2. Clinical manifestations include fever, tachypnea, increased respiratory secretions, decreased breath sounds on auscultation, and dullness to chest percussion. The chest x-ray usually demonstrates parenchymal consolidation. Overall mortality from postoperative pneumonia is 20% to 40%. Treatment consists of pulmonary support as well as pulmonary toilet and administration of appropriate antibiotics.

C. In any postoperative febrile patient, it is very important to check the wound for signs of infection, which is the most common postoperative complication. Wound infections tend to occur between postoperative days 4 and 8. Clinical symptoms include pain, swelling, erythema, tenderness, and fever. Most infections are superficial and uncomplicated and are easily treated by opening the wound, drainage of infectious contents, and local wound care. Antibiotics are indicated if cellulitis extends from the wound more than 1 cm.

E. Although intraabdominal abscess may be a cause of postoperative fevers, it usually occurs 7 to 10 days after surgery. Patients will also have complaints of abdominal pain, as well as leukocytosis. An abdominal CT scan should be obtained, and if an abscess is identified, a percutaneous drain should be placed. IV antibiotics should also be instituted and adjusted according to culture results.

121. E. The celiac axis is one of three midline branches off the abdominal aorta that supplies the gastrointestinal organs. It arises at the lower portion of T12 and supplies the organs of the foregut, mainly the abdominal esophagus, stomach, duodenum to the ampulla of Vater, liver, spleen, pancreas, and gallbladder. It has three primary branches: splenic artery, common hepatic artery, and the left gastric artery.

A. The gastroduodenal artery is the first branch of the common hepatic artery. It runs posterior to the bulb of the duodenum and may be involved in posterior duodenal ulcers. It supplies the duodenum and head of the pancreas via the pancreaticoduodenal arteries.

B. The superior mesenteric artery is the second midline branch of the abdominal aorta. It originates at the level of the first lumbar vertebral body and runs behind the neck of the spleen and anterior to the third portion of the duodenum as well as the left renal vein. It mainly supplies the midgut, the duodenum starting at the ampulla of Vater, jejunum, ileum, cecum, appendix, ascending colon, and two-thirds of the transverse colon.

C. The inferior mesenteric artery is the third and final midline branch of the abdominal aorta. It originates at the level of the third lumbar vertebra and supplies the hindgut, including a third of the transverse colon, descending colon, rectum, and superior third of the anus.

D. The inferior phrenic arteries are paired branches of the aorta originating right after the aorta enters the abdomen via the aortic hiatus. They supply the abdominal side of the diaphragm as well as the adrenal glands.

122. C. Encapsulated bacteria such as *Streptococcus pneumoniae*, *Hemophilus influenzae*, and *Meningococcus* are destroyed by the immunologic function within the spleen. Therefore, patients who have undergone splenectomy are more susceptible to infection from these organisms. Infection by these organisms can result in a fatal infection known as overwhelming postsplenectomy infections (OPSI). Children are more susceptible than adults to this complication. Prophylaxis against these organisms with vaccination should be undertaken if possible prior to splenectomy.

A, B, D, E. Although individuals are more vulnerable to developing sepsis from bacteria after splenectomy, these organisms are not the most commonly identified.

123. A. The abdominal CT in Figure 5-123B reveals a splenic vein thrombosis with extension into the portal vein (see arrow). This is a known complication of splenectomy and should be treated with anticoagulation.

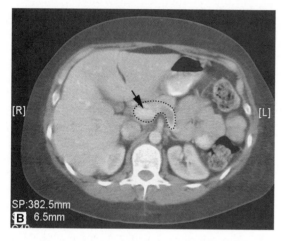

Figure 5-123B • Image Courtesy of the University of Utah School of Medicine, Salt Lake City, Utah.

B. In the abdominal CT seen here, there is no evidence of an abscess, and since there is no evidence of OPSI, antibiotics would not be indicated.

C. An exploratory laparotomy may be considered if there is a worry that there may be a bowel injury, bowel obstruction, or bleeding, but in the case of thrombosis, exploration is not indicated.

D. This choice lists possible adjunct therapies to anticoagulation therapy. Used alone, they would not effectively treat splenic and portal vein thrombosis.

E. Providing no treatment is inappropriate because this process has a significant morbidity and mortality if left untreated.

124. C. An infection of a yet undiagnosed source should be high on the differential diagnosis of unexplained or sudden hyperglycemia in a patient being given TPN. Individuals with glucose intolerance may not be able to handle the glucose load from TPN. Frequent blood glucose checks and administration of an insulin sliding scale are important during TPN administration. The hyperglycemia can usually be well controlled by appropriate calculation of carbohydrate requirements and addition of insulin to the TPN.

A. Pharmacy error is always a consideration, but unlikely after a stable period on TPN.

B. Short gut syndrome is unlikely since in this case the intestinal tract is not being used to deliver nutrition.

D. Pancreatitis is an unlikely cause of hyperglycemia without the presence of other clinical symptoms of pancreatitis.

E. Occult diabetes mellitus would most likely be noted very early after TPN was instituted.

125. D. The caloric and protein requirements of an injured person needed to meet metabolic demands increase substantially depending on the severity of the injury. An average individual requires 0.8 to 1.0 g/kg/day of protein intake. An individual requires 1.0 to 1.2 g/kg/day for mild stress, 1.3 to 1.5 g/kg/day for moderate stress, and 1.5 to 2.5 g/kg/day for severe stress. A large burn is a severe stress, and the protein intake requirement for this case would increase to 1.5 to 2.5 g/kg/day.

A. 0.5 to 0.8 g/kg/day is not enough protein for even a healthy individual.

B. 0.8 to 1.0 g/kg/day is the requirement for a healthy individual.

C. 1.0 to 1.5 g/kg/day is the requirement for a mildly to moderately stressed individual.

E. 2.5 to 3.5 g/kg/day is too much protein for even a severely stressed individual.

126. B. A zinc deficiency may result in diarrhea, dermatitis, and alopecia, as well as poor wound healing.

A. Selenium deficiency is associated with a reversible cardiomyopathy.

C. Anemia, leukopenia, and neutropenia result from a deficiency in copper.

D. Manganese deficiency is associated with dizziness, bone problems, reduced growth of hair and nails, weakness, hearing problems, weight loss, abnormal gait, and skin problems.

E. The hallmark of chromium deficiency is insulin-resistant hyperglycemia.

127. **B.** Increasing the daily caloric intake will cause an increase in the CO_2 production. Overfeeding, giving too much, will result in hypercapnia, which may impair the ability to wean from mechanical ventilation because the patient will "tire" from trying to breathe off the excess CO_2.

   A. Although overfeeding can result in hyperglycemia, this does not contribute to the patient's ventilatory failure.

   C. Hypophosphatemia can cause muscle weakness, which may affect the patient's ability to wean from a ventilator. In this case, however, the patient has a normal phosphate level.

   D. Pancreatitis may have associated pulmonary complications such as pleural effusions and ARDS. In this case, the chest x-ray is normal, so this is an unlikely cause in this patient.

   E. Respiratory alkalosis occurs when excessive CO_2 is removed via respiration by the patient, that is, hyperventilation. The opposite is true in this case. An increase of CO_2 is present because of overfeeding resulting in hypercapnia.

128. **D.** A penetrating injury to the colon with gross spillage makes this a contaminated case. Wound infection rates are associated with the level of contamination noted during the case. In a contaminated case such as this, penetrating trauma with bowel spillage, a wound infection rate of 10% 15% would be expected. The large bowel has by far the largest bacterial load and would significantly increase the risk of postoperative infection.

   A, E. Injury to the spleen and kidney put the patient at risk for bleeding, but not necessarily for a wound infection.

   B, C. Spillage from the stomach or small bowel increases the risk for wound infections but, because it does not involve the same bacterial load as the large bowel, the risk of infection is not as great.

129. **D.** The degree of contamination and time to definitive repair are the two most important factors in determining whether or not a perforating colonic injury can be repaired primarily. In cases in which there is minimal contamination and delay, primary repair of even left colon penetrating injuries is preferred.

   A, B, C, E. All of the other variables, age and history of diabetes, steroid use and prolonged surgical time, poor nutritional status and smoking, and history of cancer and chemotherapy, are all known to be immunosuppressive, but in a case of minimal contamination and delay, they would not independently preclude a primary repair.

130. **C.** Many conditions can cause a postoperative fever. A commonly used mnemonic to remember possible sources is "wind, water, wound, walking, and weird drugs." An intraabdominal abscess should be suspected in a patient on postoperative day 10, especially in a grossly contaminated surgical case, and with increasing abdominal pain. The diagnostic test of choice is a CT, and most abscesses can be treated with percutaneous drainage and IV antibiotics.

   A. Indwelling Foley catheters are foreign bodies and predispose patients to UTIs. UTIs are usually seen after postoperative day 3 and should be suspected in any patient with an indwelling urinary catheter. Obtaining a urinalysis and/or cultures will determine if there is an infection.

   B. Pneumonia must also be a consideration, especially in patients who require a ventilator for longer periods of time and in those who have undergone major abdominal procedures. Thick copious secretions, increased oxygen requirements, and decreased breath sounds are all signs of pneumonia. A chest x-ray can be helpful in determining the diagnosis.

   D. Surgery is a risk factor for developing a DVT. Compression boots used intraoperatively and while the patient is confined to bed as well as early ambulation are recommended to decrease this risk of developing a DVT.

   E. Atelectasis is responsible for over 90% of febrile episodes within the first 48 postoperative hours and, if not addressed with preventive and treatment measures, can lead to pneumonia. It is best prevented by early ambulation, frequent changes in position, coughing, and incentive spirometry.

131. **D.** Cardiogenic shock should be suspected in hypotensive patients with risk factors for coronary heart disease. Data from a pulmonary artery catheter usually reveal depressed cardiac function (cardiac index), with adequate or increased filling pressures (CVP, PCWP) and a compensatory increase in systemic vascular resistance (SVR). The underlying cause for the cardiogenic shock, such as a MI, should be determined and treated.

A. Hypovolemic shock is due to intravascular volume loss from either blood loss (trauma, surgery) or third spacing of fluids (SBO, pancreatitis). Pulmonary artery catheter readings usually demonstrate a decrease in cardiac index, decreased filling pressures (CVP, PCWP), and increased SVR.

B. Neurogenic shock is seen with spinal cord injury or anesthetic blocks. Diagnosis is based on physical exam and history. A decrease in the outflow from the sympathetic nervous system results in decreased cardiac output and decreased vascular tone (decreased CVP, PCWP, and SVR).

C. Sepsis causes disruption of the microvascular endothelium, resulting in massive third spacing of fluid and dehydration. Circulating cytokines released as a part of the inflammatory response result in fever, leukocytosis, and loss of SVR, resulting in hypotension refractory to fluid resuscitation. Pulmonary artery catheter readings in early sepsis show an increased cardiac index, with decreased PCWP and CVP, and decreased SVR.

E. Obstructive shock is seen in situations in which the blood returning to the heart is impeded, resulting in decreased cardiac output, such as in a tension pneumothorax or cardiac tamponade. The backup of blood results in elevated CVP and PCWP, with a resultant compensatory elevation of SVR.

132. C. When depressed cardiac function is the cause of hypotension, dobutamine, a β-agonist, will increase myocardial contractility leading to increased cardiac output. Patients experiencing myocardial ischemia, who are treated with dobutamine, should be monitored closely since this treatment may also increase myocardial oxygen demand resulting in further ischemia.

A. According to the Frank-Starling mechanism, increasing the preload increases cardiac contractility. However, in this patient's case, the filling pressures are adequate.

B. Transfusion is not necessary for management at this point because the underlying cause of shock is depressed cardiac function, not low intravascular volume.

D. Norepinephrine, a vasoactive drug, is the drug of choice in septic shock, as well as adequate fluid resuscitation. The potent α-agonist activity of norepinephrine provides peripheral vasoconstriction to counteract the global inflammatory response associated with septic shock. In cardiac shock, use of norepinephrine would lead to an increased cardiac contractility, but it could also cause a significant increase in afterload (SVR), further reducing cardiac output, and possibly exacerbating the shock state.

E. Nitroprusside is a potent vasodilator, which lowers blood pressure, that is useful for afterload reduction in hypertensive patients with a decreased cardiac index. The patient is already hypotensive and agents that would further lower blood pressure are not indicated in this case.

133. C. *Clostridium difficile* enterocolitis (an antibiotic-associated colitis) classically presents as acute and significant amounts of diarrhea in patients who are undergoing or have recently completed a course of antibiotic therapy. Presentation may occur up to 6 weeks after cessation of therapy. Antibiotics alter the normal intracolonic flora and permit overgrowth of *C. difficile*, a Gram-positive anaerobic bacillus. This bacterium produces an exotoxin, resulting in voluminous, foul-smelling diarrhea. In significant cases, patients may experience severe dehydration, hypotension, toxic megacolon, and possibly colonic perforation. Obtaining a stool toxin assay is the initial test that should be obtained in any patient suspected of having *C. difficile* colitis. They are inexpensive and noninvasive. Although they are less sensitive than endoscopy and may require multiple studies to increase the sensitivity, they remain the first and best initial option.

A. A serum antibody titer is not currently being used to test for *C. difficile* colitis.

B. An abdominal CT scan demonstrating a thick and edematous colonic wall with pericolonic inflammation is suggestive of colitis in general, such as ischemic, infectious, or inflammatory types.

D. Colonoscopy is an expensive and invasive procedure. If required, the diagnosis is confirmed by the endoscopic visualization of raised mucosal plaques, known as the pseudomembrane.

E. Studies have demonstrated that the majority of hospitalized patients with *C. difficile*-positive cultures are asymptomatic carriers.

134. **B.** Oral metronidazole 500 mg qid for 10 days is the first line of therapy for *C. difficile* colitis. In approximately 20% of patients, there may be a recurrence, for which the same course of treatment will give a positive response.

   A. Antidiarrheal agents should not be used in patients suspected of having *C. difficile* colitis. This can result in toxic megacolon, which is a surgical emergency and carries a high morbidity and mortality rate.
   C. Oral, not IV, vancomycin is also an effective treatment. It is most often reserved for patients who fail metronidazole therapy. The oral form of vancomycin is not absorbed in the GI tract and works within the lumen of the GI tract to kill overgrown bacteria.
   D. Cefazolin is a common cause of *C. difficile* colitis.
   E. Piperacillin-tazobactam will more likely cause, rather than treat, *C. difficile* colitis.

135. **D.** This is a critically ill woman who is in shock with obvious serious injuries. In any trauma situation, one always begins with the basics of airway, breathing, and circulation. Because this patient is critically injured, it is vital to obtain a secure airway. The first step is to intubate the patient before moving on to any other step.

   A, B. Although this patient's hypotension is very important and needs prompt attention, the airway always takes precedence over addressing any of the other issues. Often multiple tasks are being simultaneously accomplished by emergency staff members, but if not, always follow the ABCs of trauma and resuscitation.
   C. Chest x-ray is important to evaluate the chest injury but securing the airway takes priority.
   E. Placing a central line falls under circulation and is secondary to establishing an airway.

136. **E.** Flail chest occurs when a segment of the chest wall does not have continuity with the rest of the thoracic cage, and is due to multiple rib fractures with multiple fractures of individual ribs. It is a free floating or "flail" segment of ribs, which moves inward on inspiration while the rest of the chest moves outward, and the inverse with expiration, called paradoxical motion. The morbidity of a flail segment is due to an underlying lung contusion and carries a

15% mortality rate. Patients with a flail chest require intubation to maintain oxygenation.

   A. A hemothorax is blood within the pleural cavity and should be suspected with blunt and penetrating trauma to the chest. A chest x-ray will usually verify the presence of a hemothorax, and it should be drained by a tube thoracostomy.
   B. A pneumothorax can occur with both blunt and penetrating traumas. Most pneumothoraces are diagnosed by chest x-ray and are treated with a tube thoracostomy.
   C. An open pneumothorax, also known as a "sucking" chest wound, allows air to pass in and out of the pleural cavity. It is promptly treated with an occlusive dressing and tube thoracostomy in a site separate from the wound.
   D. A tension pneumothorax develops when a one-way leak allows air to enter the pleural space but prevents it from exiting. Intrapleural pressure rises causing collapse of the lung and shift of the mediastinum to the opposite side. The venous return to the heart is compromised, resulting in hypotension. This should be immediately treated with needle thoracostomy, followed by chest tube placement.

137. **C.** More than 85% of hemothoraces result from bleeding chest wall vessels such as the intercostal or internal mammary artery. An emergent exploratory thoracotomy should be considered when the initial chest tube output of blood is more than 1500 mL or the rate of output exceeds 200 mL/hour for 4 hours.

   A. The remaining 15% of traumatic hemothoraces are caused by injury to the pulmonary parenchymal or from cardiac sources.
   B. Esophageal perforation is unlikely in blunt trauma. It usually results in a pleural effusion and pneumomediastinum, not a hemothorax.
   D. Eighty-five percent of patients suffering a blunt injury to the thoracic aorta die at the scene. These patients usually present with mediastinal abnormality, such as a widened mediastinum, apical cap, loss of the AP window. Thoracic angiogram remains the gold standard in diagnosis, and prompt surgical intervention can result in 85% survival for patients who survive to the time of operation.

E. Cardiac rupture is very uncommon in blunt trauma and would result in cardiac tamponade from a mediastinal collection of blood.

138. **D. This critically ill patient may be bleeding to death from multiple injuries. Nonetheless, as in any trauma evaluation, the first step is to establish a secure airway. Intubation should be immediate before addressing other injuries. In every trauma situation, airway, breathing, and circulation always take priority, and always in that order.**

A. Although the most obvious injury, an open fracture is of low initial priority.

B. This patient may eventually need an exploratory laparotomy because of the severity of his injuries, but the airway management takes precedence.

C. Blood transfusions may be needed, but not before securing an airway via intubation.

E. Fluid resuscitation is needed and should start simultaneously with other treatments and evaluation, but always after ensuring that the airway is secure.

139. **A. The CT scan in Figure 5-139B (see arrow) demonstrates a large hepatic injury with surrounding hemoperitoneum.**

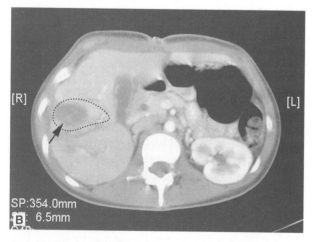

Figure 5-139B • Image Courtesy of the University of Utah School of Medicine, Salt Lake City, Utah.

B. A splenic laceration would be noted as a disruption of the splenic parenchyma with surrounding free blood.

C. Intraperitoneal bladder rupture would be noted as free fluid with excreted IV contrast in the pelvis, and with a nondistended bladder even with the Foley catheter clamped.

D. Renal devascularization injury would be noted as failure of the affected kidney to light up with IV contrast.

E. An internal iliac artery injury would present as a pelvic or retroperitoneal hematoma with an abrupt "cutoff" of contrast perfusion beyond the injury.

140. **B. Hemodynamic instability and continued blood loss in a trauma patient with a blunt hepatic injury warrants an immediate exploratory laparotomy. In hemodynamically stable trauma patients with blunt hepatic injuries, initial nonoperative management can be successful in up to 80% to 85% of cases.**

A. Angiographic embolization in hepatic injuries is not helpful, because in most cases the bleeding is venous in origin.

C. Suprapubic catheter placement would be appropriate for trauma patients who have sustained a urethral disruption.

D. Observation or nonoperative management is successful in 80% to 85% of hemodynamically stable blunt hepatic injury cases. It is inappropriate in this case because the patient is hemodynamically unstable despite adequate resuscitation measures.

141. **D. A patient who sustains burns from within a closed space, such as in a house fire, is at an extreme risk for an inhalation injury. Clinical signs of an inhalation injury include facial burns, singed nasal hairs, bronchorrhea, carbonaceous sputum, wheezing and rales, tachypnea, hoarseness, and difficulty clearing secretions. The upper airway may become obstructed secondary to edema within 48 hours of the inhalation injury. This is the main concern for this scenario.**

A. Rhabdomyolysis occurs in severe crush injuries or in injuries in which muscle is severely damaged. This would be unlikely in an 8% TBSA burn.

B. Infection of burns is a significant complication but would occur later in the course, not in the acute injury situation.

C. Significant fluid losses can occur in all burn victims. Fluid resuscitation is instituted as soon as possible, and the amount and delivery rate are based on well-described standard formulas, which take into account variables such as patient weight and burn size. The location of this patient's burns (neck and face), as well as the possibility of an inhalation injury, would make a secure airway the first priority.

E. Compartment syndrome of an extremity is a major concern in the setting of circumferential burns and is most often noted during the resuscitation phase. It is imperative that compartment pressures be measured frequently and an escharotomy is required if the pressure exceeds 30 mmHg.

142. **D. The best way to evaluate for an inhalation injury is to perform a bronchoscopy. Direct visualization of the lower airways to check for edema and for evidence of soot will establish the diagnosis and the severity of the inhalation injury.**

A. CVP monitoring is used to evaluate the fluid status and fluid requirements.

B. Urine myoglobin is an appropriate test to evaluate for rhabdomyolysis.

C. Sputum Gram stain and cultures may aid in the diagnosis of pneumonia but not in diagnosing an inhalation injury.

E. Checking compartment pressures is very important in cases of circumferential burns to extremities to evaluate for compartment syndrome.

143. **C. Gastric adenocarcinoma encompasses 90% to 95% of all gastric tumors, and it is the eighth most common cause of cancer mortality in the United States. This type of cancer is seen more frequently in males than in females (2:1 ratio), with 70% of patients being more than 50 years old. The incidence is highest in Asia and is 80 times more common in Japan than in the United States. Risk factors include diet (smoked foods, nitrosamine compounds, and low consumption of fruits and vegetables), occupational exposures (heavy metals, rubber, and asbestos), cigarette smoking, alcohol consumption, and low socioeconomic status. While the Japanese have a much higher incidence, it is believed to be related to their diet and not a genetic-based risk. Tumors can be located anywhere within the stomach.**

Thirty percent are located in the pyloric canal or antrum, 20% in the body, 37% in the cardia, and 12% in the entire stomach (Linitis plastica). Many remember the distribution as approximately "one-third in the antrum, one-third in the body, and one-third in the cardia."

A, B, D, E, F. These are all incorrect distributions of gastric tumors. See explanation for C.

144. **A. Approximately 25% of patients who have undergone a gastric resection experience "dumping syndrome." This syndrome is divided into early and late types. Early dumping syndrome occurs within 15 to 30 minutes of eating, caused by the rapid emptying of gastric contents. The hyperosmolar chyme entering the small intestine causes massive fluid shifts into the small bowel. Symptoms usually include nausea, vomiting, abdominal cramps, lightheadedness, diaphoresis, and palpitations. Most patients can eliminate this syndrome with a diet of multiple, small low-carbohydrate, high-fat, and high-protein meals.**

B. Late dumping syndrome usually occurs several hours after a meal. Symptoms are usually vasomotor and include weakness, sweating, dizziness, and flushing. They are caused by an exaggerated release of insulin from the hyperosmolar food. The subsequent hypoglycemia that develops causes the release of catecholamines.

C. Pancreatitis can occur post-gastric resection but not presenting with these symptoms.

D. Acute cholecystitis may occur post-gastric resection but more likely presents as right upper quadrant pain after meals.

E. Gastric outlet obstruction would result in immediate emesis of undigested food.

145. **C. Hypovolemic shock is due to intravascular volume loss from either blood loss (trauma, surgery) or third spacing of fluids (SBO, pancreatitis). Patients with acute pancreatitis sequester fluid in the retroperitoneum, and large volumes of IV fluids are often necessary to maintain a normal effective circulatory volume. Accurate measurement of urine output is essential in judging fluid replacement.**

A, B, D, E. See explanation to question 131 regarding neurogenic, obstructive, cardiogenic, and septic shock.

146. **A. Pulmonary artery catheter readings in hypovolemic shock usually demonstrate a decrease in cardiac index, decreased filling pressures (CVP, PCWP), and a compensatory increase in SVR, as seen in this scenario.**

    B. These values are all within normal limits.
    C. Neurogenic shock results in decreased CI, as well as decreased CVP, PCWP, and SVR.
    D. These values are more representative of cardiogenic shock, with a decreased CI, normal or elevated PCWP and CVP, and elevated SVR.
    E. Early septic shock can result in an elevated CI with a decreased CVP, PCWP, and SVR.

147. **B. Patients will usually remain asymptomatic if the hyponatremia is slow to develop down to a level of 120 mEq/L. In children, symptoms may begin to occur at a level of 130 mEq/L or if the onset of hyponatremia is rapid. Symptoms can include muscle twitching, hyperactive deep tendon reflexes, seizures, and hypertension secondary to increased ICP.**

    A, C, D, E. These are all incorrect calculations. See explanation for B.

148. **C. Central pontine myelinolysis is a unique clinical entity that occurs as a consequence of severe or prolonged hyponatremia, which is corrected too quickly. It is also called osmotic myelinolysis and the theoretical cause involves fluctuating osmotic forces that result in fluid shifting too rapidly out of the cells.**

    A, B. Edema of the cord or cerebrum does not occur as fluid is shifting out of the cells

toward the higher concentration of sodium in the blood vessels.
    D. Seizures may result from hypo- or hypernatremia and long-term neurologic consequences from seizures are unlikely.
    E. Peripheral neuropathy is unlikely to occur from hyponatremia.

149. **B. Patients with a prior history of malnutrition or an associated history of alcoholism are at greater risk for developing central pontine myelinolysis on correction of the hyponatremia.**

    A, D. A history of smoking or seizures does not contribute to increased risk of developing central pontine myelinolysis.
    C, E. It is recommended that the sodium be corrected at 2.5 mEq/L/hour or 20 mEq/L/day to prevent central pontine myelinolysis.

150. **B. Correcting a hypernatremic state too rapidly will result in rapid fluid shifts into the cells, thus leading to cerebral edema. Fluid will move from an area of lower sodium concentration to a level of higher concentration.**

    A. Clinically significant cord edema does not occur with rapid correction.
    C. CPM occurs when hyponatremia is corrected too rapidly.
    D. Seizures may occur with too rapid correction of either hyper- or hyponatremia, but it is unlikely that there would be long-term effects or injuries.
    E. Peripheral neuropathies are unlikely to occur.

BLOCK 4

The next two questions (items 151 and 152) correspond to the following vignette.

On morning rounds you enter the room of a 56-year-old male who has undergone an exploratory laparotomy for SBO 5 days ago. The patient denies having any bowel movements or flatus and has been burping up bitter secretions. On physical exam, his abdomen is distended and the surgical incision is tender and warm to touch with blanching erythema surrounding the wound edges. Over the last 24-hour period his maximum temperature was 38.9°C.

151. What is the most appropriate next step in the management of this patient?

    A. Advancing the diet
    B. Antibiotic therapy
    C. Wound exploration
    D. Exploratory laparotomy
    E. Continued observation

152. On postoperative day 5, most wounds are in which stage of wound healing?

    A. Coagulation
    B. Inflammation
    C. Proliferation
    D. Remodeling
    E. Contracture

End of Set

The next three questions (items 153 to 155) correspond to the following vignette.

A 4-year-old male is brought to your clinic by his mother. The mother tells you that while she was giving her son a bath last week she noticed and felt a "bump" on his abdomen. The child appears to be healthy and is quite active while in clinic. On physical examination, you palpate a large, firm, nontender abdominal mass. There are no other abnormal findings on physical or clinical exam. The results of a 24-hour urine demonstrated elevated levels of metanephrine and VMA.

153. What is the next most appropriate step in evaluating this patient?

    A. Abdominal ultrasound
    B. MIBG nuclear scan
    C. Abdominal MRI
    D. Intravenous pyelogram (IVP)
    E. CT scan of the abdomen and pelvis

154. What is this patient's most likely diagnosis?

    A. Neuroblastoma
    B. Wilms' tumor
    C. Hepatoblastoma
    D. Rhabdomyosarcoma
    E. Sacral teratoma

155. This patient's type of tumor classically demonstrates amplification of which protooncogene?

    A. *RET*
    B. *sis*
    C. Retinoblastoma (*Rb*)
    D. N-*myc*
    E. *ras*

End of Set

The following three questions (items 156 to 158) correspond to the following vignette.

A 25-year-old female university student presents to the clinic with a 0.8-cm pigmented lesion of her left medial thigh. According to the patient, the lesion has been present for nearly 4 years, but it seems to have increased in size over the last 3 months. The patient denies any other health problems and takes no medications. The patient grew up in California and spent a great deal of time at the beach during her adolescence.

156. Which of the following characteristics of the lesion would be most concerning?

    A. Diameter less than 6 mm
    B. Smooth, round borders
    C. Homogeneous coloring
    D. Symmetric appearance
    E. Surface elevations

157. What is the next step in obtaining a definitive diagnosis of this patient's lesion?

    A. Shave biopsy
    B. CT scan of left leg
    C. FNA
    D. Excisional biopsy
    E. Wood's lamp test

158. Which factor is most important for determining disease prognosis in this patient?

    A. Total lesion diameter
    B. Location of the lesion
    C. Depth of invasion
    D. Histologic type of melanoma
    E. Presence of superficial ulceration

End of Set

The next three questions (items 159 to 161) correspond to the following vignette.

A 76-year-old male is referred to your clinic for a history of episodic loss of vision, for up to 10 minutes, in the right eye. Over the last 3 weeks, vision loss has occurred twice and the patient describes the loss as "from the top down, like a shade being pulled over the eye." The patient denies any speech problems, memory loss, or issues with balance. Six years ago the patient had an MI treated with coronary artery stenting of the LAD. Currently the patient denies any angina, shortness of breath, or dyspnea on exertion. Medications taken include metoprolol, famotidine, aspirin, atorvastatin, and captopril. Clinic vital signs are HR 81, BP 118/78. Physical exam is significant for Hollenhorst plaques in the right eye, and a right carotid bruit.

159. What is the next most appropriate step in the evaluation of this patient?

    A. Carotid duplex ultrasound
    B. Bilateral carotid angiogram
    C. Carotid MRA
    D. CT angiogram of the carotid arteries
    E. Observation

160. What is the indication for carotid endarterectomy in a symptomatic patient such as this?

    A. Carotid artery stenosis greater than 50%
    B. Carotid artery stenosis greater than 55%
    C. Carotid artery stenosis greater than 60%
    D. Carotid artery stenosis greater than 65%
    E. Carotid artery stenosis greater than 70%

161. The patient is highly concerned about the risks of surgery. You counsel him that the most common cause of death in the immediate postoperative period following a carotid endarterectomy is

    A. Stroke
    B. Hemorrhage
    C. Pulmonary embolus
    D. MI
    E. Cranial nerve injury

End of Set

The next three questions (items 162 to 164) correspond to the following vignette.

A 40-year-old female with Crohn's disease is admitted to your service with an SBO. The patient has been treated medically with mesalamine for the last 5 years. This is the patient's fifth episode of obstruction, of which all were previously treated conservatively. Presently the patient is afebrile and hemodynamically stable. An enteroclysis is done and shown in Figure 5-162A.

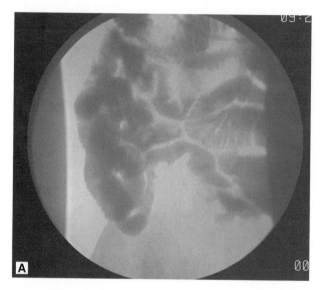

Figure 5-162A • Image Courtesy of the University of Utah School of Medicine, Salt Lake City, Utah.

162. The most likely cause of the obstruction is what process?

    A. Adhesions
    B. Perforation
    C. Fistula
    D. Abscess
    E. Stricture

163. In addition to metronidazole, what other medication is proven to facilitate perianal fistula closure in Crohn's disease?

    A. Prednisone
    B. Infliximab
    C. Sulfasalazine
    D. Cyclosporine
    E. Tacrolimus

164. Which of the following statements regarding this patient's Crohn's disease is true?

A. Surgery is the only way to cure Crohn's disease
B. Unlike ulcerative colitis, Crohn's disease does not increase the chance of colon cancer
C. The etiology of Crohn's disease is unknown
D. A patient with longstanding Crohn's disease rarely requires more than one surgical procedure for complications
E. Small bowel resection is the only way to surgically correct obstructive strictures

End of Set

The next two questions (items 165 and 166) correspond to the following vignette.

You are called to the ED to evaluate a 17-year-old male who is in obvious distress on the examination table. The patient complains of sudden, right lower abdominal and scrotal pain, beginning 3 hours ago and continuing without cessation. The patient denies change in bowel habits, fever, chills, nausea, vomiting, dysuria, or urinary frequency. The patient reports that he is healthy and has no surgical history. On examination, the patient's right scrotum is found to be swollen, red, and tender to palpation.

165. What is the most appropriate initial step to confirm your diagnosis?

    A. Abdominal ultrasound
    B. Urinalysis
    C. Pelvic CT scan
    D. KUB
    E. Testicular Doppler ultrasound

166. The patient is taken to surgery emergently. What additional procedure is indicated at this time?

    A. Inguinal hernia repair
    B. Contralateral testicular fixation
    C. Orchiectomy
    D. Cystoscopy
    E. Vasectomy

End of Set

The next two questions (items 167 and 168) correspond to the following vignette.

A 45-year-old female is referred to your clinic by her primary care physician for discussion of surgical options to control her esophageal varices. The patient has been admitted to the hospital twice in the past 2 months with an upper GI bleed. Endoscopy reveals multiple esophageal varices. The patient has portal hypertension secondary to portal vein stenosis that is a result of a portal vein injury sustained during a laparoscopic cholecystectomy. The patient has twice undergone placement of transjugular intrahepatic portosystemic shunt (TIPSS), which have ceased to function.

167. Which surgical shunt is most appropriate in this patient?

    A. TIPSS
    B. End-to-side portacaval shunt
    C. Mesocaval shunt
    D. Distal splenorenal (Warren) shunt
    E. Side-to-side portocaval shunt

168. The patient has undergone the surgical procedure 1 week after seeing you in clinic. You are called to the floor to see her on postoperative day 3 because the patient is confused and combative. You perform a neurologic exam that is nonfocal, and you note that the patient's breathing is unlabored and her vital signs are within normal limits. The patient's breath has a foul smell and her hands flap on extension. Which of the following is the most likely finding on laboratory examination?

    A. Hyponatremia
    B. Leukocytosis
    C. Hyperammonemia
    D. Elevated $PaCO_2$
    E. Hypercalcemia

End of Set

The next two questions (items 169 and 170) correspond to the following vignette.

A 62-year-old male is seen in clinic complaining of left calf pain. The patient states that the pain begins after walking a half block and the pain is relieved within 5 minutes of rest. The patient denies pain while resting or during sleep. The patient's medical and surgical history includes insulin-dependent diabetes mellitus for 12 years, MI, CAD with CABG 3 years ago, and a 45 pack/year history of smoking. Family history is unremarkable. Current medications include metoprolol, aspirin, atorvastatin, NPH insulin, and regular insulin coverage. Vital signs are T 37.8°C, HR 63, and BP 133/84. Physical exam of the neck, chest, and abdomen are normal. Peripheral pulses are as follows: 2+ carotids bilaterally without bruits, 2+ radial pulse bilaterally, 2+ femoral pulses bilaterally without bruits. The left popliteal, dorsal pedal, and posterior tibial pulses are not palpable, although there is a monophasic signal by Doppler. The right popliteal, dorsal pedal, and posterior tibial pulses are faintly palpable. Both lower extremities are cool to touch, with sluggish capillary refill, have scattered patches of scaly skin, and are devoid of hair.

169. Which of the following ankle-brachial index (ABI) values of the left lower extremity is most consistent with this patient's disease?

    A. 0.9 to 1
    B. 0.80 to 0.89
    C. 0.50 to 0.60
    D. 0.30 to 0.49
    E. less than 0.30

170. Which medical therapy is most effective in management of intermittent claudication?

    A. Smoking cessation
    B. Graded exercise program
    C. Pentoxifylline
    D. Blood pressure control
    E. Control of blood lipids

End of Set

The next two questions (items 171 and 172) correspond to the following vignette.

A 50-year-old male is referred to your office for a mass under his tongue. The patient states it has been there for about 12 months but recently it has noticeably increased in size. The patient denies previous medical problems, is not taking any medications, and has no known drug allergies. Surgical history includes an appendectomy as a teenager for appendicitis. The patient is married with two grown children and works as a manager in a local supermarket. Habits include occasional use of alcohol and chewing tobacco for 35 years. On exam the patient is found to be thin, in no apparent distress, with a regular HR of 87 and a BP of 157/92. Physical examination of the patient's head is normal except for a 1.5-cm fungating, raised, scaly, red lesion on the right underside of the tongue. On bimanual exam, you find the mass is mobile without apparent involvement of the jaw. Also noted are multiple, palpable lymph nodes in the right anterior cervical chain and no appreciable nodes on the left. There are no further abnormal findings on exam.

171. What is the most likely diagnosis?

    A. Benign cyst
    B. Adenoid cystic carcinoma
    C. Squamous cell carcinoma
    D. Lymphoepithelial lesion
    E. Mucoepidermoid carcinoma

172. What is the most appropriate treatment of this lesion?

    A. Chemotherapy
    B. Wide excision and radiation therapy
    C. Wide excision only
    D. Radiation therapy only
    E. Wide excision with radical neck dissection and radiation therapy

End of Set

The next three questions (items 173 to 175) correspond to the following vignette.

A 55-year-old female who has a 2-year history of medically treated ulcerative colitis presents to the ER with abdominal pain and a decrease in the number of daily stools. The patient states that she usually has three to four loose stools each day, but she has not had a bowel movement in 2 days. Vital signs include T 39°C, HR 115, BP 100/95, and SaO_2 94% on room air. The patient appears acutely ill with a distended and tender abdomen. No peritoneal signs are present. An abdominal CT is obtained (Figure 5-173).

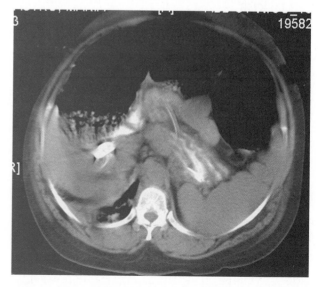

Figure 5-173 • Image Courtesy of the University of Utah School of Medicine, Salt Lake City, Utah.

173. What is the most likely diagnosis?

    A. Toxic megacolon
    B. Large bowel obstruction
    C. Sigmoid volvulus
    D. Ogilvie's syndrome
    E. Pseudomembranous colitis

174. The most appropriate initial management includes

    A. Emergent colonoscopic decompression
    B. NPO, NG decompression, IV antibiotics, IV steroids
    C. Emergent exploratory laparotomy
    D. NPO and IV antibiotics
    E. Observation

175. Characteristics of ulcerative colitis that differentiate this patient's disease from Crohn's disease include

    A. Skip lesions
    B. Linear mucosal ulcerations
    C. Noncaseating granulomas
    D. Inflammation limited to the mucosa and submucosa
    E. Involvement of the entire GI tract

End of Set

176. A 68-year-old male comes to the ED because of acute onset epigastric pain that began after shoveling his driveway. An ECG is obtained, showing ST elevation in multiple leads and elevated troponin levels, with the following vital signs: BP 95/52 and HR 108. The patient is admitted to the CCU and a cardiac catheterization shows that the patient has a 90% left main lesion, a 95% circumflex lesion, a 90% right-sided lesion, and a 100% acute marginal lesion. Hemodynamic stabilization is achieved by placement of two coronary stents and a dobutamine drip. The patient is referred to your service for coronary artery bypass grafting (CABG). In your planning of the operation, you decide to use saphenous vein for reverse vein grafts, and, in addition, you hope to use an artery as one of the grafts. Which artery is the most commonly used arterial graft in CABG?

    A. Left intercostal artery
    B. Right intercostal artery
    C. Left internal mammary artery
    D. Right internal mammary artery
    E. Left gastroepiploic artery

The next two questions (items 177 and 178) correspond to the following vignette.

A 72-year-old male is referred to your office for three-vessel coronary artery disease. The patient is otherwise healthy and takes no medications other than metoprolol and baby aspirin, which were started by his cardiologist a few weeks ago. You take him to the operating room for a planned CABG. You want to be cautious not to disrupt the conduction system of the heart during the operation.

177. Which coronary vessel usually supplies the sinus node?

    A. Left main artery
    B. Right coronary artery
    C. Circumflex coronary artery
    D. Diagonal artery
    E. Obtuse marginal artery
    F. Left anterior descending artery

178. Which vessel usually supplies the AV node?

    A. Left main artery
    B. Right coronary artery
    C. Circumflex coronary artery
    D. Diagonal artery
    E. Obtuse marginal artery
    F. Left anterior descending artery

End of Set

The next three questions (items 179 to 181) correspond to the following vignette.

Doing relatively well following cardiac bypass surgery, your 72-year-old male patient has required the ventilator for 3 days following surgery, but since being extubated he has been slowly improving. You are on morning rounds on postoperative day 6 and you notice that the WBC has gone from 8200 to 14,000. The patient had a low-grade fever of 38.5°C the previous evening and is not currently on any antibiotics. The patient does not have any indwelling central lines and the Foley catheter was previously discontinued. The most recent chest x-ray shows bilateral, mild pleural effusions. The patient complains of moderate shortness of breath, but your exam shows clear, bilateral breath sounds decreased in the bases. A left chest tube remaining from surgery is draining an appropriate amount of serous fluid. The sternal incision is without evidence of erythema or exudate, and you note that the sternum is mildly unstable compared to yesterday's exam. The patient has been ambulating up to four times a day and is eating a regular diet.

179. What may be the cause of this patient's fever and leukocytosis?

    A. Atelectasis
    B. Pneumonia
    C. UTI
    D. Mediastinitis
    E. Superficial thrombophlebitis

180. What is the most common organism for this patient's type of infection?

    A. *Klebsiella*
    B. *Streptococcus pneumonia*
    C. *Staphylococcus*
    D. *E. coli*
    E. *Enterobacter*

181. What is the best method to confirm your diagnosis?

    A. PA and lateral chest x-ray
    B. Urinalysis with culture
    C. Ultrasound the mediastinum
    D. CT scan of the chest
    E. Opening the wound

End of Set

The next three questions (items 182 to 184) correspond to the following vignette.

A 45-year-old female is referred to your clinic for evaluation of a mediastinal mass that was diagnosed after the patient sought medical help for shortness of breath. The mass was originally seen on a plain chest x-ray and confirmed by CT scan as an anterior mediastinal mass.

182. What is the most common anterior mediastinal tumor?

    A. Lymphoma
    B. Thymoma
    C. Pericardial cysts
    D. Neurogenic tumor
    E. Germ cell tumors

183. You recommend that the patient undergo mediastinoscopy for a diagnostic tissue biopsy. After a successful biopsy you recommend that she undergo anterior mediastinal exploratory surgery. What nerve is at greatest risk for injury during an anterior mediastinal exploration?

    A. Vagus nerve
    B. Facial nerve
    C. Phrenic nerve
    D. Recurrent laryngeal nerve
    E. Hypoglossal nerve

184. What systemic condition is classically associated with this patient's diagnosis?

    A. von Hippel Lindau's syndrome
    B. Myasthenia gravis
    C. von Recklinghausen disease
    D. Cystic hygromas
    E. Hashimoto's disease

End of Set

The next four questions (items 185 to 188) correspond to the following vignette.

A 42-year-old female presents to the ED with the sudden, acute onset of right-sided epigastric abdominal pain, which she experienced while eating. The abdominal pain is described as located on the right side and in her right shoulder. Vital signs are T 38.4°C, HR 118, BP 156/78, and RR 20. Physical exam reveals a flat and diffusely tender abdomen with evidence of peritonitis. The patient takes Pepcid for a history of ulcers, but she hasn't taken any for nearly a month because she has been unable to afford it. The WBC is 13,500 and all other labs are normal. You suspect that the patient may have a perforated ulcer.

185. What is the first radiographic study that you should obtain in this patient?

    A. Right upper quadrant ultrasound
    B. Flat plate of the abdomen
    C. Upright chest x-ray
    D. CT scan of the abdomen
    E. Diagnostic peritoneal lavage

186. What is the most likely source of this patient's right shoulder pain?

    A. Undiagnosed shoulder injury
    B. Psychogenic causes
    C. Radiating pancreatic irritation
    D. Referred diaphragmatic irritation
    E. Referred hepatic irritation

187. You obtain the appropriate study and confirm your suspicion. What is the next step in management of this patient?

    A. IV infusion of pantoprazole
    B. Upper endoscopy
    C. IV fluid resuscitation and pain control
    D. Exploratory laparoscopy
    E. Exploratory laparotomy

188. You perform a vagotomy to help eliminate gastric acid secretion. Why must a gastric drainage procedure be performed at the same time?

    A. To prevent dumping syndrome
    B. To prevent delayed gastric emptying
    C. To prevent alkaline reflux gastritis
    D. To bypass the duodenal perforation
    E. To prevent afferent loop syndrome

End of Set

The next two questions (items 189 and 190) correspond to the following vignette.

A 24-year-old male is referred to your office for evaluation of a soft tissue mass located on his right thigh. According to the patient, the mass has gotten much larger over the last 2 months, and it is now causing significant lower extremity pain. You are concerned this may be a soft tissue sarcoma so you obtain an MRI, which shows the mass to be 2.8 cm in diameter. An excisional biopsy of the mass is done, and the pathology confirms a malignant fibrous histiocytoma.

189. What is the most important factor in the prognosis of this patient?

    A. Tumor size
    B. Histologic grade
    C. Lymph node involvement
    D. Tumor location
    E. Patient age

190. What is the most likely site of metastasis of a sarcoma?

    A. Liver
    B. Lungs
    C. Brain
    D. Kidney
    E. Bone

End of Set

The next three questions (items 191 to 193) correspond to the following vignette.

A 31-year-old male is brought to the ER after being involved in a head-on collision that occurred during a severe winter storm. Extrication from the vehicle was a prolonged process, and the patient was intubated at the scene for respiratory distress. On arrival, the patient is found to have a secure airway, significantly decreased breath sounds on the left, and a palpable radial pulse. The secondary exam is significant for an obvious left femur fracture, and on chest x-ray you find a left pneumothorax with multiple left-sided rib fractures, with proper positioning of the endotracheal tube. You immediately place a left thoracostomy tube to relieve the pneumothorax.

191. Which of the following is an immediately life-threatening thoracic injury that should be identified on primary exam?

    A. Myocardial contusion
    B. Rib fracture
    C. Cardiac tamponade
    D. Esophageal tear
    E. Traumatic diaphragmatic disruption

192. Which of the following is the most likely associated injury for this patient?

    A. Pulmonary embolus
    B. Pulmonary contusion
    C. MI
    D. Fat embolus
    E. Tension pneumothorax

193. Which of the following treatments is most significant in relation to long-term management of this patient's pulmonary injury?

    A. Adequate pain management
    B. Surgical stabilization of rib fractures
    C. Thoracic brace for rib fractures
    D. Inferior vena cava filter for DVT prophylaxis
    E. Heparin prophylaxis for DVT

End of Set

The next two questions (items 194 and 195) correspond to the following vignette.

You are called to see a 71-year-old female in the ED being admitted for evaluation of abdominal pain. The patient describes the pain as severe and related to eating because she has lost 35 lbs over the last 6 months. The patient denies nausea or vomiting and reports normal bowel function. History includes well-controlled hypertension, atrial fibrillation, no previous abdominal surgery, and a 60 pack/year smoking history. The patient's primary care physician and a gastroenterologist have started working up the pain by obtaining an ultrasound of the gallbladder, a CT scan of the abdomen and pelvis, an HIDA scan, an upper endoscopy, and a colonoscopy, all of which are reported as normal. Physical exam reveals an abdomen that is soft, nontender, nondistended, and without peritoneal signs. The WBC is 9200 and liver function tests and electrolytes are normal.

194. What is this patient's likely diagnosis?

   A. Acute cholecystitis
   B. Biliary dyskinesia
   C. SBO
   D. Acute mesenteric ischemia
   E. Chronic mesenteric ischemia

195. What is the most likely etiology of this diagnosis?

   A. Cholelithiasis
   B. Intraabdominal adhesions
   C. Atherosclerosis
   D. Embolic disease
   E. Biliary sludge

End of Set

The response options for items 196 to 200 are the same. You will be required to select one answer for each item in the set.

   A. Gastric vascular malformation
   B. Associated with CNS trauma or tumor
   C. Squamous cell carcinoma in a chronic wound
   D. Ulcer at an anastomosis
   E. Associated with a major burn injury

For each type of ulcer, select the most appropriate description.

196. Cushing's ulcer

197. Curling's ulcer

198. Marginal ulcer

199. Dieulafoy's ulcer

200. Marjolin's ulcer

End of Set

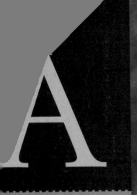

Answers and Explanations

151. C	168. C	185. C
152. C	169. C	186. D
153. E	170. A	187. E
154. A	171. C	188. B
155. D	172. E	189. B
156. E	173. A	190. B
157. D	174. B	191. C
158. C	175. D	192. B
159. A	176. C	193. A
160. A	177. B	194. E
161. D	178. B	195. C
162. E	179. D	196. B
163. B	180. C	197. E
164. C	181. D	198. D
165. E	182. B	199. A
166. B	183. C	200. C
167. D	184. B	

151. C. A surgical site infection (SSI) is the most common complication following surgery. The incidence depends on how much contamination occurs during the operative case, that is clean, clean contaminated, contaminated, or dirty case. A bacterial load of 10^5 colony-forming units per gram of tissue usually results in a wound infection. Other variables play a role in the development of a wound infection, including the duration of operative procedure, improper skin preparation, poor surgical technique, and the nutritional status of the patient. Presentation of an infected wound usually occurs between days 5 to 7 postoperatively. Erythema, induration, pain on palpation, and purulent drainage are often seen. The initial treatment of choice is opening the wound and debriding the purulent material. In abdominal wounds, the underlying fascia should be thoroughly investigated to verify that it is intact. Most infections do not require antibiotics, but they are indicated if cellulitis extends more than 1 cm from the wound edge, or if the patient is immunocompromised.

   A. Clinically this patient appears to have an ileus and diet should be limited.
   B. The standard treatment for a wound infection is opening the wound with indications for antibiotic therapy, as in the explanation for C.
   D. Given the above scenario, there is no indication for exploratory laparotomy. If the fascia was not found to be intact, then an exploratory laparotomy with wound closure would be warranted.
   E. Observation will only result in delayed treatment.

152. C. Proliferation occurs from day 3 through day 21 and is characterized by the production of fibrous collagenous tissue. Fibroblasts are the predominate cell type and deposit extracellular matrix, mainly collagen.

   A. Coagulation occurs in the first hour of the wound healing process. Platelets, the coagulation cascade, and the injured vessel all work simultaneously to obtain hemostasis at the site of injury.
   B. The inflammation stage begins shortly after the creation of the wound and continues until approximately the third day. An inflammatory reaction results in the migration to the wound of polymorphonuclear (PMN) leukocytes, which begin debriding the wound. By 48 hours, macrophages have become the predominate cell in the wound and are responsible for the complex cellular interrelationships necessary in normal healing.
   D. The remodeling stage lasts from 21 days to 2 years after injury. During this phase, the collagen fibers become more organized and cross-linked. The strength of the tissue continues to increase over time, but it will never return to what it was prior to injury.
   E. Contracture is caused by the myofibroblasts within the wound that decrease the size of the wound.

153. E. If an abdominal tumor is suspected, the initial diagnostic test should be a CT scan of the abdomen and pelvis. This will help determine the extent of disease, invasion into surrounding structures, and lymph node involvement.

   A. An abdominal ultrasound is a reasonable choice, but it will not provide as detailed a look at the current intraabdominal process as a CT would.
   B. MIBG scan is used in identifying bony metastases, not as a primary survey of the suspected tumor.
   C. An MRI scan would be more reasonable in patients with abdominal tumors and neurologic symptoms to assess for involvement of the spinal canal or cord.
   D. The extent and detail of the tumor cannot be adequately assessed with an IVP.

154. A. Neuroblastomas are the most common extracranial solid tumors seen in children. This type of tumor originates from neural crest cells and is found most frequently in the abdomen. They may occur anywhere neural crest cells migrate during development, mainly along the sympathetic plexus. Diagnosis is usually made near 2 years of age, with males being affected slightly more frequently than females. The tumor is most often discovered by parents while they are bathing the child. Ninety-five percent of these tumors actively secrete catecholamines, and the diagnosis is made by sending the child's urine for homovanillic acid (HVA) and VMA. Treatment consists of a combination of surgery, radiation, and chemotherapy determined by the stage of the tumor.

B. Although very similar to the presentation of a neuroblastoma, a Wilms' tumor originates from the kidney. The urine catecholamine screen in this case will be negative. This tumor usually presents in children between 2 and 4 years old, and it is seen as an asymptomatic abdominal mass associated with hypertension and hematuria. A CT scan of the abdomen is the study of choice for further evaluation. This tumor is often associated with other abnormalities such as aniridia, hemihypertrophy, and Beckwith-Wiedemann's syndrome. Treatment is also dictated by stage and may include surgery, chemotherapy, and radiation therapy.

C. A hepatoblastoma is a malignant tumor of the liver presenting within the first 3 years of life. The child usually has abdominal distention with a right upper quadrant mass, which moves with respiration. Serum α-fetoprotein level is elevated in more than 90% of cases. Treatment consists of surgical resection.

D. Rhabdomyosarcoma is a highly malignant striated muscle sarcoma seen in children. Although it can be found in the abdomen, it is most commonly seen in the head and neck. Diagnosis is confirmed by tissue biopsy and treatment consists of a combination of surgery, chemotherapy, and radiation.

E. The sacrococcygeal area is the most frequent site of teratomas in children, followed by the mediastinum. In adults, the most common location of teratomas is the gonads, followed by the mediastinum. The tumors can continue in all three germ layers in a mature state, and when cystic they can contain mature teeth and hair.

155. D. The protooncogene, N-*myc,* is found on the short arm of chromosome 2. Amplification occurs in 25% of neuroblastoma cases, and it is associated with advanced stage of disease and a poorer prognosis.

A. The *RET* protooncogene is associated with multiple endocrine neoplasia (MEN) syndrome II.

B. The *sis* protooncogene is often overexpressed in osteosarcoma.

C. The retinoblastoma tumor suppressor gene is associated with both retinoblastoma and osteosarcoma.

E. Point mutations of the *ras* protooncogene are seen in a variety of cancers including lung, colon, and pancreatic cancer.

156. E. In evaluating a suspicious skin mole, you can remember the characteristics of melanoma with the mnemonic "ABCD." A = asymmetry of the mole, B = borders that are irregular, C = color variegation, and D = diameter greater than 6 mm. The incidence of melanoma has tripled in the last three decades. Risk factors include severe sunburn before age 18, giant congenital nevus syndrome, family history of melanoma, multiple dysplastic nevi syndrome, and Caucasian race. Early detection significantly improves the results of treatment.

A, B, C, D. Diameter less than 6 mm, smooth, round borders, homogenous coloring, and symmetric appearance are all characteristics of normal skin nevi.

157. D. Any suspicious skin lesion should be biopsied. A full-thickness excisional biopsy allows the pathologist to most accurately determine the depth of the lesion. A rim of 1 to 3 mm of normal tissue should be included when performing the biopsy.

A. There is no role for shave biopsies in lesions suspicious of melanoma because the depth of the lesion cannot be adequately assessed.

B. There is no indication for a radiographic study at this point for determining the diagnosis.

C. An FNA should not be used to diagnose primary skin lesions. This procedure is helpful in the diagnosis of nodal disease.

E. A Wood's lamp test is more appropriate in the diagnosis of a fungal infection.

158. C. Tumor depth is the most accurate index of metastatic potential of a melanoma. Breslow's classification of staging is determined by tumor thickness as measured by pathologists and is as follows: 1.0 mm or less, 1.01 to 2.00 mm, 2.01 to 4.00 mm, and over 4.00 mm. The greater the depth involved with tumor, the higher the risk of regional and distant metastasis as well as local recurrence.

A. Although the width of the lesion may make obtaining clear margins difficult, as with facial lesions, it is the depth of the lesion that primarily determines prognosis.

B. In terms of location, acral lentiginous melanoma usually occurs on the palms, soles, and under the nails, and is the most aggressive form of melanoma; but the most important prognostic features include ulceration and depth of the lesion.

D. Depth is the most important prognostic indicator in all histologic types of melanoma.

E. Although ulceration of the lesion is a poor prognostic indicator, depth is more important.

159. A. This patient history is consistent with a transient ischemic attack (TIA), an episode of neurologic dysfunction lasting less than 24 hours with no residual deficit. Amaurosis fugax is a transient blindness of one eye classically described as a "shade closing over the eye." These symptoms are concerning for atherosclerotic carotid artery disease. A carotid duplex ultrasound is the best noninvasive test to identify carotid artery stenosis. It can provide an approximate percentage of stenosis, nature of the plaque, and any surface irregularity.

B. An angiogram is an invasive test not used for screening purposes. At one time it was indicated before performing a carotid endarterectomy; currently, many surgeons will proceed with surgery if sufficient information is available from the carotid duplex studies.

C, D. Although both of these tests adequately evaluate the carotid arteries, they are more expensive and less reliable in determining carotid artery disease.

E. Observation is an inappropriate choice in a patient with symptomatic disease that requires treatment.

160. A. The indication for carotid endarterectomy has been well studied by multicenter, prospective, randomized clinical trials. The Asymptomatic Carotid Atherosclerosis Study (ACAS) demonstrated a reduction of stroke when carotid endarterectomy was used instead of medical therapy in asymptomatic patients with 60% or greater carotid stenosis, from approximately 10% to 5% over 5 years. Surgery in patients with asymptomatic carotid stenosis is debated in the vascular literature, and many factors should be considered before surgery is recommended. The North American Symptomatic Carotid Endarterectomy Trial (NASCET) showed a significant reduction of stroke in patients with greater than 70% carotid stenosis randomized to CEA compared to those treated medically. The stroke rate over 2 years following endarterectomy was lowered to 9% from 26%. Subsequent data have supported endarterectomy for symptomatic, greater than 50%, carotid disease.

A, B, D, E. These are all erroneous percentages. See explanation for C.

161. D. Patients with atherosclerotic carotid stenosis have a high likelihood of having coronary artery disease. A thorough history and physical, including cardiac review of systems, is important in the initial evaluation. Further cardiac testing may be necessary prior to surgery because postoperative MI is the leading cause of death following surgery.

A. Stroke is the most devastating complication of a carotid endarterectomy, and it occurs in fewer than 5% of patients undergoing this procedure.

B. Hemorrhage may occur postoperatively as the procedure is often performed under full heparinization. This is a rare occurrence that can lead to fatal airway compromise if not diagnosed early.

C. The risk of pulmonary embolus is slightly increased in patients with accompanying peripheral vascular disease because of increased immobility. However, this is not the most common cause of postoperative death.

E. The hypoglossal nerve crosses superficial to the carotid artery near its bifurcation. Traction may result in the deviation of the tongue toward the side of injury. The vagus nerve may also be injured resulting in vocal cord paralysis and hoarseness due to loss of the recurrent laryngeal nerve.

162. E. Ninety percent of all patients with Crohn's disease will eventually require an operation, with intestinal obstruction being the most common indication. Small bowel strictures occur secondary to acute edema or chronic fibrosis and produce the narrowing seen on this study (note arrow in Figure 5-162B). Unfortunately, surgery is not curative, and recurrence is inevitable. Therefore, preservation of intestinal length is of utmost importance during surgery. Some strictures can be treated with stricturoplasty in an effort to conserve bowel length.

A, B, C, D. Adhesions, perforations, fistulas, and abscesses are also indications for operation in patients with Crohn's disease. However, strictures remain the most common cause of obstruction and are the only answer consistent with the films shown.

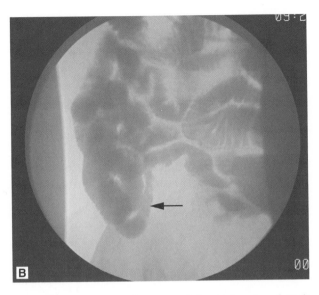

Figure 5-162B. • Image Courtesy of the University of Utah School of Medicine, Salt Lake City, Utah.

163. **B. Studies have shown that infliximab (Remicade), a chimeric monoclonal antibody against TNF-α, resulted in a higher rate (46%) of fistula closure compared to placebo (13%).**

A. Prednisone is used during active flares of Crohn's disease. It is superior to placebo over a short period of time. Steroid use should be limited because of multiple side effects, and it has not been found to improve healing in Crohn's associated fistulas.

C. Sulfasalazine is also proven in the treatment of active Crohn's disease as well as maintaining remission. It plays a limited role in perirectal fistulas.

D. Cyclosporine is an immunosuppressive agent shown to be effective in the treatment of Crohn's disease. It works quickly and is helpful in reducing use of steroids. It is not indicated for fistula closure.

E. Tacrolimus is an immunosuppressive drug that is used in transplant patients not with Crohn's.

164. **C. The etiology of Crohn's disease continues to be elusive despite extensive research. Although this disease is most likely due to autoimmune or infectious causes, no primary abnormality is consistently present.**

A. Unfortunately, there is no cure for Crohn's disease. It is managed medically unless surgery is indicated, most commonly because of obstruction, fistula, perforation with abscess formation, or malignancy.

B. Both Crohn's disease and ulcerative colitis (UC) increase the patient's risk of colon cancer. The risk with UC, however, is higher than with Crohn's.

D. Over 90% of Crohn's patients will require surgery, and a repeat operation is required in about 30% of these patients.

E. Preservation of intestinal length is extremely important in the surgical management of Crohn's disease. Patients who undergo surgery for strictures may be treated with resection or stricturoplasty. If the stricture is 12 cm or longer, or if an abscess or fistula is present, resection with primary anastomosis is recommended. If the stricture is less than 12 cm, or there are multiple strictures, stricturoplasty should be performed.

165. **E. A patient presenting with a unilateral swollen, tender scrotum has testicular torsion until proven otherwise. It typically occurs in adolescent males who present with a sudden onset of unilateral scrotal pain. Nausea and vomiting often accompany this pain, which is unrelenting and relieved by nothing. Irreversible testicular ischemia occurs within 4 hours; therefore, prompt diagnosis and treatment are mandatory. Testicular Doppler ultrasound can help assess the testicular blood flow. A lack of blood flow to the testicles confirms the diagnosis. Manual detorsion may be attempted, however, immediate exploration is the definitive treatment.**

A. An abdominal ultrasound has no role in the initial evaluation of testicular pain.

B. A urinalysis is nonspecific and is typically negative for blood or leukocytes in testicular torsion.

C. A noncontrast CT scan may be used in the initial workup of kidney stones but is not the first test to confirm testicular torsion.

D. This is an important tool in the initial workup of suspected kidney stones but not testicular torsion.

166. **B.** Testicular torsion is usually a result of a congenital defect of the gubernaculum of the testis that allows the testicle to rotate, also known as the "bell clapper" deformity. It is often bilateral, and contralateral testicular fixation should be performed at the same time the testicular torsion is corrected.

   A, D, E. Inguinal hernia repair, cytoscopy, and vasectomy are not indicated at this time.

   C. Orchiectomy may be performed if the testicle remains ischemic following detortion.

167. **D.** The operation chosen should stop the variceal hemorrhage and have a low risk of encephalopathy. The distal splenorenal (Warren) shunt consists of a ligation of the distal splenic vein, or the point closest to the junction with the superior mesenteric vein. This end is anastomosed end-to-side with the left renal vein. The coronary vein is completely ligated at the junction with the portal vein. This selectively diverts the blood flow away from the varices via the spleen and short gastrics. Portal flow from the small and large intestine remains intact, reducing the rate of encephalopathy.

   A. TIPS is an inappropriate option because the patient has already undergone two failed TIPS procedures.

   B, C, E. Unlike the Warren shunt, these are nonselective shunts and therefore have a higher risk of hepatic encephalopathy.

168. **C.** This patient most likely is suffering from a portal-systemic encephalopathy (hepatic encephalopathy). This is a neuropsychiatric syndrome caused by the shunting of portal blood directly to the systemic circulation without first passing through the liver. The liver metabolizes and detoxifies digestive products from the intestines through the portal vein. If these toxins bypass the liver, via a portosystemic shunt, the effect on the brain produces a clinical syndrome. Signs of this syndrome include personality change, impaired consciousness, confusion, fetor hepaticus, asterixis, and agitation. If left untreated, the patient eventually progresses to a comatose state. The toxic substances are not known and the patient's serum ammonia level is usually high.

   A. Hyponatremia causes a change in mental status and can eventually result in seizure activity. Patients on IV fluids should be monitored carefully. Correction to above 125 mmol/dL usually resolves the problem.

   B. Septic patients may present with mental status changes. A leukocytosis or leucopenia may be noted in these patients. This patient does not demonstrate any other signs of sepsis.

   D. Hypercarbia is a common cause of mental status changes, especially in postoperative patients receiving narcotics. It should always be included on the differential and, if suspected, is easily detected by an ABG.

   E. Hypercalcemia, as seen in primary hyperparathyroidism or metastatic cancer to the bone, usually results in a depressed mood and difficulty concentrating. It can also cause psychosis, but this is unlikely in the acute setting.

169. **C.** Claudication is seen in peripheral arterial occlusive disease. It is defined as exercise-induced discomfort in a particular muscle group due to ischemia. The pain often subsides within 5 minutes of exercise cessation. The pain is associated with tissue hypoxia when the demand for oxygen during exercise cannot be met. Risk factors include tobacco use, hypercholesterolemia, hypertension, diabetes mellitus, age, and male gender. Physical exam reveals a lack of distal pulses, thinning of the skin, loss of hair, and thickness of the nails. The ABI is a noninvasive test to help determine the extent of peripheral vascular disease. It measures the ratio of the ankle pressure to the highest brachial pressure. A ratio of 0.5 to 0.6 is usually seen with claudication.

   A. A ratio of 0.9 to 1 is a normal value.

   B. A ratio of 0.8 to 0.89 is consistent with mild insufficiency, usually asymptomatic.

   D. A ratio of 0.3 to 0.49 is usually observed in patients complaining of rest pain.

   E. A ratio of less than 0.3 is seen in patients who have limb ischemia and tissue loss.

170. **A.** Seventy-five to eighty percent of patients with claudication will remain stable and can be treated medically. Conservative measures consist of smoking cessation, along with a graded exercise program. Abstinence from tobacco has the largest impact on halting progression of peripheral vascular disease (PVD).

B, E. Graded exercise programs and control of blood lipids are also important aspects of medical management of PVD, but stopping smoking is the most effective initial step.

C. Pentoxifylline is a rheologic agent that increases the flexibility of erythrocytes and decreases platelet aggregation in peripheral vessels, resulting in decreased blood viscosity. It may have some benefit in the medical treatment of PVD.

D. Blood pressure control will not effect claudication management, but it will improve overall health issues.

171. **C. Carcinoma of the tongue usually develops in males with a history of alcohol and tobacco abuse and is most commonly squamous cell carcinoma (SCC). Most tumors occur on the lateral or ventral surface of the tongue and frequently present with invasion of the inner table of the mandible. Over 50% of patients present with metastases to the cervical lymph nodes, as in this case.**

A, B, D, E. Benign cysts, adnoid cystic carcinoma, lymphoepithelial lesions, and mucoepidermal carcinoma are all lesions of the salivary glands and should be included in the workup of an oral mass. Given the patient's history and physical findings, SCC is the most likely diagnosis.

172. **E. Surgical excision offers the best chance for cure. Negative margins should be the goal in every cancer surgery. Lymph nodes that are clinically involved are always treated with a neck dissection. Radiation therapy is often added to obtain local control. Most surgeons prefer radiation therapy to be administered postoperatively, when it seems to have a better response rate.**

A. Chemotherapy without debulking the tumor is inadequate treatment.

B. Wide excision and radiation therapy would be a valid option, but this patient has a clinically suspicious lymph node warranting a neck dissection.

C, D. Wide excision only and radiation therapy only are options in management; however, they should be combined with a radical neck dissection.

173. **A. Toxic megacolon occurs in approximately 10% of patients with UC and has a mortality rate approaching 40%. It should be suspected in patients with known UC complaining of severe abdominal pain and distention, with a dilated transverse colon (greater than 9 cm) on plain films. Fever and tachycardia usually accompany these findings. The CT shown (see Figure 5-173) shows massive colonic dilatation.**

B. Large bowel obstructions account for only 15% of intestinal obstructions. They are most commonly caused by colorectal cancer (65%), diverticulitis (20%), volvulus (10%), and miscellaneous causes (10%). Although this entity should be considered, the patient's history of UC should place toxic megacolon higher on the differential.

C. Although volvulus can be a cause of large bowel obstruction, it is usually seen in older, debilitated patients.

D. Ogilvie's syndrome, or pseudoobstruction, is a paralytic ileus of the large intestine. Risk factors include severe blunt trauma, orthopedic trauma or procedures, cardiac disease, acute neurologic disease, and acute metabolic derangements. This condition is dangerous because the cecum can expand up to 10 to 12 cm and possibly perforate.

E. *Clostridium difficile* enterocolitis patients may also develop toxic megacolon. This is associated with prior antibiotic usage. It is a serious condition that could lead to colonic perforation. Treatment is the same as mentioned below. In addition, the patient should be started on metronidazole.

174. **B. Initial treatment consists of bowel rest and decompression. Prompt administration of IV steroids should be initiated as well as broad-spectrum IV antibiotics. If the patient's clinical situation does not improve within the next 48 hours, surgical intervention with an abdominal colectomy with creation of an ileostomy is indicated.**

A. Emergent colonic decompression should not be attempted as it may lead to colonic perforation.

C. If peritoneal signs exist, an emergent laparotomy should be the primary therapy. Initial therapy is usually conservative.

D. Actions such as making the patient NPO and giving IV antibiotics should be undertaken; taken alone, however, they are inadequate.

E. Observation is unacceptable and would most certainly lead to the patient's demise.

175. **D.** UC is an inflammatory bowel disease primarily limited to the colon and rectum. It usually presents between the ages of 15 and 40 years. The cause is unknown, but felt to be immunologic. The disease is limited to the mucosa and submucosa and progresses continuously, commencing from the rectum. Medical treatment is much like that for Crohn's disease, consisting of sulfasalazine, steroids, and immunosuppressive agents. Unlike Crohn's disease, UC can be cured surgically with the entire removal of the colon and rectum. Indications for surgery include hemorrhage, toxic megacolon, obstruction, dysplasia, and failure of medical management.

   A, B, C, E. Skip lesions, lineal mucosal ulcerations, noncaseating granulomas, and involvement of the entire GI tract are all characteristics of Crohn's disease.

176. **C.** The left internal mammary artery is the most commonly used arterial graft and most often grafted to the left anterior descending artery. Other arteries that may be used are the gastroepiploic arteries, the inferior epigastric arteries, or the radial artery. The saphenous vein is commonly used in conjunction with the internal mammary artery.

   A, B. Intercostal arteries are not used for grafting in CABG.
   D. The right internal mammary artery may be used, but not as commonly as the left.
   E. The gastroepiploic arteries may be used as well, but not as commonly. They are options if a patient does not have other available conduits, such as the saphenous vein.

177. **B.** The sinus node receives its blood supply from the right coronary artery over 95% of the time. All other arteries listed are part of the left coronary system.

   A. The left main coronary artery bifurcates into the left anterior descending and the circumflex arteries.
   C. The circumflex is a branch of the left main artery.
   D. The diagonal artery is a branch of the left anterior descending artery.
   E. The obtuse marginal is a branch of the circumflex artery.
   F. The left anterior descending is a branch of the left main artery.

178. **B.** Like the sinus node, the AV node receives its blood supply from the right coronary artery more than 95% of the time. All other arteries listed are part of the left coronary system.

   A. The left main coronary artery bifurcates into the left anterior descending and the circumflex arteries.
   C. The circumflex is a branch of the left main artery.
   D. The diagonal artery is a branch of the left anterior descending artery.
   E. The obtuse marginal is a branch of the circumflex artery.
   F. The left anterior descending is a branch of the left main artery

179. **D.** Acute suppurative mediastinitis is a sternal infection with a high mortality rate, which may occur after a median sternotomy performed for open heart surgery. This infection usually presents with fever, chest pain, leukocytosis, and tachycardia, as well as with evidence of sternal instability and possible serous drainage from the wound.

   A. Atelectasis is a common cause of postoperative fever, but it would not explain the sternal instability and leukocytosis.
   B. Pneumonia is high on the list of postoperative sources of fever, especially after a prolonged intubation. In this scenario, the patient has done well since the time of extubation and his chest x-ray and clinical chest exam do not support a diagnosis of pneumonia.
   C. A UTI is unlikely to be the source of infection since there is no indwelling Foley catheter. The sternal instability remains a more likely explanation for fever and leukocytosis.
   E. A superficial thrombophlebitis may cause a slight elevation in the WBC and possibly a fever, but the exam presented offers no evidence of superficial thrombophlebitis, such as localized tenderness or erythema along a vessel.

180. **C.** The most likely cause of mediastinitis is *Staphylococcus*, either from *S. aureus* or *S. epidermidis.* These two organisms account for 75% of cases of mediastinitis. The remaining cases are caused by Gram-negative organisms.

A, D, E. *Klebsiella, E. coli,* and *Enterobacter* are all Gram-negative organisms that could cause mediastinitis, but are less common.

B. *S. pneumoniae* is an unlikely organism to cause mediastinitis.

181. D. Mediastinitis is most commonly diagnosed with clinical and laboratory findings, as described in previous answers. Suspicion can be confirmed by obtaining a CT scan of the chest. Anterior mediastinal gas or a mediastinal abscess may be seen radiographically.

A. A chest x-ray is unlikely to reveal evidence of mediastinitis.

B. A urinalysis with a culture will obviously be diagnostic for a UTI, but in the scenario presented it will not be diagnostic for mediastinitis.

C. An ultrasound of the mediastinum is not likely to reveal evidence of mediastinitis, unless an abscess is present. This procedure is also operator dependent and less reliable than a CT scan.

E. Opening and exploring the mediastinal wound should be done in the operating room after the diagnosis of mediastinitis is confirmed. Debridement of the infection with subsequent irrigation is required, followed by closure of the wound, with possible muscle flap over the sternum.

182. B. Overall, mediastinal tumors are rare, but the most common anterior mediastinal tumor is thymoma at a rate of 30%, followed by lymphoma (25%), and germ cell tumors (15%).

A. Lymphoma occurs in the anterior and middle mediastinal compartments at a 25% rate.

C. Pericardial cysts occur in the middle mediastinal compartment at a 35% rate.

D. Neurogenic tumors comprise 50% of posterior mediastinal tumors.

E. Germ cell tumors comprise 15% of anterior mediastinal tumors.

183. C. The phrenic nerves are at highest risk for being injured because of their proximity to anterior mediastinal structures.

A, B, D, E. The vagus, facial, recurrent laryngeal, and hypoglossal nerves are all more likely to be injured during neck surgery, rather than during mediastinal operations.

184. B. Thirty to fifty percent of patients with a thymoma will have myasthenia gravis, but only 10% of patients with myasthenia gravis will have thymomas.

A. Von Hippel-Lindau's syndrome is an autosomal-dominant inherited familial cancer syndrome associated with a variety of benign and malignant tumors.

C. Von Recklinghausen disease or generalized neurofibromatosis is associated with café au lait pigmentation and neurofibromas of the GI tract.

D. Cystic hygromas or lymphangiomas are benign endothelial-lined cystic masses most commonly found in the neck, axilla, and mediastinum, and are seen most commonly in children.

E. Hashimoto's disease is an autoimmune disorder, usually seen in middle-aged women with hypothyroidism.

185. C. The first study to obtain in suspected viscous perforation is an upright chest x-ray. This is likely to show free air under the diaphragm (Figure 5-185), which virtually dictates a direct trip to the operating room for an exploratory laparotomy.

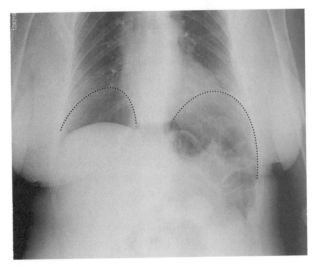

Figure 5-185 • Image Courtesy of the University of Utah School of Medicine, Salt Lake City, Utah.

A. Ultrasound in this situation is unhelpful. It is unlikely to reveal free air, which is characteristic of a perforated duodenal ulcer.

B. A flat plate x-ray of the abdomen is not as likely to show free air as an upright abdominal or chest film.

D. An abdominal CT scan would reveal evidence of free air, however, it is more time consuming and expensive, and may allow oral contrast to spill into the peritoneal cavity from the perforation.

E. A diagnostic peritoneal lavage may reveal evidence of peritonitis, but it is invasive, time consuming, and not routinely used in this situation.

186. **D. The diaphragm is innervated by the phrenic nerves, originating at spinal levels C3, C4, and C5, which explains the referred diaphragmatic irritation to the shoulder region. Perforation of a duodenal ulcer occurs on the right side of the abdomen causing irritation of the right hemidiaphragm.**

A, B. Both undiagnosed shoulder injury and psychogenesis are possible, but less likely causes of this patient's shoulder pain when associated with a likely perforation.

C. Patients with pancreatic irritation typically complain of pain radiating to their back.

E. Hepatic irritation usually does not cause pain. The diaphragm may become irritated with some hepatic processes, but it is a very unlikely choice in this acute scenario.

187. **E. Evidence of free air on an upright chest x-ray in conjunction with peritoneal signs warrants an emergent exploratory laparotomy.**

A. Pantoprazole is a proton pump inhibitor, which is useful in treating ulcer disease but not free perforation.

B. An upper endoscopy is useful in diagnosing ulcers, but in this case it is not appropriate and potentially hazardous after ulcer perforation.

C. Fluid resuscitation and pain control are very important and necessary; however, this patient needs to be taken to the operating room emergently to continue fluid resuscitation.

D. Although laparoscopy may be used to diagnose the duodenal perforation, most surgeons would not be able to adequately treat a perforated duodenal ulcer without an open laparotomy.

188. **B. The pylorus and "antral pump" of the stomach are under parasympathetic control from the vagus nerve. Performing a vagotomy will inhibit pyloric relaxation and antral contractions and cause delayed gastric emptying. Therefore, a drainage procedure must be performed to allow proper emptying of stomach.**

A, C, E. Dumping syndrome, alkaline reflux gastritis, and afferent loop syndrome are all complications of surgical management of peptic ulcer disease, which will not be helped with a gastric drainage procedure.

D. Bypass procedures are not used in the surgical treatment of perforated duodenal ulcers.

189. **B. Histologic grade of the primary lesion is the most important prognostic factor of soft tissue sarcomas.**

A, D. A tumor size of less than 5 cm and tumor location in a distant extremity predict a more favorable outcome, but the grade of the tumor remains the most important factor.

C. Lymph node involvement is uncommon in soft tissue tumors, which tend to metastasize via the bloodstream rather than the lymphatics.

E. Increased age is associated with poor prognosis, but not compared with the significance of the histologic grade.

190. **B. The most common site, and often the only site, of metastasis is the lungs. Metastatic disease most often occurs hematogenously, and the overall incidence of lymph node involvement is only 5%. Surgical resection of the pulmonary metastases has been shown to increase patient survival.**

A, C, D, E. The liver, brain, kidney, and bone are possible, but unlikely, locations for metastatic disease from soft tissue sarcomas.

191. **C. The thorax contains multiple vital anatomic structures, which, if injured, may lead to patient demise. Some are immediately life threatening, whereas others are life threatening if not identified in a thorough and methodical workup. The immediately life-threatening injuries, called the "6 quick killers" are airway obstruction, tension pneumothorax, open pneumothorax, flail chest, massive hemothorax, and cardiac tamponade.**

A. A myocardial contusion may be a "later" life-threatening event, which is diagnosed by ECG and with an echo, not usually diagnosed on the primary trauma exam.

B. Rib fractures are not necessarily life threatening, but they may lead to life-threatening conditions such as tension pneumothorax or a significant pulmonary contusion.

D. An esophageal tear is uncommon in blunt trauma and would most likely not be noted on a primary trauma exam.

E. A traumatic diaphragmatic disruption usually occurs on the left side of the chest and is most often diagnosed by an abdominal or chest x-ray.

192. B. Because of this patient's multiple rib fractures, he is at significant risk for developing a significant pulmonary contusion beneath the site of rib trauma.

A. The majority of trauma patients are at an increased risk for developing DVTs and require proactive and preventative treatment. In this scenario, a pulmonary contusion is the more likely associated injury.

C. An MI without myocardial contusion is unlikely in a 31-year-old male.

D. Patients such as this, with long bone fractures, are at an increased risk for fat emboli, but the more likely risk is for an associated pulmonary contusion.

E. A tension pneumothorax is a potential complication of rib fractures. The risk has been minimized by proper management of the initially identified pneumothorax by placement of a thoracostomy tube.

193. A. Proper management of rib fractures includes adequate pain control and aggressive pulmonary support. Placement of an epidural catheter for pain control is often required to allow patients to perform their pulmonary exercises. This is necessary to prevent further pulmonary deterioration or development of pneumonia, both of which have significant associated morbidity and mortality.

B. Surgical stabilization of rib fractures is not routinely performed.

C. Placement of a thoracic brace is not indicated, since this would increase the work of breathing.

D. Placement of an IVC filter may be indicated for pulmonary embolus prophylaxis, but not for pulmonary contusion.

E. Trauma patients are at an increased risk for developing DVT for which systemic prophylaxis is indicated when the patient is deemed safe to receive heparin.

194. E. Chronic mesenteric ischemia causes postprandial abdominal pain, which often results in weight loss mainly because association with pain makes the patients reluctant to eat. This diagnosis is less common, and thus other more common causes of abdominal pain and weight loss must be ruled out. Figure 5-194A shows stenosis of the celiac axis and absence of the superior mesenteric artery. On delayed views (Figure 5-194B), you see collaterals filling the superior mesenteric artery via the middle colic artery.

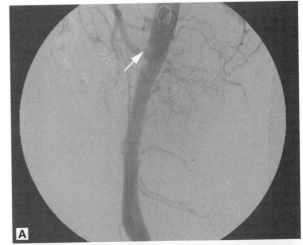

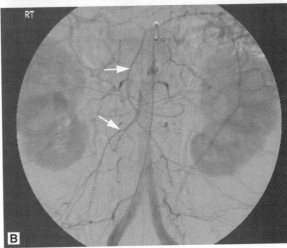

Figure 5-194A and B • Images Courtesy of the University of Utah School of Medicine, Salt Lake City, Utah.

A, B. Acute cholecystitis and biliary dyskinesia are unlikely choices with the patient history and previously normal HIDA scan and right upper quadrant ultrasound.

C. Without a history of a previous abdominal surgery or nausea and vomiting, and normal bowel function, SBO is a very unlikely presentation for bowel obstruction.

D. Acute mesenteric ischemia normally presents with sudden acute abdominal pain with signs of peritonitis. This patient's history of 35-lb weight loss is more consistent with a chronic intestinal ischemia picture.

195. C. Although acute mesenteric ischemia is usually due to embolic disease, chronic mesenteric ischemia is usually caused by mesenteric atherosclerosis involving two or all three mesenteric vessels. This patient has classic chronic symptoms with a history of hypertension and smoking.

A. Cholelithiasis is associated with acute cholecystitis.

B. Intraabdominal adhesions are associated with SBO, or a history of previous abdominal surgery.

D. Embolic disease is usually associated with acute mesenteric ischemia.

E. Biliary sludge is associated with acalculous cholecystitis or biliary dyskinesia.

196. B. Cushing's ulcer is peptic ulcer disease or gastritis associated with CNS tumor or head trauma.

197. E. Curling's ulcer is peptic ulcer disease or gastritis associated with a major burn injury.

198. D. Marginal ulcer is an ulcer at an anastomosis after prior gastric surgery.

199. A. Dieulafoy's ulcer is a gastric vascular malformation. Necrosis in the overlying mucosa results in recurrent hematemesis.

200. C. Marjolin's ulcer is associated with an SCC in a chronic wound.

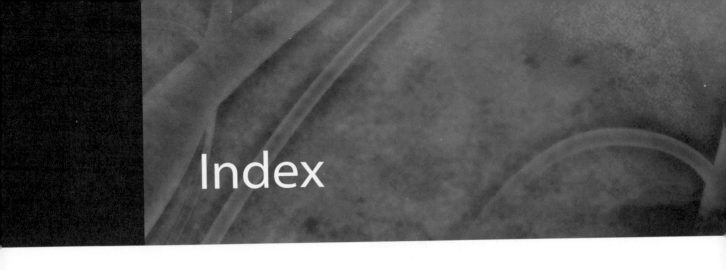

Index

Index note: Page numbers with an *f* indicate figures; those with a *t* indicate tables on designated page; page references in **bold** indicate discussion of the subject in the Answers and Explanations sections